Transmucosal Absorption Enhancers in the Drug Delivery Field

Transmucosal Absorption Enhancers in the Drug Delivery Field

Special Issue Editors

Luca Casettari
Sam Maher
Lisbeth Illum

MDPI • Basel • Beijing • Wuhan • Barcelona • Belgrade

MDPI

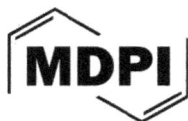

Special Issue Editors
Luca Casettari
University of Urbino Carlo Bo
Italy

Sam Maher
Royal College of Surgeons
in Ireland
Ireland

Lisbeth Illum
Independent Researcher
UK

Editorial Office
MDPI
St. Alban-Anlage 66
4052 Basel, Switzerland

This is a reprint of articles from the Special Issue published online in the open access journal *Pharmaceutics* (ISSN 1999-4923) from 2018 to 2019 (available at: https://www.mdpi.com/journal/pharmaceutics/special_issues/transmucosal_absorption_enhancers).

For citation purposes, cite each article independently as indicated on the article page online and as indicated below:

LastName, A.A.; LastName, B.B.; LastName, C.C. Article Title. *Journal Name* **Year**, *Article Number, Page Range.*

ISBN 978-3-03921-848-6 (Pbk)
ISBN 978-3-03921-849-3 (PDF)

Contents

About the Special Issue Editors

Luca Casettari is an Associate Professor in Pharmaceutical Technology leading his own research group at the University of Urbino Carlo Bo (Italy). He obtained his PhD in Pharmaceutical and Chemistry Sciences in 2010 and a Hospital Pharmacy specialization in 2015. His current research aims to develop novel strategies of drug delivery systems to facilitate and increase the absorption of drugs in various disease states to overcoming physiological barriers, and thus providing practical solutions for current healthcare problems. Moreover, his group synthetizes and characterizes new materials ranging from sugar-based surfactants to biodegradable polymers. These novel materials are then employed to formulate innovative pharmaceutical dosage forms, particularly in the nanomedicine field. He has published more than 60 papers (Tcit > 1000, H-index 17) in peer-reviewed international journals and co-founded two spin-off university companies.

Sam Maher is a senior lecturer in Pharmaceutics in the School of Pharmacy and Biomolecular Sciences at the Royal College of Surgeons in Ireland (RCSI). He has worked in the area of oral drug delivery over the last 15 years with positions in the Veterinary Sciences Centre in University College Dublin and the UCD Conway Institute. In 2012, he joined RCSI, and continues to research strategies to enhance oral absorption of poorly absorbed drugs using physical peptide hydrophobisation, lipoidal vehicles, intestinal devices and intestinal permeation enhancers. He has co-authored 34 peer reviewed publications and has a H Index of 18.

Lisbeth Illum was the founder and Managing Director of DanBioSyst UK Ltd, a drug delivery technology company which was sold successfully to West Pharmaceutical Services in 1996 and later to Archimedes Lab Ltd. She was also a co-founder of Phaeton Ltd, a drug delivery company, which was sold in 2003. She was the CEO of Critical Pharmaceuticals Ltd a drug delivery company (sustained release injectable and nasal technologies). She was awarded her M. Pharm, Ph. D and D.Sc. from the Royal Danish School of Pharmacy in 1972, 1978 and 1988, respectively. Her research expertise is in the area of transmucosal drug delivery systems for peptide, proteins and other difficult to deliver drugs. She has published more than 350 scientific papers, co-edited four books, edited various special journal issues and filed more than 45 patent families on novel drug delivery systems. Furthermore, she has lectured extensively throughout the world at conferences and workshops. She is presently working as a consultant for the pharmaceutical industry and as an expert witness in patent litigation cases, mainly in the US, whilst also fulfilling her duties as a Fellow of the AAPS and CRS and a special Professor at the Dept Pharmaceutical Sciences and Dept. of Chemistry at University of Nottingham She is or has been on the Editorial Boards of 12 scientific journals.

pharmaceutics

MDPI

Editorial

Transmucosal Absorption Enhancers in the Drug Delivery Field

Sam Maher [1,*], Luca Casettari [2,*] and Lisbeth Illum [3,*]

1   School of Pharmacy, Royal College of Surgeons in Ireland, St. Stephens Green, Dublin 2, Ireland
2   Department of Biomolecular Sciences, University of Urbino Carlo Bo, Piazza del Rinascimento 6, 61029 Urbino (PU), Italy
3   IDentity, 19 Cavendish Crescent North, The Park, Nottingham NG7 1BA, UK
*   Correspondence: sammaher@rcsi.com (S.M.); luca.casettari@uniurb.it (L.C.); lisbeth.illum@illumdavis.com (L.I.)

Received: 10 July 2019; Accepted: 11 July 2019; Published: 15 July 2019

Abstract: Drug delivery systems that safely and consistently improve transport of poorly absorbed compounds across epithelial barriers are highly sought within the drug delivery field. The use of chemical permeation enhancers is one of the simplest and widely tested approaches to improve transmucosal permeability via oral, nasal, buccal, ocular and pulmonary routes. To date, only a small number of permeation enhancers have progressed to clinical trials, and only one product that includes a permeation enhancer has reached the pharmaceutical market. This editorial is an introduction to the special issue entitled *Transmucosal Absorption Enhancers in the Drug Delivery Field* (https://www.mdpi.com/journal/pharmaceutics/special_issues/transmucosal_absorption_enhancers). The guest editors outline the scope of the issue, reflect on the results and the conclusions of the 19 articles published in the issue and provide an outlook on the use of permeation enhancers in the drug delivery field.

Keywords: permeation enhancers; absorption modifying excipients; oral delivery; nasal delivery; ocular delivery; vaginal delivery; transmucosal permeation

---

1. Introduction

Developing delivery strategies to assist movement of compounds across functionally conserved and structurally diverse epithelial barriers challenges drug delivery scientists. The most successful strategy to overcome poor permeation across epithelia, to date, has been to chemically modify the active compound to enable increased passive transport across non-injected epithelial routes. In cases where chemical modification is not feasible or unlikely to appreciably alter bioavailability, there may be no alternative but to formulate the active in an injectable dosage form, at considerable cost to manufacturers and inconvenience to patients. This is currently the case for many therapeutic macromolecules, including peptides, proteins and nucleic acids. Much of the early emphasis within the delivery field has focused on non-invasive administration of insulin; while it remains a major scientific challenge, oral delivery of other peptides, including GLP-1 receptor agonists may be preferable development candidates for Type II diabetes. Insulin is an affordable model peptide with established tools for qualitative and quantitative analysis, but there is interest in shifting towards development of smaller derivatised peptides [1] and cyclized peptides [2] that exhibit physicochemical properties that are more amenable to transmucosal permeation. Chemical engineering of poorly permeable macromolecules can improve potency, lengthen half-life, increase passive transcellular permeation and limit enzymatic degradation; these improved features may reduce the overall amount of active that is required to be shepherded across the epithelium. This may ultimately reduce the demand on the delivery system that is tasked with improving permeation across the epithelial barrier.

Peptides and other macromolecules are not the only targets for assisted permeation across biological barriers. A percentage of marketed small molecule drugs, that exhibit low and variable bioavailability (Biopharmaceutics Classification System (BCS) Class III drugs), may show improved efficacy in second generation formulations containing delivery platforms. Additionally, successful delivery platforms may help to relax constraints on discovery screening of compounds that are predicted to exhibit low bioavailability, thereby enriching the pharmaceutical pipeline.

Inclusion of a chemical permeation enhancer (PE), sometimes referred to as an absorption modifying excipient (AME), in a dosage form is considered a simple approach to improve absorption across biological barriers. The most widely tested use of PEs today is in oral, nasal, pulmonary and buccal applications and to a lesser extent via rectal, ocular and vaginal routes. Altering the integrity of an epithelial barrier is met with caution within the field; especially as a wide range of potentially noxious compounds are included in PE categories (e.g., toxins [3]). Not all substances that alter barrier integrity can be considered candidate PEs, and it is only candidate PEs that are already used to improve delivery in marketed products that can be termed an AME. In reality however, only a small number of PEs have progressed to clinical testing, the majority of these having a history of safe use in humans (e.g., FDA-allowed excipients (ethylenediaminetetraacetic acid), to food additives (fatty acids), and endogenous secretions (e.g., bile acids)). Even in oral formulations that have advanced in clinical trials, the persistence of generally low and variable drug absorption hampers progress. Ongoing research attempts to address this problem through (i) identification of safer and more selective PEs that are not associated with some of the in vitro cytotoxicity that is observed with ionizable surfactants and chelating agents [4], and (ii) by investigating the impediments to translation of established PEs that have demonstrated promising enhancement action in pre-clinical delivery models.

This Special Issue presents an insight in to some of the current research on PEs. Research topics include assessment of natural, semi-synthetic and fully synthetic PEs in pulmonary, ocular, buccal, intestinal, vaginal and nasal delivery. Themes discussed in this issue include: bioassays to assess the effect of PEs on barrier integrity, identification of novel PEs, co-application of PEs with micro-and nano- encapsulation, comparison of mechanisms underpinning PEs that have been investigated in clinical trials, as well as a discussion of the technical challenges that continue to impede translation. Topics are broadly grouped as enteral (oral) or non-enteral (nasal, pulmonary and vaginal). As most PE applications pertain to oral and nasal routes of administration, reviews by Ghadiri et al. (nasal/pulmonary [5]), and Maher et al. (oral [6]) provide a current outlook on promising new developments by these major routes. Contributing authors also reviewed PEs by category [7].

2. Application of PEs via Enteral Routes

Delivery of peptides and proteins via the oral route is one of the key challenges in the delivery field. At present there are nine peptides administered by the oral route on the market, seven of which act locally, and only two are intended to reach systemic targets [8]. One of these two peptides is cyclised and lipophilic (cyclosporin) and so, only one conventional linear hydrophilic peptide (Desmopressin, 1069 Da) is marketed for systemic delivery via the oral route. Desmopressin is formulated in an immediate release tablet (0.2 mg, Desmotabs®, Ferring Pharmaceuticals, Saint-Prex, Switzerland), and has a bioavailability (BA) of only 0.16%. Additionally, concomitant ingestion with food decreases the extent of absorption by 40% [9]. The study of PEs in oral delivery is largely driven by the ambition to reformulate marketed injectables, but, unless an equivalent oral dosage form has a similar cost to the injectable formulation or has "extended value" over the injection (in terms of safety and/or efficacy), the patient may not be eligible for reimbursement, depending on the national healthcare system. In the absence of reimbursement for the oral tablet, patients may be unwilling to pay for the oral formulation, although there are exceptions (e.g., patients with needle phobia). Cost and reimbursement issues were several of the reasons behind the commercial failure of the first inhaled insulin (Exubera®) [10].

Evidence of enhancement of oral absorption of marketed injectable drugs provided a foundation for oral delivery of peptide analogues that exhibit high potency and long biological half-lives from the injected route (e.g., semaglutide with sodium salcaprozate (SNAC) [1] or stable insulin analogues with sodium caprate (C_{10})) [11]. That is not to say that some therapeutic peptides that are currently marketed in injectable and/or nasal formulations cannot be developed into commercially successful oral formulations. In 2015, the FDA agreed to accept the filing of a New Drug Application (NDA) for once daily oral salmon calcitonin (sCT) (TBRIA^{TM}, Tarsa Therapeutics USA, Philadelphia, PA, USA). Additionally, Chiasma (Ness Ziona, Israel) is currently conducting a Phase 3 trial termed OPTIMAL (Octreotide capsules vs. Placebo Treatment In MultinationAL centres) for oral octreotide. In pre-clinical testing, several PEs categories have been extensively tested in oral delivery models, including surfactants, bile salts, chelating agents, toxins, and tight junction (TJ) modulators.

Maher et al. [6] provides a critical assessment of PEs in oral delivery. This review emphasizes the need to look beyond insulin to smaller peptides that may be more amenable to oral delivery, summarizes selected PEs in early development (e.g., choline geranate (CAGE) [12], permeant inhibitor of phosphatase (PIP) peptide 640 (PIP 640) [13]) and promising new formulations in the clinic [14], and explores some of the physiological challenges to translation of PEs in oral delivery. After a period of unsuccessful clinical trials and/or discontinuation of oral peptide programmes (e.g., salmon calcitonin (sCT) with Nordic Biosciences (Herlev, Denmark)/Novartis (Basel, Switzerland), there has been cause for optimism with positive clinical trial data emerging for selected peptide dosage forms, for example sCT with Tarsa Therapeutics (Philadelphia, PA, USA), octreotide with Chiasma and semaglutide with Novo Nordisk (Bagsværd, Denmark) [15], and ongoing effort to engineer stable peptides that are more amenable to oral delivery [2]. The lessons learned in unsuccessful clinical trials (reviewed in [16,17]) have also helped investigators identify the impediments to clinical translation, which has led to greater focus on formulation of PEs and efforts to translate promising pre-clinical data into an effective oral formulation that suitably co-presents the PE and the active in high concentrations at the intestinal epithelium. The article by Maher et al. also provides a commentary on the value of using simulated intestinal fluid in pre-clinical PE testing, an update on PE safety, and the lack of predictive power using certain animal models.

The review article by Twarog et al. [18] provides the first analysis of a head-to-head comparison between C_{10} and SNAC, two of the most widely tested PEs in oral delivery. Distinct mechanisms of action have been proposed for each based on in vitro data, although there remains uncertainty around their mechanisms at higher doses used in vivo. This article highlights the extensive history of clinical testing of both compounds, as well as the importance of both the selection of poorly permeable active and the design of the formulation. As things currently stand, SNAC has progressed further than C_{10}, having gained approval for oral delivery of vitamin B_{12} as a medical food (Eligen®-Vitamin B_{12}, Emisphere, Roseland, NJ, USA) and has completed Phase III studies in oral formulation of semaglutide with Novo Nordisk [19].

A number of novel PEs are discussed in this Issue, including tryptophan [20], lactose esters [21], sodium dilauramidoglutamide lysine [22] and ammonium mysristoyl chitosan [23]. Kamei et al. [20] performed a comprehensive study assessing the enhancement action of tryptophan, a hydrophobic amino acid that plays a key functional role in the action of cell penetrating peptides (CPPs) in pre-clinical delivery models. In rat ileal instillations, L-tryptophan improved bioavailability of insulin from 0.1% to 18.7% without causing mucosal injury. Other hydrophobic amino acids (isoleucine, proline, and phenylalanine) had no effect on insulin absorption. Further studies are required to elucidate the mechanism of enhancement action and to understand why this amino acid is effective in rat studies, but apparently not in Caco-2 monolayers.

Lucarini et al. [21] performed a preliminary structure activity relationship on a panel of synthetic fatty acid lactose esters (hydrophobic chain lengths of C_{10}, C_{12}, C_{14} and C_{16}). The authors recorded a decrease in the critical micelle concentration (CMC) for longer hydrophobic chain lengths, and an increase in cytotoxicity in Caco-2 and Calu-3 monolayers. At concentrations below the IC_{50} (half the maximum inhibitory concentration), there was no alteration to transepithelial electrical resistance

(TEER) in Caco-2 monolayers, although there was a partial TEER reduction in lung epithelial cells; suggesting that Calu-3 cells may be more sensitive to the action of lactose esters [21].

Silva et al. [23] synthesized an amphiphilic quaternary ammonium chitosan derivative and assessed its capacity to improve solubility and in vitro permeability of the lipophilic small molecule, curcumin. Permeation of curcumin from micelles was assessed in Caco-2 monolayers and a tri-culture model (Caco-2, HT29 and Raji B cells). The study showed only a modest effect of the derivative on permeation enhancement, but the concept of using cationic amphiphilic agents for combined solubilization and permeation enhancement is worthy of further investigation. Additionally, this study highlights how mixed cell cultures can impact interpretation of how PEs alter barrier integrity.

Haasbroek et al. [24] investigated how natural extracts from *Aloe vera* interact with intestinal epithelial cells. The study found whole leaf and gel extracts of *Aloe vera* contain considerable quantities of the acidifiers, citric acid and malic acid, which have previously demonstrated enhancement action [4]. Extracts caused a partial reduction in TEER and a two- to three- fold increase in permeation of fluorescein isothiocyanate (FITC) dextran 4 kDa (FD4) in Caco-2 monolayers. Confocal analysis of monolayers showed that FD4 was localized at the paracellular space, and that there was disruption of filamentous actin, a scaffolding protein that holds tight junctions in place. While this study does not provide definitive evidence of a paracellular effect over a transcellular effect, or elucidate the mechanistic steps leading to alteration in barrier integrity, the data shows that FD4 diffuses along the paracellular route.

Bocsik et al. [25] performed a detailed evaluation of the interaction of the 18-mer CPP, PN159, with Caco-2 monolayers. This study highlights the difficulty of elucidating how PEs alter intestinal permeability. PN159 increased permeability and modulated the localization of TJ proteins. There was binding to claudins -4, and -7 at concentrations below a threshold for cytotoxicity in Caco-2 monolayers. Nevertheless, there was evidence of ultrastructural aberration and leakage of an extracellular dye into cells, suggesting a degree of transcellular perturbation. The authors therefore concluded that PN159 has a dual mode of action. It would be interesting to see if the paracellular mechanism can be uncoupled from cell penetrating effects via substitution of amino acid responsible for cell perturbation. Irrespective of the mode of action, PN159 caused a rapid reduction in TEER over 5 to 15 min that was partially recovered over 6 h and completely recovered after 24 h. There was a concomitant increase in permeability of fluorescent dextrans in the molecular weight range of 4–40 kDa.

Alama et al. [22] performed mode of action studies on SLG-30, a Gemini surfactant (so called for their distinctive chemical structure: hydrocarbon tail 1—ionic head group 1—spacer—ionic head group 2—hydrocarbon tail 2). In a head-to-head comparison, SLG-30 improved absorption of carboxyfluorescein in rat intestinal loop instillations by an order of magnitude more than two established PEs (sodium laurate and sodium glycocholate). Fluorescence anisotropy of brush border membrane vesicles showed that SLG-30 altered the membrane fluidity in the protein portion of enterocyte membrane as well as the inner leaflet of the plasma membrane. Concurrently, there was a significant reduction in the total cell expression of claudin-1 (57%) and claudin-4 (64%). These data emphasize how surfactant alteration to membrane architecture may directly influence TJ proteins and permeability via the paracellular route.

A detailed understanding of how PEs alter permeability is an important aspect in PE selection, and there is often conflicting data within the scientific literature. Danielsen and Hansen [26] performed mode of action studies on two surfactants (sodium cholate and dodecylmaltoside (DDM)) in a jejunal mucosal explant [26]. This delivery model involved short-term culture of jejunal tissue segments in organ culture dishes with cell culture media. Sodium cholate and DDM caused leakage of Lucifer Yellow into epithelial cells as well as paracellular penetration of Texas Red dextran (3 kDa). At low concentrations (2 mM), there was no evidence of histological damage by light microscopy, although there was evidence of ultrastructural aberration by electron microscopy and histological damage was recorded at higher concentrations (10 mM). Both surfactants preferentially extracted non-lipid raft domains of the plasma membrane, suggesting these substances might cause perturbation at specific regions of the membrane rather than indiscriminate perturbation.

An extensive volume of literature has outlined the potential application of nanoparticles in a wide range of delivery applications. The initial premise that untargeted nanoparticles can facilitate significant translocation across the intestinal epithelium has not been forthcoming. There is demand to discover targeting ligands that can improve nanoparticle uptake such as through endogenous transporters on the mucosal surface (e.g., vitamin B_{12} [27]). Yong et al. [28] sought to determine if transferrin-mediated endocytosis can facilitate translocation of targeted polystyrene nanoparticles across Caco-2 monolayers. This study showed that polystyrene nanoparticles coated with an adsorbed layer of transferrin improved cellular uptake in non-polarized Caco-2 cells by 5-fold compared to the uncoated nanoparticles. In polarized Caco-2 monolayers, there was a 16-fold higher uptake of transferrin coated nanoparticles compared to non-polarized cells. There was also a 23-fold increase in permeation of transferrin coated nanoparticles compared to the non-coated particles. The authors conclude that the transferrin transport system may have potential application for both regional and systemic delivery of nanomedicines.

3. Application of PEs via Non-Enteral Routes

The nasal drug delivery technology market is expected to exceed $64 B by the year 2021 [29]. Nasal administration is among the most successful approaches for the systemic delivery of macromolecules. A number of small peptides are marketed in intranasal formulations, including; pritorelin (362 Da), oxytocin (1 kDa), desmopressin (1 kDa), buserelin (1.2 kDa), gonadorelin (1.2 kDa), nafarelin (1.4 kDa) and sCT (3.8 kDa) [30]. The largest of these peptides, sCT (Miacalcin®, Novartis, Switzerland), has a BA of approximately 1–3% with large variability (0.3–30%) [31]. None of these nasal peptide products contain a PE except for Miacalcin®, which contains benzalkonium chloride—a cationic surfactant that alters nasal permeability at selected concentrations [32]. PEs are commonly tested for nasal delivery of larger peptides and proteins (e.g., insulin, human growth hormone, interferon). Example PE categories for nasal delivery include; chitosan [31], non-ionic surfactants [33,34], CPPs [35,36], thiolated polymers [37], and cyclodextrins [38]. The non-ionic surfactants together represent the most clinically advanced PEs in nasal delivery (e.g., polyethylene glycol stearates and alkyl maltosides). DDM and tetradecyl maltoside (TDM) are constituents of Intravail™ (Aegis, San Diego, USA acquired by Neurelis, San Diego, CA, USA), a delivery platform that has been approved for use to assist nasal absorption of sumatriptan (Tosymra™, Dr Reddy's, Hyderabad, India) [33]. In this Issue, Ghadiri et al. [5] discuss strategies for exploitation of PEs for improvement of intranasal and pulmonary delivery of macromolecules. PEs were grouped into five major categories; (i) surfactants, (ii) cyclodextrins, (iii) protease inhibitors, (iv) cationic polymers and (v) tight junction modulators. An overview of other approaches that may be used to improve permeability via the nasal and pulmonary routes is also provided. Additionally, promising PEs that have progressed to clinical testing are listed.

In their article, Pearson et al. continued the evaluation of the soluble non-ionic surfactant PE, polyethylene glycol (15)-hydroxystearate (Solutol® HS15, recently re-branded as Kolliphor® HS15, BASF, Ludwigshafen am Rhein, Germany) as part of the CriticalSorb™ delivery platform (Critical Pharma, Nottingham, UK) [34,39]. This PE previously showed promising enhancement action in rats, where nasal BA of parathyroid hormone 1-34 (PTH1-34) was improved from 7.8% to 78% [40]. The current article examined intranasal administration of PTH1-34 in sheep (200 mcg) and humans (90 mcg) as either a liquid (containing 7.5% *w/v* Solutol® HS15) or dry powder (40% *w/w* Solutol® HS15). Overall, the promising PK data previously observed in rats were not replicated in large animals or humans. Nasal BA of PTH1-34 was 1.4% for the liquid and 1% for the dry powder in the ovine model. When the nasal spray was tested in seven healthy human volunteers, there were five non-responders. Mean BA was 0.26%, a value that increased to 1% when the non-responders were excluded. These values were considerably lower than the nasal BA of 3% observed in a previous Phase I study of human growth hormone (hGH) administered with Solutol® HS15 in a dry powder formulation [41]. The nasal formulation caused mild irritation to the nasal cavity of sheep, but not in human subjects, which could be due to dose differences. Scintigraphy performed in humans showed the nasal spray was deposited in anterior segment of the nasal cavity, which may not be optimal for absorption of PTH1-34, and the authors acknowledge that BA may be improved if local residence time can be increased. Overall, further studies are necessary to determine the clinical potential of Solutol® HS15 in nasal drug delivery.

Rassu et al. [42] assessed the effect of combining methyl-β-cyclodextrin (MβD) and chitosan chloride on nasal permeability of the model hydrophilic compound, N^6-cyclohexyladenoside. Here, insufflation of spray-dried microparticles in rats improved BA in the order of [1:0] MβD:chitosan (BA: 36%) > [1:1] MβD:chitosan (BA: 12.8%) and [0:1] MβD:chitosan (BA: 1.85%) showing that the combination of the two PEs did not accentuate the enhancement action. The ADME data for these formulations compared favorably to an aqueous suspension of N^6-cyclohexyladenoside administered via drops, which was below detectable levels in plasma of rats. There was also an undetectable level of N^6-cyclohexyladenoside in cerebrospinal fluid. Interestingly, all test formulations containing PE also increased transport of N^6-cyclohexyladenoside into cerebrospinal fluid, suggesting elevation in nose-to-brain transport.

Emulsomes are colloidal vesicular structures where a lipid core is coated with a phospholipid bilayer; thus, combining the properties of liposomes and simple emulsions. Additionally, excipients used in the preparation of emulsomes are often shown to alter epithelial permeability in pre-clinical animal models. El-Zaafarany et al. [43] describe the nasal delivery of oxcarbazepine loaded in emulsomes that were dispersed in a thermoresponsive gel. The emulsome in this formulation was composed of phosphatidylcholine: triolein (3:1) and polysorbate 80. There was comparable release of oxcarbazepine from the emulsomes and thermoresponsive gel over 8 h, but slower release from the gel over 24 h. In a previous study [44], intranasal administration of the emulsome thermogel to rats had a major impact on mean residence time (MRT) and oxcarbazepine area under the plasma concentration curve ($AUC_{0-48 h}$) relative to either a suspension or solution dosage form. Additionally, there was a higher concentration of oxcarbazepine in the brain for a sustained period when administered in the combination of emulsomes with the thermoresponsive gel system.

Bento et al. [45] assessed a co-adjuvant strategy to improve nasal vaccine administration of recombinant hepatitis B surface antigen (HBsAg). The strategy involves combining a mast cell activator (C48/80) and a chitosan nanoparticle with adsorbed antigen, the rationale being that the immune potentiator activates the adaptive immune response while the nanoparticles improve immunogenicity of antigens. Loading efficiency for C48/80 chitosan nanoparticles (500 nm) was less than 20%, which was attributed to repulsion of cargo. There was considerable variation in the amount of model test antigen adsorbed to the particle surface (bovine serum albumen (BSA): ~90%, ovalbumin: ~70% and myoglobin: ~10%), possibly due to differences in the extent of protein ionisation. There was internalization of BSA-FITC in RAW 264.7 macrophages as measured by confocal microscopy. Intranasal administration of C48/80 loaded chitosan nanoparticles coated with HBsAg to C57BL/6 mice led to a higher anti-HBsAg IgG titer than another comparative nanoparticle (poly-ε-caprolactone [46]) by day 42.

Bruinsmann et al. [47] developed a chitosan coated lipid-core nanocapsules for nose-to-brain delivery of simvastatin, a BCS Class II small molecule statin with potential neuroprotective actions [48]. The cationic lipid nanocapsules consisted of sorbitan monostearate and medium chain triglycerol surrounded by poly-ε-caprolactone and coated with low (21 kDa) or high (152 kDa) *Mw* chitosan. Mean particle size measurements for simvastatin loaded nanocapsules ranged between 163 to 168 nm for the low *Mw* chitosan form and 161 to 210 nm for the high molecular weight forms. The higher *Mw* nanocapsules had a slightly higher zeta potential (34 mV versus 29 mV in 10 mM NaCl), higher mucin weight ratios suggesting more efficient mucoadhesion and exhibited slightly slower release of simvastatin (31%) compared to the low *Mw* (37%) and solution control (56%). There was an increase in simvastatin permeation in human nasal epithelial cells and isolated rabbit nasal mucosa with both chitosan nanocapsule prototypes. Permeation of simvastatin in rabbit nasal mucosa was 1.7-fold higher for the low *M*w chitosan capsules, which was attributed to differences in the physicochemical properties. Overall, more efficient mucoadhesion could improve localization of nanocapsules.

Ocular drug delivery can broadly be considered in terms of topical, peri-ocular, or intra-ocular administration. The most common route of administration is topical delivery where medicaments are directly applied to the cornea, sclera and conjunctiva for local or regional actions. Delivery to peri-ocular or intra-ocular targets via either the cornea or blood retinal barrier is difficult even for highly permeable actives. The cornea is a widely accessible epithelial surface, although drug transport across this barrier is arguably more challenging than via other epithelia. Aside from a relatively short residence time, there is likely to be legitimate concerns regarding the use of any additive that causes transmucosal perturbation. Moiseev et al. [49] comprehensively reviews the categories of PE (sometimes termed penetration enhancers via this route) assessed in ophthalmic delivery. This article includes an outline of ocular physiology and selected conditions where PEs may have potential application. A detailed description of major PE categories is provided: including cyclodextrins, chelating agents, crown ethers, CPPs, bile acids/salts, and a range of soluble and insoluble surfactants. The authors conclude that penetration enhancers act by modulating the tear film or epithelial integrity. While penetration enhancers may assist permeation of actives, it remains to seen whether the active can diffuse to intraocular or periocular targets for conditions such as age-related macular degeneration or diabetic retinopathy.

While PEs primarily act to improve systemic absorption of poorly permeable actives, which can be achieved by enzyme inhibition, mucoadhesion and direct alteration to barrier integrity, these same functions may assist penetration of actives into tumors. Ci et al. [50] assessed the effect of a hydrogel containing cationic nanocrystals of imatinib/TPGS coated with polydopamine, to improve localization and penetration in a model of cervical cancer. The introduction of a cationic coating (polydopamine) inverted the zeta potential of imatinib nanocrystals from −9.27 mV to +27.25 mV and improved binding to mucin. The cationic charge enables mucoadhesion, and as cationic polymers have been shown to alter permeability, there is potential for improved transport with polydopamine. In the current study, the nanocrystals of imatinib had greater cellular uptake and improved anti-tumor efficacy in a murine orthotopic cervicovaginal cancer tumor model.

4. Review by PE Category

Promising PEs are also reviewed by category. The article by Peterson et al. is a useful guide to PEs from natural sources, which the authors collectively refer to as bioenhancers [7]. The article summarizes application of bioenhancers in buccal, nasal, oral and pulmonary routes of administration, and provides information on source, model of action, test delivery model and payloads. This comprehensive review discusses a wide range of phytochemicals that have not been previously reviewed in such detail, including *aloe vera*, black cumin, caraway, curcumin, diosmin and emodin.

5. An Outlook on PEs in the Delivery Field

PEs have been extensively tested via oral and nasal routes, and to a lesser extent via pulmonary, buccal, ocular and vaginal routes. As articles within this Issue highlight, there are challenges that impact translation of promising data observed in pre-clinical animal models into effective oral dosage forms in humans. The hurdle for investigators is to understand and control the action of PEs in dynamic environments observed in the GI tract, nasal cavity, lungs and oral cavity, preferably in animal models and humans. Co-localization of PE and active may help to replicate promising action that is observed in static delivery models. It may be that improving the effectiveness of PEs requires engineering technologies that co-localize the active and PE at the target epithelium. A focus on the final formulation requires convergence between formulation science, delivery science and engineering [51]. As academic research shifts from PEs towards nanoparticles and devices, there is less emphasis on addressing these hurdles to translation. This Issue also highlights that current emphasis in research on PEs remains on discovery of novel PEs that improve on potency, efficacy and safety of established candidates. However, improving these qualities may not negate issues related to co-delivery in dynamic environments. While discovery of new PEs that act via intricate and elegant paracellular mechanisms without evidence of mucosal perturbation is attractive, these PEs remain in preclinical research and have yet to be licensed to Pharma due to the higher risks: They have not improved upon the efficacy of leading PEs that have established safety records in humans.

An additional highlight of this Issue is the evolving nature of the target drug. Non-invasive delivery of insulin was long considered the pinnacle of the drug delivery field, whereas today emphasis has switched to GLP-1 agonists and other peptides. This is not only because they are smaller and more amendable for transmucosal delivery, but also because they may have a higher therapeutic index. An oral insulin formulation may eventually progress, as major manufacturers report data on novel insulin analogues with improved stability in GI fluids and longer half-lives [11]. The importance of oral insulin is immediately recognized as a key challenge to the scientific community [52], but it is worth emphasizing there is unquestionable demand for practical, non-invasive delivery systems for other poorly permeable macromolecules, development of which could help to shape the future pharmaceutical pipeline with leads that are safer and more effective than conventional small molecules. As most marketed therapeutic peptides are small, stable and often cyclised, then it may be more pertinent to initially focus on developing prototype delivery systems and formulations for these target peptides. This may be difficult, as cost of more contemporary peptides and availability of suitable analytical methods can limit options available to academic investigators.

Funding: This research received no external funding.

Conflicts of Interest: Lisbeth Illum was Chief Executive Officer of Critical Pharmaceuticals Ltd (Nottingham, UK) until the end of 2011.

References

1. Buckley, S.T.; Baekdal, T.A.; Vegge, A.; Maarbjerg, S.J.; Pyke, C.; Ahnfelt-Ronne, J.; Madsen, K.G.; Scheele, S.G.; Alanentalo, T.; Kirk, R.K.; et al. Transcellular stomach absorption of a derivatized glucagon-like peptide-1 receptor agonist. *Sci. Transl. Med.* **2018**, *10*. [CrossRef] [PubMed]
2. Nielsen, D.S.; Shepherd, N.E.; Xu, W.; Lucke, A.J.; Stoermer, M.J.; Fairlie, D.P. Orally Absorbed Cyclic Peptides. *Chem. Rev.* **2017**, *117*, 8094–8128. [CrossRef] [PubMed]
3. Fasano, A.; Nataro, J.P. Intestinal epithelial tight junctions as targets for enteric bacteria-derived toxins. *Adv. Drug Deliv. Rev.* **2004**, *56*, 795–807. [CrossRef] [PubMed]
4. Maher, S.; Mrsny, R.J.; Brayden, D.J. Intestinal permeation enhancers for oral peptide delivery. *Adv. Drug Deliv. Rev.* **2016**, *106*, 277–319. [CrossRef] [PubMed]
5. Ghadiri, M.; Young, P.M.; Traini, D. Strategies to Enhance Drug Absorption via Nasal and Pulmonary Routes. *Pharmaceutics* **2019**, *11*. [CrossRef]
6. Maher, S.; Brayden, D.J.; Casettari, L.; Illum, L. Application of Permeation Enhancers in Oral Delivery of Macromolecules: An Update. *Pharmaceutics* **2019**, *11*. [CrossRef]
7. Peterson, B.; Weyers, M.; Steenekamp, J.H.; Steyn, J.D.; Gouws, C.; Hamman, J.H. Drug Bioavailability Enhancing Agents of Natural Origin (Bioenhancers) that Modulate Drug Membrane Permeation and Pre-Systemic Metabolism. *Pharmaceutics* **2019**, *11*, 33. [CrossRef] [PubMed]
8. Lewis, A.L.; Richard, J. Challenges in the delivery of peptide drugs: an industry perspective. *Ther. Deliv.* **2015**, *6*, 149–163. [CrossRef]
9. Health Products Regulatory Authority of Ireland, Summary of Product Characteristics: Nordurine 0.2 mg Tablets. Available online: http://www.hpra.ie/img/uploaded/swedocuments/LicenseSPC_PA1009-017-002_08022017094138.pdf (accessed on 28 June 2019).
10. Heinemann, L. The failure of exubera: are we beating a dead horse? *J. Diabetes Sci. Technol.* **2008**, *2*, 518–529. [CrossRef]
11. Halberg, I.B.; Lyby, K.; Wassermann, K.; Heise, T.; Zijlstra, E.; Plum-Morschel, L. Efficacy and safety of oral basal insulin versus subcutaneous insulin glargine in type 2 diabetes: a randomised, double-blind, phase 2 trial. *Lancet Diabetes Endocrinol.* **2019**, *7*, 179–188. [CrossRef]

12. Banerjee, A.; Ibsen, K.; Brown, T.; Chen, R.; Agatemor, C.; Mitragotri, S. Ionic liquids for oral insulin delivery. *Proc. Natl. Acad. Sci. USA* **2018**, *115*, 7296–7301. [CrossRef] [PubMed]

13. Almansour, K.; Taverner, A.; Eggleston, I.M.; Mrsny, R.J. Mechanistic studies of a cell-permeant peptide designed to enhance myosin light chain phosphorylation in polarized intestinal epithelia. *J. Control Release* **2018**, *279*, 208–219. [CrossRef] [PubMed]

14. Davies, M.; Pieber, T.R.; Hartoft-Nielsen, M.L.; Hansen, O.K.H.; Jabbour, S.; Rosenstock, J. Effect of Oral Semaglutide Compared With Placebo and Subcutaneous Semaglutide on Glycemic Control in Patients With Type 2 Diabetes: A Randomized Clinical Trial. *JAMA* **2017**, *318*, 1460–1470. [CrossRef] [PubMed]

15. Aguirre, T.A.S.; Teijeiro-Osorio, D.; Rosa, M.; Coulter, I.S.; Alonso, M.J.; Brayden, D.J. Current status of selected oral peptide technologies in advanced preclinical development and in clinical trials. *Adv. Drug Deliv. Rev.* **2016**, *106*(Part B), 223–241. [CrossRef]

16. Karsdal, M.A.; Henriksen, K.; Bay-Jensen, A.C.; Molloy, B.; Arnold, M.; John, M.R.; Byrjalsen, I.; Azria, M.; Riis, B.J.; Qvist, P.; et al. Lessons learned from the development of oral calcitonin: the first tablet formulation of a protein in phase III clinical trials. *J. Clin. Pharmacol.* **2011**, *51*, 460–471. [CrossRef]

17. Karsdal, M.A.; Riis, B.J.; Mehta, N.; Stern, W.; Arbit, E.; Christiansen, C.; Henriksen, K. Lessons learned from the clinical development of oral peptides. *Br. J. Clin. Pharmacol.* **2015**, *79*, 720–732. [CrossRef]

18. Twarog, C.; Fattah, S.; Heade, J.; Maher, S.; Fattal, E.; Brayden, D.J. Intestinal Permeation Enhancers for Oral Delivery of Macromolecules: A Comparison between Salcaprozate Sodium (SNAC) and Sodium Caprate (C10). *Pharmaceutics* **2019**, *11*. [CrossRef] [PubMed]

19. Knudsen, L.B.; Lau, J. The Discovery and Development of Liraglutide and Semaglutide. *Front. Endocrinol.* **2019**, *10*, 155. [CrossRef]

20. Kamei, N.; Tamiwa, H.; Miyata, M.; Haruna, Y.; Matsumura, K.; Ogino, H.; Hirano, S.; Higashiyama, K.; Takeda-Morishita, M. Hydrophobic Amino Acid Tryptophan Shows Promise as a Potential Absorption Enhancer for Oral Delivery of Biopharmaceuticals. *Pharmaceutics* **2018**, *10*. [CrossRef]

21. Lucarini, S.; Fagioli, L.; Cavanagh, R.; Liang, W.; Perinelli, D.R.; Campana, M.; Stolnik, S.; Lam, J.K.W.; Casettari, L.; Duranti, A. Synthesis, Structure(-)Activity Relationships and In Vitro Toxicity Profile of Lactose-Based Fatty Acid Monoesters as Possible Drug Permeability Enhancers. *Pharmaceutics* **2018**, *10*. [CrossRef]

22. Alama, T.; Kusamori, K.; Morishita, M.; Katsumi, H.; Sakane, T.; Yamamoto, A. Mechanistic Studies on the Absorption-Enhancing Effects of Gemini Surfactant on the Intestinal Absorption of Poorly Absorbed Hydrophilic Drugs in Rats. *Pharmaceutics* **2019**, *11*. [CrossRef]

23. Silva, D.S.; D, M.D.S.; Almeida, A.; Marchiori, L.; Campana-Filho, S.P.; Ribeiro, S.J.L.; Sarmento, B. N-(2-Hydroxy)-propyl-3-trimethylammonium, O-Mysristoyl Chitosan Enhances the Solubility and Intestinal Permeability of Anticancer Curcumin. *Pharmaceutics* **2018**, *10*. [CrossRef]

24. Haasbroek, A.; Willers, C.; Glyn, M.; du Plessis, L.; Hamman, J. Intestinal Drug Absorption Enhancement by Aloe vera Gel and Whole Leaf Extract: In Vitro Investigations into the Mechanisms of Action. *Pharmaceutics* **2019**, *11*, 36. [CrossRef]

25. Bocsik, A.; Grof, I.; Kiss, L.; Otvos, F.; Zsiros, O.; Daruka, L.; Fulop, L.; Vastag, M.; Kittel, A.; Imre, N.; et al. Dual Action of the PN159/KLAL/MAP Peptide: Increase of Drug Penetration across Caco-2 Intestinal Barrier Model by Modulation of Tight Junctions and Plasma Membrane Permeability. *Pharmaceutics* **2019**, *11*. [CrossRef] [PubMed]

26. Danielsen, E.M.; Hansen, G.H. Probing the Action of Permeation Enhancers Sodium Cholate and N-dodecyl-beta-D-maltoside in a Porcine Jejunal Mucosal Explant System. *Pharmaceutics* **2018**, *10*. [CrossRef]

27. Chalasani, K.B.; Russell-Jones, G.J.; Jain, A.K.; Diwan, P.V.; Jain, S.K. Effective oral delivery of insulin in animal models using vitamin B12-coated dextran nanoparticles. *J. Control. Release* **2007**, *122*, 141–150. [CrossRef]

28. Yong, J.M.; Mantaj, J.; Cheng, Y.; Vllasaliu, D. Delivery of Nanoparticles across the Intestinal Epithelium via the Transferrin Transport Pathway. *Pharmaceutics* **2019**, *11*, 298. [CrossRef] [PubMed]

29. Nasal Drug Delivery Technology Market Expected to Reach US$ 64 Billion By 2021. Available online: https://www.marketwatch.com/press-release/nasal-drug-delivery-technology-market-expected-to-reach-us-64-billion-by-2021-2018-12-20 (accessed on 28 June 2019).

30. Rohrer, J.; Lupo, N.; Bernkop-Schnurch, A. Advanced formulations for intranasal delivery of biologics. *Int. J. Pharm.* **2018**, *553*, 8–20. [CrossRef]

31. Hinchcliffe, M.; Jabbal-Gill, I.; Smith, A. Effect of chitosan on the intranasal absorption of salmon calcitonin in sheep. *J. Pharm. Pharmacol.* **2005**, *57*, 681–687. [CrossRef]

32. Bortolotti, F.; Balducci, A.G.; Sonvico, F.; Russo, P.; Colombo, G. In vitro permeation of desmopressin across rabbit nasal mucosa from liquid nasal sprays: the enhancing effect of potassium sorbate. *Eur. J. Pharm. Sci.* **2009**, *37*, 36–42. [CrossRef]

33. Maggio, E.T. Intravail: highly effective intranasal delivery of peptide and protein drugs. *Expert Opin. Drug Deliv.* **2006**, *3*, 529–539. [CrossRef] [PubMed]

34. Lewis, A.L.; Jordan, F.; Illum, L. CriticalSorb™: enabling systemic delivery of macromolecules via the nasal route. *Drug Deliv. Transl. Res.* **2013**, *3*, 26–32. [CrossRef] [PubMed]

35. Kamei, N.; Nielsen, E.J.; Khafagy el, S.; Takeda-Morishita, M. Noninvasive insulin delivery: the great potential of cell-penetrating peptides. *Ther. Deliv.* **2013**, *4*, 315–326. [CrossRef] [PubMed]

36. Kristensen, M.; Nielsen, H.M. Cell-penetrating peptides as tools to enhance non-injectable delivery of biopharmaceuticals. *Tissue Barriers* **2016**, *4*, e1178369. [CrossRef]

37. Jain, A.; Hurkat, P.; Jain, A.; Jain, A.; Jain, A.; Jain, S.K. Thiolated Polymers: Pharmaceutical Tool in Nasal Drug Delivery of Proteins and Peptides. *Int. J. Pept. Res. Ther.* **2018**. [CrossRef]

38. Merkus, F.W.; Verhoef, J.C.; Marttin, E.; Romeijn, S.G.; van der Kuy, P.H.; Hermens, W.A.; Schipper, N.G. Cyclodextrins in nasal drug delivery. *Adv. Drug Deliv. Rev.* **1999**, *36*, 41–57. [CrossRef]

39. Shubber, S.; Vllasaliu, D.; Rauch, C.; Jordan, F.; Illum, L.; Stolnik, S. Mechanism of mucosal permeability enhancement of CriticalSorb(R) (Solutol(R) HS15) investigated in vitro in cell cultures. *Pharm. Res.* **2015**, *32*, 516–527. [CrossRef]

40. Williams, A.J.; Jordan, F.; King, G.; Lewis, A.L.; Illum, L.; Masud, T.; Perkins, A.C.; Pearson, R.G. In vitro and preclinical assessment of an intranasal spray formulation of parathyroid hormone PTH 1-34 for the treatment of osteoporosis. *Int. J. Pharm.* **2018**, *535*, 113–119. [CrossRef]

41. Lewis, A.L.; Jordan, F.; Patel, T.; Jeffery, K.; King, G.; Savage, M.; Shalet, S.; Illum, L. Intranasal Human Growth Hormone (hGH) Induces IGF-1 Levels Comparable With Subcutaneous Injection With Lower Systemic Exposure to hGH in Healthy Volunteers. *J. Clin. Endocrinol. Metab.* **2015**, *100*, 4364–4371. [CrossRef]

42. Rassu, G.; Ferraro, L.; Pavan, B.; Giunchedi, P.; Gavini, E.; Dalpiaz, A. The Role of Combined Penetration Enhancers in Nasal Microspheres on In Vivo Drug Bioavailability. *Pharmaceutics* **2018**, *10*. [CrossRef]

43. El-Zaafarany, G.M.; Soliman, M.E.; Mansour, S.; Cespi, M.; Palmieri, G.F.; Illum, L.; Casettari, L.; Awad, G.A.S. A Tailored Thermosensitive PLGA-PEG-PLGA/Emulsomes Composite for Enhanced Oxcarbazepine Brain Delivery via the Nasal Route. *Pharmaceutics* **2018**, *10*. [CrossRef]

44. El-Zaafarany, G.M.; Soliman, M.E.; Mansour, S.; Awad, G.A. Identifying lipidic emulsomes for improved oxcarbazepine brain targeting: In vitro and rat in vivo studies. *Int. J. Pharm.* **2016**, *503*, 127–140. [CrossRef] [PubMed]

45. Bento, D.; Jesus, S.; Lebre, F.; Gonçalves, T.; Borges, O. Chitosan Plus Compound 48/80: Formulation and Preliminary Evaluation as a Hepatitis B Vaccine Adjuvant. *Pharmaceutics* **2019**, *11*, 72. [CrossRef]

46. Jesus, S.; Soares, E.; Costa, J.; Borchard, G.; Borges, O. Immune response elicited by an intranasally delivered HBsAg low-dose adsorbed to poly-epsilon-caprolactone based nanoparticles. *Int. J. Pharm.* **2016**, *504*, 59–69. [CrossRef] [PubMed]

47. Bruinsmann, F.A.; Pigana, S.; Aguirre, T.; Souto, G.D.; Pereira, G.G.; Bianchera, A.; Fasiolo, L.T.; Colombo, G.; Marques, M.; Pohlmann, A.R.; et al. Chitosan-Coated Nanoparticles: Effect of Chitosan Molecular Weight on Nasal Transmucosal Delivery. *Pharmaceutics* **2019**, *11*. [CrossRef]

48. Wood, W.G.; Eckert, G.P.; Igbavboa, U.; Muller, W.E. Statins and neuroprotection: a prescription to move the field forward. *Ann. N. Y. Acad. Sci.* **2010**, *1199*, 69–76. [CrossRef] [PubMed]

49. Moiseev, R.V.; Morrison, P.W.J.; Steele, F.; Khutoryanskiy, V.V. Penetration enhancers in ocular drug delivery. *Pharmaceutics* **2019**, *11*, 321. [CrossRef]

50. Ci, L.-Q.; Huang, Z.-G.; Lv, F.-M.; Wang, J.; Feng, L.-L.; Sun, F.; Cao, S.-J.; Liu, Z.-P.; Liu, Y.; Wei, G.; et al. Enhanced Delivery of Imatinib into Vaginal Mucosa via a New Positively Charged Nanocrystal-Loaded in Situ Hydrogel Formulation for Treatment of Cervical Cancer. *Pharmaceutics* **2019**, *11*, 15. [CrossRef] [PubMed]

51. Traverso, G.; Kirtane, A.R.; Schoellhammer, C.M.; Langer, R. Convergence for Translation: Drug-Delivery Research in Multidisciplinary Teams. *Angew. Chem. Int. Ed. Engl.* **2018**, *57*, 4156–4163. [CrossRef]

52. Mathieu, C. Oral insulin: time to rewrite the textbooks. *Lancet Diabetes Endocrinol.* **2019**, *7*, 162–163. [CrossRef]

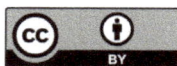

pharmaceutics

MDPI

Article

Probing the Action of Permeation Enhancers Sodium Cholate and N-dodecyl-β-D-maltoside in a Porcine Jejunal Mucosal Explant System

E. Michael Danielsen * and Gert H. Hansen

Department of Cellular and Molecular Medicine, The Panum Institute, Faculty of Health Sciences, University of Copenhagen, 2200 Copenhagen, Denmark; gerth@sund.ku.dk
* Correspondence: midan@sund.ku.dk; Tel.: +45-3532-7786

Received: 28 August 2018; Accepted: 28 September 2018; Published: 2 October 2018

Abstract: The small intestinal epithelium constitutes a major permeability barrier for the oral administration of therapeutic drugs with poor bioavailability, and permeation enhancers (PEs) are required to increase the paracellular and/or transcellular uptake of such drugs. Many PEs act as surfactants by perturbing cell membrane integrity and causing permeabilization by leakage or endocytosis. The aim of the present work was to study the action of sodium cholate (NaC) and N-dodecyl-β-D-maltoside (DDM), using a small intestinal mucosal explant system. At 2 mM, both NaC and DDM caused leakage into the enterocyte cytosol of the fluorescent probe Lucifer Yellow, but they also blocked the constitutive endocytotic pathway from the brush border. In addition, an increased paracellular passage of 3-kDa Texas Red Dextran into the lamina propria was observed. By electron microscopy, both PEs disrupted the hexagonal organization of microvilli of the brush border and led to the apical extrusion of vesicle-like and amorphous cell debris to the lumen. In conclusion, NaC and DDM acted in a multimodal way to increase the permeability of the jejunal epithelium both by paracellular and transcellular mechanisms. However, endocytosis, commonly thought to be an uptake mechanism that may be stimulated by PEs, was not involved in the transcellular process.

Keywords: intestinal permeation enhancers; sodium cholate (NaC); N-dodecyl-β-D-maltoside (DDM); small intestine; enterocyte; brush border

---

1. Introduction

The small intestinal brush border has two equally important, but mutually conflicting bodily functions to take care of: (1) to digest and absorb dietary nutrients, and (2) to prevent harmful luminal agents from gaining access to the body. Whereas the digestive/absorptive capacity of enterocytes is optimized by the large apical surface expansion represented by numerous microvilli [1,2], the unusually high glycolipid content of the apical membrane bilayer favors the formation of "lipid raft" domains [3–5]. The ensuing membrane robustness not only renders the brush border relatively resistant to noxious luminal agents, but also proves a challenge to overcome in the pharmacological quest for permeation enhancers (PEs) suitable for oral administration of drugs with otherwise poor bioavailability [6]. Surfactants represent a large and chemically diverse group of PEs, and as amphiphilic compounds, they have a capacity to adsorb to the cell membrane bilayer, thereby rendering it more fluid and causing it to expand, leading to a loss of integrity and an increase in permeability [6,7]. At higher concentrations, PEs may cause membrane solubilization, and ultimately, buckling and lysis of the cell membrane itself [6]; ideally however, PE action should strike the optimal balance between achieving adequate drug absorption from the gut without compromising mucosal integrity [8]. Functionally, intestinal PEs may act to increase transcellular pathways and/or the paracellular permeability by the opening of tight junctions between adjacent epithelial cells. Regarding the former, permeabilization is thought to be achieved by generating pores or leaks in the cell membrane, or by engaging one of several possible endocytotic mechanisms [6,9,10].

Bile salts are a distinct group of chemically related endogenous compounds engaged in assimilation of dietary fat [11]. Their role in this process may be likened to that of other types of surfactants, and they have long attracted considerable interest as potential PEs in drug absorption, as evidenced by their listing in several patents of oral peptide delivery systems [6,12–14]. Another class of widely-used soluble surfactant PEs is alkyl maltosides, of which members like bile salts are included in some formulations currently undergoing preclinical testing for oral drug delivery [6,15].

The aim of the present work was to compare how a bile salt, sodium cholate (NaC), and an alkyl maltoside, N-dodecyl-β-D-maltoside (DDM) affect the different cellular uptake pathways of a number of fluorescent polar and lipophilic probes, using a small intestinal mucosal organ culture model. This experimental setup is simple to use and offers a more in-vivo-like alternative to commonly-used epithelial cell lines such as Caco-2 [16]. Using this model, we have previously been able to visualize directly how other types of PEs, including lauroyl-carnitine, monocaprin, the ethoxylate $C_{12}E_9$, and melittin interact with the epithelium to affect uptake of polar and lipophilic probes [17–19]. At a concentration of 2 mM (~0.1%), NaC and DDM both exhibited multimodal actions as PEs, i.e., increased paracellular, as well as transcellular, permeability, without causing excessive damage to the integrity of the epithelium. At the ultrastructural level, NaC and DDM disrupted the normally ordered hexagonal organization of microvilli of the brush border and led to the extrusion of vesicle-like and amorphous cell debris to the lumen. Otherwise, overall cell morphology, including tight junctions and basolateral cell membranes, appeared intact, implying that the brush border is the primary target of both PEs.

2. Materials and Methods

2.1. Materials

Sodium cholate hydrate (NaC, MW 409 Da) and N-dodecyl-β-D-maltoside (DDM, MW 511 Da) were supplied by Sigma-Aldrich (Copenhagen, Denmark; www.sigmaaldrich.com), Lucifer yellow CH ammonium salt (LY), a fixable analog of the FM lipophilic styryl dye FM 1-43 FX (FM), Texas Red Dextran (MW 3000 Da, lysine fixable) (TRD), ProLong antifade reagent with DAPI, and a monoclonal antibody to Na+/K+-ATPase (α-chain) by Thermo Scientific (Roskilde, Denmark; www.thermodanmark.dk), a rabbit antibody to intestinal alkaline phosphatase (IAP) was from AbD Serotec (Copenhagen, Denmark; www.bio-rad-antibodies.com), and a mouse anti-rat early endosome antigen-1 (EEA-1) antibody by BD Transduction Laboratories (Lyngby, Denmark; www.bdbiosciences.com). A rabbit antibody to pig intestinal aminopeptidase N (ApN) was prepared as previously described [20].

2.2. Animals

Animal experimentation included in this work was performed only by licensed staff at the Department of Experimental Medicine, the Panum Institute, University of Copenhagen, and was covered by license 2012-15-2934-00077 issued to the Dept. of Experimental Medicine, the Panum Institute, University of Copenhagen. A total of six animals were used in this study.

Segments of porcine jejunum, taken about 2 m from the pylorus of overnight fasted, postweaned animals, were surgically removed from the anaesthetized animals. After excision of the tissue, the animals were sacrificed by an injection with pentobarbital/lidocaine (1 mg/kg bodyweight). As this study contained no further animal experimentation, no specific approval by an ethics committee was required.

2.3. Organ Culture of Porcine Jejunal Mucosa

Organ culture of small intestinal mucosa was performed essentially as described previously [16,21]. Briefly, after excision from the animals, jejunal segments of ~20 cm in length were quickly opened longitudinally and immersed in ice-cold RPMI medium. Mucosal tissue specimens weighing ~0.1 g were excised with a scalpel and placed on metal grids in organ culture dishes, to which 1 mL of pre-warmed RPMI medium was added. The dishes were placed in an incubator kept at 37 °C, and after 15 min of preincubation, reagents were added to the RPMI medium at the following concentrations: NaC and DDM (2 mM or 10 mM), LY (0.5 mg/mL), FM dye (10 μg/mL), and TRD (50 μg/mL). The explants were cultured in the presence of the reagents for 1 h in the dark, and after culture they were carefully rinsed in fresh RPMI medium and immersed in a fixative overnight at 4 °C.

2.4. Fluorescence Microscopy

Explants were fixed at 4 °C overnight in 4% paraformaldehyde in 0.1 M sodium phosphate, pH 7.2 (buffer A). Following fixation and a quick rinse in buffer A, the explants were immersed overnight in 25% sucrose in buffer A before they were mounted in Tissue-Tek and sectioned (~7 μm thick sections cut parallel to the crypt-villus axis) at −19 °C in a Leica CM1850 cryostat. For immunolabeling, the sections were incubated for 1 h at room temperature with antibodies to EEA-1 (diluted 1: 100), Na$^+$/K$^+$-ATPase (diluted 1:100) or aminopeptidase N (diluted 1:5000) in 50 mM Tris-HCl, 150 mM NaCl, 0.5% ovalbumin, 0.1% gelatin, 0.2% teleostan gelatin, 0.05% Tween 20, 0.05% Triton X-100, pH 7.2 (buffer B). Incubation with Alexa-conjugated secondary antibodies (diluted 1:200 in buffer B) was for 1 h at room temperature. Controls with omission of primary antibodies were routinely included in the labeling experiments.

All sections were finally mounted in antifade mounting medium containing DAPI, and examined in a Leica DM 4000B microscope (Leica, Wetzlar, Germany) fitted with a Leica DFC495 digital camera. Images were obtained using Leica HCX PL Fluotar objectives with the following magnification/numerical aperture: 20×/0.40, 40×/0.65, 63×/0.90, and 100×/1.30. The following filter cubes were used: I3 (band pass filter, excitation 450–490 nm), TX2 (band pass filter, excitation 560/40 nm), and A4 (band pass filter, excitation 360/40 nm).

Hematoxylin-eosin (HE) staining of fixed tissue sections was performed according to a standard protocol.

2.5. Transmission Electron Microscopy

For transmission electron microscopy, cultured explants were fixed in 3% glutaraldehyde (v/v), 2% (w/v) paraformaldehyde in buffer A overnight at 4 °C. After a rinse in buffer A, the explants were post-fixed in 1% osmium tetroxide in buffer A for 1 h at 4 °C, dehydrated in acetone and finally embedded in Epon (an epoxy resin). Ultrathin sections were cut in a Pharmacia LKB Ultrotome III, and stained with 1% (w/v) uranyl acetate in H_2O and lead citrate. All sections were finally examined in a Zeiss EM 900 electron microscope (Zeiss, Oberkochen, Germany) equipped with a Mega View II camera.

2.6. Preparation of Microvillus Membrane Vesicles and Treatment with NaC and DDM

Brush border microvillus membrane vesicles were prepared from pig jejunal mucosa by the divalent cation precipitation method [22]. Briefly, the mucosa was scraped from the gut and homogenized in 10 volumes of 2 mM Tris-HCl, 50 mM mannitol, pH 7.1, containing 10 μg/mL aprotinin and leupeptin. After centrifugation at 500× g, 5 min, $MgCl_2$ was added to the supernatant (final concentration: 10 mM), and after 10 min on ice, the preparation was centrifuged at 1.500× g, 10 min. The resulting supernatant was collected and centrifuged at 48.000× g, 30 min, to yield a pellet of microvillus membrane vesicles (stored at −20 °C until use).

For subsequent treatments with NaC or DDM, microvillus vesicles (~1 mg/mL) were resuspended in 25 mM HEPES-HCl, 150 mM NaCl, pH 7.1, and samples of 75 μL were mixed with 25 μL of NaC or DDM to obtain a final concentration in the range of 0–10 mM. After 15 min incubation at 37 °C and rapid cooling on ice, the membrane suspensions were centrifuged at $20.000\times g$, 20 min, to yield a membrane pellet and a supernatant of solubilized protein. Both fractions were collected and subjected to SDS/PAGE in 10% gels, electrotransfered onto Immobilon membranes and stained for protein with Coomassie brilliant blue, as described in Section 2.8.

2.7. Detergent Resistant Membrane (DRM) Analysis of Microvillus Membranes by Sucrose Gradient Ultracentrifugation

One milliliter of microvillus membrane vesicles, prepared as described above, was resuspended in HEPES-buffer, pH 7.2. The membranes were then treated with NaC, DDM or Triton X-100 (all at a concentration of 1%) for 10 min on ice. A DRM analysis of the microvillus membranes was performed by sucrose density gradient ultracentrifugation by a method previously described [23,24]. Briefly, centrifugation was performed in a SW40 Ti rotor (Beckman Instruments, Palo Alto, CA) for 20–22 h at 35.000 rpm (g_{max} = $217.000\times g$), and after centrifugation, the gradient was fractionated into a pellet and 12 fractions of 1 mL. Protein from each of the soluble fractions was isolated by acetone precipitation before analysis by SDS/PAGE.

2.8. SDS/PAGE and Immunoblotting

Samples were denatured by boiling for 3 min in the presence of 1% SDS and 10 mM dithiothreitol, and subjected to SDS/PAGE in 10% gels as described [25]. After electrophoresis and electrotransfer of proteins onto Immobilon PVDF membranes, immunoblotting was performed with antibodies to IAP (1: 1000 dilution), followed by horseradish peroxidase-coupled secondary antibodies (1: 2000 dilution). An electrochemiluminescence (ecl) reagent was used according to the manufacturers (GE Healthcare, www.gehealthcare.com) protocol to develop the blots. After immunoblotting, total protein was stained with Coomassie brilliant blue R250 (0.2% dissolved in an ethanol/H_2O/acetic acid mixture (50:43:7).

3. Results

3.1. Microvillus Membrane-Solubilizing Effects of NaC and DDM

Chemically, NaC and DDM belong to the large class of surfactant PEs of which the main common functional characteristic is the ability to adsorb to cell membranes, and thereby, to modify their physical and biological properties (Figure 1). In order to evaluate the membrane solubilizing effect on the intestinal brush border and to select optimal working concentrations of NaC and DDM for subsequent culture experiments, the concentration-dependency of their ability to release proteins from microvillus vesicles was first established. As shown in Figure 2, NaC had hardly any solubilizing effect above background levels at concentrations up to 2 mM, but at 5 and 10 mM, an increasing release of microvillus proteins was achieved. Both integral membrane proteins, such as the 150 kDa ApN, and the major microvillus cytoskeleton protein actin (42 kDa) appeared in the supernatant, indicating both membrane disruption and leakage. For DDM, microvillus solubilization was detectable already at 1 mM, consistent with the comparatively lower CMC-value for this PE (Figure 2).

NaC   **DDM**

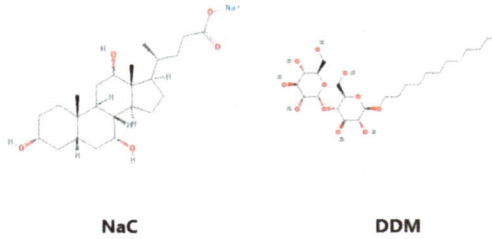

Figure 1. The chemical structure of NaC and DDM. (The images were downloaded from the PubMed Open Chemistry Data Base (https://www.ncbi.nlm.nih.gov/Structure/pdb/2MLT)).

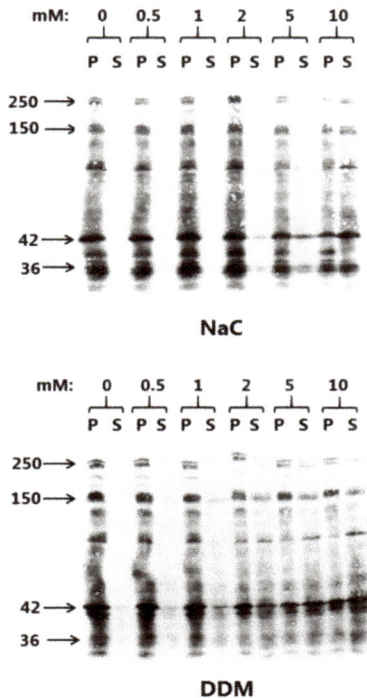

NaC

DDM

Figure 2. Solubilization of microvillus membrane vesicles with NaC or DDM at concentrations ranging from 0–10 mM as described in Methods. After centrifugation, the pellet (P) and supernatant (S) fractions were subjected to SDS/PAGE and proteins visualized by staining with Coomassie brilliant blue. Arrows indicate the molecular mass-values of the brush border proteins sucrase-isomaltase (250 kDa), ApN (150 kDa), actin (42 kDa), and annexin A2 (36 kDa).

The ability to resist solubilization by detergents/surfactants at low temperature is the biochemical hallmark of liquid-ordered membrane domains (i.e., lipid rafts) [5,26]. Thus, in the glycolipid-rich intestinal brush border, many of the major digestive hydrolases resist solubilization by the detergent Triton X-100, which is indicative that they reside in lipid rafts [24]. The 67-kDa IAP, linked to the extracellular leaflet of the membrane by a glycolipid anchor, is a well-known lipid raft marker [23], and as shown in Figure 3, this protein predominantly partitions in the floating DRM fractions of the sucrose gradient when using the "classical" detergent Triton X-100 for solubilization. An essentially similar DRM distribution for IAP was likewise observed for NaC, as well as for DDM, although relatively more of the enzyme appeared to be soluble. In addition, the profile of total microvillus protein also resembled that obtained with Triton X-100 (data not shown). This experiment thus indicates that the "non raft" domains of the brush border, i.e., those relatively enriched in phospholipids and poor in glycolipids, are those most vulnerable to the action of both PEs.

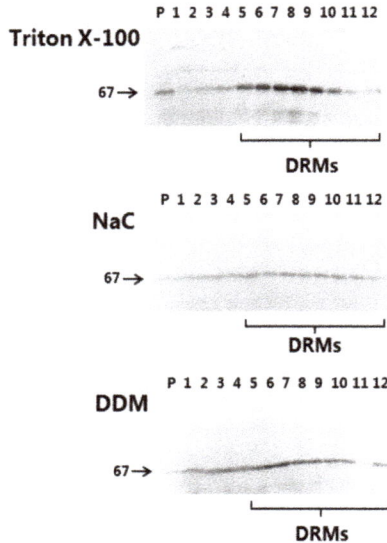

Figure 3. DRM analysis of microvillus membrane vesicles. Microvillus membrane vesicles were prepared and solubilized with either 1% Triton X-100, NaC or DDM on ice, followed by sucrose gradient ultracentrifugation, gradient fractionation, SDS/PAGE and immunoblotting for IAP (67 kDa). "P" indicates the pellet fraction, fractions 1-2 contain solubilized protein and fractions 4–12 contain DRMs.

3.2. Effects of NaC and DDM on Mucosal Morphology in Cultured Mucosal Explants

Organ culture of mucosal explants is an ideal model system for investigating the direct, short-term effects of luminal compounds, and we have recently used it with a number of other types of permeation enhancers [17–19]. In subsequent mucosal organ culture experiments, NaC and DDM were both used at 2 and 10 mM in order to study cell-permeating effects under relative mild, as well as under more membrane damaging, conditions. Both concentrations (corresponding to 0.86% and 4.3% for NaC, and 1.0% and 5.1% for DDM, respectively) are well within the range of concentrations previously used by other investigators [6].

As shown in Figure 4, exposure to either NaC or DDM at a concentration of 2 mM for 1 h caused no gross overall deterioration of the mucosal morphology. Villus height was preserved and the integrity of the epithelium generally upheld; only occasionally could foci of exfoliation be detected, typically at the tip of the villi. In contrast, at a concentration of 10 mM, both PEs caused extensive denudation at the tip of the villi, which are the most exposed and sensitive areas of the mucosal epithelium. Further down along the sides of the villi and in the generative crypts, the epithelium was generally well preserved.

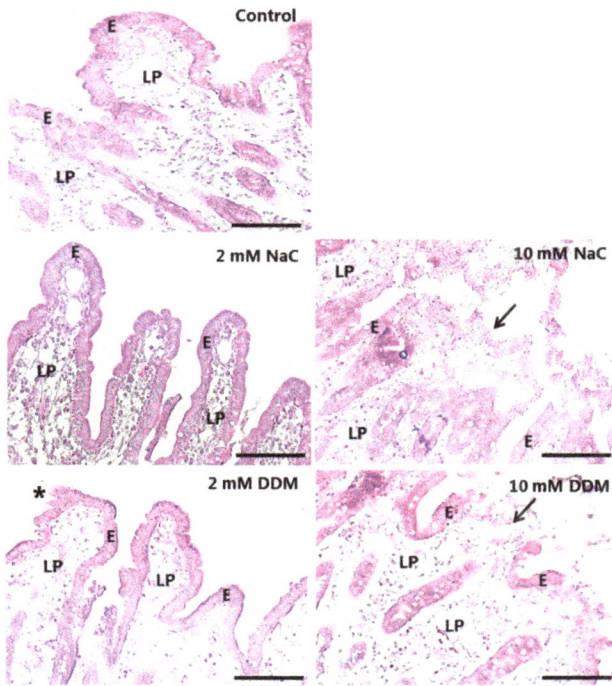

Figure 4. HE-stained sections of mucosal explants cultured for 1 h in the absence (control) or presence of 2 mM or 10 mM of NaC/DDM, as described in Methods. The villus organization and epithelium were generally well preserved at 2 mM of both surfactants, although foci of exfoliation was occasionally observed (asterisk). At 10 mM, both NaC and DDM caused extensive denudation, particularly near the tips of the villi (arrows), whereas the epithelium along the sides of the villi and in the crypts were generally better preserved. Enterocytes (E) and lamina propria (LP) are indicated. Bars: 100 μm.

3.3. Effects of NaC and DDM on Permeability of Lucifer Yellow

LY is a small fluorescent polar tracer (MW 444 Da) with little or no permeability through normal cell membranes. It has previously been used to assess paracellular permeability in Caco-2 monolayers [27], and we have used it in the mucosal organ culture system for studying damage to epithelial cell integrity under various conditions [18,19,28]. As shown in Figure 5, little or no staining of the cytosol was seen in enterocytes of control explants, indicating well-preserved membrane integrity with little or no leakage through the cell membrane. Likewise, the brush border was devoid of staining by LY. However, an array of distinct subapical punctae was indicative of an uptake by constitutive endocytosis from the brush border. These punctae were EEA-1-positive, thus representing a subpopulation of early endosomes in the terminal web region of the enterocytes that we have previously termed "TWEEs" (Terminal Web Early Endosomes) [29]. The underlying lamina propria was strongly stained by LY in the control, and widespread stripy lateral staining along the enterocytes was indicative of a paracellular passage across the epithelium. Both NaC and DDM caused a diffuse staining of the enterocyte cytosol, indicating a leakage through the cell membrane. However, only some enterocytes appeared to be thus affected, resulting in a characteristic mosaic staining pattern of the epithelium; occasionally, single exfoliating cells were detected as well (Figure 5). The brush border marker ApN was confined to the apical surface in the presence of both PEs, indicating that no gross membrane disruption had occurred. However, noticeably, both NaC and DDM prevented the appearance of the LY-positive TWEEs, implying a blocked uptake via constitutive endocytosis.

At a concentration of 10 mM, both NaC and DDM caused widespread leakage of LY into all enterocytes, although the localization of both the apical (ApN) -and basolateral marker (Na^+/K^+-ATPase) was seemingly unaffected in areas where the epithelium was still intact (Figure 6).

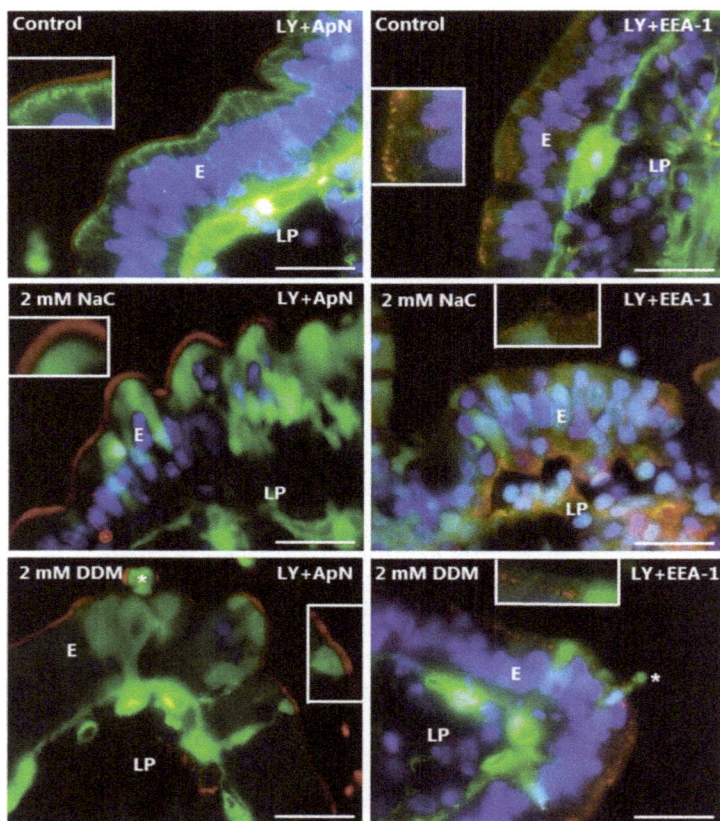

Figure 5. Permeability of the mucosal epithelium probed with LY at 2 mM concentration of PEs. Sections of mucosal explants cultured for 1 h with LY in the absence or presence of 2 mM NaC or DDM, respectively. In addition, the sections were immunolabeled for ApN, a brush border enzyme, or for EEA-1, a marker for early endosomes. In the controls, a string of EEA-1-positive subapical punctae shows uptake of LY into apical early endosomes of the enterocytes, whereas the cytosol is only weakly labeled. Lateral labeling and strong staining of the lamina propria are also seen, indicating a paracellular passage of LY through the tight junctions. At 2 mM, both NaC and DDM frequently caused LY to enter the enterocyte cytosol, indicating a leakage through the cell membrane, but endocytic uptake was not observed. Asterisks indicate enterocytes in the process of exfoliation. Inserts show enlarged image details. Bars: 20 μm.

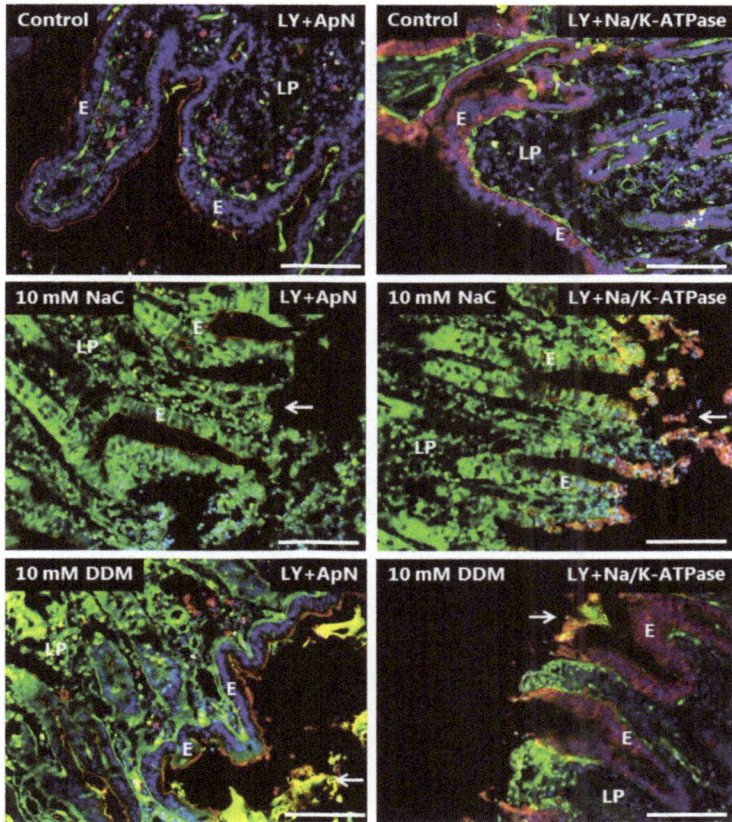

Figure 6. Permeability of the mucosal epithelium probed with LY at 10 mM concentration of PEs. Sections of mucosal explants cultured for 1 h with LY in the absence or presence of 10 mM NaC or DDM, respectively. In addition, the sections were immunolabeled for ApN, or Na^+/K^+-ATPase, a basolateral cell membrane marker. Both NaC and DDM caused extensive denudation at the tips of the villi (arrows), but epithelial integrity with preservation of cell membrane polarity was maintained along the sides of the villi. However, all enterocytes had taken up LY into the cytosol. Bars: 20 μm.

3.4. Effects of NaC and DDM on Permeability of Texas Red Dextran and FM 1-43 FX

The TRD used in this study is polar like LY, but of higher MW (3000 Da), and is a commonly used probe for cellular uptake studies [30]. Unlike LY, it labeled the brush border of control enterocytes, but was only taken up sparsely into TWEEs in comparison with LY, implying a poor accessibility to the bottom part of the microvilli from where endocytosis occurs (Figure 7). TRD stained the lamina propria, but only weakly compared with LY, and a lateral staining along the enterocytes was barely visible, which was indicative of limited paracellular diffusion through the tight junctions. Binding to the brush border was unaffected by NaC and DDM, but no or little uptake into TWEEs was detected (Figure 7). However, both PEs greatly increased the staining of the lamina propria, and a stripy lateral labeling along the enterocytes was now clearly visible, implying a higher paracellular permeability of TRD.

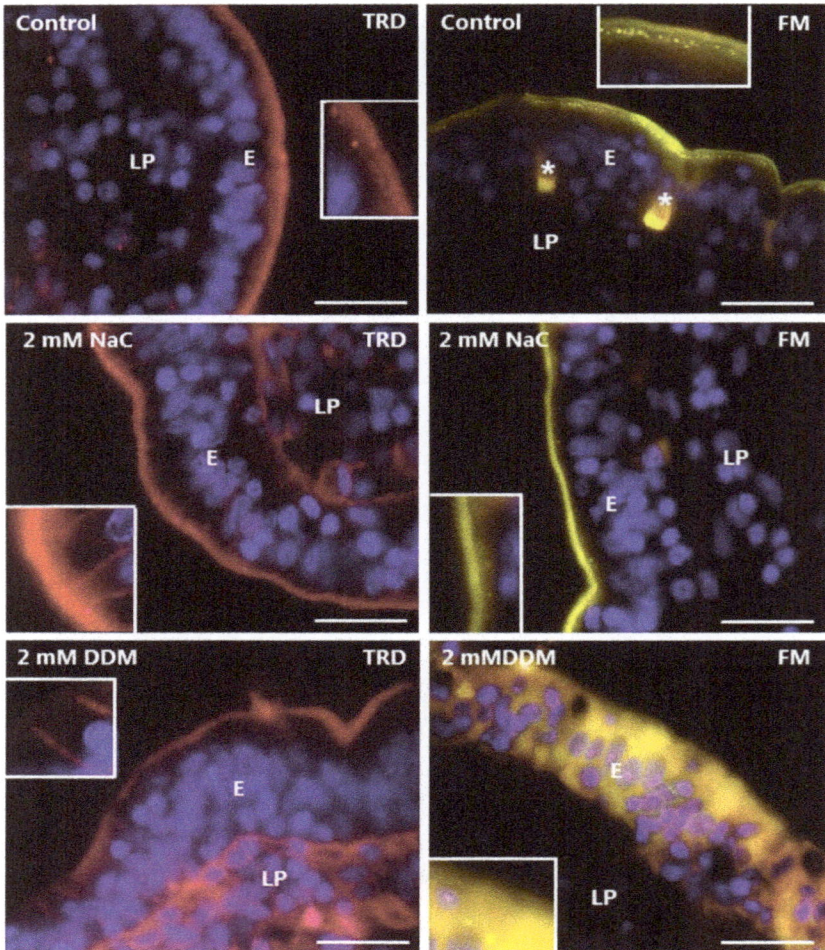

Figure 7. Permeability of the mucosal epithelium probed with TRD and FM. Sections of mucosal explants cultured for 1 h with TRD or FM in the absence or presence of 2 mM NaC or DDM, respectively. In the control, TRD bound to the enterocyte brush border, but only few and weakly-stained TRD-positive supapical punctae were observed. In addition, a faint labeling of the lamina propria was detectable. NaC and DDM both greatly increased the lateral TRD-labeling and accumulation of the probe in the lamina propria without affecting TRD-binding at the brush border, but little if any leakage was seen into the cytosol of the enterocytes. Like TRD, FM strongly labeled the enterocyte brush border, and also appeared in bright subapical punctae in the control. The brush border labeling was generally unaffected by both surfactants, but subapical punctae were sparse. Occasionally, FM was absent from the brush border, but leaked into the cytosol of enterocytes, as shown for DDM, but no staining of the lamina propria was observed. (Asterisks show goblet cells labeled by FM and inserts show enlarged image details.) Bars: 20 μm.

FM is a non-toxic, water-soluble and lipophilic probe (MW 560 Da) that only becomes fluorescent when incorporated into cell membranes [31], and as shown in Figure 7, it strongly labeled the entire brush border of control enterocytes together with goblet cells. In addition, it was efficiently taken up into TWEEs like LY, as earlier reported [29]. However, in contrast to LY, FM did not stain the lamina propria or the basolateral sides of the enterocytes, indicating that this lipophilic probe, despite its small size, is incapable of paracellular passage through the tight junctions. FM labeling of the brush border was generally not affected by NaC or DDM, but the uptake into TWEEs was greatly diminished (Figure 7). Lamina propria and lateral staining with FM was not detected in the presence of the PEs; however, as seen with LY, leakage into the cytosol of enterocytes was occasionally observed.

In summary, the results obtained with LY, TRD and FM documented both paracellular and transcellular mechanisms of action of both NaC and DDM. The data are consistent with the PEs interacting with/inserting into the brush border membrane, resulting in functional leaks in the bilayer that allow passage of both small polar (LY) and lipophilic (FM) compounds. In addition, the ability of the apical cell membrane to engage in endocytosis was largely abolished by both PEs. This effectively excludes the possibility that they act as PEs by stimulating luminal endocytotic uptake.

3.5. Effects of NaC and DDM on the Ultrastructure of the Enterocyte Brush Border

Transmission electron microscopy was employed to study in closer detail the direct action of NaC and DDM on the morphology of the enterocytes. As shown in Figure 8A, the brush border of enterocytes from control explants in longitudinal sections from the mid-villus area consisted of a regular array of uniform microvilli of about 1.2–1.3 μm in length with actin rootlets extending into the subapical terminal web region. Microvillus length gradually increases in enterocytes along the villi as enterocytes move towards the extrusion zone at the tip, but microvillus diameter normally remains unchanged at ~0.1 μm throughout the crypt-villus migration, as shown in cross sections (Figure 8D). NaC (2 mM) did not affect the overall columnar shape of enterocytes or microvillus length in the brush border (Figure 8B). However, in cross sections, the normally ordered, hexagonal alignment of microvilli was less dense and frequently disrupted, and microvilli of smaller diameter were scattered amongst seemingly normal microvilli (Figure 8E). In addition, bulbous protrusions were occasionally observed at the tip of the microvilli (Figure 9A). Membrane-enveloped spherical bodies containing electron-dense material and with a diameter of about 0.3 μM were frequently observed interspaced between the microvilli, and in some cases they were surrounded by small (~50 nm) vesicles seemingly attached to their surface. (Figure 9B,C).

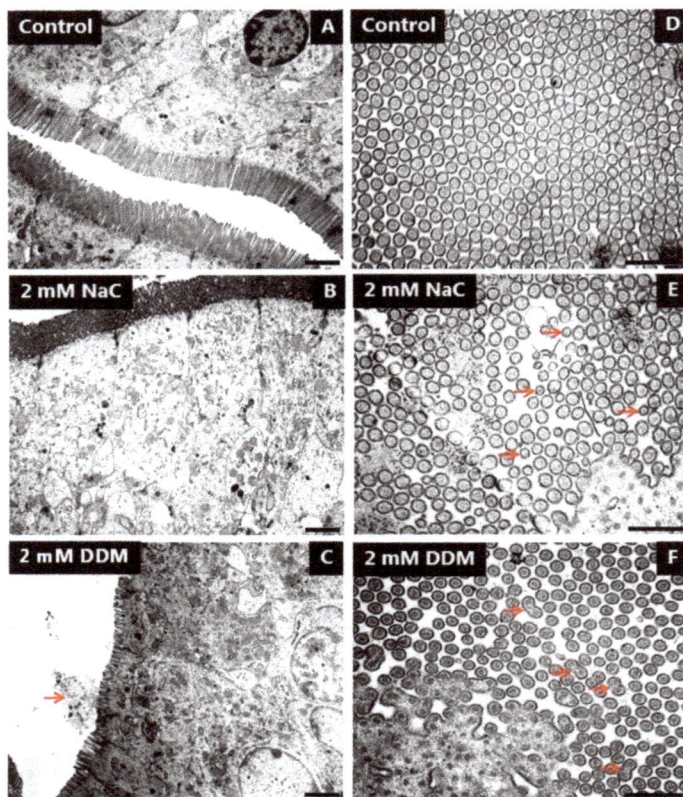

Figure 8. Effects of NaC and DDM on brush border ultrastructure. Electron micrographs showing longitudinal (**A–C**) and cross sections (**D–F**) of the brush border. (Arrows indicate apparent leakage into the lumen of cellular debris from the brush border in (**C**), microvilli with diminished diameter in (**E**) and fused microvilli in (**F**).) Bars: 1 μm (**A–C**); 0.5 μm (**D–F**).

Enterocytes were also generally well preserved after exposure to DDM (2 mM), but in contrast to NaC, DDM caused a marked shortening of the microvilli of villus enterocytes (Figure 8C). The effect was variable, but frequently cells with microvilli as short as 0.5 μm were observed. Although one must be cautious interpreting such data because, as mentioned above, microvillus length generally increases as enterocytes move along the crypt-villus axis, stunted microvilli like those seen with DDM are normally found only at the bottom of the crypts. In cross sections, the microvilli were of normal diameter, but as with NaC, the hexagonal alignment was less dense and organized than in the control. However, longitudinal fusion of pairs of microvilli was occasionally observed (Figure 8F). Noticeably, variation in microvillus length sometimes even occurred between neighboring cells (Figure 9D). At high magnification, microvesiculation of single microvilli was evident, and the tips of the microvilli often appeared flat instead of the normal rounded shape of a cap (Figure 9E). In areas near the bottom of the villi, vesicle-like structures and amorphous material, probably leaking through the brush border (Figure 8C), accumulated in the narrow cleft between opposing villi (Figure 9F). This phenomenon was observed both with NaC and DDM.

In contrast to the brush border, the tight junctions and meandering lateral cell membranes were seemingly unaffected by both PEs at 2 mM (data not shown). Taken together, the electron microscopy data therefore strongly indicate that the brush border is the primary target of both NaC and DDM. The lesions induced by NaC and DDM were similar, but not identical, implying that the two PEs cause disruption of the membrane organization by different mechanisms.

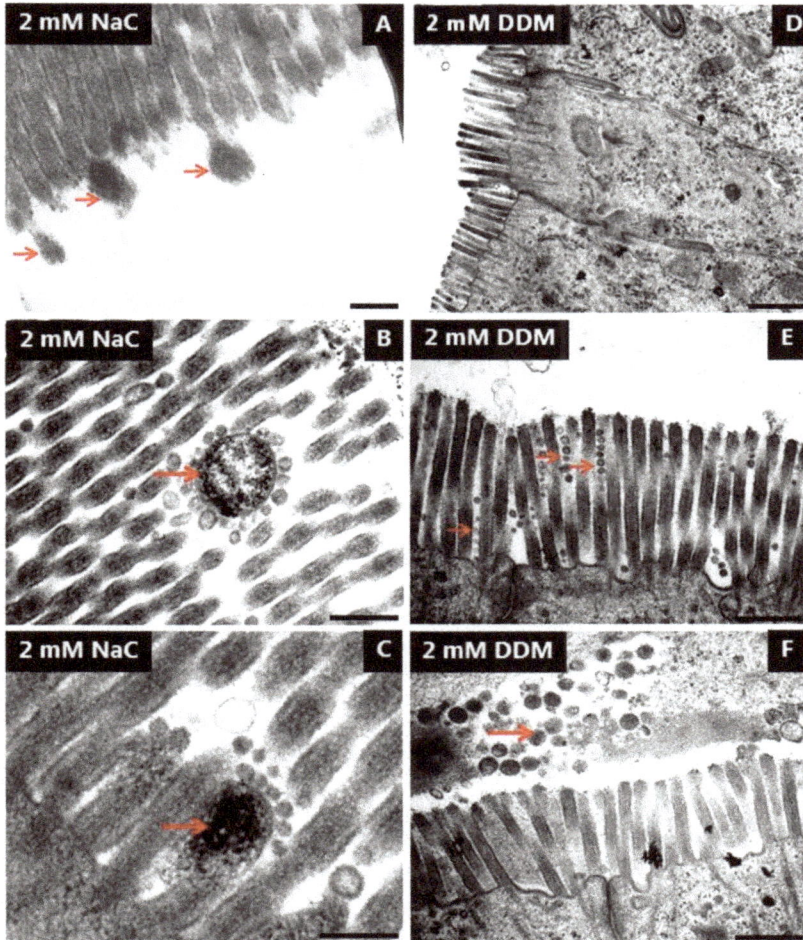

Figure 9. Effects of NaC and DDM on brush border ultrastructure. Electron micrographs showing different lesions in the brush border induced by NaC or DDM. Arrows indicate bulbous protrusions from single microvilli in (**A**), electron dense bodies with small vesicles attached in (**B**) and (**C**), microvesiculated, single microvilli in (**E**) and accumulated cellular debris in the lumen in (**F**). Bars: 0.2 μm (**A–C**); 1 μm (**D**); 0.5 μm (**E,F**).

4. Discussion

Surfactants belonging to the bile salt or alkyl maltoside classes of compounds all have a long history as PEs, but with regard to the intestinal permeation enhancement, they have so far been tested mainly either in epithelial cell models, most often Caco-2 cells, or in colonic tissue [6,32,33]. For this reason, we thought it worthwhile to reinvestigate the PE action of NaC and DDM in a jejunal mucosal explant system. The jejunum is the region of the intestine where endogeneous bile salts normally aid assimilation of poorly-soluble dietary constituents and where the brush border membrane presumably is optimally equipped to withstand the action of luminal surfactants under physiological conditions.

In elucidating the PE action of a specific compound, it is essential to clarify the mechanism whereby epithelial permeabilization is achieved, i.e., whether a paracellular and/or transcellular route is facilitated [34,35]. Bile salts and alkyl maltosides are commonly classified as multimodal in their action, i.e., acting both via para and transcellular mechanism(s) [6,36], and the results of the present work agree well with this classification. Hypothetically, transcellular permeabilization may occur by endocytosis by one or more of several clathrin-dependent or independent molecular mechanisms known to internalize cell membrane and cargo to the cellular endosomal system. In enterocytes, apical endocytosis of cargo might be succeeded by trancytosis, leading to a complete crossing of the epithelial barrier [9,37,38]. In this context, the main conclusion of the present work is that neither NaC nor DDM achieved transcellular permeability by stimulating apical endocytotic uptake. In contrast, both largely abolished the constitutive endocytosis of polar (LY) and lipophilic (FM) probes that normally operates at the brush border and which can be readily visualized by these fluorescent compounds. Instead, transcellular permeabilization occurred by rendering the apical cell membrane leaky. The sometimes mosaic appearance of leaky enterocytes adjacent to unaffected cells together with the selective leakiness to the 444 Da LY, but not the 3-kDa TRD, implies that disruption of the membrane bilayer was not too extensive. This agrees well with the electron microscopy data, showing a reasonably well-preserved microvillus ultrastructure. Nevertheless, the partial break-up of the uniform hexagonal organization of microvilli and the appearance of scattered, abnormally thin (NaC) or fused (DDM) microvilli are direct visual evidence of PE-induced membrane damage. Some of the lesions observed in this study resemble those previously reported for intestinal brush borders of myosin-1a gene knockout mice, including disorganization of microvilli and bulbous protrusions from the microvillus tips [39]. Myosin-1a is a motor protein that links the microvillus actin cytoskeleton with the cell membrane and, amongst other functions, is responsible for the mechanical stabilization of the microvillus structure [1,2]. If PEs like NaC are able to disrupt this link, it could be the triggering event that ultimately leads to the observed morphological changes of the brush border. This suggests a stochastic process of disruption where single, affected microvilli form microvesicles and break up, followed by membrane resealing. Given the fact that the brush border architecture expands the apical surface area of the enterocyte roughly ten times compared to a "flat" cell surface [40], it harbors a large membrane reservoir for use in repair of damaged microvilli. Interestingly, microvillus microvesiculation in the rat and mouse has been proposed to be the result of a Ca^{2+}-induced, villin-dependent severing of the actin filaments [41], and the subsequent release of vesicles into the lumen as a physiological process in the gut host defense aimed to deploy catalytic activities into the intestinal lumen [39,42,43]. Microvillus microvesiculation was very rarely observed in cultured control explants in this study on porcine jejunum, but the induction of this process by DDM may nevertheless reflect an uncontrolled triggering of a natural process.

In recent studies, other types of surfactant PEs (lauroyl-carnitine, monocaprin and the ethoxylate $C_{12}E_9$) were found to permeabilize the brush border mainly by inducing microvillus microvesiculation and/or longitudinal fusion of microvilli [18], and the amphipathic cell penetrating peptide melittin caused a marked elongation both of microvilli and their actin rootlets [19]. Nevertheless, despite apparent differences in modes of microvillus disruption, these different types of PE agents all resulted in membrane leakage of LY as well as inhibition of apical endocytosis. Collectively, we infer from these observations that although the mechanism of action of the different types of membrane-interacting agents seems to vary, they possess a similar functionality as PEs. The common endocytosis-inhibiting effect may seem intriguing, and we are not certain of its cause. It could be ascribed simply to energy depletion by leakage of ATP or loss of essential other small molecules/ions, but local changes in membrane fluidity and lipid raft structure might also be sufficient to interfere with endocytosis even in areas where the microvillus architecture remains intact. The latter explanation

Pharmaceutics **2018**, *10*, 172

is supported by the DRM analysis showing that "non raft" areas of the microvillus membrane are preferentially targeted by NaC and DDM.

5. Conclusions

In the present work, we studied the action of a bile salt (NaC) and an alkyl maltoside (DDM) on the different luminal uptake pathways across the intestinal epithelium, using a jejunal mucosal organ culture model. Both PEs increased the paracellular and transcellular pathways for polar fluorescent probes, but of note, one common uptake mechanism, endocytosis, was virtually blocked. Instead, leakage through the brush border membrane occurred. Ultrastructurally, lesions of the brush border included microvillus microvesiculation, shortening, longitudinal fusion of microvilli, and the formation and extrusion of dense bodies. A DRM analysis of microvillus membrane vesicles indicated that both NaC and DDM, like the nonionic detergent Triton X-100, preferentially extract the "non-raft" domains of the lipid bilayer, thereby decreasing the fluidity of the remaining membrane.

Author Contributions: Conceptualization, E.M.D.; Methodology, E.M.D., G.H.H.; Investigation, E.M.D.; G.H.H.; Writing-Original Draft Preparation, E.M.D.; Writing-Review & Editing, E.M.D., G.H.H.; Project Administration, E.M.D.; Funding Acquisition, E.M.D.

Funding: The Research was funded by a grant from Læge Sofus Carl Emil Friis og hustru Olga Doris Friis legat.

Acknowledgments: Karina Rasmussen is thanked for excellent technical assistance.

Conflicts of Interest: The authors declare no conflict of interest.

References

1. Crawley, S.W.; Mooseker, M.S.; Tyska, M.J. Shaping the intestinal brush border. *J. Cell Biol.* **2014**, *207*, 441–451. [CrossRef] [PubMed]
2. Delacour, D.; Salomon, J.; Robine, S.; Louvard, D. Plasticity of the brush border—The yin and yang of intestinal homeostasis. *Nat. Rev. Gastroenterol. Hepatol.* **2016**, *13*, 161–174. [CrossRef] [PubMed]
3. Christiansen, K.; Carlsen, J. Microvillus membrane vesicles from pig small intestine. Purity and lipid composition. *Biochim. Biophys. Acta* **1981**, *647*, 188–195. [CrossRef]
4. Danielsen, E.M.; Hansen, G.H. Lipid rafts in epithelial brush borders: Atypical membrane microdomains with specialized functions. *Biochim. Biophys. Acta* **2003**, *1617*, 1–9. [CrossRef] [PubMed]
5. Simons, K.; Ikonen, E. Functional rafts in cell membranes. *Nature* **1997**, *387*, 569–572. [CrossRef] [PubMed]
6. Maher, S.; Mrsny, R.J.; Brayden, D.J. Intestinal permeation enhancers for oral peptide delivery. *Adv. Drug Deliv. Rev.* **2016**, *106*, 277–319. [CrossRef] [PubMed]
7. Lichtenberg, D.; Robson, R.J.; Dennis, E.A. Solubilization of phospholipids by detergents. Structural and kinetic aspects. *Biochim. Biophys. Acta* **1983**, *737*, 285–304. [CrossRef]
8. McCartney, F.; Gleeson, J.P.; Brayden, D.J. Safety concerns over the use of intestinal permeation enhancers: A mini-review. *Tissue Barriers* **2016**, *4*, e1176822. [CrossRef] [PubMed]
9. Lundquist, P.; Artursson, P. Oral absorption of peptides and nanoparticles across the human intestine: Opportunities, limitations and studies in human tissues. *Adv. Drug Deliv. Rev.* **2016**, *106*, 256–276. [CrossRef] [PubMed]
10. Sanchez-Navarro, M.; Garcia, J.; Giralt, E.; Teixido, M. Using peptides to increase transport across the intestinal barrier. *Adv. Drug Deliv. Rev.* **2016**, *106*, 355–366. [CrossRef] [PubMed]
11. Shiau, Y.F. Mechanisms of intestinal fat absorption. *Am. J. Physiol.* **1981**, *240*, G1–G9. [CrossRef] [PubMed]
12. Aungst, B.J. Absorption enhancers: Applications and advances. *AAPS J.* **2012**, *14*, 10–18. [CrossRef] [PubMed]
13. Fasinu, P.; Pillay, V.; Ndesendo, V.M.; du Toit, L.C.; Choonara, Y.E. Diverse approaches for the enhancement of oral drug bioavailability. *Biopharm. Drug Dispos.* **2011**, *32*, 185–209. [CrossRef] [PubMed]
14. Yewale, C.; Patil, S.; Kolate, A.; Kore, G.; Misra, A. Oral Absorption Promoters: Opportunities, Issues, and Challenges. *Crit. Rev. Ther. Drug Carr. Syst.* **2015**, *32*, 363–387. [CrossRef]

15. Petersen, S.B.; Nolan, G.; Maher, S.; Rahbek, U.L.; Guldbrandt, M.; Brayden, D.J. Evaluation of alkylmaltosides as intestinal permeation enhancers: Comparison between rat intestinal mucosal sheets and Caco-2 monolayers. *Eur. J. Pharm. Sci.* **2012**, *47*, 701–712. [CrossRef] [PubMed]

16. Lorenzen, U.S.; Hansen, G.H.; Danielsen, E.M. Organ Culture as a Model System for Studies on Enterotoxin Interactions with the Intestinal Epithelium. *Methods Mol. Biol.* **2016**, *1396*, 159–166. [PubMed]

17. Danielsen, E.T.; Danielsen, E.M. Glycol chitosan: A stabilizer of lipid rafts in the intestinal brush border. *Biochim. Biophys. Acta* **2017**, *1859*, 360–367. [CrossRef] [PubMed]

18. Danielsen, E.M.; Hansen, G.H. Intestinal surfactant permeation enhancers and their interaction with enterocyte cell membranes in a mucosal explant system. *Tissue Barriers* **2017**, *5*, e1361900. [CrossRef] [PubMed]

19. Danielsen, E.M.; Hansen, G.H. Impact of cell-penetrating peptides (CPPs) melittin and Hiv-1 Tat on the enterocyte brush border using a mucosal explant system. *Biochim. Biophys. Acta* **2018**, *1860*, 1589–1599. [CrossRef] [PubMed]

20. Hansen, G.H.; Sjostrom, H.; Noren, O.; Dabelsteen, E. Immunomicroscopic localization of aminopeptidase N in the pig enterocyte. Implications for the route of intracellular transport. *Eur. J. Cell Biol.* **1987**, *43*, 253–259. [PubMed]

21. Danielsen, E.M.; Sjostrom, H.; Noren, O.; Bro, B.; Dabelsteen, E. Biosynthesis of intestinal microvillar proteins. Characterization of intestinal explants in organ culture and evidence for the existence of pro-forms of the microvillar enzymes. *Biochem. J.* **1982**, *202*, 647–654. [CrossRef] [PubMed]

22. Booth, A.G.; Kenny, A.J. A rapid method for the preparation of microvilli from rabbit kidney. *Biochem. J.* **1974**, *142*, 575–581. [CrossRef] [PubMed]

23. Brown, D.A.; Rose, J.K. Sorting of GPI-anchored proteins to glycolipid-enriched membrane subdomains during transport to the apical cell surface. *Cell* **1992**, *68*, 533–544. [CrossRef]

24. Danielsen, E.M. Involvement of detergent-insoluble complexes in the intracellular transport of intestinal brush border enzymes. *Biochemistry* **1995**, *34*, 1596–1605. [CrossRef] [PubMed]

25. Laemmli, U.K. Cleavage of structural proteins during the assembly of the head of bacteriophage T4. *Nature* **1970**, *227*, 680–685. [CrossRef] [PubMed]

26. Brown, D.A. Lipid rafts, detergent-resistant membranes, and raft targeting signals. *Physiology* **2006**, *21*, 430–439. [CrossRef] [PubMed]

27. Hanani, M. Lucifer yellow—An angel rather than the devil. *J. Cell. Mol. Med.* **2012**, *16*, 22–31. [CrossRef] [PubMed]

28. Danielsen, E.M.; Hansen, G.H.; Rasmussen, K.; Niels-Christiansen, L.L. Permeabilization of enterocytes induced by absorption of dietary fat. *Mol. Membr. Biol.* **2013**, *30*, 261–272. [CrossRef] [PubMed]

29. Hansen, G.H.; Rasmussen, K.; Niels-Christiansen, L.L.; Danielsen, E.M. Endocytic trafficking from the small intestinal brush border probed with FM dye. *Am. J. Physiol. Gastrointest. Liver Physiol.* **2009**, *297*, G708–G715. [CrossRef] [PubMed]

30. Woodcroft, B.J.; Hammond, L.; Stow, J.L.; Hamilton, N.A. Automated organelle-based colocalization in whole-cell imaging. *Cytom. A* **2009**, *75*, 941–950. [CrossRef] [PubMed]

31. Bolte, S.; Talbot, C.; Boutte, Y.; Catrice, O.; Read, N.D.; Satiat-Jeunemaitre, B. FM-dyes as experimental probes for dissecting vesicle trafficking in living plant cells. *J. Microsc.* **2004**, *214*, 159–173. [CrossRef] [PubMed]

32. Lucarini, S.; Fagioli, L.; Cavanagh, R.; Liang, W.; Perinelli, D.R.; Campana, M.; Stolnik, S.; Lam, J.K.W.; Casettari, L.; Duranti, A. Synthesis, Structure(-)Activity Relationships and In Vitro Toxicity Profile of Lactose-Based Fatty Acid Monoesters as Possible Drug Permeability Enhancers. *Pharmaceutics* **2018**, *10*, 81. [CrossRef] [PubMed]

33. Lucarini, S.; Fagioli, L.; Campana, R.; Cole, H.; Duranti, A.; Baffone, W.; Vllasaliu, D.; Casettari, L. Unsaturated fatty acids lactose esters: Cytotoxicity, permeability enhancement and antimicrobial activity. *Eur. J. Pharm. Biopharm.* **2016**, *107*, 88–96. [CrossRef] [PubMed]

34. Blikslager, A.T.; Moeser, A.J.; Gookin, J.L.; Jones, S.L.; Odle, J. Restoration of barrier function in injured intestinal mucosa. *Physiol. Rev.* **2007**, *87*, 545–564. [CrossRef] [PubMed]

35. Odenwald, M.A.; Turner, J.R. The intestinal epithelial barrier: A therapeutic target? *Nat. Rev. Gastroenterol. Hepatol.* **2017**, *14*, 9–21. [CrossRef] [PubMed]

36. Moghimipour, E.; Ameri, A.; Handali, S. Absorption-Enhancing Effects of Bile Salts. *Molecules* **2015**, *20*, 14451–14473. [CrossRef] [PubMed]

37. Doherty, G.J.; McMahon, H.T. Mechanisms of endocytosis. *Annu. Rev. Biochem.* **2009**, *78*, 857–902. [CrossRef] [PubMed]
38. Mrsny, R.J. Strategies for targeting protein therapeutics to selected tissues and cells. *Expert Opin. Biol. Ther.* **2004**, *4*, 65–73. [CrossRef] [PubMed]
39. Tyska, M.J.; Mackey, A.T.; Huang, J.D.; Copeland, N.G.; Jenkins, N.A.; Mooseker, M.S. Myosin-1a is critical for normal brush border structure and composition. *Mol. Biol. Cell* **2005**, *16*, 2443–2457. [CrossRef] [PubMed]
40. Helander, H.F.; Fandriks, L. Surface area of the digestive tract—Revisited. *Scand. J. Gastroenterol.* **2014**, *49*, 681–689. [CrossRef] [PubMed]
41. Mooseker, M.S.; Graves, T.A.; Wharton, K.A.; Falco, N.; Howe, C.L. Regulation of microvillus structure: Calcium-dependent solation and cross-linking of actin filaments in the microvilli of intestinal epithelial cells. *J. Cell Biol.* **1980**, *87*, 809–822. [CrossRef] [PubMed]
42. McConnell, R.E.; Higginbotham, J.N.; Shifrin, D.A., Jr.; Tabb, D.L.; Coffey, R.J.; Tyska, M.J. The enterocyte microvillus is a vesicle-generating organelle. *J. Cell Biol.* **2009**, *185*, 1285–1298. [CrossRef] [PubMed]
43. Shifrin, D.A., Jr.; Tyska, M.J. Ready . . . aim . . . fire into the lumen: A new role for enterocyte microvilli in gut host defense. *Gut Microbes* **2012**, *3*, 460–462. [CrossRef] [PubMed]

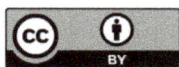

pharmaceutics

MDPI

Article

Mechanistic Studies on the Absorption-Enhancing Effects of Gemini Surfactant on the Intestinal Absorption of Poorly Absorbed Hydrophilic Drugs in Rats

Tammam Alama [1], Kosuke Kusamori [2], Masaki Morishita [1], Hidemasa Katsumi [1], Toshiyasu Sakane [3] and Akira Yamamoto [1,*]

[1]   Department of Biopharmaceutics, Kyoto Pharmaceutical University, Misasagi, Yamashina-Ku, Kyoto 607-8414, Japan; abowaleed87@gmail.com (T.A.); morishita@mb.kyoto-phu.ac.jp (M.M.); hkatsumi@mb.kyoto-phu.ac.jp (H.K.)
[2]   Laboratory of Biopharmaceutics, Faculty of Pharmaceutical Sciences, Tokyo University of Science, 2641 Yamazaki, Noda, Chiba 278-8510, Japan; kusamori@rs.tus.ac.jp
[3]   Department of Pharmaceutical Technology, Kobe Pharmaceutical University, Higashinada-ku, Kobe 658-8558, Japan; sakane@kobepharma-u.ac.jp
*   Correspondence: yamamoto@mb.kyoto-phu.ac.jp; Tel.: +81-75-595-4661; Fax: +81-75-595-4761

Received: 12 January 2019; Accepted: 28 March 2019; Published: 7 April 2019

Abstract: Generally, the use of absorption enhancers might be the most effective approaches to ameliorate the enteric absorption of poorly absorbed substances. Among numerous absorption enhancers, we already reported that a gemini surfactant, sodium dilauramidoglutamide lysine (SLG-30) with two hydrophobic and two hydrophilic moieties, is a novel and promising adjuvant with a high potency in improving the absorption safely. Here, we examined and elucidated the absorption-improving mechanisms of SLG-30 in the enteric absorption of substances. SLG-30 increased the intestinal absorption of 5(6)-carboxyfluorescein (CF) to a greater level than the typical absorption enhancers, including sodium glycocholate and sodium laurate, as evaluated by an *in situ* closed-loop method. Furthermore, SLG-30 significantly lowered the fluorescence anisotropy of dansyl chloride (DNS-Cl), suggesting that it might increase the fluidity of protein sections in the intestinal cell membranes. Moreover, SLG-30 significantly lowered the transepithelial-electrical resistance (TEER) values of Caco-2 cells, suggesting that it might open the tight junctions (TJs) between the enteric epithelial cells. Additionally, the levels of claudin-1 and claudin-4 expression decreased in the presence of SLG-30. These outcomes propose that SLG-30 might improve the enteric transport of poorly absorbed substances through both transcellular and paracellular routes.

Keywords: absorption enhancer; gemini surfactant; intestinal absorption; poorly absorbed drug; Caco-2 cells

---

1. Introduction

The enteric epithelium represents a physical barrier for the intestinal absorption of most substances to the systemic-circulation. It is well-established that the enteric epithelium acts as an impervious barrier against many pathogens and toxins through its complicated structure, although it can permit the intestinal absorption of nutrients [1]. The most important barrier against the permeability of drugs is the brush-border membranes of the enteric epithelial cells, which can restrict the passage of drugs through cells into the systemic circulation. The other important barrier is the tight junction between the adjacent cells, which is an aqueous route for compounds of molecular weight less than 500 Da [2–4]. These two barriers are considered great hurdles when some drugs are transported across the intestinal epithelial cells, assuming that drugs could survive the harsh environment and the decomposition in the gastrointestinal tract [5,6]. Therefore, the major routes for drugs to be absorbed by the intestinal cells are the transcellular and paracellular routes [7–9]. This could be a serious problem for a wide range of newly discovered and synthesized drugs, especially peptide and protein drugs, which also suffer from enzymatic deterioration [10] in the gastrointestinal tract before reaching the enteric cell membrane.

A variety of systems have been tested to improve the enteric absorption of poorly absorbed substances [1]. Of all these approaches, the use of absorption enhancers is a promising way to improve the enteric absorption of poorly absorbed substances [11–20]. It was reported that typical absorption enhancers involving medium chain fatty acids (e.g., sodium laurate, sodium caprate, and sodium caprylate) could improve the absorption of poorly absorbed substances such as antibiotics, peptide and protein drugs, and bisphosphonates [11–20]. However, most of the typical absorption-enhancers usually prompt irritation along with damage to enteric membranes.

Gemini surfactants are a new type of absorption enhancers with a rather different structure than the typical ones [21]. The structure is composed of two hydrophilic heads connected with a linker and two hydrophobic tails. This structure makes the CMC values of gemini-type surfactants lower than the CMC values of typical surfactants with an equal chain length [21]. However, the effects of gemini surfactants on the enteric absorption of substances and how they improve absorption are seldom studied.

We previously reported SLG-30, a gemini surfactant, increased the enteric absorption of hydrophilic poorly absorbed substances [22]. As shown in Figure 1, the hydrophilic heads of SLG-30 have two amino acid derivatives, i.e., two glutamic acid moieties, linked through a lysine spacer, and two hydrophobic chains of twelve carbons each [23]. We showed that SLG-30 might be safe *in vitro* and *in vivo* and may be a very efficient absorption enhancer, which can possibly be used as an adjuvant in oral formulations for increasing the enteric absorption of poorly absorbed hydrophilic substances. However, we did not compare the effectiveness of SLG-30 with that of typical absorption enhancers regarding the enteric absorption of substances. Moreover, the absorption-enhancing mechanisms of SLG-30 in improving the enteric absorption of poorly absorbed substances were not clearly understood.

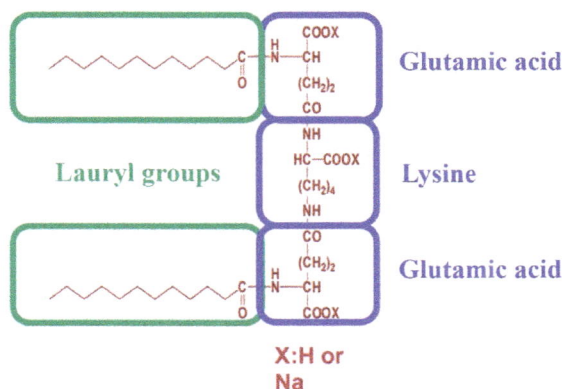

Figure 1. The chemical structure of a gemini surfactant, SLG-30. The hydrophilic moiety of this surfactant has two derivatives of amino acid, i.e., two glutamic acid moieties, linked through a lysine spacer, while the hydrophobic moieties are lauric acid.

The purpose of this study was to study the difference between SLG-30, a gemini surfactant, with typical absorption enhancers, including sodium glycocholate and sodium laurate, regarding absorption-enhancing performance. Furthermore, we also examined and clarified the possible absorption-enhancing mechanisms of SLG-30 on the enteric absorption of substances.

2. Materials and Methods

2.1. Materials

Male Wistar rats, weighing 250–300 g, were purchased from SLC, Inc. (Hamamatsu, Shizuoka, Japan). SLG-30 was kindly supplied by Asahi Kasei Chemicals Co. (Tokyo, Japan). CF was obtained from Eastman Kodak Co. (Rochester, NY, USA). LDH-Cytotoxicity Test Wako, sodium glycocholate (NaGC), sodium laurate, and tma-DPH (1-(4-(trimethylamino)phenyl)-6-phenylhexa-1,3,5-hexatriene-p-toluenesulfonate) were purchased from Wako Pure Chemical Industries, Ltd. (Osaka, Japan). DPH (1,6-diphenyl-1,3,5-hexatriene) and Hank's balanced salt solution (HBSS) were purchased from Sigma-Aldrich Chemical Co. (St. Louis, MO, USA). Dansyl chloride (DNS-Cl) was purchased from Santa Cruz Biotechnology, Inc. (Dallas, Texas, USA). Anti-claudin-1, anti-β-actin (rabbit monoclonal antibodies), and goat anti-rabbit IgG HRP-linked antibodies were purchased from Cell Signaling Technology® (Danvers, MA, USA). Anti-claudin-4 (mouse monoclonal antibodies) and rabbit anti-mouse IgG HRP-linked antibodies were purchased from Invitrogen™ (Carlsbad, CA, USA). Chemi-Lumi One Ultra kit, Dulbecco's modified Eagle medium (DMEM) with 4500 mg/L glucose, nonessential amino acids (MEM–NEAA), antibiotic–antimycotic mixture stock (10,000 U/mL penicillin, 10,000 μg/mL streptomycin, and 25 μg/mL amphotericin B in 0.85% sodium chloride), and 0.25% trypsin-1 mM EDTA solution were purchased from Nacalai Tesque Inc. (Kyoto, Japan). Human colon adenocarcinoma-derived Caco-2 cell line was purchased from Dainippon Sumitomo Pharma Co., Ltd. (Osaka, Japan). Fetal bovine serum (FBS) was purchased from Gibco® Life Technologies (Grand Island, NE, USA). All other reagents used in the experiments were of analytical grade.

2.2. In Vivo Enteric Absorption Studies

The enteric absorption of CF was examined by an *in situ* closed-loop method, as reported previously [22,24]. The experiments were carried out in accordance with the guidelines of the Animal Ethics Committee at Kyoto Pharmaceutical University. The protocols were approved by this Committee (permit number: 16-12-069, permit date: 14 April 2016). The rats were starved overnight for approx. 16 h pre-dosing, but water was freely available. After inducing anesthesia with sodium pentobarbital which was administered intraperitoneally at a dose of 32 mg/kg body weight, the rats were placed under a heat lamp to maintain a body temperature at around 37 °C, and the intestines were exposed using a midline-abdominal incision. After the bile duct was ligated, the intestines were washed with phosphate buffered saline (PBS, pH 7.4), and the remaining buffer solution was expelled with air. Enteric cannulation was performed at both ends using polyethylene tubing, and the distal parts of the small intestines were clipped by forceps. The dosing solutions (3 mL) with or without absorption enhancers kept at 37 °C, were directly introduced into the lumen of the enteric loop through a cannulated opening in the proximal part of the small enteric loop, which was then closed by clipping with another forceps. The jugular vein was exposed, and approx. 0.3 mL of blood was collected via a direct puncture into heparinized syringes at predetermined time intervals up to 240 min. The samples were immediately centrifuged at 12,000 rpm ($15,000 \times g$) for a period of 5 min to obtain the plasma fraction, which was stored on ice for further analysis. CF fluorescence signals in these plasma samples were detected after the treatment with the same volume of acetonitrile using a fluorescence spectrophotometer, Powerscan1 HT supplied by BioTek Instruments (Winooski, VT, USA) at an excitation wavelength of 485 nm and an emission wavelength of 535 nm. There was no significant background fluorescence in the plasma when the fluorescence intensities of CF were determined in this study. The peak drug concentrations (C_{max}) and the time to reach the peak drug concentrations (T_{max}) in the plasma were directly determined from the plasma concentration–time profiles. The area under the curve (AUC) was calculated by the trapezoidal method from pre-dose (time zero) till the administration of the final sample. The absorption enhancement ratios of CF, with or without absorption enhancers, were calculated as follows:

$$\text{Absorption enhancement ratio} = AUC_{\text{with enhancer}} / AUC_{\text{control without enhancer}}$$

2.3. Preparation of Brush Border Membrane Vesicles (BBMVs)

To prepare BBMVs, we followed the methods as reported previously [25–27] with a slight modification. Briefly, an *in situ* small intestinal loop was prepared in each rat, as mentioned above, and then, PBS (pH 7.4) was administered into the loop. The fat was trimmed off from the small intestine and mesentery. Then, the whole small intestine was soaked in ice-cold PBS (pH 7.4). The small intestine was divided into 10 cm segments. Mucosa was scraped out with a slide glass from each of these segments and used for subsequent studies. BBMVs were prepared by the divalent cation precipitation method using $MgCl_2$ in the presence of ethylenebis (oxyethylenenitrilo) tetraacetic acid (EGTA) [25–27]. Briefly, the collected mucosa was homogenized in a buffer containing mannitol (300 mM), EGTA (5 mM), and Tris (pH 7.4) (12 mM) by using a tissue homogenizer. An aqueous solution of 10 mM magnesium chloride was added to the homogenate. The homogenate was centrifuged at $3000\times g$ for 15 min. The supernatant was then centrifuged at $32,000\times g$ for 30 min. The pellet was resuspended in a buffer containing mannitol (300 mM), EGTA (5 mM), and Tris (pH 7.4) (12 mM) by using a 26-G needle. The protein concentration was determined by the BCA method using bovine serum albumin as a standard, and the final concentration was adjusted to 1 mg/ml in each Eppendorf tube. The samples were frozen by liquid nitrogen and kept at −80 °C for further studies.

2.4. Measurement of Membrane Fluidity by Fluorescence Polarization

The BBMVs (100 µg protein) were incubated with 1 µM DPH, with 0.5 µM tma-DPH or with 5 µM DNS-Cl in HEPES-Tris buffer (25 mM HEPES, 5.4 mM KCl, 1.8 mM $CaCl_2$, 0.8 mM $MgSO_4$, 140 mM NaCl, 5 mM glucose, pH 7.4 adjusted by 1 M Tris) in the dark at 37 °C for 30 min [25,28]. Then, various concentrations (0.1% v/v, 0.25% v/v, 0.5% v/v, and 1.0% v/v) of SLG-30 were added. Then, the samples were incubated in the dark for 1 min at 37 °C. For the control group, the same procedure was carried out by adding the HEPES-Tris buffer only. The fluorescence intensities and the steady-state polarization of fluorescence expressed as the fluorescence anisotropy, r, of the labeled membrane vesicles were measured at 37 °C. The excitation and emission wavelengths were λ_{ex} = 360 nm, and λ_{em} = 430 nm for DPH and tma-DPH and λ_{ex} = 380 nm and λ_{em} = 480 nm for DNS-Cl. The measurements were carried out by using a Hitachi Spectrofluorometer (F-2000 Spectrofluorometer, Hitachi Seisakusho Corp, Yokohama, Japan) equipped with a polarizer set.

The fluorescence anisotropy (r) was calculated using the following equation:

$$r = \frac{I_V - I_H}{I_V + 2I_H}$$

where I_V and I_H respectively represent the perpendicular and parallel fluorescence intensities to the polarized excitation plane [29].

2.5. Measurement of Transepithelial Electrical Resistance (TEER) and the Transport of CF Using Caco-2 cell Monolayers

Caco-2 cells (passage 45) were cultured in 175-cm^2 culture flask (Thermo Fisher Scientific™, Waltham, MA, USA). The culture medium consisted of DMEM containing 10% FBS, 0.1 mM MEM–NEAA, 2 mM glutamine, 100 U/mL penicillin, and 100 µg/mL streptomycin [30]. Cells were cultured in a humidified atmosphere of 5% CO_2 at 37 °C. The culture medium was changed every two days. When the cultured Caco-2 cells became sub-confluent, they were seeded onto 12-mm Transwell® with 0.4-µm pore polycarbonate membrane inserts (Corning Inc., New York, NY, USA) at a density of 1×10^5 cells/insert. The transepithelial transport studies were performed when the transepithelial electrical resistance (TEER) values were more than 500 $\Omega \cdot cm^2$ (i.e., after 21 days) [17,18]. Briefly, after removing the incubation medium by aspiration, the apical and basal sides were washed thrice by Hank's Balanced Salt (HBSS) solution (pH 7.4). The cells were incubated in HBSS (pH 6.0) for the apical side and HBSS (pH 7.4) for the basal side for 20 min at 37 °C. HBSS supplemented with 1 mg/mL glucose was used in all cell culture experiments. After removing the washing solution by aspiration, 500 μL of 10 μM CF in a HBSS (pH 6.0) solution with or without various concentrations (0.001% v/v, 0.01% v/v, 0.025% v/v, 0.05% v/v, and 0.1% v/v) of SLG-30, 0.1% (w/v) and 1% (w/v) NaGC or 0.05% (w/v) sodium laurate were added to the apical side at zero time, whereas precisely 1500 μL of HBSS (pH 7.4) was added to the basal side at 37 °C. The cells were kept at 37 °C and 5% CO_2 and were continuously agitated on a shaker during the transport experiments.

The TEER values were measured by Millicell® (ERS-2 Volt-Ohm Meter, Billerica, MA, USA) at the predetermined times up to 24 h, and the initial values were considered as 100%. The samples from the basal side were withdrawn at predetermined time points up to 24 h. The samples were replaced with an equal volume of HBSS (pH 7.4). CF was determined as previously mentioned. The apparent permeability coefficients P_{app} (cm/s) for the transported CF was determined by the following equation:

$$P_{app} = \frac{dX_R}{dt} \times \frac{1}{A} \times \frac{1}{C_0}$$

where P_{app} is the apparent permeability coefficient in centimeters per second, X_R is the amount of CF in moles in the receptor side, $\frac{dX_R}{dt}$ is the flux across the monolayer, A is the diffusion area (i.e., in square centimeters), and C_0 is the initial concentration of CF in the donor side in moles per milliliter.

2.6. Assessment of Caco-2 Cell Damage

After the transport studies were over, the solution on the apical side of each well was collected. Cell injury caused by SLG-30 was determined by tracking the LDH release [31,32]. The cell precipitate and the monolayers left on the filters were solubilized with 1% (v/v) Triton X-100. The solutions from apical sides and the lysates were centrifuged for 7 min at 200× g at a temperature of 4 °C. The activities of LDH in the supernatant were measured. (LDH$_{release}$) stands for the activity of the LDH released into the apical side in the existence of SLG-30. (LDH$_{cell}$) stands for the activity of the LDH obtained from the cell lysate. LDH$_{released}$% was calculated by the following equation:

$$LDH_{release}\% = LDH_{release} \times 100/(LDH_{release} + LDH_{cells})$$

2.7. Western Blotting

Western blotting was performed by the method described previously with slight modifications [33,34]. Three male Wistar rats weighing 250 g were prepared to perform an *in situ* closed-loop method on the small intestine, as mentioned above. A control study, a treatment study, and a pretreatment study were conducted on the first, second, and third rat, respectively. For the control study, only PBS solution (pH 7.4) was administered into the small intestine, and then, the rat was sacrificed, while for the treatment study, SLG-30 was administered for 1 h, and then, the rat was sacrificed without washing the SLG-30 out. The pretreatment study was performed by administrating SLG-30 for 1 h then washing it out with PBS solution (pH 7.4), followed by sacrificing the rat after 4 h. The small intestine (60 cm) of three rats was taken and treated, as mentioned above, for extracting the BBMVs. The total protein amount of each sample was adjusted to 30 μg.

The expression levels of proteins from the claudin family, in the homogenate of the small intestine membrane, were evaluated by western blotting. Briefly, equal amounts of protein samples (30 μg protein) were mixed with an SDS buffer solution and electrophoretically separated on SDS-polyacrylamide (15%) gels. The separated proteins were transferred to a polyvinylidene difluoride (PVDF) membrane. After blocking in 5% skim milk in Tris-buffered saline (pH 7.4) for 1 h at room temperature, the PVDF membrane was incubated overnight in a blocking buffer with diluted (1:1000) monoclonal antibodies for claudin-1, claudin-4, and β-actin at 4 °C. Subsequently, the PVDF membrane was washed three times using Tris-buffered saline containing 0.05% Tween 20 (TTBS), followed by incubation with peroxidase-conjugated anti-rabbit IgG antibody for claudin-1 and β-actin, and with peroxidase-conjugated anti-rabbit IgG antibody for claudin-4 for 1 h at room temperature. The signals were visualized by luminescence imaging (Fujifilm Luminescent Image Analyzer LAS4000 System, Tokyo, Japan). The intensity of each signal was corrected using the values obtained from the β-actin bands, and the relative protein intensity was expressed as the fold change compared to the relative protein intensity in the normal group.

2.8. Statistical Analysis

The results are expressed as the mean ± S.E. of at least three experiments. The statistical significance between groups was analyzed using Dunnett's test; $p < 0.05$ was regarded to be significant. Significance levels are denoted (**) $p < 0.01$, (*) $p < 0.05$, and (n.s.) not significantly different. The number of experiments is indicated by n.

3. Results

3.1. In Vivo Comparative Study between SLG-30 and Typical Surfactants Including Sodium Glycocholate and Sodium Laurate

First, the effects of 0.5% (v/v) SLG-30 and 1% (w/v) sodium glycocholate (NaGC) on the enteric absorption of CF were examined by an *in situ* closed-loop method, and the effectiveness of SLG-30 was compared with that of NaGC (a typical absorption enhancer). As Figure 2 shows, the enteric absorption of CF was significantly improved in the existence of 0.5% (v/v) SLG-30, and the $AUC_{0\rightarrow240}$ of CF was 16 times higher than that of the control group, as opposed to 4.5 times in the presence of 1% (w/v) NaGC. The absorption improvement of CF in the existence of 0.5% (v/v) SLG-30 was about 3.5 times higher than that in the existence of 1% (w/v) NaGC (Table 1). As shown in Figure 1, SLG-30 contains two moieties of fatty acid (lauric acid). Therefore, in order to clarify whether SLG-30 is effective as a whole compound or whether the effectiveness is related to lauric acid, a degradation product of SLG-30, we also studied the absorption improvement effect of 0.5% (w/v) sodium laurate in the small intestines by the *in situ* closed-loop method. We found that the T_{max} of CF in the case of sodium laurate-treated samples is approximately 15 min. Thereafter, the concentrations of CF decreased quickly and continuously until the end of the experiment. Contrarily, SLG-30 greatly increased the concentrations of CF until T_{max} (180 min), followed by a decrease, as revealed in Figure 2 and Table 1. The absorption improvement ratio of CF for SLG-30 was approximately 6 times higher than that of sodium laurate.

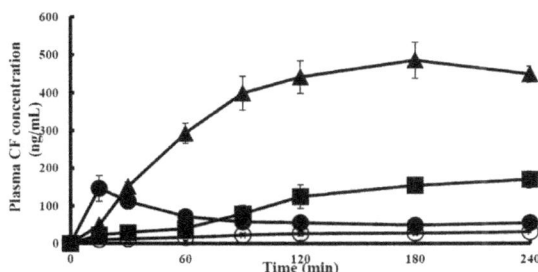

Figure 2. The profile of concentration vs. time course of 5(6)-carboxyfluorescein (CF) in the plasma after an enteric administration with SLG-30, a gemini surfactant, or typical absorption enhancers including sodium glycocholate and sodium laurate by an *in situ* closed-loop method. The results are expressed as the mean ± S.E. ($n = 3$). Keys: (○) Control, (▲) 0.5% (v/v) SLG-30, (●) 0.5% (w/v) sodium laurate, and (■) 1% (w/v) sodium glycocholate.

Table 1. A summary of the pharmacokinetic parameters of CF (0.5 mg/kg) after its administration with 0.5% (*v/v*) SLG-30, 0.5% (*w/v*) sodium laurate, and 1% (*w/v*) sodium glycocholate into rat small intestines by an in situ closed-loop method.

Absorption Enhancer	Conc.	C_{max} (ng/mL)	T_{max} (min)	$AUC_{0\to240}$ (ng·min/mL)	Enhancement Ratio
Control	-	-	-	5450 ± 700	-
SLG-30	0.5% (*v/v*)	487 ± 4	180 ± 0	87,200 ± 6000 **	16.0
Sodium laurate	0.5% (*w/v*)	375 ± 2	15 ± 0	14,700 ± 1950	2.7
Sodium glycocholate	1% (*w/v*)	172 ± 2	180 ± 0	24,500 ± 3700 *	4.5

The results are expressed as the mean ± S.E. (*n* = 3). ** $p < 0.01$, * $p < 0.05$, when compared with the control group.

3.2. Effects of SLG-30 on the Membrane Fluidity of Small Intestines in Rats

One of the important absorption-enhancing mechanisms of absorption enhancers is that they increase the membrane fluidity of the enteric membrane, thereby increasing the enteric absorption of poorly absorbed substances through a transcellular route. To examine the effect of SLG-30 on the enteric membrane fluidity, DPH, tma-DPH, and DNS-Cl, which can bind to different portions of the lipid bilayers (i.e., inner, outer, and protein portion, severally) were used as fluorescence probes in this study. Any decrease in the fluorescence anisotropy of these markers represents an increase in the membrane fluidity of BBMVs. Figure 3A–C shows that cholesterol, used as a positive control, increased the fluorescence anisotropy, which indicates a decrement in the membrane fluidity of BBMVs. Figure 3A shows that SLG-30 slightly decreased the fluorescence anisotropy of DPH compared to that of the control group. However, as Figure 3B shows, SLG-30 did not decrease, but significantly increased the tma-DPH fluorescence anisotropy. However, SLG-30 significantly reduced the fluorescence anisotropy of DNS-Cl in a dose dependent pattern (** $p < 0.01$ vs. control group) (Figure 3C). These findings propose that the membrane fluidity in the protein section of the enteric membranes could be significantly augmented by SLG-30, while it also slightly augmented the membrane fluidity in the inner section of the lipid bilayers.

(A)

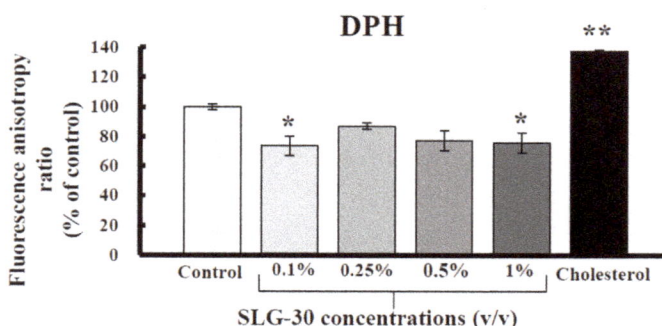

Figure 3. *Cont.*

(B)

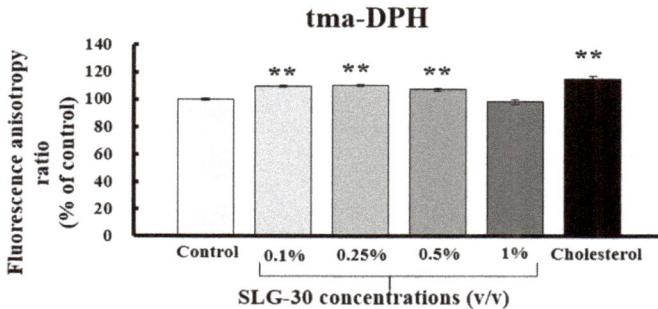

(C)

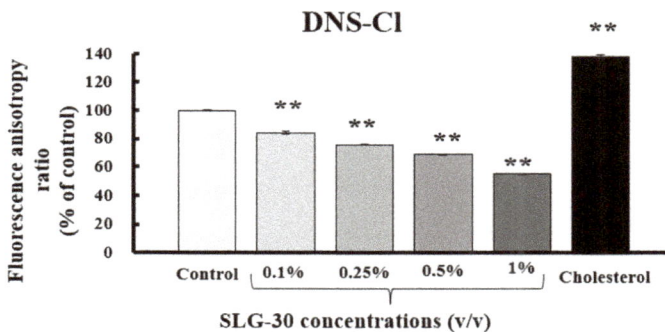

Figure 3. The effect of SLG-30 on the membrane fluidity of brush-border membrane vesicles (BBMVs). DPH (**A**), tma-DPH (**B**), and DNS-Cl (**C**) were used as fluorescein probes of inner lipid bilayers, outer lipid bilayers, and the protein portion of the enteric membranes. The absolute concentrations of DPH, tma-DPH, and DNS-Cl were 1 μM, 0.5 μM, and 5 μM, respectively. The results are expressed as the mean $\pm$ S.E. ($n = 4$). ** $p < 0.01$, n.s. not significantly different when compared with the control.

3.3. Effect of SLG-30 on TEER and Transport of CF in Caco-2 Cell Monolayers

We also estimated the effects of SLG-30 on the TEER values and the transport of poorly absorbed substances through the paracellular route by using Caco-2 cell monolayers. CF solutions in HBSS with or without various concentrations of SLG-30 (i.e., 0.001% *v/v*, 0.01% *v/v*, 0.025% *v/v*, 0.05% *v/v*, and 0.1% *v/v*) were added to the apical side of the cells and incubated at 37 °C. As shown in Figure 4A, a significant decrease in the TEER values was noticed in the presence of SLG-30 at all concentrations studied, including the lowest concentration of 0.001% (*v/v*), in the first hour. The TEER values did not recover to the baseline (without removing SLG-30) for the higher concentrations, but they started to recover for the lower concentrations. In contrast to the TEER results, as shown in Figure 5, the transport of CF significantly increased after 24 h upon coadministration with SLG-30 at all concentrations. The enhancement ratios of the CF transport were 6, 7, 9, 11, and 12 times higher than the control group for SLG-30 concentrations of 0.001% (*v/v*), 0.01% (*v/v*), 0.025% (*v/v*), 0.05% (*v/v*), and 0.1% (*v/v*), respectively.

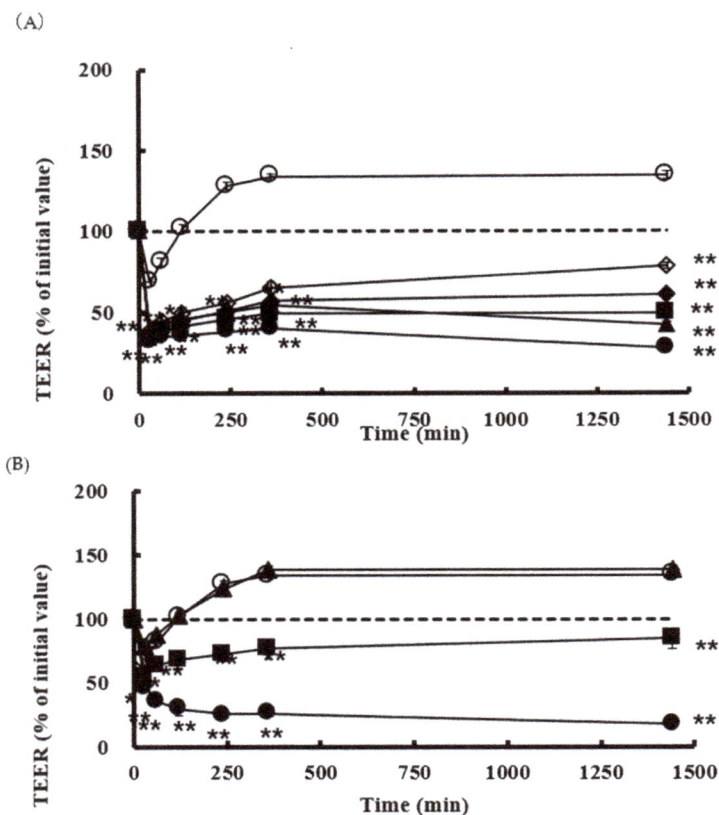

Figure 4. The TEER values in the existence of (**A**) SLG-30 and (**B**) sodium glycocholate and sodium laurate in Caco-2 cell monolayers. The results are expressed as the mean $\pm$ S.E. ($n = 3$). ** $p < 0.01$, n.s. not significantly different when compared with the control. Keys for Figure 4A: ($\bigcirc$) Control, ($\diamond$) 0.001% (v/v) SLG-30, ($\blacklozenge$) 0.01% (v/v) SLG-30, ($\blacksquare$) 0.025% (v/v) SLG-30, ($\blacktriangle$) 0.05% (v/v) SLG-30, and ($\bullet$) 0.1% (v/v) SLG-30. Keys for Figure 4B: ($\bigcirc$) Control, ($\blacktriangle$) 0.1% (w/v) sodium glycocholate, ($\blacksquare$) 1% (w/v) sodium glycocholate, and ($\bullet$) 0.05% (w/v) sodium laurate.

Parallel studies were performed with 0.1% (w/v) and 1% (w/v) NaGC and with 0.05% (w/v) sodium laurate. Figure 4B shows that TEER values were significantly reduced in the presence of 0.05% (w/v) sodium laurate without recovering to the baseline within the period of the experiment. In the case of 1% (w/v) NaGC, the TEER values significantly decreased then recovered to the baseline at the end of the experiment. Almost no effect was seen with 0.1% (w/v) NaGC on the TEER values. As shown in Figure 5, 0.05% (w/v) sodium laurate significantly increased (94 times) the transport of CF as compared to that observed in the control group; 1% (w/v) NaGC also significantly increased the transport of CF to a lesser extent than SLG-30 (i.e., 5 times higher than the control group). Further, 0.1% (w/v) NaGC had an insignificant effect on the transport of CF through Caco-2 cells (Figure 5).

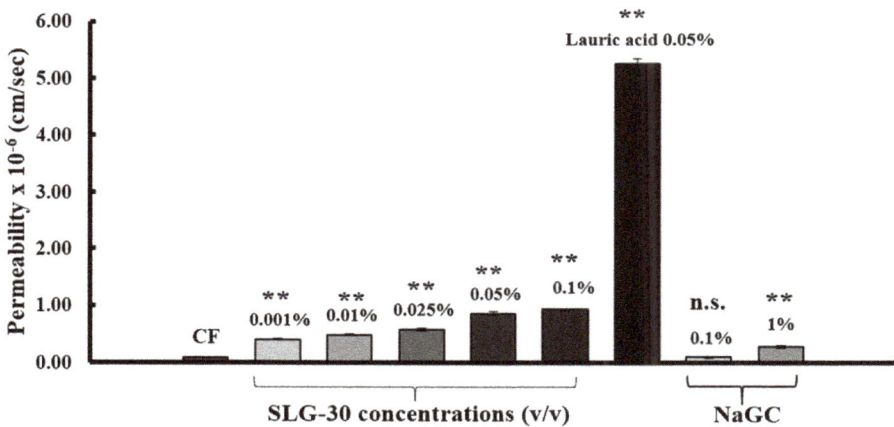

Figure 5. The permeability of CF in the presence of SLG-30, sodium glycocholate, and sodium laurate across Caco-2 cell monolayers: The results are expressed as the mean $\pm$ S.E. ($n = 3$). ** $p < 0.01$, n.s. not significantly different when compared with the control.

3.4. Assessment of Caco-2 Cells Injury

To assess the membrane injury of Caco-2 cells caused by SLG-30, sodium laurate, and NaGC, the LDH activities were measured right after the transport studies. The solutions were collected from the apical sides of wells and then centrifuged at 200× g for 7 min at 4 °C. The activity of the released LDH was measured in the supernatant (LDH$_{release}$). As shown in Figure 6A, the activity of LDH released from Caco-2 cells did not increase after the treatment with SLG-30 as compared to that in the control group. In contrast, the activity of LDH released significantly increased after the treatment with 0.05% (w/v) sodium laurate. Neither 0.1% (w/v) nor 1% (w/v) of NaGC increased the release of LDH. These findings proposed that SLG-30 did not cause serious injury to the cell membranes. Figure 6B shows the relationship between the effects of SLG-30 and typical absorption enhancers on the CF permeability across Caco-2 cells on one side and their toxic effects on the other side. While the absorption-improving effect of SLG-30 is concentration-dependent, we found no serious injury to enteric membrane irrespective of SLG-30 concentrations.

3.5. Estimation of Claudin Proteins by Western Blotting

As described above, SLG-30 might open the tight junctions of the intestinal epithelium, thus increasing the movement of substances through the paracellular route. However, the mechanism by which SLG-30 might open the tight junctions was not elucidated. Therefore, we finally evaluated the expression levels of claudin-1 and claudin-4 by western blotting. Figure 7A shows the bands of western blotting for claudin-1 and claudin-4 after a treatment with 0.5% (v/v) SLG-30. The treatment with 0.5% (v/v) SLG-30 decreased the intensity of the claudin-1 and claudin-4 bands by 57% and 64%, respectively, as shown in Figure 7B,C. The expression levels of claudin-1 and claudin-4 were about 64% and 45% less than the control, respectively, after the pretreatment study.

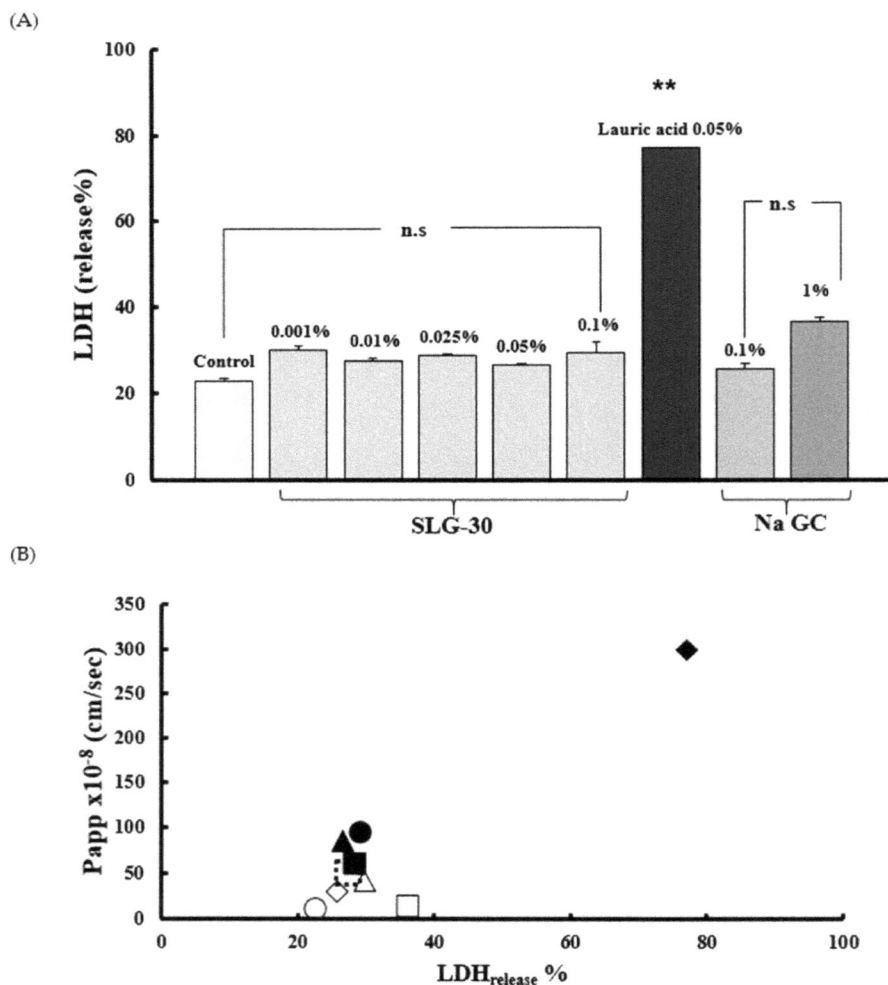

Figure 6. (**A**) The evaluation of the membrane toxicity of Caco-2 cells monolayers in the existence of SLG-30, sodium glycocholate, and sodium laurate and (**B**) the relationship between the effects of SLG-30 and typical absorption enhancers on the CF permeability across Caco-2 cells and their toxic effects: The results are expressed as the mean ± S.E. ($n = 6$). ** $p < 0.01$, n.s. not significantly different when compared with the control. Keys for Figure 6B: (○) Control, (Δ) 0.001% (*v/v*) SLG-30, (◻) 0.01% (*v/v*) SLG-30, (■) 0.025% (*v/v*) SLG-30, (▲) 0.05% (*v/v*) SLG-30, (●) 0.1% (*v/v*) SLG-30. (◇) 0.1% (*w/v*) sodium glycocholate, (◻) 1% (*w/v*) sodium glycocholate, and (◆) 0.05% (*w/v*) sodium laurate.

(A)

(B)   (C)

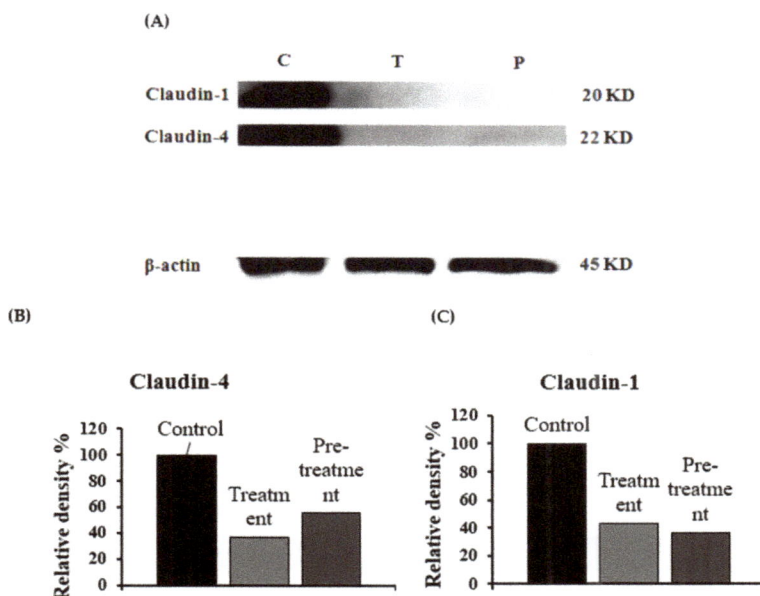

Figure 7. Western blot images of claudin-1 and claudin-4 (**A**): The expression levels of claudin-1 (**B**) and claudin-4 (**C**) in the rat small intestine were quantitatively calculated after a treatment with 0.5% (*v*/*v*) SLG-30 for 1 h. Control, without treatment; treatment, treatment with 0.5% (*v*/*v*) SLG-30 for 1 h; and pretreatment, pretreatment for 1 h. The proteins were extracted after 4 h.

4. Discussion

SLG-30 is a gemini surfactant with good surface-active properties and it is different from typical surfactants of similar chain lengths [21]. In this study, the efficacy of SLG-30 in improving enteric absorption was compared with that of a typical absorption enhancer. We used 1% (*w*/*v*) NaGC, a typical bile salt, as a typical absorption enhancer. Previously, it was proposed that bile acids interact with cell membranes to form reverse micelles, which act as a channel to increase permeation [35]. On the other hand, previous reports demonstrated the inhibition of insulin hydrolysis in different mucosal homogenates of rats by 1% (*w*/*v*) NaGC (a protease inhibitor) [36]. As shown in Figure 2, 1% (*w*/*v*) NaGC improved the absorption of CF from the small intestine to a much lower range than SLG-30. As shown in Table 1, the $AUC_{0 \to 240}$ value of CF in the presence of 0.5% *v*/*v* SLG-30 is 3.5 times greater than that in the presence of 1% (*w*/*v*) NaGC. These findings suggested that the absorption-enhancing effect of SLG-30, a gemini surfactant, is more potential than typical absorption enhancers.

We also studied the absorption-improving effect of sodium laurate, as a typical absorption enhancer and a major component of SLG-30 molecule. From Figure 2, we conclude that the effect of sodium laurate on the enteric absorption of CF was quite low and rapid, probably because sodium laurate itself was absorbed into the bloodstream due to its low molecular weight (approximately 288 Da), leading to a decrease in the concentration of sodium laurate at the site of absorption. This could explain the lower T_{max} observed for sodium laurate than for SLG-30. Table 1 also shows the difference between the $AUC_{0 \to 240}$ values of CF in the presence of SLG-30 and sodium laurate. Therefore, SLG-30 by itself, rather than sodium laurate, a degradation product of SLG-30, could improve the enteric absorption of poorly absorbable substances. These results provided three outcomes: firstly, the superiority of the enteric absorption-enhancing effects SLG-30 over typical absorption enhancers. Secondly, SLG-30 was effective as a whole compound and not because of lauric acid moieties present in the SLG-30 molecule. Finally, SLG-30 was stable in the intestines and was not degraded to its basic components.

In this study, we examined and elucidated the absorption-enhancing mechanisms of SLG-30 in improving the enteric absorption of poorly absorbed substances. Of all the absorption-enhancing mechanisms, an increase in the membrane fluidity is one of the most important mechanisms of action of many absorption enhancers. Labeling the cell membrane with fluorescent compounds allows the tracking of membrane fluidity changes by fluorescence polarization techniques [25,28]. Enteric BBMVs were used to study the membrane lipid fluidity in the presence of SLG-30. This was done by measuring the fluorescence intensities and calculating the fluorescence anisotropies of DPH, tma-DPH, and DNS-Cl [37,38]. As shown in Figure 3A, SLG-30 slightly decreased the anisotropy of DPH; meanwhile, it decreased the anisotropy of DNS-Cl in a dose-dependent pattern, as shown in Figure 3C. These results suggested that SLG-30 has a great effect on the protein portion of the cell membrane with a mild effect on the inner portion between the phospholipids bilayers. However, it did not have an effect on the outer portion of the phospholipid bilayers, as indicated in Figure 3B.

Caco-2 cell monolayers were used in this study to understand the mechanism by which SLG-30 could improve the absorption of chemical compounds and peptides. Caco-2 monolayers are more susceptible to the cytotoxic influences of permeation enhancers than whole enteric tissue [39,40]. For this reason, we used low concentrations of SLG-30, i.e., 0.0001% (v/v), 0.001% (v/v), 0.025% (v/v), 0.05% (v/v), and 0.1% (v/v), and a low concentration of CF (10 μM). When SLG-30 was added at concentrations used in *in vivo* studies, the cells were detached and severely injured. The TEER values usually decreased when the tight junctions between the adjacent cells were opened. In the present study, SLG-30 at all concentrations, significantly decreased the TEER values, suggesting that this enhancer might open the tight junctions, even at low concentrations, thereby increasing the transport of CF. The TEER values did not recover to the baseline when high concentrations of SLG-30 were used, while in the *in vivo* absorption studies, we noticed that the concentrations of CF in the plasma decreased [22]. This distinction might be explained by the nature of Caco-2 cells, which are more sensitive than the enteric cells and have a lower ability to remove any substance away from the cell surface than in vivo enteric cells [12,40].

In the present work, we also compared the effects of typical absorption enhancers and SLG-30 on Caco-2 cells. As shown in Figure 5B, the effects of NaGC were consistent with the results of previous report [24] and with the *in vivo* studies. NaGC at a concentration of 1% (w/v) might also open the tight junctions to an extent lower than SLG-30. The cumulative amounts of CF (Figure 7) after using 1% (w/v) NaGC was also less than that obtained after using 0.001% (v/v) of SLG-30, thus confirming the superiority of SLG-30 over NaGC. Figure 4B also indicates that sodium laurate significantly decreased the TEER values without recovering and, with a significant cumulative amount of CF (Figure 5), even more than that of 0.1% (v/v) SLG-30, while in the in vivo studies, the absorption enhancement ratio for SLG-30 was better than that of sodium laurate. This discrepancy can be partially explained by the highly toxicity effects of sodium laurate on Caco-2 cells. As Figure 6A shows, the amount of LDH released from Caco-2 cells was significant, and sodium laurate might cause a disintegration of Caco-2 cell monolayers and a rupture of cell membranes which led to a high permeability of CF to the basal side.

We previously reported the *in vivo* safety of SLG-30, as an absorption enhancer for the enteric epithelium [22]. The results of toxicity studies on Caco-2 cells (Figure 6A) also confirm the safety of SLG-30 on the intestinal epithelium. Apparently, SLG-30 might loosen the tight junctions to an extent enough for drug permeability but not enough to cause cell detachment, as in the case of sodium laurate, or to cause damage to the cell membrane, as suggested by the normal release of LDH.

Many previous studies have suggested the importance of claudin family proteins (molecular masses of approx. 23 kDa) to tight junctions to function properly [41,42]. Occludin family proteins are also important tight junction components. However, the deletion of occludin did not cause a disturbance of the TJs barrier function [43], and whether occludin is a major part of TJs remains unclear.

Claudins, which have molecular weight of approx. 23 kDa, comprise a multigene family consisting of more than 20 members. In our experiment, we studied the levels of claudin-1 and claudin-4 after treatment with 0.5% (v/v) SLG-30. The expression levels of both claudin-1 and claudin-4 were impaired (Figure 7A), suggesting that the loosening of TJs might be connected to the decrease in the levels of these proteins and that SLG-30 increased enteric transport of substances through the paracellular route. The pretreatment studies indicated that these proteins levels recovered, although at different rates, which could explain the partially reversible effects of SLG-30 [22]. It seems that the tight junctions might need more than 4 h for recovery. However, other proteins involved in TJs should be tested, including occludin and ZO-1, and further studies are required to understand the underlying mechanism of the decrease in these protein levels.

These findings also suggested that SLG-30 might enhance the enteric absorption of substances through a paracellular route in addition to a transcellular route.

5. Conclusions

Comparative studies conducted *in vivo* and *in vitro* showed that SLG-30, a gemini surfactant, had a greater absorption-improving effect than typical absorption enhancers, including NaGC and sodium laurate. Furthermore, the study also suggested that SLG-30 was stable in the intestines and acted as a whole compound to ameliorate the enteric absorption of poorly absorbed substances. The *in vitro* evaluation of membrane damage results confirmed the safety of SLG-30 on the enteric membrane. SLG-30 might also improve absorption through the transcellular route by changing the membrane fluidity. In addition, *in vitro* mechanistic studies suggested that SLG-30 might affect tight junctions by decreasing the levels of claudin-1 and claudin-4; thus, SLG-30 might open TJs and enhance the permeability through the paracellular route.

Author Contributions: Conceptualization, A.Y.; methodology, T.A. and A.Y.; software, T.A.; validation, T.A. and H.K.; formal analysis, T.A.; investigation, T.A., K.K., and M.M.; resources, A.Y.; data curation, T.A. and H.K..; writing—original draft preparation, T.A.; writing—review and editing, H.K., T.S., and A.Y.; visualization, T.A.; supervision, A.Y.; project administration, A.Y.; funding acquisition, A.Y.

Funding: The authors would like to express their sincere gratitude to Al-Baath University (Syria) for the financial support.

Conflicts of Interest: The authors declare no conflict of interest.

References

1. Beg, S.; Swain, S.; Rizwan, M.; Irfanuddin, M.; Malini, D.S. Bioavailability enhancement strategies: Basics, formulation approaches and regulatory considerations. *Curr. Drug Deliv.* **2011**, *8*, 691–702. [CrossRef]
2. Adson, A.; Raub, T.J.; Burton, P.S.; Barsuhn, C.L.; Hilgers, A.R.; Audus, K.L.; Ho, N.F. Quantitative approaches to delineate paracellular diffusion in cultured epithelial cell monolayers. *J. Pharm. Sci.* **1994**, *83*, 1529–1536. [CrossRef]
3. Antosova, Z.; Mackova, M.; Kral, V.; Macek, T. Therapeutic application of peptides and proteins: Parenteral forever? *Trends Biotechnol.* **2009**, *27*, 628–635. [CrossRef]
4. Mitic, L.L.; Anderson, J.M. Molecular architecture of tight junctions. *Annu. Rev. Physiol.* **1998**, *60*, 121–142. [CrossRef] [PubMed]
5. Fricker, G.; Drewe, J. Current concepts in intestinal peptide absorption. *J. Pept. Sci.* **1996**, *2*, 195–211. [CrossRef] [PubMed]
6. Salamat-Miller, N.; Johnston, T.P. Current strategies used to enhance the paracellular transport of therapeutic polypeptides across the intestinal epithelium. *Int. J. Pharm.* **2005**, *294*, 201–216. [CrossRef] [PubMed]
7. Fix, J.A.; Engle, K.; Porter, P.A.; Leppert, P.S.; Selk, S.J.; Gardner, C.R.; Alexander, J. Acylcarnitines: Drug absorption-enhancing agents in the gastrointestinal tract. *Am. J. Physiol.* **1986**, *251*, G332–G340. [CrossRef]
8. Lee, V.H.L.; Yamamoto, A. Penetration and enzymatic barriers to peptide and protein absorption. *Adv. Drug Deliv. Rev.* **1989**, *4*, 171–207. [CrossRef]

9. Nellans, H.N. (B) Mechanisms of peptide and protein absorption. *Adv. Drug Deliv. Rev.* **1991**, *7*, 339–364. [CrossRef]

10. Pauletti, G.M.; Okumu, F.W.; Borchardt, R.T. Effect of size and charge on the passive diffusion of peptides across Caco-2 cell monolayers via the paracellular pathway. *Pharm. Res.* **1997**, *14*, 164–168. [CrossRef]

11. Aungst, B.J. Absorption enhancers: Applications and advances. *AAPS J.* **2012**, *14*, 10–18. [CrossRef] [PubMed]

12. Yamamoto, A.; Uchiyama, T.; Nishikawa, R.; Fujita, T.; Muranishi, S. Effectiveness and toxicity screening of various absorption enhancers in the rat small intestine: Effects of absorption enhancers on the intestinal absorption of phenol red and the release of protein and phospholipids from the intestinal membrane. *J. Pharm. Pharmacol.* **1996**, *48*, 1285–1289. [CrossRef] [PubMed]

13. Yamamoto, A.; Tatsumi, H.; Maruyama, M.; Uchiyama, T.; Okada, N.; Fujita, T. Modulation of intestinal permeability by nitric oxide donors: Implications in intestinal delivery of poorly absorbable drugs. *J. Pharmacol. Exp. Ther.* **2001**, *296*, 84–90. [PubMed]

14. Gao, Y.; He, L.; Katsumi, H.; Sakane, T.; Fujita, T.; Yamamoto, A. Improvement of intestinal absorption of water-soluble macromolecules by various polyamines: Intestinal mucosal toxicity and absorption-enhancing mechanism of spermine. *Int. J. Pharm.* **2008**, *354*, 126–134. [CrossRef]

15. Gao, Y.; He, L.; Katsumi, H.; Sakane, T.; Fujita, T.; Yamamoto, A. Improvement of intestinal absorption of insulin and water-soluble macromolecular compounds by chitosan oligomers in rats. *Int. J. Pharm.* **2008**, *359*, 70–78. [CrossRef] [PubMed]

16. Lin, Y.; Fujimori, T.; Kawaguchi, N.; Tsujimoto, Y.; Nishimi, M.; Dong, Z.; Katsumi, H.; Sakane, T.; Yamamoto, A. Polyamidoamine dendrimers as novel potential absorption enhancers for improving the small intestinal absorption of poorly absorbable drugs in rats. *J. Control. Release* **2011**, *149*, 21–28. [CrossRef]

17. Nakaya, Y.; Takaya, M.; Hinatsu, Y.; Alama, T.; Kusamori, K.; Katsumi, H.; Sakane, T.; Yamamoto, A. Enhanced oral delivery of bisphosphonate by novel absorption enhancers: Improvement of intestinal absorption of alendronate by *N*-acyl amino acid and *N*-acyl taurates and their absorption-enhancing mechanisms. *J. Pharm. Sci.* **2016**, *105*, 3680–3690. [CrossRef]

18. Alama, T.; Katayama, H.; Hirai, S.; Ono, S.; Kajiyama, A.; Kusamori, K.; Katsumi, H.; Sakane, T.; Yamamoto, A. Enhanced oral delivery of alendronate by sucrose fatty acids esters in rats and their absorption-enhancing mechanisms. *Int. J. Pharm.* **2016**, *515*, 476–489. [CrossRef]

19. Dahlgren, D.; Roos, C.; Johansson, P.; Tannergren, C.; Lundqvist, A.; Langguth, P.; Sjöblom, M.; Sjögren, E.; Lennernäs, H. The effects of three absorption-modifying critical excipients on the *in vivo* intestinal absorption of six model compounds in rats and dogs. *Int. J. Pharm.* **2018**, *547*, 158–168. [CrossRef]

20. Maher, S.; Mrsny, R.J.; Braydenc, D.J. Intestinal permeation enhancers for oral peptide delivery. *Adv. Drug Deliv. Rev.* **2016**, *106*, 277–319. [CrossRef]

21. Hait, S.K.; Moulik, S.P. Gemini surfactants: A distinct class of self- assembling molecules. *Curr. Sci. Gemini Surfactants* **2002**, *82*, 1101–1111.

22. Alama, T.; Kusamori, K.; Katsumi, H.; Sakane, T.; Yamamoto, A. Absorption-enhancing effects of gemini surfactant on the intestinal absorption of poorly absorbed hydrophilic drugs including peptide and protein drugs in rats. *Int. J. Pharm.* **2016**, *499*, 58–66. [CrossRef]

23. Kaneko, D.; Olsson, U.; Sakamoto, K. Self-assembly in some *N*-lauroyl-L-glutamate/water Systems. *Langmuir* **2002**, *18*, 4699–4703. [CrossRef]

24. Yamamoto, A.; Taniguchi, T.; Rikyuu, K.; Tsuji, T.; Fujita, T.; Murakami, M.; Muranishi, S. Effects of various protease inhibitors on the intestinal absorption and degradation of insulin in rats. *Pharm. Res.* **1994**, *11*, 1496–1500. [CrossRef]

25. Bhor, V.M.; Sivakami, S. Regional variations in intestinal brush border membrane fluidity and function during diabetes and the role of oxidative stress and non-enzymatic glycation. *Mol. Cell. Biochem.* **2003**, *252*, 125–132. [CrossRef]

26. Ganapathy, V.; Mendicino, J.F.; Leibach, F.H. Transport of glycyl-L-proline into intestinal and renal brush border vesicles from rabbit. *J. Biol. Chem.* **1981**, *256*, 118–124.

27. Prabhu, R.; Balasubramanian, K.A. A novel method of preparation of small intestinal brush border membrane vesicles by polyethylene glycol precipitation. *Anal. Biochem.* **2001**, *289*, 157–161. [CrossRef]

28. Koga, K.; Kusawake, Y.; Ito, Y.; Sugioka, N.; Shibata, N.; Takada, K. Enhancing mechanism of Labrasol on intestinal membrane permeability of the hydrophilic drug gentamicin sulfate. *Eur. J. Pharm. Biopharm.* **2006**, *64*, 82–91. [CrossRef]

29. Ohyashiki, T.; Sakata, N.; Matsui, K. A decrease of lipid fluidity of the porcine intestinal brush-border membranes by treatment with malondialdehyde. *J. Biochem.* **1992**, *111*, 419–423. [CrossRef]

30. Hidalgo, I.J.; Raub, T.J.; Borchardt, R.T. Characterization of the human colon carcinoma cell line (Caco-2) as a model system for intestinal epithelial permeability. *Gastroenterology* **1989**, *96*, 736–749. [CrossRef]

31. Choksakulnimitr, S.; Masuda, S.; Tokuda, H.; Takakura, Y.; Hashida, M. *In vitro* cytotoxicity of macromolecules in different cell culture systems. *J. Control. Release* **1995**, *34*, 233–241. [CrossRef]

32. Quan, Y.S.; Hattori, K.; Lundborg, E.; Fujita, T.; Murakami, M.; Muranishi, S.; Yamamoto, A. Effectiveness and toxicity screening of various absorption enhancers using Caco-2 cell monolayers. *Biol. Pharm. Bull.* **1998**, *21*, 615–620. [CrossRef]

33. Sugibayashi, K.; Onuki, Y.; Takayama, K. Displacement of tight junction proteins from detergent-resistant membrane domains by treatment with sodium caprate. *Eur. J. Pharm. Sci.* **2009**, *36*, 246–253. [CrossRef]

34. Takizawa, Y.; Kishimoto, H.; Kitazato, T.; Tomita, M.; Hayashi, M. Changes in protein and mRNA expression levels of claudin family after mucosal lesion by intestinal ischemia/reperfusion. *Int. J. Pharm.* **2012**, *426*, 82–89. [CrossRef]

35. Gordon, G.S.; Moses, A.C.; Silver, R.D.; Flier, J.S.; Carey, M.C. Nasal absorption of insulin: Enhancement by hydrophobic bile salts. *Proc. Natl. Acad. Sci. USA* **1985**, *82*, 7419–7423. [CrossRef]

36. Yamamoto, A.; Hayakawa, E.; Lee, V.H. Insulin and proinsulin proteolysis in mucosal homogenates of the albino rabbit: Implications in peptide delivery from nonoral routes. *Life Sci.* **1990**, *47*, 2465–2474. [CrossRef]

37. Rinken, A.; Harro, J.; Engström, L.; Oreland, L. Role of fluidity of membranes on the guanyl nucleotide-dependent binding of cholecystokinin-8S to rat brain cortical membranes. *Biochem. Pharmacol.* **1998**, *55*, 423–431. [CrossRef]

38. Schedl, H.P.; Christensen, K.K.; Clark, E.D.; Buettner, G.R. Surface charge, fluidity, and calcium uptake by rat intestinal brush-border vesicles. *Biochim. Biophys. Acta Biomembr.* **1995**, *1234*, 81–89. [CrossRef]

39. Aungst, B.J. Intestinal permeation enhancers. *J. Pharm. Sci* **2000**, *89*, 429–442. [CrossRef]

40. Chao, A.C.; Nguyen, J.V.; Broughall, M.; Griffin, A.; Fix, J.A.; Daddona, P.E. *In vitro* and *in vivo* evaluation of effects of sodium caprate on enteral peptide absorption and on mucosal morphology. *Int. J. Pharm.* **1999**, *191*, 15–24. [CrossRef]

41. Morita, K.; Furuse, M.; Fujimoto, K.; Tsukita, S. Claudin multigene family encoding four-transmembrane domain protein components of tight junction strands. *Proc. Natl. Acad. Sci. USA* **1999**, *96*, 511–516. [CrossRef] [PubMed]

42. Sonoda, N.; Furuse, M.; Sasaki, H.; Yonemura, S.; Katahira, J.; Horiguchi, Y.; Tsukita, S. Clostridium perfringens enterotoxin fragment removes specific claudins from tight junction strands: Evidence for direct involvement of claudins in tight junction barrier. *J. Cell Biol.* **1999**, *147*, 195–204. [CrossRef] [PubMed]

43. Balda, M.S.; Whitney, J.A.; Flores, C.; González, S.; Cereijido, M.; Matter, K. Functional dissociation of paracellular permeability and transepithelial electrical resistance and disruption of the apical-basolateral intramembrane diffusion barrier by expression of a mutant tight junction membrane protein. *J. Cell Biol.* **1996**, *134*, 1031–1034. [CrossRef] [PubMed]

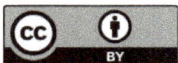

pharmaceutics

MDPI

Article

Dual Action of the PN159/KLAL/MAP Peptide: Increase of Drug Penetration across Caco-2 Intestinal Barrier Model by Modulation of Tight Junctions and Plasma Membrane Permeability

Alexandra Bocsik [1], Ilona Gróf [1,2], Lóránd Kiss [1,3], Ferenc Ötvös [4], Ottó Zsíros [5], Lejla Daruka [2,6], Lívia Fülöp [7], Monika Vastag [8], Ágnes Kittel [9], Norbert Imre [7], Tamás A. Martinek [7], Csaba Pál [6], Piroska Szabó-Révész [10] and Mária A. Deli [1,*]

[1] Institute of Biophysics, Biological Research Centre, Hungarian Academy of Sciences, H-6726 Szeged, Hungary; bocsik.alexandra@brc.mta.hu (A.B.); ilona.grof@brc.mta.hu (I.G.); kiss.lorand@med.u-szeged.hu (L.K.)
[2] Doctoral School in Biology, Faculty of Science and Informatics, University of Szeged, H-6726 Szeged, Hungary; daruka.lejla@brc.mta.hu
[3] Department of Pathophysiology, University of Szeged, H-6701 Szeged, Hungary
[4] Institute of Biochemistry, Biological Research Centre, Hungarian Academy of Sciences, H-6726 Szeged, Hungary; otvos.ferenc@brc.mta.hu
[5] Plant Biology, Biological Research Centre, Hungarian Academy of Sciences, H-6726 Szeged, Hungary; zsiros.otto@brc.mta.hu
[6] Synthetic and Systems Biology Unit, Institute of Biochemistry, Biological Research Centre, Hungarian Academy of Sciences, H-6726 Szeged, Hungary; pal.csaba@brc.mta.hu
[7] Department of Medical Chemistry, University of Szeged, H-6720 Szeged, Hungary; fulop.livia@med.u-szeged.hu (L.F.); imre.norbert@med.u-szeged.hu (N.I.); martinek.tamas@med.u-szeged.hu (T.A.M.)
[8] Division of Pharmacology and Drug Safety Research, Gedeon Richter Plc., H-1103 Budapest, Hungary; m.vastag@richter.hu
[9] Institute of Experimental Medicine, Hungarian Academy of Sciences, H-1450 Budapest, Hungary; kittel@koki.hu
[10] Department of Pharmaceutical Technology, University of Szeged, H-6720 Szeged, Hungary; revesz@pharm.u-szeged.hu
*   Correspondence: deli.maria@brc.mta.hu; Tel.: +36-62-599602

Received: 10 December 2018; Accepted: 5 February 2019; Published: 10 February 2019

Abstract: The absorption of drugs is limited by the epithelial barriers of the gastrointestinal tract. One of the strategies to improve drug delivery is the modulation of barrier function by the targeted opening of epithelial tight junctions. In our previous study the 18-mer amphiphilic PN159 peptide was found to be an effective tight junction modulator on intestinal epithelial and blood–brain barrier models. PN159, also known as KLAL or MAP, was described to interact with biological membranes as a cell-penetrating peptide. In the present work we demonstrated that the PN159 peptide as a penetration enhancer has a dual action on intestinal epithelial cells. The peptide safely and reversibly enhanced the permeability of Caco-2 monolayers by opening the intercellular junctions. The penetration of dextran molecules with different size and four efflux pump substrate drugs was increased several folds. We identified claudin-4 and -7 junctional proteins by docking studies as potential binding partners and targets of PN159 in the opening of the paracellular pathway. In addition to the tight junction modulator action, the peptide showed cell membrane permeabilizing and antimicrobial effects. This dual action is not general for cell-penetrating peptides (CPPs), since the other three CPPs tested did not show barrier opening effects.

Keywords: absorption enhancer; antimicrobial peptide; Caco-2; claudin; cell-penetrating peptide (CPP); drug delivery; intestinal epithelial cells; KLAL; PN159; tight junction modulator

1. Introduction

The oral administration of medicines is the most common method in drug therapy because of its easy administration and good patient compliance. However, the absorption of several drugs is limited in the gastrointestinal tract by the barriers composed of epithelial cell layers [1]. Since the non-invasive delivery of orally administered hydrophilic drugs or biopharmaceuticals to the systemic circulation is still a challenge, several strategies and molecules have been investigated as penetration enhancers, including biosurfactants, sucrose esters and peptides [1–3].

Tight junctions (TJs) between epithelial cells form the anatomical basis of the intestinal barrier which is one of the main biological barriers in our organism and the body's largest interface with the external environment [1]. These TJs, located in the apical regions of cells, close the intercellular gap and thus determine the paracellular permeability and the tightness of the epithelial barriers [1, 4]. The absorption level and rate across biological barriers depends on the composition of cellular membranes, the anatomical structures, and the expression pattern of TJ proteins and transporters in the cell membrane [5]. TJs are complex structures composed of integral membrane proteins including among others the occludin protein and the claudin family [6].

One of the basic strategies to improve drug delivery is the modulation of barrier function by the targeted opening of TJs [1] Peptides which act directly on TJs and modulate their permeability are potential candidates to increase the absorption of hydrophilic or large therapeutic molecules in a non-invasive manner [1,7]. In our recent work six TJ modulator peptides acting on different targets were compared using culture models of the intestinal and the blood-brain barriers [8]. All the six peptides induced reversible opening of TJs but barrier selectivity and differences in efficacy were observed. We found the PN159 as the most effective TJ modulator peptide on both barrier models [8]. This peptide was identified as a TJ modulator on cultured human bronchial epithelial cell layers in 2005 [4]. PN159 peptide effectively increased the permeability of respiratory epithelium both in culture and animal experiments [9]. The specific target proteins of the peptide were unknown, but we demonstrated that PN159 interacts with the extracellular loops of integral membrane TJ proteins claudin-1 and -5 [8].

The amino acid sequence of the 18-mer PN159, KLALKLALKALKAALKLA-amide, contains several KLA motifs, and therefore it is also named as KLA or KLAL peptide [10]. The other name of this peptide is MAP, which stands for model amphipathic peptide [11,12]. The structure of the lipid vesicle-bound PN159 peptide is mostly α-helical [10] and strongly interacts with biological membranes [10,13]. Cell-penetrating peptides (CPPs) are a group of short natural or synthetic peptides with 5–30 amino acids, which by crossing cellular membranes can transport into cells a wide range of small and macromolecules, including nucleic acids, proteins, imaging agents [14]. Based on their physical-chemical properties, CPPs can be classified into groups. The most investigated CPPs belong to the amphipathic class. These peptides contain hydrophilic and hydrophobic motifs and are especially rich in lysine, arginine, leucine and alanine. Examples include the PN159 peptide [10,11]; the cyclic φ-peptide [15] and Pep-1 [16]. Among the cationic CPPs penetratin [17] or polyarginine peptides [18] are extensively investigated.

CPPs are structurally similar to antimicrobial peptides, which are important defense elements of the innate immunity, and accordingly, they show an antimicrobial effect against pathogens [19]. Bacterial resistance is a growing clinical problem, as it was highlighted by the Infectious Diseases Society of America publishing the list of ESKAPE pathogens (*Enterobacter species, Staphylococcus aureus, Klebsiella pneumoniae, Acinetobacter baumannii, Pseudomonas aeruginosa* and *Enterococcus faecium*) [20]. This group of microbes causes the large majority of nosocomial infections throughout the world. The combat antibiotic resistance, CPPs can be promising alternative molecules, since increased sensitivity (collateral sensitivity) for antimicrobial peptides were found in antibiotic-resistant *Escherichia coli* strains [21].

As a culture model of the intestinal epithelial barrier, we used in our study the Caco-2 human cell line resembling the epithelium of the small intestine both from structural and functional aspects [22]. The cells have polarized cell morphology, grow in monolayer, possess microvilli, form TJs, express nutrient and efflux transporters, and show good correlation with in vivo data [23,24]. Caco-2 epithelial cells are routinely used in drug permeability studies [24,25].

Crucial parameters for absorption enhancers include their safety, reversibility and efficacy. There are no data available about the effectiveness and safety of PN159 peptide on the intestinal barrier, so our primary goal was to test the TJ modulator peptide for these aspects. Therefore, the aim of the study was to (i) determine the influence of long-time and concentration-dependent effects of treatments with PN159 peptide on intestinal epithelial cell viability, barrier function and recovery; (ii) test the effect of PN159 peptide on drug penetration across the intestinal barrier model; (iii) identify further potential targets of this TJ modulator peptide by molecular modelling; (iv) measure the cell uptake of the PN159 in intestinal epithelial cells and its antimicrobial activity on ESKAPE pathogens; and (iv) test other CPPs for the TJ modulator effect.

2. Materials and Methods

2.1. Materials

All reagents were purchased from Sigma-Aldrich Ltd. (Budapest, Hungary) except for those specifically mentioned.

2.2. Peptide Synthesis

PN159 peptide (KLALKLALKALKAALKLA-amide) [4,10], and Pep-1 (Chariot) peptide (KETWWETWWTEWSQPKKKRKV-amide) were synthesized manually on a 0.5 mmolar scale with the use of standard Fmoc-chemistry on a Rink-amide resin. Couplings were performed in DMF with three-fold excess of DCC, HOBt, and Fmoc-amino acids for 3 h at ambient temperature. In the case of octaarginine (RRRRRRRR-amide, R8) three-fold excess of HATU and six-fold excess of DIPEA was used. Fmoc deprotection was performed in 20% piperidine/DMF mixture for 20 min. The peptides were cleaved from the resin by incubating them with the mixture of TFA/water/triisopropylsilane (48:1:1 volume ratio), precipitated with diethyl-ether and lyophilized. Crude peptides were purified using a Shimadzu semi-preparative high-performance liquid chromatography (HPLC) instrument equipped with a Phenomenex JupiterC18 column, in the following solvent system: (A) 0.1% aqueous TFA and (B) 0.1% TFA in 80% aqueous acetonitrile, in a linear gradient mode. Analysis and purity control were carried out on an analytical HPLC instrument (HP Model 1100 liquid chromatograph equipped with a Phenomenex Jupiter C18 column). Quality control of the peptides was done by performing mass spectrometric measurements on a FinniganTSQ-7000 triple quadrupole mass spectrometer in positive ion mode.

The cyclic φ-peptide (cyclo[CGGFWRRRRGE(εAca)G])was also synthesized manually on a 0.5 mmolar scale with the use of Boc-chemistry on a MBHA-HCl resin, by applying a native chemical ligation strategy. Couplings were performed in DMF with three-fold excess of DIC, HOBt, and Boc-amino acids for 3 h at ambient temperature. Boc deprotection was performed in TFA/DCM (1:1 volume ratio) mixture for 20 min. The peptide was cleaved from the resin by the standard HF method. Native chemical ligation was performed with 2% thiophenol in an ammoniumacetate solution (0.1 M) at room temperature for 12h. Cyclic crude peptide was purified and analyzed as described above.

2.3. Cell Culture

The human Caco-2 intestinal epithelial cell line was purchased from ATCC (cat.no. HTB-37). Caco-2 cells were grown in DMEM/HAM's F-12 culture medium with stable glutamine

(Life Technologies, Gibco, Carlsbad, CA, USA) supplemented with 10% fetal bovine serum (Life Technologies, Gibco, Carlsbad, CA, USA and 50 µg/mL gentamycin in a humidified incubator with 5% CO_2 at 37 °C. All plastic surfaces were coated with 0.05% rat tail collagen in sterile distilled water before cell seeding.

2.4. Peptide Treatment

The PN159 peptide stock solution (5 mM) was prepared freshly in sterile DMSO. Treatment solutions were further diluted in Ringer-Hepes (150 mM NaCl, 6 mM $NaHCO_3$, 5.2 mM KCl, 2.2 mM $CaCl_2$, 0.2 mM $MgCl_2$, 2.8 mM D-glucose, 5 mM Hepes; pH 7.4) or cell culture medium. Final concentrations of the peptide in treatment solutions were as follows: 1, 3, 10, 30 and 100 µM for cell viability assays; 1, 3, 10 and 30 µM for the barrier integrity assays and 10 µM for the recovery measurements.

The stock solutions of the three reference CPPs were the following: Pep-1: 1 mM in distilled water (DW); R8: 1 mM in DW; φ-peptide, 5 mM in DW and 2.5% DMSO. The 100 µM working solutions were dissolved in cell culture medium or Ringer–Hepes buffer. We prepared all solutions freshly in sterile conditions.

2.5. MTT Assay

For the cell viability assays Caco-2 epithelial cells were seeded to 96-well plates at the density of 6×10^3 cells/well (Orange Scientific) and cultured for 3-5 days. Confluent cultures were treated with PN159 peptide (1, 3, 10, 30 and 100 µM) in phenol red free DMEM (Life Technologies, Gibco, Carlsbad, CA, USA) for 1-h. This viability assay was performed at three different time points: (i) immediately after the 1-h treatment, (ii) at one-day recovery, (iii) at one-week recovery. To determine 100% toxicity, cells were incubated with 1 mg/mL Triton X-100 detergent. After treatment the medium was changed and 0.5 mg/mL MTT (3-(4,5-dimethyltiazol-2-yl)-2,5-diphenyltetrazolium bromide) solution was added to the cells for 3 h. During the incubation cells were kept in a CO_2 incubator. The metabolic activity of cells is reflected by the conversion of the yellow MTT dye to purple formazan. Formazan crystals were dissolved in DMSO and the amount of converted dye was determined by measuring absorbance at 595 nm wavelength with a microplate reader (Fluostar Optima, BMG Labtechnologies, Ortenberg, Germany). Cell viability and/or metabolic activity was calculated as percentage of dye conversion by non-treated cells.

2.6. Impedance Measurement

Kinetics of epithelial cell reaction to PN159 peptide treatment was monitored by impedance measurement at 10 kHz (RTCA-SP instrument, ACEA Biosciences, San Diego, CA, USA). Impedance measurement is non-invasive, label-free and real time, and linearly correlates with adherence, growth, number and viability of cells [2,26]. For background measurements 50 µL cell culture medium was added to the wells, then cells were seeded at a density of 6×10^3 cells/well to the coated 96-well plates with integrated gold electrodes (E-plate 96, ACEA Biosciences). Cells were cultured for 5–7 days in a CO_2 incubator at 37 °C and monitored every 10 min until the end of experiments. Cells were treated with PN159 peptide solutions at 1, 3, 10, 30 and 100 µM concentrations at the beginning of the plateau phase of growth and the effects were followed for 1-h or 24 h. To measure cell recovery, peptide solutions were changed to culture medium and the impedance was monitored for one week. Culture medium was changed every 2 days. Caco-2 cells were also treated with the three selected CPPs, Pep-1, R8 and φ-peptide, at 100 µM concentrations at the beginning of the plateau phase of cell growth for 24-h. Triton X-100 detergent (1 mg/mL) was used as a reference compound to induce cell death. Cell index was defined as R_n-R_b at each time point of measurement, where R_n is the cell-electrode impedance of the well when it contains cells and R_b is the background impedance of the well with the medium alone.

2.7. Measurement of the Electrical Resistance of Caco-2 Cell Layers

For the measurement of barrier integrity Caco-2 cells were seeded onto culture inserts (Transwell 3460, polyester membrane, 0.4 µm pore size, Corning Costar) and cultured for three weeks [2,24]. Transepithelial electrical resistance (TEER) reflects the tightness of the intercellular junctions. TEER was measured by an EVOM volt-ohmmeter (World Precision Instruments, Sarasota, FL, USA) combined with STX-2 electrodes, and was expressed relative to the surface area of the monolayers ($\Omega \times cm^2$). Resistance of cell-free inserts (130 $\Omega \times cm^2$) was subtracted from the measured values. TEER values were measured before and right after permeability experiments). TEER values indicated the integrity and paracellular permeability of cell layers for ions. The TEER of Caco-2 monolayers was 1302 $\pm$ 49 $\Omega \times cm^2$ (mean $\pm$ SD; $n = 46$) after 3 weeks culturing. For the recovery experiment, after changing the 10 µM peptide solutions to culture medium, TEER was monitored for one day.

2.8. Penetration of Marker and Drug Molecules across Caco-2 Cell Layers

In the permeability experiments inserts with Caco-2 cell layers grown for 3 weeks were transferred to 12-well plates containing 1.5 mL Ringer–Hepes buffer in the lower (basal or acceptor) compartments. In the upper or apical compartments culture medium was replaced by 0.5 mL buffer containing peptide solutions: PN159 peptide at 1, 3, 10 and 30 µM concentrations and CPPs at 100 µM concentration. Permeability marker molecules albumin (1 mg/mL; Mw: 65 kDa) labeled with Evans blue (167.5 µg/mL) and fluorescein (10 µg/mL; Mw: 376 Da) were added 30 min later. The incubation with permeability markers in the presence of PN159 peptide lasted for 30 min. In case of CPPs the incubation time with fluorescein was 1-h. Samples were collected from both compartments and the concentrations of the marker molecules were determined by a fluorescence multi-well plate reader (Fluostar Optima; excitation wavelength: 485 nm, emission wavelength: 535 nm in the case of fluorescein and excitation wavelength: 584 nm, emission wavelength: 680 nm in the case of Evans-blue labeled albumin). Fluorescein isothiocyanate (FITC)-labelled dextran marker molecules (Table 1) were used at 1 mM concentrations, and fluorescence intensities of collected samples were measured using a Fluorolog FL3-22 (Horiba Jobin Yvon, Paris, France) spectrofluorometer using 492 nm excitation wavelength, 515 nm emission wavelength, and 0.5 s integration time. Drugs were used at 10 µM concentrations and samples were measured by HPLC as described below. The apparent permeability coefficients (P_{app}) were calculated as described previously [8,24]. Briefly, cleared volume was calculated from the concentration difference of the tracer in the basal compartments ($\Delta[C]_B$) after 30 min and apical compartments at 0 h ($[C]_A$), the volume of the basal compartment (V_B; 1.5 mL) and the surface area available for permeability (A; 1.1 cm^2).

Table 1. The amino acid sequences of the tested cell-penetrating peptides.

CPPs	Amino Acid Sequence	References
PN159 (KLAL/MAP)	KLALKLALKALKAALKLA-amide	[4,10]
Pep-1	KETWWETWWTEWSQPKKKRKV-amide	[16]
R8	RRRRRRRR-amide	[18]
φ-peptide	cyclo[CGGFWRRRGE(εAca)G]	[15]

2.9. High-Performance Liquid Chromatography (HPLC) Analytical Procedures

Analytical measurements were performed on a Merck-Hitachi LaChrom HPLC system equipped with an ultraviolet (UV) and fluorescence detector (Merck, Darmstadt, Germany). All reagents used were of analytical reagent grade. Atenolol and verapamil were determined by using a Gemini C18 column (150 $\times$ 3 mm, 5 µm, 110 Å; Phenomenex Inc., Torrance, CA, USA) operated at 0.5 mL/min flow rate, maintained at 35°C. For atenolol measurements isocratic elution was applied with a mixture of 300 mL methanol, 400 mL 100 mM ammonium acetate, 20 mL 10% ammonium-hydroxide and 2 mL 0.1 M ethylenediaminetetraacetic acid. The mobile phase for verapamil consisted of 350 mL methanol with 250 mL 20 mM ammonium acetate and 2 mL 10% trifluoroacetic acid with isocratic elution, at 0.5 mL/min flow rate. UV detection for atenolol was performed at 270 nm while for verapamil the 230 nm wavelength was adjusted. The calibration curve was linear ($r^2 = 0.9999$) over a range of 0.01–1.5 μM for atenolol. The calibration curve for verapamil also showed a good linearity within the examined concentration range of 0.01–1 μM ($r^2 = 0.9952$). In both cases 10μL sample was injected into the chromatographic system. Samples at higher than 1 μM atenolol and verapamil concentrations were 10× diluted with Ringer–Hepes solution.

HPLC measurement of quinidine was performed using a YMC Pack Pro C18 column (RS 150 × 2.1 mm, 5 μm, 80 Å; YMC America Inc., Allentown, PA, USA) equipped with a guard column operated at 0.2 mL/min flow rate. The chromatographic column was maintained at 40 °C and the 5 μL sample was injected onto the column. The elution of quinidine was performed with a buffer containing a mixture of 100 mL methanol, 250 mL 0.1% ammonium acetate, and 4 mL 10% trifluoroacetic acid. Quinidine was quantified at 250/430 nm excitation/emission wavelengths. The calibration curve was linear over the quantitation range of 0.01–1 μM ($r^2 = 0.9984$).

HPLC measurement of cimetidine was performed using a Gemini NX column (150 × 4.6 mm, 3 μM) equipped with a guard column operated at 0.8 mL/min flow rate. The column temperature was maintained at 40 °C and a 20 μL sample was injected onto the chromatographic system. A buffer comprising of 15% acetonitrile and 85% 100 mM ammonium acetate was utilized for the isocratic elution of cimetidine. UV detection was set at 228 nm. The calibration curve was linear ($r^2 = 0.9999$) over the range of 0.01–10 μM.

2.10. Electron Microscopy

Cells grown on culture inserts were treated with 10 μM PN159 peptide for 30 min and fixed immediately after treatment or after a 1-day recovery. Cells were briefly washed with phosphate-buffered saline (PBS) and fixed with 3% paraformaldehyde containing 0.5% glutaraldehyde in cacodylate buffer (pH 7.4) for 30 min at 4 °C. After washing with the buffer several times, cells were postfixed in 1% OsO$_4$ for 20 min. Following a rinse with distilled water, the cells were block stained with 1% uranyl acetate in 50% ethanol for 20 min, dehydrated in graded ethanol and after the last step of dehydration inserts were placed in the 1:1 mixture of ethanol and Taab 812 (Taab; Aldermaston, Berks, UK) for 10 min at 30°C. Finally, the membranes of the culture inserts with the cells were removed from their support and embedded in Taab 812. Polymerization was performed overnight at 60°C. Ultrathin sections were cut perpendicularly for the membrane using a Leica EM UC6 ultramicrotome (Nussloch, Germany) and picked up on formvar-coated single-slot copper grids. The sections were examined using a Hitachi 7100 transmission electron microscope (Hitachi Ltd., Tokyo, Japan) and a side-mounted Veleta CCD camera (Olympus Soft Imaging Solutions). Altogether, 105 non-overlapping images from the 3 groups at the same magnification were analyzed for the presence or absence of tight junctions (control group $n = 28$; PN159 group $n = 42$; recovery group $n = 35$).

2.11. Immunohistochemistry

Morphological changes in interepithelial junctions after treatment with different concentrations of CPPs (100 μM) and PN159 peptide (1, 3, 10, 30 and 100 μM) were followed by immunostaining for claudin-1 integral membrane tight junction protein, β-catenin and zonula occludens protein-1 (ZO-1) cytoplasmic linker proteins. F-actin was stained by fluorescently labeled phalloidin. Treatments lasted for 1 h. After peptide treatment cell layers were washed with PBS and fixed with a 1:1 mixture of ice cold acetone and methanol for 2 min. Cells were blocked with 3% bovine serum albumin in PBS and incubated with primary antibodies mouse anti-claudin-1 and -4, rabbit anti-ZO-1 and rabbit anti-β-catenin (Life Technologies, Carlsbad, CA, USA) overnight. Fluorescent Atto 647N-phalloidin (ATTO-TEC GmbH, Germany) lasted for 1 h. Incubation with Alexa Fluor-488-labeled anti-mouse and anti-rabbit secondary antibodies (Life Technologies, Invitrogen, USA) lasted for 1 h. Bis-benzimide dye (Hoechst 33342) was used to stain cell nuclei. After mounting (Fluoromount-G; Southern Biotech,

Birmingham, AL, USA) the samples staining was visualized by a Leica TCS SP5 confocal laser scanning microscope (Leica Microsystems GmbH, Wetzlar, Germany) and Visitron spinning disk confocal system (Visitron Systems GmbH, Puchheim, Germany).

2.12. Circular Dichroism (CD) Spectroscopy

Far-UV circular dichroism (CD) spectra of the peptides were recorded at 25°C temperature on a J-810 spectropolarimeter (JASCO International Co. Ltd., Tokyo, Japan). The CD spectra were measured between 260 nm and 185 nm with an optical pathlength of 1 mm, at a peptide concentration of 0.1 mg/mL in Milli-Q water diluted directly from powder. The bandwidth was 2 nm and data pitch 0.5 nm, the scan speed was set to 100 nm/min and the integration time was 1 sec. Ten spectra were accumulated and plotted. The data were analyzed by CDSSTR method [27]. To test the thermostability of the peptide structure the CD spectra were recorded between 25 °C and 55 °C temperature with a ramp rate of 5 °C/min on a JASCO J-810 spectropolarimeter by using a Peltier sample holder. The CD spectra were measured immediately between 260 and 185 nm with an optical pathlength of 1 mm, the peptide concentration was 0.1 mg/mL in Milli-Q water. The bandwidth was 2 nm and data pitch 1 nm, the scan speed was set to 100 nm/min, and the integration time was 1 sec. Five spectra were accumulated and plotted.

2.13. Molecular Modelling

Protein structures were obtained by homology modeling using the MODELLER program package [28]. First, the structure of mouse claudin-15 was completed by homology modelling because its X-ray structure file is lacking the fragment of residues from 34 to 41 [29]. Human claudins 1, 4 and 7 were homology modeled using the completed mouse claudin-15 as a template. The protein homology models were further relaxed by a short (400 ns) molecular dynamics simulation in which the proteins were embedded in a 95 by 95 Å POPC bilayer-water system containing 150 mM NaCl. Molecular dynamics simulations were performed by the program NAMD [30], using the CHARMM27 molecular force field with CMAP correction. The results were visualized by VMD v1.9.1. [31]. The docking studies were performed by the CABS docking server [32] and the resulting C-alpha traces were reconstructed by MODELLER using the python script supplied by the server homepage.

2.14. Visualization of the Uptake of PN159 Peptide in Caco-2 Cells

The Caco-2 cells were grown on glass bottomed petri dishes coated with collagen to visualize the cellular uptake of the Bodipy FL maleimide labeled (BODIPY FL *N*-(2-aminoethyl) maleimide, Thermo Fischer, Waltham, MA, USA) PN159 peptide. The cells were treated with peptide at concentrations of 1, 3 and 10 μM for 5 min. To stain the cell nuclei the H33342dye (1 μg/mL) was used before peptide treatment for 10 min. After peptide incubation the living cells were washed three times with Ringer–Hepes buffer supplemented with 1%fetal bovine serum (FBS) and examined immediately with a Visitron spinning disk confocal system.

In the case of the co-localization analysis the labeled PN159 peptide was used in 10 μM for 5 min. Then the cellular uptake cells were fixed and immunohistochemistry was performed for claudin-4. The samples were mounted and visualized by a Leica TCS SP5 confocal laser-scanning microscope.

2.15. Determination of Minimum Inhibitory Concentration (MIC) on Microbial Pathogens

We tested the spectrum of activity of PN159 on a set of five sensitive ESKAPE pathogens: *Staphylococcus aureus* (ATCC 29213), *Klebsiella pneumoniae* (ATCC 10031), *Acinetobacter baumannii* (ATCC 17978), *Pseudomonas aeruginosa* (ATCC 27853), *Enterobacter cloacae spp. cloacae* (ATCC 13047); and one vancomycin resistant ESKAPE pathogen, *Enterococcus faecium* (ATCC 700221). The MIC of PN159 on the 6 sensitive and resistant ESKAPE pathogenic strains was determined in cation-adjusted Muller–Hinton broth. For *Enterococcus faecium*, which does not grow in Muller-Hinton broth, Brain-Heart-Infusion broth was used. Minimum inhibitory concentrations (MICs) were determined by using a standard serial broth dilution technique [33]. Briefly, 11-step serial dilutions were prepared in 96-well microtiter plates with three biological replicates per strain. Pathogens were inoculated into each well at a density of 5×10^5 bacteria/mL, and the plates were incubated at 37 °C. Plates were shaken at 300 rpm during incubation for 18 h. Cell growth was monitored by measuring the optical density (OD600 value, Synergy 2 microplate reader BioTek Instruments Inc, Winooski, VT, USA). MIC was defined as complete growth inhibition (i.e., OD600 < 0.05). As reference compounds we tested the antimicrobial activity of three bactericidal drugs with different modes of action. Cefoxitin inhibits the cell wall synthesis, gentamicin (Applichem GmbH, Darmstadt, Germany) is a 30S ribosomal subunit inhibitor, while ciprofloxacin is a gyrase inhibitor. The highest tested concentrations were 100 µg/mL in the case of cefoxitin and gentamicin, and 10 µg/mL for ciprofloxacin.

2.16. Statistical Analysis

For statistical analysis Graph Pad Prism 5.0 software (Graph Pad Software Inc., San Diego, CA, USA) was used. All data presented are means ± SD. Values were compared using analysis of variance followed by Dunnett's test. Changes were considered statistically significant at $p < 0.05$. All measurements were repeated three times and the number of parallel samples was minimum three.

3. Results

3.1. Concentration-Dependent Effect of PN159 Peptide on Epithelial Cell Viability

The colorimetric endpoint MTT test was performed after a 1-h treatment with different PN159 peptide concentrations at three different time points: (i) immediately after the 1-h treatment, (ii) at one-day recovery and (iii) at one-week recovery (Figure 1A). Low concentrations of the peptide (1–10 µM) did not decrease cell viability, while cell damage was found at higher, 30 and 100 µM concentrations. The cytotoxic effect of PN159 at 100 µM concentration was not reversible after one day or even one week. The kinetics of PN159 effects on Caco-2 cells were followed by real-time impedance measurements after 1-h (Figure 1B) or one-day treatment (Figure 1C). In both conditions only the two highest peptide concentrations decreased the cell impedance indicating cell damage, similarly to the results of the MTT assay.

Based on both tests, PN159 peptide treatment for 1-h was non-toxic at 10 µM or lower concentrations, reversible at 30 µM and toxic at the highest 100 µM concentration. The results obtained by MTT test and impedance measurement on Caco-2 cells were similar (Figure 1) and indicated that all the used concentrations of PN159 peptide were safe, except the 100 µM. Because of its toxicity, the 100 µM concentration was not used in further experiments.

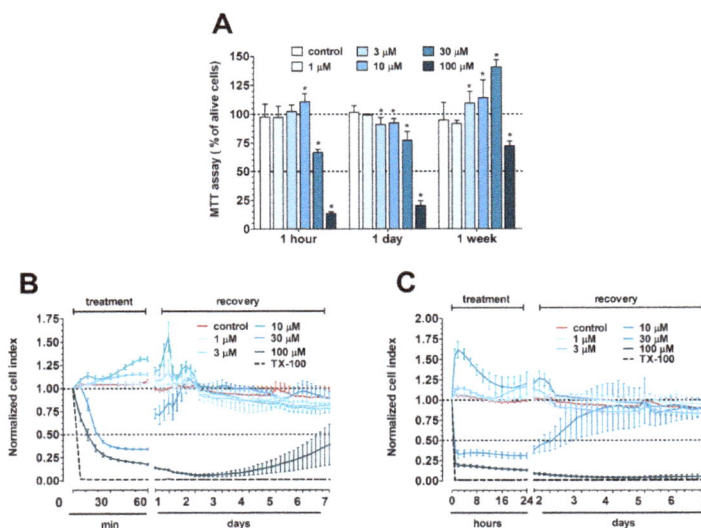

Figure 1. (**A**) MTT assay after 1-h treatment with PN159 peptide on Caco-2 cells followed by 1-h, 1-day or 1-week recovery. The MTT values are given as percent of the control group (100% viability). Values are presented as means ± SD, n = 3–8. Statistical analysis: analysis of variance (ANOVA) followed by Dunnett test, $p < 0.05$ as compared with the control groups. (**B**) Impedance measurements after 1-h treatment and (**C**) 1-day treatment followed by a recovery phase of 1-week. The effects of PN159 peptide on the impedance were shown as normalized cell index. Values are presented as means ± SD, n = 3–8.

3.2. Concentration-Dependent Effect of PN159 Peptide on Intestinal Epithelial Barrier Integrity

All tested concentrations of the PN159 peptide significantly decreased the resistance of epithelial cell layers after a 1-h treatment (Figure 2A). The two highest concentrations, 10 and 30 μM, opened the paracellular barrier the most, causing 80–90% decrease in TEER. In concordance, these two highest concentrations of PN159 showed the most effective permeability enhancer activity for both fluorescein and albumin (Figure 2B). Because the peptide was safe for the cells but effectively opened the barrier at 10 μM, this concentration was selected to reveal the kinetics of the reversibility of barrier opening, and to investigate its effects on drug penetration.

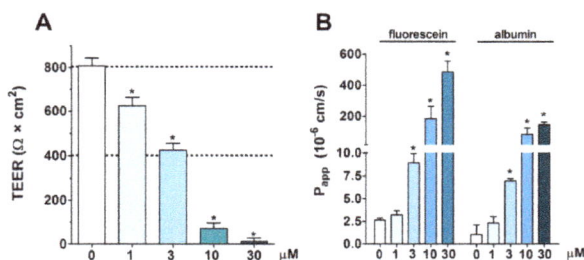

Figure 2. Effect of 1-h PN159 treatment on barrier integrity of Caco-2 cell layers. (**A**) Transepithelial electrical resistance (TEER). (**B**) Permeability for fluorescein and albumin marker molecules (P$_{app}$ A-B 10^{-6} cm/s). Values are presented as means ± SD, n = 3–8. Statistical analysis: ANOVA followed by Dunnett's test, $p < 0.05$ as compared with the control groups.

3.3. Reversible Effect of PN159 Peptide on the Opening of the Paracellular Cleft

The effect of PN159 peptide was very rapid, the electrical resistance dropped already to 42% of the control value after 1-min treatment (Figure 3A). The decrease of TEER continued until the end of the 30-min treatment (5 min: 16%, 15 min: 2.7%, 30 min: 1.4% of the control value). After the removal of the peptide the barrier function of Caco-2 cells was restored about 44% of the control value at six hours and a complete recovery could be observed at the 20 h timepoint. Intact TJs providing the morphological basis of barrier functions were visualized between Caco-2 epithelial cells in the control group by transmission electron microscopy, but no junctions were observed following treatment with PN159 peptide (Figure 3B). The disappearance of intercellular TJs was reversible, because after 1-day recovery the ultrastructure of epithelial junctions became similar to control cells. No open TJs were observed in the control or recovery groups by checking the electron micrographs (28–42 images/groups).

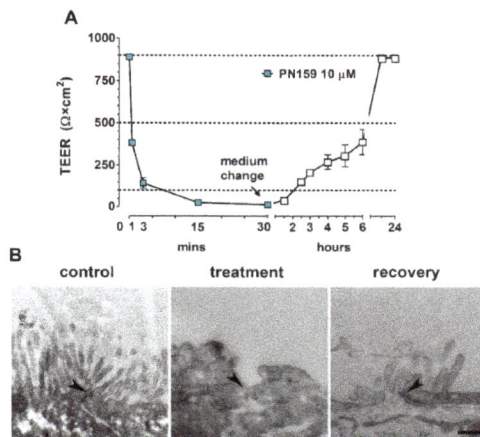

Figure 3. Reversible effect of PN159 peptide (10 µM, 30-min treatment, 24-h recovery) on Caco-2 cells. (**A**) Kinetic analysis of transepithelial electrical resistance (TEER) after PN159 peptide treatment. (**B**) Transmission electron micrographs of cell–cell connections (arrowheads); bar = 400 nm.

3.4. Effects of PN159 Peptide on the Penetration of Dextran Marker Molecules and Drugs

All these previous functional and morphological results pointed to the TJ opening effect of PN159 in Caco-2 cells which potentially can be exploited to increase drug penetration across the intestinal barrier. The permeability of Caco-2 monolayers was measured in the apical to basal (intestine to blood) direction for four water-soluble dextran marker molecules of different sizes (4–40 kDa) and four drugs, the hydrophilic atenolol and cimetidine, and the lipophilic quinidine and verapamil (Table 2). All four drugs are substrates of active efflux transporters [24]. The apparent permeability coefficients of the large fluorescein isothiocyanate-labeled dextran (FD) macromolecules were very low in control conditions but they were elevated by 159-400 fold following PN159 treatment. The highest increase was measured in the case of FD-40, the largest macromolecule. In control conditions the permeability of atenolol and cimetidine was the lowest from the tested molecules, while the highest penetration was measured for quinidine and verapamil on Caco-2 cells. PN159 treatment caused more than 30-fold change for atenolol and cimetidine which penetrate slowly across the cells layers. The peptide increased about 2 fold the permeability of the intestinal culture model for the lipophilic quinidine and verapamil, which already showed a good penetration.

Table 2. Apparent permeability coefficients of dextran marker molecules and drugs in the apical-basal direction (P_{app} A-B, 10^{-6} cm/s) in control and PN159 treated cultures. The differences between control and treated groups were expressed in fold changes. FD, fluorescein isothiocyanate-labeled dextran.

Markers and Drug	Control	PN159	Fold Change
FD-4	0.021 ± 0.001	4.2 ± 0.1	200.0
FD-10	0.025 ± 0.010	4.8 ± 0.7	192.0
FD-20	0.022 ± 0.002	3.5 ± 1.0	159.0
FD-40	0.015 ± 0.003	6.0 ± 0.3	400.0
atenolol	1.2 ± 0.3	36.3 ± 1.9	30.0
cimetidine	0.9 ± 0.2	34.5 ± 4.5	38.3
quinidine	45.0 ± 13.3	72.6 ± 2.4	1.6
verapamil	46.2 ± 3.9	86.7 ± 18.8	1.9

3.5. The Effect of PN159 Peptide on the Staining of Junctional Proteins and F-Actin

The concentration-dependent effects of the peptide on epithelial barrier integrity in Caco-2 cells were confirmed by the immunostaining of junctional proteins claudin-1, ZO-1 and β-catenin, and the labeling of the actin cytoskeleton (F-actin) (Figure 4). The 1 μM concentration of the peptide caused a slight effect on cell morphology. At higher than 3 μM concentrations significant changes were observed both in the junctional protein pattern and in the actin cytoskeleton organization. Claudin-1 was the junctional protein most sensitive to the peptide treatment. PN159 at a concentration of 10 μM caused a drastic change in actin cytoskeleton and epithelial junctional morphology, with a visible opening of intercellular junctions.

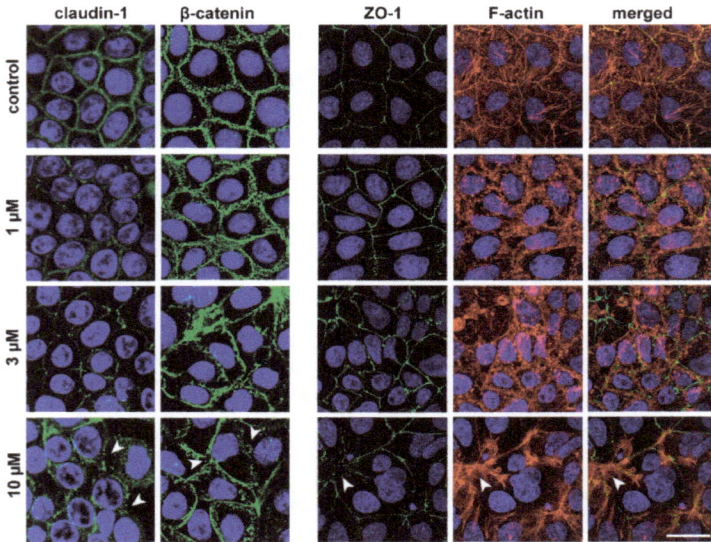

Figure 4. Effects of PN159 peptide on junctional morphology of Caco-2 cells. Immunostaining for claudin-1, β-catenin and zonula occludens-1 (ZO-1) junctional proteins and fluorescent staining for F-actin are shown in control conditions or after 1-hour peptide treatment. Green color: immunostaining for ZO-1, β-catenin and claudin-1. Blue color: staining of cell nuclei. Red color staining of F-actin. Bar = 20 μm. Arrowheads indicate the opened junctions between the cells.

3.6. Molecular Modeling of Human Claudin Proteins and Docking of PN159 Peptide

According to the CD spectra obtained, the secondary structure of PN159 peptide contains 11% α-helix, 31% β-sheet, 24% turns and 34% unordered structure (Figure 5A). This secondary structure of PN159 peptide was stable between 25 and 55 °C (Figure 5B). In concordance with the result of CD spectra, similar secondary structure motifs were found by molecular modeling (Figure 5C).

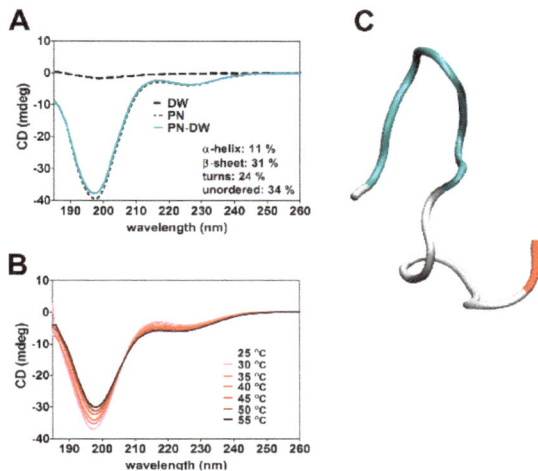

Figure 5. (**A**) Circular dichroism (CD) spectroscopy of PN159 peptide at 25 °C. (**B**) Thermostability measurement of the peptide structure. (**C**) Structure of PN159 by molecular modeling. Blue color: turn motifs; White color: coil-coil motifs; Red color: C-terminal region.

Claudin protein structures were obtained by homology modeling using the MODELLER program package (Figure 6A). Docking of PN159 peptide to full length homology modeled human claudin-1, -3, -4, and -7 monomers, highly expressed in Caco-2 cells [34] was performed on the CABS server (Figure 6B). Favorable docking poses located around extracellular loops ECL1 and ECL2 were sought by both energetic and geometric considerations and analyzed in all docking trajectories. Docking energies ("total energy") were decomposed to "ligand energy", "interaction energy" and "receptor energy" parts (Table 3). Correct docking poses were expected to have low values not only for the total energies, but as low as possible for all energy components simultaneously. Thus, the "ligand energy", "interaction energy" and "total energy" values were investigated. Based on the modeling, energetically highly favorable interactions were found between PN159 and the ECLs of claudin-1, -4 and -7, but not for claudin-3 (Table 3). Docked poses of PN159 with ECLs of claudin-1, -4 and -7 are shown on Figure 6B.

Table 3. Docking energy components of PN159 to selected human claudin monomers. E_{tot}, total energy; E_{lig}, ligand energy; E_{int}, interaction energy.

Energy	Claudin-1	Claudin-3	Claudin-4	Claudin-7
E_{lig}	−34	−17	−61	−32
E_{int}	−63	−59	−79	−186
E_{tot}	−1228	−1163	−1229	−1798

The amino acid sequence of ECL1 and ECL2 of the three claudins which showed interaction with the TJ modulator peptide were compared and the most important amino acids which interact with PN159 were identified (Figure 6C). Four residues in ECL1, the polar Q44 and S/N/D53, the hydrophobic V55 and L71, and in ECL2 the polar N/Q156 participate in major interactions with the peptide. Q44 and V55 residues of claudin-1 and -7 form a binding pocket for L11 of the peptide, and the same two residues of claudin-4 bind L6 and K9 (Figure 6C). The polar S/N/D53 and L71 of claudin-4 and -7 interact with K5, while the same amino acids of claudin-1 bind K12. The N/Q156 amino acid of ECL2 of all three claudins interacts with lysine: in the case of claudin-1 this is L17 of PN159, for claudin-4 L2, and for claudin-7 L6, L8, L15, L17. Based on the docking results, lysine, especially K1 and K5 and leucine L6 and L17 of PN159 interact with all three claudins examined (Figure 6D). After docking of the peptide disappearance of β-strands in ECLs of claudins was observed (Figure 6B), which seems to be correlated with the strength of interaction (Table 3). Comparing the docking energy values of PN159 to claudins the following rank order in the strength of interaction can be established: claudin-3 < claudin-1 < claudin-4< claudin-7. The energy values from modeling are shown in Table 3.

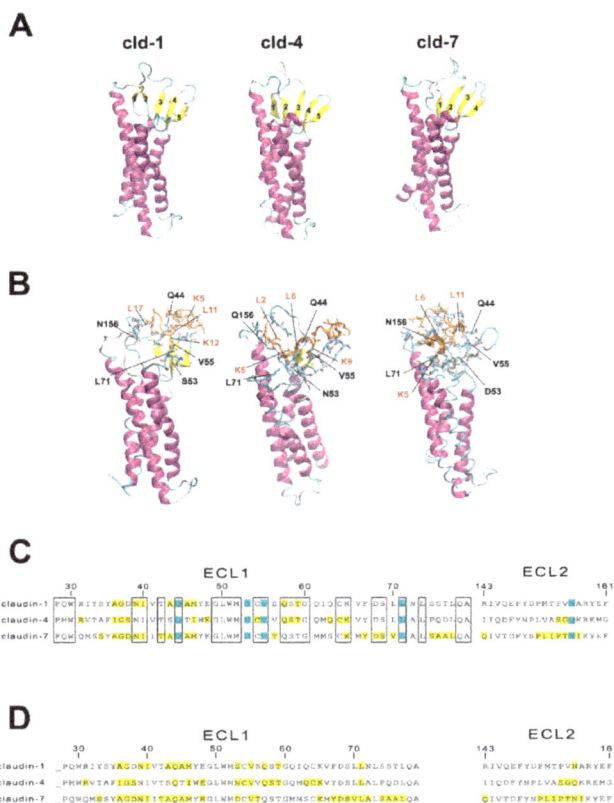

Figure 6. (**A**) Modeling human claudin-1, -4, -7 proteins. (**B**) Docking of PN159 peptide to claudin proteins. Interacting residues are shown as sticks. Orange color: PN159 peptide; Yellow color: β-strands; purple color: α-helices of claudins. (**C**) Amino acid sequence of ECL1 and ECL2 of human claudin monomers 1, 4 and 7. Conserved amino acids are indicated in the boxes. The amino acids which interact with PN159 according to docking studies are marked by yellow and light blue. Blue color indicates interaction between the amino acids of claudins and PN159 peptide at the same position in all three claudins. ECL: extracellular loop. (**D**) Interaction between PN159 peptide and human claudin monomers 1, 4 and 7. Amino acids of PN159 peptide which interact with the claudins according to docking.

3.7. Cell-Penetrating Effect and Uptake of PN159 Peptide in Epithelial Cells

Besides the junctional effects, changes in the cell membrane integrity were also examined by ethidium homodimer-1 (856.77 Da) staining of Caco-2 epithelial cells after 24-h treatments in the concentration range of 1 to 10 μM. Only the highest PN159 concentration caused plasma membrane entry of the red fluorescent dye, which stained cell nuclei (Figure 7A).

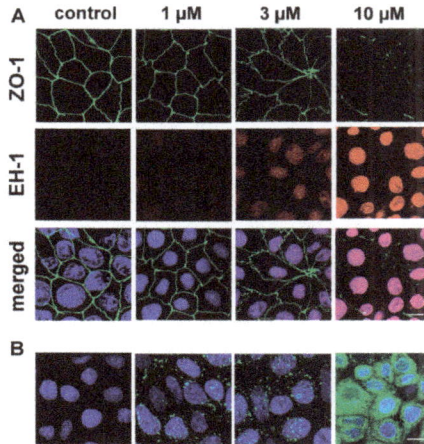

Figure 7. (**A**) Fluorescent staining of juntional protein zonula occludens-1 and double staining of cell nuclei in Caco-2 cells after 1-h treatment with PN159 peptide. Green color: immunostaining for ZO-1. Red color: staining by ethidium homodimer-1 (EH-1), indicating increased membrane permeability.Blue color: staining of all cell nuclei by H33342. Bar = 10 μm. (**B**) Confocal microscopy images of living Caco-2 epithelial cells incubated with Bodipy FL labeled PN159 peptide in different concentrations for 5 min at 37°C. Green color: BodipyFL-PN159 peptide. Blue color: staining of cell nuclei. Bar = 10 μm.

The uptake of the fluorescently labeled PN159 peptide, reflected by the green fluorescent signal, was visualized by confocal microscopy (Figure 7B). In Caco-2 cells treated with 1 and 3 μM concentrations, the peptide was detectable in the cytoplasm as green dots. The cellular uptake of the peptide in cells incubated with 10 μM concentration was more pronounced.

We confirmed the interaction of PN159 peptide with claudin-4 junctional protein by a co-localization analysis. The labeled peptide was visible in the cytoplasm and also in the cell membrane at the level of intercellular junctions immunolabeled for claudin-4 (Figure 8).

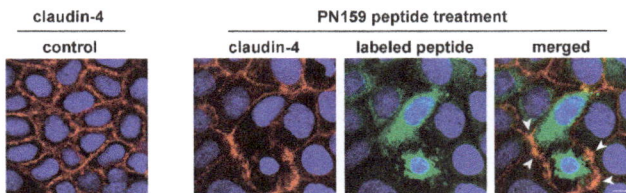

Figure 8. Caco-2 cells were treated with Bodipy FL labeled PN159 peptide (5 min), then fluorescent immunostaining of junctional protein claudin-4 and staining of cell nuclei were performed. Red color: immunostaining for claudin-4. Green color: Bodipy FL labeled PN159 peptide. Blue color: staining of cell nuclei by H33342. Bar = 10 μm. Arrowheads indicate co-localization of claudin-4 and the labeled PN159 peptide.

3.8. Antimicrobial Effect of PN159

We tested the antimicrobial activity of PN159 peptide on six ESKAPE pathogens (Table 4) at a wide range of concentration (0.8 to 70 μM). Among the tested bacteria *Acinetobacter baumannii* and *Enterococcus faecium* were the two most sensitive strains with MIC values below 5 μM. The concentration of PN159 to inhibit the growth of *Staphylococcus aureus* and *Klebsiella pneumoniae* was around 10 μM, which was in similar range where peptide effects were seen on human epithelial cells. The peptide was still effective on the vancomycin-resistant *Enterobacter cloacae* and on *Pseudomonas aeruginosa*, but at 10-times higher concentrations than in the case of the most sensitive pathogens.

As compared to the reference bactericidal antibiotic cefoxitin, PN159 was more effective in the case of *Acinetobacter baumannii*, *Enterococcus faecium*, *Enterobacter cloacae* and *Pseudomonas aeruginosa*. Gentamicin and ciprofloxacin showed strong antimicrobial activity for all ESKAPE pathogens, except *Enterococcus faecium*. This strain was resistant for all investigated antibiotics, however, PN159 efficiently inhibited its growth (Table 4).

Table 4. Antibacterial activity of PN159 peptide, cefoxitin, gentamicin and ciprofloxacin antibiotics on ESKAPE pathogens. ATCC numbers are added in brackets. MIC (μM), minimal inhibitory concentration.

ESKAPE Pethogens (ATCC)	PN159	Cefoxitin	Gentamicin	Ciprofloxacin
Acinetobacter baumannii (17978)	3.6	222.6	0.6	0.94
Enterococcus faecium (700221)	4.4	>222.6	>143.9	>30.18
Staphylococcus aureus (29213)	9.2	6.9	1.1	1.89
Klebsiella pneumonia (10031)	13.8	3.5	0.6	0.06
Enterobacter cloacae (13047)	31.0	>222.6	1.1	0.06
Pseudomonas aeruginosa (27853)	46.4	>222.6	2.3	1.89

3.9. The Effect of Cell-Penetrating Peptides on Intestinal Barrier Integrity

The kinetics of the effects of three other CPPs on Caco-2 cells were followed by real-time impedance measurements (Figure 9A). The R8 and φ-peptides decreased the cell impedance during the 24-h monitoring which indicates a cell reaction. Changes in cell index without cytotoxic effects most probably are caused by an increase in plasma membrane ionic permeability. There was no major influence of CPPs on barrier integrity (Figure 9B,C) as compared to the effect of PN159. We observed a slightly decreased TEER in the case of R8 and φ-peptide and only the φ-peptide caused an elevated permeability for the fluorescein marker molecule. Based on these results the investigated CPPs have no significant opening effect on the intercellular junctions, which was also verified by immunostaining for junctional proteins (Figure 9D).

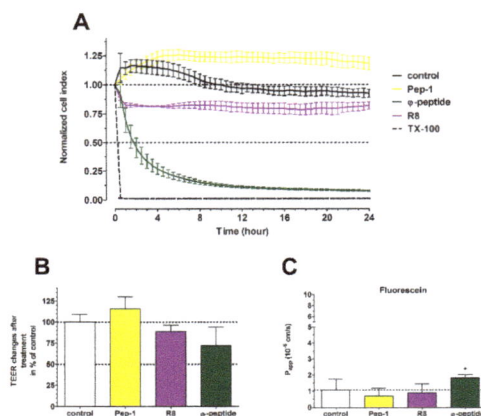

Figure 9. *Cont.*

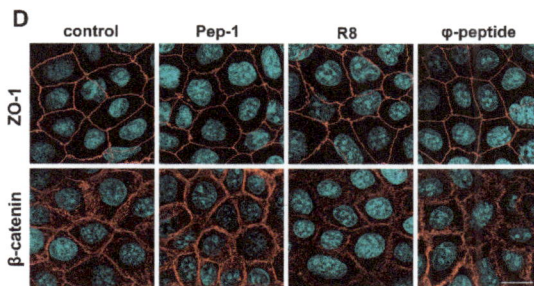

Figure 9. (A) Effects of different cell-penetrating peptides (CPPs; 100 μM, 24 h) on Caco-2 cells followed by impedance measurements. The effects of peptides on the impedance were shown as normalized cell index. Values are presented as means ± SD, *n* = 3−8. **(B)** Evaluation of barrier integrity on Caco-2 cell layers by measurement of transepithelial electrical resistance (TEER) after 1-h CPP treatment. **(C)** Caco-2 cell layer permeability for fluorescein marker molecule (P_{app} A-B 10^{-6} cm/s) after 1-h CPP treatment. **(D)** Effects of CPPs on junctional morphology of Caco-2 cells. Immunostaining for zonula occludens-1 (ZO-1) and β-catenin junctional proteins in control conditions and after 1-h peptide treatment. Red color: immunostaining for ZO-1 and β-catenin. Blue color: staining of cell nuclei. Bar = 20 μm.

4. Discussion

We investigated for the first time the dual, TJ modulator and cell membrane actions of the PN159 peptide. PN159 was described as a TJ modulator and permeability-enhancing peptide on airway epithelial cell layers in vitro and in vivo [4], and in our previous comparative work we found it also very effective on culture models of the blood–brain and intestinal barriers [8]. The same peptide, known also as KLAL or MAP was extensively studied for its cell membrane action as a CPP [10–12,35]. However, the identity of the differently named molecule was not previously known for the researchers of the two fields. We demonstrated, that beside the cell-penetrating and antimicrobial effects, PN159 is a TJ modulator on intestinal epithelial cells and by molecular modeling new members of the claudin family were identified as its potential targets.

4.1. TJ Modulator Effect of PN159: Safety, Concentration Dependence and Reversibility

All the presented functional and morphological results point to the safe, concentration-dependent and reversible TJ opening effect of PN159 in Caco-2 cells. The effect of the peptide on epithelial cell viability was investigated for one and 24 h. We found that the peptide has no effect on cell metabolism measured by MTT test or on impedance kinetics and can be considered as safe up to 10 μM. The changes seen after higher, 30 μM concentration were fully reversible. The 100 μM concentration of PN159 caused irreversible changes in both parameters on intestinal epithelial cells after either 1-h or one-day treatment. Using respiratory epithelial tissue (EpiAirway model) and MTT assay, PN159 was found to be safe at concentrations up to 100 μM for a 1-h treatment [9]. The difference between the sensitivity of the epithelial models and also the sensitivity of the applied methods may explain the dissimilarity of these data.

We found a marked concentration-dependence of the TJ modulator effect. With the most sensitive method, TEER, we could determine that 1 μM PN159 already opened the paracellular cleft for ions, while higher concentrations gradually decreased TEER. This TJ modulation by the effective but safe 10 μM concentration of the peptide was fast, within minutes, but after removal of the peptide a full recovery was seen. This opening and complete recovery of the intestinal TJ structure was verified by electron microscopy in the present study and by immunohistochemistry for TJ proteins both in this and our previous work [8]. A similar concentration-dependent and reversible effect of PN159 on TEER was found on airway epithelial tissue, too [4].

The concentration dependence of the TJ modulator effect of the peptide was also detected in the permeability assay for a small and a large hydrophilic marker, fluorescein and albumin. A similarly high permeability increase with a full reversibility was measured for the same markers on both Caco-2 and blood–brain barrier culture models with the 10 μM concentration of PN159 peptide [8]. This action of the peptide was verified by the immunostaining of junctional proteins with higher concentrations causing bigger alterations in junctional protein intensity and distribution. Other claudin-specific TJ modulator peptides act similarly on junctional protein staining as well as on permeability of epithelial and endothelial cells [36,37].

In addition, the opening of the paracellular pathway in Caco-2 monolayers was measured by four dextran markers with size between 4 and 40 kDa. The apparent permeability coefficients of the large dextran macromolecules were very low in control conditions. PN159 treatment (10 μM) elevated the dextran penetration by 159- to 400-fold. The highest increase was measured in the case of the largest, FD-40 marker. The concentration dependency of the permeability increasing effect of PN159 was also observed on the EpiAirway model, but in the concentration range of 25 to 100 μM. The elevation of the permeability was 10- to 30-fold for FD-4 [4] and for peptide hormones with the same size [9].

To study the effect of PN159 on drug penetration, we tested two hydrophilic and two lipophilic drugs, which are substrates of active efflux transporters [24,38]. The permeability of hydrophilic atenolol and cimetidine was very low, while high penetration was measured for the lipophilic quinidine and verapamil on Caco-2 cells in agreement with our previous study [24]. PN159 treatment caused more than 30-fold permeability elevation for atenolol and cimetidine which penetrate slowly across the cell's layers. The peptide increased about 2-fold the permeability of the intestinal culture model for the lipophilic quinidine and verapamil, which already showed a high penetration. The permeability of the slightly lipophilic plant alkaloid, galantamine (287 Da), a substrate of P-glycoprotein, was also increased 2 to 3-fold by PN159 in airway epithelial tissue model [9] confirming the peptide's penetration enhancer effect.

4.2. Tight Junction (TJ)Modulator Effect of PN159: Interaction with Claudins

In our previous study, binding of PN159 in the micromolar range to epithelial claudin-1 and endothelial claudin-5 was demonstrated by affinity measurements and confirmed by docking studies [8]. In this report we describe an additional two intestinal epithelial junctional proteins, claudin-4 and -7 which are highly expressed in Caco-2 cells [34], as potential targets of the peptide by molecular docking. All these results suggest that PN159 peptide may open cell–cell junctions by acting on claudins, the most prominent family of integral membrane junctional proteins. C-CPE and C1C2 tight junction modulator peptides were also described to target claudins. C-CPE is a fragment of *Clostridium perfringens* enterotoxin which directly binds claudin subtypes including claudin-3 and -4 and induces disintegration of tight junctions [39]. The peptidomimetic C1C2 which contains the C-terminal half of ECL1 of claudin-1 predominantly binds to claudin-1 and -5, opens the paracellular barrier in cultured cells and causes cytosolic distribution of claudin-1, -2, -3, -4, and -5 [36]. What is common in the action of these three TJ modulator peptides is that they have specific interactions with conserved amino acids of claudins [8,40], however, these peptides do not share any similarity in their amino acid sequence. The secondary structure of C1C2 consists of β-sheet stabilized by α-helix [40], the claudin-binding domain of C-CPE is a nine-stranded β-sandwich [41], while according to our CD measurements and molecular modelling PN159 also contains β-sheet in addition to α-helix. This structural similarity between the three different but claudin-targeting peptides may be linked to the TJ modulator effect.

4.3. Cell Penetration and Antimicrobial Effect of PN159

We observed a concentration-dependent cellular uptake of PN159 on intestinal barrier cells as reflected in the confocal microscope images. PN159 has a fast uptake in human melanoma cells, treatment with 1 μM concentration already causing detectable entry of the peptide into the cells, in concordance with our results [12]. The cellular uptake of PN159 was also verified on other four cell lines [42]. After treatment with a concentration of 10 μM, the peptide entered the cytoplasm of cells without cytotoxic effects, similar to our data.

Most of the CPPs have antimicrobial activity due to their structural properties, especially the cationic and the amphipathic membrane active peptides [13]. Based on literature data the amphipathic PN159 effectively inhibited the growth of different microorganisms, like *Escherichia coli, Staphylococcus epidermidis, Bacillus megaterium, Saccharomyces cerevisiae* [10,19,43]. In this study we demonstrated the antimicrobial activity of PN159 peptide in the concentration range of 3–46 μM on clinically relevant ESKAPE pathogens. As compared to the reference antibiotics, PN159 was more effective in the inhibition of the growth of *Acinetobacter baumannii, Enterococcus faecium, Enterobacter cloacae* and *Pseudomonas aeruginosa*. (Table 4).

Comparing our results with data from the literature, another amphipathic antimicrobial peptide, melittin, inhibited the growth of *Escherichia coli* and *Micrococcus luteus* [44] and was also tested against three of the ESKAPE pathogens. *Acinetobacter baumannii* and *Pseudomonas aeruginosa* were more sensitive for melittin treatment, than *Klebsiella pneumoniae:* for the inhibition of growth of *Klebsiella pneumoniae* more than 100 μM melittin was needed [45], while in our study around 10 μM PN159 was already effective.

PN159, as a model amphipathic CPP peptide, strongly interacts with biological membranes due to its physical-chemical properties. As a CPP, PN159 enters epithelial cells [42], enhances the membrane penetration of molecules and exerts antimicrobial effects [10,11]. Because PN159 binds different claudins and interacts specifically with their conserved amino acids, it acts as a TJ modulator [8]. It is an open question, however, if the plasma membrane and the TJ modulator actions of PN159 are connected or not.

4.4. TJ Modulator Effect of Other CPPs?

Based on these results we asked the question whether this TJ modulator ability is a unique effect of PN159 among the CPPs or not. Therefore, we have tested two other amphipathic CPPs, the widely used Pep-1 [16] and the cyclic φ-peptide [15], and one cationic CPP, R8 peptide [18] on the barrier integrity of Caco-2 monolayers. None of the tested CPPs had a TJ modulator effect similar to PN159. There was no change in the TEER values and only the φ-peptide increased the permeability of fluorescein. Since no effect was seen on junctional staining in epithelial cells treated with φ-peptide, the increase in permeability and decrease in the cell layer impedance may be linked to the cell membrane action of this CPP [15]. As we demonstrated by our modeling results, PN159 peptide interacts with conserved residues of the claudins investigated (Figure 6) suggesting its ability for specific interactions [8]. The amino acid sequence of PN159 results in an amphipathic helix structure [10], which is not characteristic of the other CPPs investigated in our paper. From the other three investigated peptides, R8 and φ-peptide have positively charged arginine clusters (Table 1) and are considered as clearly cationic CPPs [17]. Pep-1 also contains a positively charged amino acid cluster and is rich in tryptophan repeats (Table 1). Neither PN159 contains clusters of arginine or positively charged amino acids, nor tryptophan (Table 1). While we have not found a CPP with a TJ modulator effect in the current study, we cannot exclude that other membrane active peptides can have such dual action. The amphipathic antimicrobial peptide melittin enhanced the paracellular permeability for dextran marker molecules on Caco-2 cells [46]. The opening of TJs by melittin was mediated, at least partially, by the prostaglandin signaling pathway [46].

5. Conclusions

We demonstrated that PN159 (KLAL/MAP) peptide as a penetration enhancer has a dual action on intestinal epithelial cells. The peptide safely and reversibly enhances the permeability of model molecules and drugs through intestinal epithelial cell layers by opening the intercellular junctions. We identified claudin-4 and -7 junctional proteins by docking studies as potential binding partners and targets of the peptide in the opening of the paracellular pathway. In addition to the tight junction modulator action, the peptide has a concentration-dependent cellular uptake and cell membrane permeabilizing effect, which can also contribute to its penetration-enhancing effect. This dual action is not general for cell-penetrating peptides, since the other three CPPs tested did not show barrier opening effects. Therefore, we propose the investigation of CPPs for testing their effect on paracellular permeability.

Author Contributions: Conceptualization, M.A.D., A.B. and T.A.M.; methodology, A.B., I.G. and L.K.; formal analysis, A.B. and F.Ö.; investigation, A.B., I.G., L.K., O.Z., L.D., M.V. and Á.K.; resources, L.F., N.I., T.A.M., C.P., P.S.-R. and M.A.D.; data curation, A.B. and I.G.; writing—original draft preparation, A.B., M.A.D.; writing—review and editing, A.B., I.G., L.K., F.Ö., O.Z., L.D., L.F., M.V., Á.K., N.I., T.A.M., C.P., P.S.-R. and M.A.D.; visualization, A.B., Á.K. and F.Ö.; supervision, M.A.D., P.S.-R., T.A.M., and C.P.; funding acquisition, M.A.D., T.A.M., M.V. and C.P.

Funding: This research was funded by the National Research, Development and Innovation Office of Hungary, grant number GINOP-2.2.1-15-2016-00007.

Acknowledgments: The help of Zoltán Kóta during the experiments is gratefully acknowledged. We are grateful to Zsombor Kapás for his help in the preparation of the figures. The European Research Council H2020-ERC-2014-CoG 648364—Resistance Evolution (C.P.).

Conflicts of Interest: The authors declare no conflict of interest. The funders had no role in the design of the study; in the collection, analyses, or interpretation of data; in the writing of the manuscript, or in the decision to publish the results.

References

1. Deli, M.A. Potential use of tight junction modulators to reversibly open membranous barriers and improve drug delivery. A review. *Biochim. Biophys. Acta* **2009**, *1788*, 892–910. [CrossRef] [PubMed]
2. Kiss, L.; Hellinger, É.; Pilbat, A.M.; Kittel, Á.; Török, Z.; Füredi, A.; Szakács, G.; Veszelka, S.; Sipos, P.; Ózsvári, B.; et al. Sucrose esters increase drug penetration, but do not inhibit p-glycoprotein in caco-2 intestinal epithelial cells. *J. Pharm. Sci.* **2014**, *103*, 3107–3119. [CrossRef] [PubMed]
3. Perinelli, D.R.; Vllasaliu, D.; Bonacucina, G.; Come, B.; Pucciarelli, S.; Ricciutelli, M.; Cespi, M.; Itri, R.; Spinozzi, F.; Palmieri, G.F.; et al. Rhamnolipids as epithelial permeability enhancers for macromolecular therapeutics. *Eur. J. Pharm. Biopharm.* **2017**, *119*, 419–425. [CrossRef] [PubMed]
4. Johnson, P.H.; Quay, S.C. Advances in nasal drug delivery through tight junction technology. A review. *Expert. Opin. Drug Deliv.* **2005**, *2*, 281–298. [CrossRef] [PubMed]
5. Chiba, H.; Osanai, M.; Murata, M.; Kojima, T.; Sawada, N. Transmembrane proteins of tight junctions. A review. *Biochim. Biophys. Acta* **2008**, *1778*, 588–600. [CrossRef] [PubMed]
6. Krause, G.; Winkler, L.; Mueller, S.L.; Haseloff, R.F.; Piontek, J.; Blasig, I.E. Structure and function of claudins. A review. *Biochim. Biophys. Acta* **2008**, *1778*, 631–645. [CrossRef] [PubMed]
7. Tscheik, C.; Blasig, I.E.; Winkler, L. Trends in drug delivery through tissue barriers containing tight junctions. *Tissue Barriers* **2013**, *1*, e24565. [CrossRef] [PubMed]
8. Bocsik, A.; Walter, R.F.; Gyebrovszki, A.; Fülöp, L.; Blasig, I.; Dabrowski, S.; Ötvös, F.; Tóth, A.; Rákhely, G.; Veszelka, S.; et al. Reversible opening of intercellular junctions of intestinal epithelial and brain endothelial cells with tight junction modulator peptides. *J. Pharm. Sci.* **2016**, *105*, 754–765. [CrossRef] [PubMed]
9. Chen, S.C.; Eiting, K.; Cui, K.; Leonard, A.K.; Morris, D.; Li, C.Y.; Farber, K.; Sileno, A.P.; Houston, M.E., Jr.; Johnson, P.H.; et al. Therapeutic utility of a novel tight junction modulating peptide for enhancing intranasal drug delivery. *J. Pharm. Sci.* **2006**, *95*, 1364–1371. [CrossRef] [PubMed]
10. Dathe, M.; Schümann, M.; Wieprecht, T.; Winkler, A.; Beyermann, M.; Krause, E.; Matsuzaki, K.; Murase, O.; Bienert, M. Peptide helicity and membrane surface charge modulate the balance of electrostatic and hydrophobic interactions with lipid bilayers and biological membranes. *Biochemistry* **1996**, *35*, 12612–12622. [CrossRef]
11. Oehlke, J.; Scheller, A.; Wiesner, B.; Krause, E.; Beyermann, M.; Klauschenz, E.; Melzig, M.; Bienert, M. Cellular uptake of an alpha-helical amphipathic model peptide with the potential to deliver polar compounds into the cell interiornon-endocytically. *Biochim. Biophys. Acta* **1998**, *1414*, 127–139. [CrossRef]

12. Hällbrink, M.; Florén, A.; Elmquist, A.; Pooga, M.; Bartfai, T.; Langel, U. Cargo delivery kinetics of cell-penetrating peptides. *Biochim. Biophys. Acta* **2001**, *1515*, 101–109. [CrossRef]

13. Arouri, A.; Dathe, M.; Blume, A. The helical propensity of KLA amphipathic peptides enhances their binding to gel-state lipid membranes. *Biophys. Chem.* **2013**, *180–181*, 10–21. [CrossRef] [PubMed]

14. Copolovici, D.M.; Langel, K.; Eriste, E.; Langel, Ü. Cell-penetrating peptides: Design, synthesis, and applications. A review. *ACS Nano* **2014**, *8*, 1972–1994. [CrossRef] [PubMed]

15. Qian, Z.; LaRochelle, J.R.; Jiang, B.; Lian, W.; Hard, R.L.; Selner, N.G.; Luechapanichkul, R.; Barrios, A.M.; Pei, D. Early endosomal escape of a cyclic cell-penetrating peptide allows effective cytosolic cargo delivery. *Biochemistry* **2014**, *53*, 4034–4046. [CrossRef]

16. Morris, M.C.; Deshayes, S.; Heitz, F.; Divita, G. Cell-penetrating peptides: From molecular mechanisms to therapeutics. A review. *Biol. Cell* **2008**, *100*, 201–217. [CrossRef]

17. Guidotti, G.; Brambilla, L.; Rossi, D. Cell-Penetrating Peptides: From Basic Research to Clinics. A review. *Trends Pharmacol. Sci.* **2017**, *38*, 406–424. [CrossRef]

18. He, L.; Sayers, E.J.; Watson, P.; Jones, A.T. Contrasting roles for actin in the cellular uptake of cell penetrating peptide conjugates. *Sci. Rep.* **2018**, *8*, 7318. [CrossRef]

19. Palm, C.; Netzereab, S.; Hällbrink, M. Quantitatively determined uptake of cell-penetrating peptides in non-mammalian cells with an evaluation of degradation and antimicrobial effects. *Peptides* **2006**, *27*, 1710–1716. [CrossRef]

20. Boucher, H.W.; Talbot, G.H.; Bradley, J.S.; Edwards, J.E.; Gilbert, D.; Rice, L.B.; Scheld, M.; Spellberg, B.; Bartlett, J. Bad bugs, no drugs: No ESKAPE! An update from the Infectious Diseases Society of America. A review. *Clin. Infect. Dis.* **2009**, *48*, 1–12. [CrossRef]

21. Lázár, V.; Martins, A.; Spohn, R.; Daruka, L.; Grézal, G.; Fekete, G.; Számel, M.; Jangir, P.K.; Kintses, B.; Csörgő, B.; et al. Antibiotic-resistant bacteria show widespread collateral sensitivity to antimicrobial peptides. *Nat. Microbiol.* **2018**, *3*, 718–731. [CrossRef] [PubMed]

22. Artursson, P.; Palm, K.; Luthman, K. Caco-2 monolayers in experimental and theoretical predictions of drug transport. *Adv. Drug Deliv. Rev.* **2001**, *46*, 27–43. [CrossRef]

23. Hubatsch, I.; Ragnarsson, E.G.; Artursson, P. Determination of drug permeability and prediction of drug absorption in Caco-2 monolayers. *Nat. Protoc.* **2007**, *2*, 2111–2119. [CrossRef] [PubMed]

24. Hellinger, E.; Veszelka, S.; Tóth, A.E.; Walter, F.; Kittel, Á.; Bakk, M.L.; Tihanyi, K.; Háda, V.; Nakagawa, S.; Duy, T.D.; Niwa, M.; et al. Comparison of brain capillary endothelial cell-based and epithelial (MDCK-MDR1, Caco-2, and VB-Caco-2) cell-based surrogate blood-brain barrier penetration models. *Eur. J. Pharm. Biopharm.* **2012**, *82*, 340–351. [CrossRef] [PubMed]

25. Roka, E.; Vecsernyes, M.; Bacskay, I.; Félix, C.; Rhimi, M.; Coleman, A.W.; Perret, F. para-Sulphonato-calix[n]arenes as selective activators for the passage of molecules across the Caco-2 model intestinal membrane. *Chem. Commun.* **2015**, *51*, 9374–9376. [CrossRef] [PubMed]

26. Kürti, L.; Veszelka, S.; Bocsik, A.; Dung, N.T.; Ozsvári, B.; Puskás, L.G.; Kittel, A.; Szabó-Révész, P.; Deli, M.A. The effect of sucrose esters on a culture model of thenasal barrier. *Toxicol. In Vitro* **2012**, *26*, 445–454. [CrossRef] [PubMed]

27. Dichroweb, on-line Analysis for Protein Circular Dichroism spectra. Available online: dichroweb.cryst.bbk.ac.uk/html/home.shtml (accessed on 10 December 2015).

28. Sali, A.; Blundell, T.L. Comparative protein modelling by satisfaction of spatial restraints. *J. Mol. Biol.* **1993**, *234*, 779–815. [CrossRef] [PubMed]

29. Suzuki, H.; Nishizawa, T.; Tani, K.; Yamazaki, Y.; Tamura, A.; Ishitani, R.; Dohmae, N.; Tsukita, S.; Nureki, O.; Fujiyoshi, Y. Crystal structure of a claudin provides insight into the architecture of tight junctions. *Science* **2014**, *344*, 304–307. [CrossRef]

30. Phillips, J.C.; Braun, R.; Wang, W.; Gumbart, J.; Tajkhorshid, E.; Villa, E.; Chipot, C.; Skeel, R.D.; Kalé, L.; Schulten, K. Scalable molecular dynamics with NAMD. *J. Comput. Chem.* **2005**, *26*, 1781–1802. [CrossRef]

31. Humphrey, W.; Dalke, A.; Schulten, K. VMD: Visual molecular dynamics. *J. Mol. Graph.* **1996**, *14*, 33–38. [CrossRef]

32. Kurcinski, M.; Jamroz, M.; Blaszczyk, M.; Kolinski, A.; Kmiecik, S. CABS-dock web server for the flexible docking of peptides to proteins without prior knowledge of the binding site. *Nucleic. Acids. Res.* **2015**, *43*, W419–W424. [CrossRef] [PubMed]

33. Wiegand, I.; Hilpert, K.; Hancock, R.E. Agar and broth dilution methods to determine the minimal inhibitory concentration (MIC) of antimicrobial substances. *Nat. Protoc.* **2008**, *3*, 163–175. [CrossRef] [PubMed]

34. Veszelka, S.; Tóth, A.; Walter, F.R.; Tóth, A.E.; Gróf, I.; Mészáros, M.; Bocsik, A.; Hellinger, É.; Vastag, M.; Rákhely, G.; Deli, M.A. Comparison of a Rat Primary Cell-Based Blood-Brain Barrier Model With Epithelial and Brain Endothelial Cell Lines: Gene Expression and Drug Transport. *Front. Mol. Neurosci.* **2018**, *11*, 166. [CrossRef] [PubMed]

35. Erbe, A.; Kerth, A.; Dathe, M.; Blume, A. Interactions of KLA amphipathic model peptides with lipid monolayers. *ChemBioChem* **2009**, *10*, 2884–2892. [CrossRef] [PubMed]

36. Staat, C.; Coisne, C.; Dabrowski, S.; Stamatovic, S.M.; Andjelkovic, A.V.; Wolburg, H.; Engelhardt, B.; Blasig, I.E. Mode of action of claudin peptidomimetics in the transient opening of cellular tight junction barriers. *Biomaterials* **2015**, *54*, 9–20. [CrossRef] [PubMed]

37. Dithmer, S.; Staat, C.; Müller, C.; Ku, M.C.; Pohlmann, A.; Niendorf, T.; Gehne, N.; Fallier-Becker, P.; Kittel, Á.; Walter, F.R.; Veszelka, S.; et al. Claudin peptidomimetics modulate tissue barriers for enhanced drug delivery. *Ann. N. Y. Acad. Sci.* **2017**, *1397*, 169–184. [CrossRef] [PubMed]

38. Hellinger, E.; Bakk, M.L.; Pócza, P.; Tihanyi, K.; Vastag, M. Drug penetration model of vinblastine-treated Caco-2 cultures. *Eur. J. Pharm. Sci.* **2010**, *41*, 96–106. [CrossRef] [PubMed]

39. Sonoda, N.; Furuse, M.; Sasaki, H.; Yonemura, S.; Katahira, J.; Horiguchi, Y.; Tsukita, S. Clostridium perfringens enterotoxin fragment removes specific claudins from tight junction strands: Evidence for direct involvement of claudins in tight junction barrier. *J. Cell Biol.* **1999**, *147*, 195–204. [CrossRef]

40. Dabrowski, S.; Staat, C.; Zwanziger, D.; Sauer, R.S.; Bellmann, C.; Günther, R.; Krause, E.; Haseloff, R.F.; Rittner, H.; Blasig, I.E. Redox-sensitive structure and function of the first extracellular loop of the cell-cell contact protein claudin-1: Lessons from molecular structure to animals. *Antioxid. Redox. Signal* **2015**, *22*, 1–14. [CrossRef]

41. Veshnyakova, A.; Piontek, J.; Protze, J.; Waziri, N.; Heise, I.; Krause, G. Mechanism of Clostridium perfringens enterotoxin interaction with claudin-3/-4 protein suggests structural modifications of the toxin to target specific claudins. *J. Biol. Chem.* **2012**, *287*, 1698–1708. [CrossRef]

42. Mueller, J.; Kretzschmar, I.; Volkmer, R.; Boisguerin, P. Comparison of cellular uptake using 22 CPPs in 4 different cell lines. *Bioconjug. Chem.* **2008**, *19*, 2363–2374. [CrossRef] [PubMed]

43. Bagheri, M.; Beyermann, M.; Dathe, M. Immobilization reduces the activity of surface-bound cationic antimicrobial peptides with no influence upon the activity spectrum. *Antimicrob. Agents Chemother.* **2009**, *53*, 1132–1141. [CrossRef] [PubMed]

44. Maher, S.; McClean, S. Investigation of the cytotoxicity of eukaryotic and prokaryotic antimicrobial peptides in intestinal epithelial cells in vitro. *Biochem. Pharmacol.* **2006**, *71*, 1289–1298. [CrossRef] [PubMed]

45. Lam, S.J.; O'Brien-Simpson, N.M.; Pantarat, N.; Sulistio, A.; Wong, E.H.; Chen, Y.Y.; Lenzo, J.C.; Holden, J.A.; Blencowe, A.; Reynolds, E.C.; et al. Combating multidrug-resistant Gram-negative bacteria with structurally nanoengineered antimicrobial peptide polymers. *Nat. Microbiol.* **2016**, *1*, 16162. [CrossRef] [PubMed]

46. Maher, S.; Feighery, L.; Brayden, D.J.; McClean, S. Melittin as an epithelial permeability enhancer I: Investigation of its mechanism of action in Caco-2 monolayers. *Pharm. Res.* **2007**, *24*, 1336–1345. [CrossRef] [PubMed]

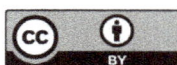

pharmaceutics

MDPI

Review

Intestinal Permeation Enhancers for Oral Delivery of Macromolecules: A Comparison between Salcaprozate Sodium (SNAC) and Sodium Caprate (C$_{10}$)

Caroline Twarog [1], Sarinj Fattah [1], Joanne Heade [1], Sam Maher [2], Elias Fattal [3] and David J. Brayden [1,*]

[1]   UCD School of Veterinary Medicine and UCD Conway Institute, University College Dublin, Belfield, Dublin 4, Ireland; caroline.twarog@ucdconnect.ie (C.T.); sarinj.fattah@ucd.ie (S.F.); joanne.heade@ucdconnect.ie (J.H.)
[2]   School of Pharmacy, Royal College of Surgeons in Ireland, St. Stephen's Green, Dublin 2, Ireland; sammaher@rcsi.ie
[3]   School of Pharmacy, Institut Galien, CNRS, Univ. Paris-Sud, Univ. Paris-Saclay, 92290 Châtenay-Malabry, France; elias.fattal@u-psud.fr
*   Correspondence: david.brayden@ucd.ie; Tel.: +3531-716-6013

Received: 21 January 2019; Accepted: 11 February 2019; Published: 13 February 2019

Abstract: Salcaprozate sodium (SNAC) and sodium caprate (C$_{10}$) are two of the most advanced intestinal permeation enhancers (PEs) that have been tested in clinical trials for oral delivery of macromolecules. Their effects on intestinal epithelia were studied for over 30 years, yet there is still debate over their mechanisms of action. C$_{10}$ acts via openings of epithelial tight junctions and/or membrane perturbation, while for decades SNAC was thought to increase passive transcellular permeation across small intestinal epithelia based on increased lipophilicity arising from non-covalent macromolecule complexation. More recently, an additional mechanism for SNAC associated with a pH-elevating, monomer-inducing, and pepsin-inhibiting effect in the stomach for oral delivery of semaglutide was advocated. Comparing the two surfactants, we found equivocal evidence for discrete mechanisms at the level of epithelial interactions in the small intestine, especially at the high doses used in vivo. Evidence that one agent is more efficacious compared to the other is not convincing, with tablets containing these PEs inducing single-digit highly variable increases in oral bioavailability of payloads in human trials, although this may be adequate for potent macromolecules. Regarding safety, SNAC has generally regarded as safe (GRAS) status and is Food and Drug Administration (FDA)-approved as a medical food (Eligen®-Vitamin B$_{12}$, Emisphere, Roseland, NJ, USA), whereas C$_{10}$ has a long history of use in man, and has food additive status. Evidence for co-absorption of microorganisms in the presence of either SNAC or C$_{10}$ has not emerged from clinical trials to date, and long-term effects from repeat dosing beyond six months have yet to be assessed. Since there are no obvious scientific reasons to prefer SNAC over C$_{10}$ in orally delivering a poorly permeable macromolecule, then formulation, manufacturing, and commercial considerations are the key drivers in decision-making.

Keywords: oral macromolecule delivery; oral peptides; sodium caprate; salcaprozate sodium; epithelial permeability; epithelial transport

1. Introduction

Despite an increasing trend in drug discovery and development in favor of biologics (macromolecules), poor oral availability remains a major impediment to even more widespread application. One group of macromolecules, peptides and proteins, are especially advocated due to excellent specificity, selectivity, safety, and efficacy. Indeed, a combined ~240 were marketed since the 1980s [1]. Of that list, 12% have <60 amino acids, designating approximately 30 peptides from that total [2]. Over 90% of peptides are injectable formulations, with just 4% delivered orally, and even lower percentages delivered via the skin and airway routes [2]. Recent progress was made toward the development of oral formulations for peptides where there are scientific, patient acceptability, and commercial arguments for non-injectable alternatives, especially for those that are used chronically and require frequent dosing (e.g., glucagon-like peptide 1 (GLP-1) analogs) [3]. The oral route offers greater patient compliance and can generate large market sales for molecules working indirectly on the same overall biological target, even if overall efficacy is lower than parenteral options. This is the case for oral dipeptidyl peptidase 4 (DPP-4) small-molecule inhibitors in competition with injectable GLP-1 peptide analogs [4]. Oral administration of peptides is limited by local conditions within the gastro-intestinal (GI) tract except for two relatively low-molecular-weight (LMW) examples designed for systemic delivery: a microemulsion of cyclosporin (Neoral®, Novartis, Switzerland) and a conventional solid-dose formulation of desmopressin (Minirin®, Ferring, USA) [5]. However, these examples are exceptions based on the atypical macrocycle structures of the two peptides, yielding oral bioavailabilities (BA) of 30–40% for lipophilic cyclosporine in Neoral® and just 0.17% for the highly potent hydrophilic desmopressin, Minirin® [6].

2. Challenges for Oral Delivery of Macromolecules

Oral administration of hydrophilic macromolecules with a molecular weight (MW) above 1000 Da remains a challenge due to susceptibility to pH and gastric/small intestinal enzymes, as well as low intestinal epithelial membrane permeability. The low permeability results from minimal passive or carrier-mediated transcellular permeation across phospholipid bilayers, as well as restricted paracellular transport via tight junctions. If they were small molecules, peptides would likely be assigned to Class III of the biopharmaceutics classification system (BCS), typically exhibiting high aqueous solubility (but not always) and low intestinal permeability. It is noteworthy that, even in the example of cyclosporine where the fraction absorbed (f_{abs}) is high, sensitivity to intestinal cytochrome P450 metabolism and P-glycoprotein efflux reduce the BA [7]; its primary problem is intestinal wall metabolism, not permeability. Other variables also impact the feasibility of oral delivery of macromolecules. If the plasma half-life ($t_{\frac{1}{2}}$) is too short, it will not be economically viable to administer a peptide candidate in multiple daily oral doses, where safety, efficacy, and variability issues would also arise. Similarly, a large therapeutic index (TI) is important in the context of selecting potent macromolecules as oral candidates, since efficacy and safety need to be addressed at the low and variable BA values that may be achieved even with successful oral formulations.

Investigators attempted to address pre-systemic degradation and poor permeation in the same formulation. A common approach is to combine peptidase inhibitors with absorption-modifying excipients (AMEs) or chemical permeation enhancers (PEs). These are usually formulated in enteric-coated dosage forms [6], although those formulated with salcaprozate sodium (SNAC), the leading candidate PE of the Eligen® technology (Emisphere, NJ, USA), do not seem to require coating [8]. In addition to avoiding degradation by gastric enzymes and low pH, enteric-coated capsules and tablets avoid dilution and premature release of both PE and macromolecule in the stomach. Furthermore, coatings can assist in promoting co-release of both in high concentrations at the same region to maximize intestinal permeability [9], a formulation goal to maximize payload delivery. Incorporation of PEs in conventional oral dosage forms is considered a relatively basic technology approach to address macromolecule permeability [10]. However, the ease with which PEs can be incorporated into delivery systems without the need for sophisticated and costly formulation made them more commercially attractive compared to, for example, nanotechnology [11] and device-based systems [12]. The majority of formulations currently in clinical trials for oral peptides are, therefore, based on PEs, whereas most nanotechnology and device-based systems remain in preclinical research [6]. This scenario may change if PE-based formulations only prove efficacious and commercially viable for exceptions: highly potent, stable, long-$t_{\frac{1}{2}}$ molecules of relatively low MW, and with a large TI.

3. Intestinal Permeation Enhancers

Numerous compounds including surfactants, bile salts, bacterial toxins, chelating agents, and medium-chain fatty acids (MCFA) proved to be effective PEs for poorly permeable molecules in in vitro and in vivo studies [10,13]. A comprehensive analysis of the majority of intestinal PEs from these classes that are used with peptides is available [10]. PEs that increase permeability across Caco-2 monolayers, isolated intestinal tissue mucosae, and in rodent models may also improve oral BA in humans, but this is not guaranteed since such studies are predominantly based on admixtures with payloads, not oral formulations. Furthermore, scale-up of the final formulation, PE dose, dilution, spreading, and release of both PE and payload during transit in the human GI tract, as well as the influence of enzymes, bile salts, and lipids in human intestinal fluids, must all be taken into account when attempting to make oral BA predictions for humans from preclinical studies. There are currently over 50 clinical trials in which PEs were shown to increase oral absorption of poorly permeable molecules, mostly achieved using surfactants [14]. The most widely tested PEs in these trials include Eligen® carriers, MCFAs, acyl carnitines, bile salts, and ethylenediaminetetraacetic acid (EDTA) [15]. The MCFA, sodium caprate (C_{10}), and the C_8 derivative, salcaprozate sodium (SNAC), are of particular interest as they had over 20 years of development in proprietary delivery platforms and have been tested in human trials more than any other PEs. C_{10} was originally developed as the main component of an oral solid-dosage form (GIPET™, Gastro-Intestinal Permeation Enhancement Technology) by Elan Pharma (Dublin, Ireland), and then, following licensing, by Merrion Pharmaceuticals (Dublin, Ireland) for oral peptide delivery, and by Ionis Pharmaceuticals (Carlsbad, CA, USA) for oral delivery of antisense oligonucleotides. SNAC was developed by Emisphere (NJ, USA) as the lead agent of its Eligen® carrier technology. Novo Nordisk (Bagsværd, Denmark) licensed both GIPET™ and Eligen® to assess with their insulin and GLP-1 analogs, ultimately opting to focus on an SNAC tablet formulation with their highly potent, stable, long-$t_{\frac{1}{2}}$ (160 h) injectable GLP-1 analog, semaglutide, for advanced clinical development, while abandoning GIPET™, along with further attempts to create an oral insulin.

4. Introducing C_{10}

C_{10} is the sodium salt of capric acid, an aliphatic saturated 10-carbon MCFA (Figure 1A). Fatty acids are ubiquitous nutrients liberated in high quantities during digestion of glycerides in the GI tract. They are also present in low mM concentrations in various nutrient sources, including milk. C_{10} is approved as a food additive in both the United States (US) and European Union (EU) and there are no daily limits on consumption; it was recently concluded that its presence in food should have no impact on human health [16]. C_{10} was a component of an approved rectal suppository of ampicillin (Doktacillin®, Meda, Solna, Sweden) [17]. It was since assessed in clinical trials by Merrion Pharma as oral solid-dosage forms (GIPET™) for the delivery of a wide range of poorly permeable actives, including small molecules (e.g., zoledronic acid, alendronate) and macromolecules (insulin, desmopressin, acyline, and antisense oligonucleotides) [18]. C_{10} is a soluble anionic surfactant, sensitive to changes in pH and ionic strength. At pH values 1–3 units below its pKa (~5) in gastric fluid, it exists in the non-ionized, insoluble, and inactive capric acid form. At acidic pH values, the surfactant can reduce surface tension, but does not exhibit detergent action. At pH values 1–3 units above its pKa (i.e., values that typically occur in the small intestine), C_{10} exists in an ionized soluble form with detergent capacity. Like many other efficient detergents, it does not form micelles efficiently owing to repulsion between the charged hydrophilic head groups. The resulting high concentration of free monomeric surfactant enables epithelial plasma membrane interaction and confers a transcellular element to its mode of action. The critical micellar concentration (CMC) value of C_{10}, like other ionizable surfactants, varies depending on the medium composition. Micelles form at lower concentrations in higher-ionic-strength buffers because the counter-ions in media interact closely with anionic head groups. Thus, varying the ionic strength alters the free monomeric concentration of C_{10} in the small intestine.

5. Introducing SNAC

SNAC is a synthetic *N*-acetylated amino-acid derivative of salicylic acid (Figure 1B). It was discovered as part of a screen to identify carrier-based PEs that could "chaperone" poorly permeable payloads across the intestine [19]. The carrier library of over 1500 compounds was collectively termed Eligen®, and it formed the portfolio of Emisphere Technologies. SNAC is the most extensively tested carrier and the only PE approved in an oral formulation designed to improve oral BA, albeit with a small molecule, cyanocobalamin/SNAC [20]. It is important to note that this oral form of vitamin B_{12} was approved under the regulatory pathway for medical foods, which does not have to meet the standards required for drug approvals, although the regulatory requirements for medical foods are still much higher than those of dietary supplements [21]. Emisphere obtained generally recognized as safe (GRAS) status for SNAC, which was a requirement for developing cyanocobalamin/SNAC for the medical food regulatory pathway. Having GRAS status for this PE may have somewhat mitigated some of the perceived risks associated with the oral semaglutide program at Novo Nordisk. In the 1990s, initial focus on SNAC was aimed at developing an oral formulation of the poorly permeable macromolecule, heparin [22]. In other preclinical studies, it also improved intestinal permeation of peptides (salmon calcitonin (sCT) and insulin) [23], along with poorly permeable small molecules (e.g., cromolyn) [24]. SNAC was tested in many formats: taste-masked liquids, tablets, and soft gelatin capsules. Similar to C_{10}, SNAC can be blended with the active pharmaceutical ingredient (API) using conventional processes, which makes manufacturing uncoated oral tablet dosage forms economic and relatively easy to scale.

It remains unclear if the high concentrations of SNAC required to improve small intestinal epithelial permeation relate to membrane perturbation, membrane fluidization, payload solubility changes, or tight junction openings, or whether it is a chaperone system that improves transcellular permeation via hydrophobization of the payload through non-covalent linkages. Of these factors and, unlike C_{10}, there is less direct evidence for tight junction involvement in the mechanism of SNAC than the other factors; hence, its common designation is as a transcellular PE. Common features are that C_{10} and SNAC are weak acids that display amphiphilicity and surface activity. However, there is a structural difference between them arising from the greater distribution of hydrophilic functional groups in the salicylamide region of SNAC, as evident from its higher polar surface area (89.5 Å^2) compared to C_{10} (40.1 Å^2) [25,26]. It follows that the hydrophobic region of SNAC should be less efficient at inserting into phospholipid membranes than C_{10} [27]. This may be one of the reasons why higher concentrations of SNAC than C_{10} are needed to improve permeation.

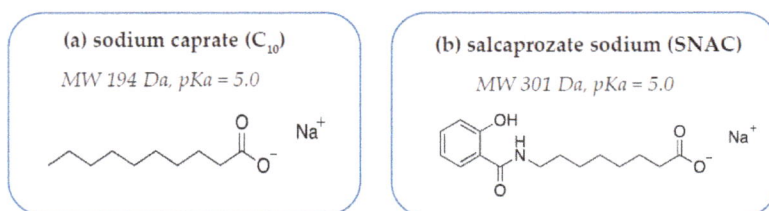

Figure 1. Structures of (a) sodium caprate (C_{10}) and (b) salcaprozate sodium (SNAC).

6. How Do SNAC and C_{10} Alter GI Permeability?

6.1. Challenges in Determining Mechanism of Action

PEs can improve permeability via a combination of mechanisms. Such mechanisms include opening tight junctions to increase paracellular permeability, decreasing mucus viscosity, inhibition of epithelial efflux pumps, complexation/hydrophobization of payload, increasing membrane fluidity, and (indirectly) via peptidase inhibition. The various mechanisms of action of C_{10} and SNAC were studied using cell biology and physicochemical techniques including membrane fluorescence, Western blotting, electrophoretic mobility, molecular imaging, and physical analysis. More recent approaches to the study of the interactions between PEs and payloads use surface plasmon resonance [28], as well as accelerated capillary electrophoresis, and isothermal titrated calorimetry (ITC) [29]; however, these techniques are mostly restricted to simple physiological buffers rather than bio-relevant intestinal fluids. In particular, a concern is that intricate mechanisms determined in in vitro assays might not reflect the true mechanism, because the PE concentrations used in vitro are typically lower than the efficacious doses used in vivo. There is, therefore, uncertainty regarding the actual local concentrations of PE and payload at the small intestinal epithelial wall in a particular region due to variability in dissolution, spreading, and dilution in the human GI lumen during transit.

6.2. C_{10} Mode of Action

The mode of action of C_{10} was studied at great lengths in a range of delivery models. In summary, concentrations that lead to alteration to permeability coefficients or oral BA are associated with mild mucosal damage and other hallmarks of transcellular perturbation. At low concentrations, increases in permeability of hydrophilic small molecules across Caco-2 monolayers using relatively low concentrations of C_{10} (2.5 mM) can be uncoupled from loss of monolayer integrity, accompanied by reversible reductions in transepithelial electrical potential (TEER) [27,30], indicative of a paracellular mechanism. The higher concentrations required to alter permeability in isolated rat and human intestinal tissue mucosae are associated with transcellular perturbation [31,32]. Mode-of-action studies at higher concentrations (8–13 mM) in Caco-2 monolayers also allude to a paracellular mechanism involving activation of membrane-bound phospholipase C [33–35]. The resulting increase in inositol 1,4,5-triphosphate (IP3) leads to an increase in intracellular calcium (Ca^{2+}), which in turn activates calmodulin and myosin light-chain kinase (MLCK). This event triggers the contraction of the peri-junctional actomyosin ring (PAMR) [36], permitting increased tight junction (TJ) permeability.

Nonetheless, these studies involving pharmacological inhibitors are not definitive proof of a discrete paracellular effect. Impedance spectroscopy in HT29/B6 human intestinal monolayers also supports the dataset showing that C_{10} acts via a paracellular mechanism; this was associated with removal or redistribution of the TJ proteins claudin 5 and tricellulin [37]. However, in the absence of data supporting the absence of transcellular perturbation (a dye uptake assay), the data from this study do not provide conclusive evidence for a paracellular mode of action either. It is impossible to ignore the evidence from a wide range of studies that C_{10} also disrupts cell membranes at 8–13 mM. C_{10} also caused Caco-2 cell leakage of intracellular ATP from Caco-2 cells [33], a likely consequence of plasma membrane perturbation. One interpretation is that cells respond to the initial membrane perturbation challenge by C_{10} with compensating intracellular signaling processes involved in mucosal repair, beginning with disbandment of TJs, and concluded by epithelial resealing [38].

Some of the strongest evidence in favor of a mechanism driven primarily by perturbation, however, comes from high content image analysis in live Caco-2 cells. C_{10} (2.5 mM) increased intracellular Ca^{2+} in Caco-2 cells prior to the plasma membrane permeability changes detected at 8.5 mM [27]. C_{10} (8.5–13 mM) altered both plasma and mitochondrial membrane integrity, indicative of perturbation; importantly, these were the minimum concentrations needed to induce a permeability increase. The elucidation of the primary mode of action as membrane perturbation was clarified by the capacity of C_{10} to preferentially displace claudins 4 and 5 from lipid rafts in MDCK cells, consistent with surfactant properties [39]. Other evidence comes from a recent surfactant screen using isolated rat intestinal mucosae in Ussing chambers, where C_{10} caused a concentration-dependent increase in epithelial histology damage [40]. Given the close association between permeation enhancement and mucosal perturbation in tissue and animal models, it was, therefore, not surprising that the cyto-protectant prostaglandin analog, misoprostol, prevented both the C_{10}-induced increase in flux of hydrophilic markers across Caco-2 monolayers and cell damage [41]. From these arguments, it is likely that the high concentrations of C_{10} used in tablets also cause a degree of mild reversible mucosal perturbation in vivo, not unlike that seen with aspirin, alcohol, and spicy foods [42]. In a study of a human rectal formulation of ampicillin with C_{10}, there was evidence of mild and reversible mucosal perturbation [17], although the data were confounded by the hyper-osmolarity of the formulation. While it is not possible to conclude that mucosal perturbation of the relatively static rectal mucosal compartment extrapolates directly to the small intestine where transit is relatively fast, it is likely that C_{10} causes mild and reversible regional perturbation within a short period at the high concentrations exposed to the small intestinal epithelium prior to its almost complete absorption within minutes.

There is a lack of understanding of the physicochemical aspects of how C_{10} interacts with mixed micelles in the small intestine in the fasted and fed states. Above its CMC of 25 mM in physiological buffer [27], C_{10} forms micelles and there is a distinct ratio of monomer to micellar-bound material, as highlighted in a recent study on alkyl maltosides [43]. In simulated intestinal buffers, it is uncertain whether the payload is incorporated into or adsorbs onto colloidal structures (e.g., mixed micelles, vesicles, lipid droplets), or whether it admixes with the C_{10} monomer. There is resulting confusion over which format the payload permeates. Thus, while one envisages a paracellular permeation route for polar macromolecules due to hydrophilicity, a transcellular pathway may also be available if C_{10}-entrapped vesicles and mixed micelles adsorb payload. Figure 2 is a composite of the possible multiple effects of C_{10} on intestinal epithelia.

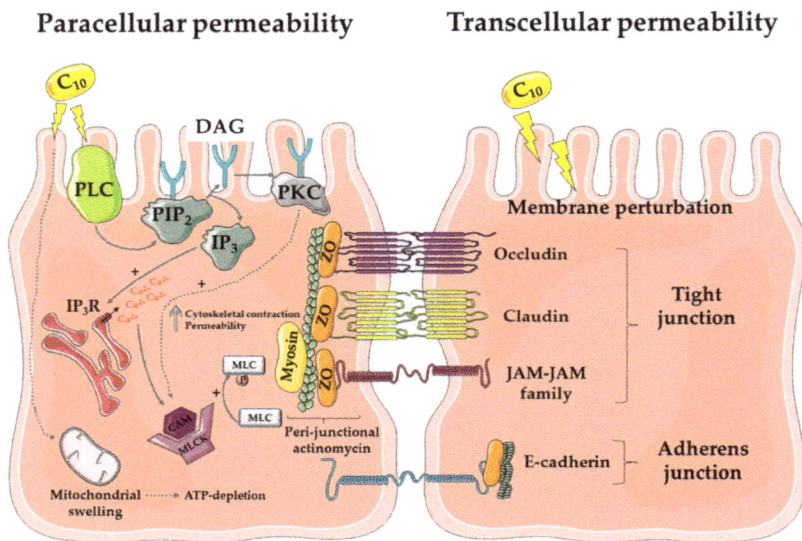

Figure 2. Mode of action of C_{10}. The diagram represents the proposed mechanism of action of C_{10} via paracellular flux (**left**) and transcellular perturbation (**right**) to induce drug permeability across the intestinal mucosa. Abbreviations: PLC: phospholipase C; PIP$_2$: phosphatidylinositol 4,5-bisphosphate; DAG: di-acyl glycerol; PKC: protein kinase C; IP$_3$R: inositol triphosphate receptor; MLC: myosin light chain, CAM: calmodulin; ZO: zonula occludens; JAM: junctional adhesion molecule. Image created using a template from Servier Medical Art under a Creative Commons Attribution License.

6.3. SNAC Mode of Action

A different mode of action to that of C_{10} was proposed to explain how SNAC improves intestinal permeability. In the 1990s, Emisphere scientists proposed that SNAC improves passive transcellular permeation via hydrophobization. The hypothesis was that dipole–dipole non-covalent interaction between the carrier and structural moieties of the payload caused a conformational change in the latter, leading to exposure of hydrophobic regions that favor transcellular permeation. The interaction between SNAC and heparin [22,44] and with insulin [45] was, therefore, thought to be based on increased lipophilicity through hydrogen bonding and/or hydrophobic interactions, permitting dissolution of the complex in lipid bilayers. In support of this hypothesis, SNAC at a concentration of 17 mg/mL improved the permeation of insulin, but not that of radiolabeled mannitol across Caco-2 monolayers, suggesting that the effect was neither related to opening tight junctions nor to a decline in barrier integrity, and this interpretation was supported by confocal microscopy [45]. Higher concentrations of SNAC (50 mg/mL) that were more reflective of concentrations used in in vivo studies, however, caused complete loss of TEER and a 36-fold increase in [^{3}H]-mannitol permeability in Caco-2 monolayers [44], data that do not permit definitive conclusions to be made regarding mechanism since such high concentrations compromised the Caco-2 model. In isolated rat jejunal mucosae mounted in Ussing chambers, SNAC (33–66 mM) boosted the flux of a polar marker molecule, 6-carboxy-fluorescein (6-CF), but not that of [^{3}H]-mannitol across the epithelium and without reducing TEER values [46]. The authors argued that SNAC was indeed exploiting a transcellular pathway and not tight junctions to allow permeation of the hydrophilic polar ionized molecule (6-CF) and, somewhat controversially, they suggested that SNAC was reducing the charge on CF, thereby improving the capacity to partition in the epithelium. Similar to the Caco-2 study [44], when SNAC was added to jejunal mucosae at a concentration of 165 mM, TEER dropped and the permeability coefficient (Papp) of [^{3}H]-mannitol was increased [46], denoting a compromising event. Other Caco-2 studies also support a transcellular mechanism; Malkov et al. [47] detected intracellular signal increases ascribed to fluorescently labeled heparin and in the presence of SNAC, whereas immunohistochemistry data indicated that there were no changes of F-actin or the actinomycin ring during heparin flux. Ding et al. [48] used ITC and Fourier-transform infrared (FTIR) spectroscopy to study the interaction between cromolyn and SNAC, and concluded that the aromatic ring of SNAC inserted between those of cromolyn via its 2-hydroxybenzamide motif, leading to an increase in hydrophobicity of the complex and a reduction in cromolyn hydration. Lactate hydrogenase release (LDH) measurements indicated that the increased cromolyn fluxes across Caco-2 monolayers in the presence of SNAC were not associated with cell damage.

Despite the elegance of the purported complex mechanism (Figure 3) of how SNAC might increase transcellular flux of multiple payloads, the hypothesis is problematic in several respects. If Eligen® carriers acted solely using dipole–dipole interactions via hydrophobization (and not an electrostatic interaction), it would be difficult to envisage a significant increase in passive permeation since the retention of ionized functional groups would impede passive movement across phospholipid bilayers.

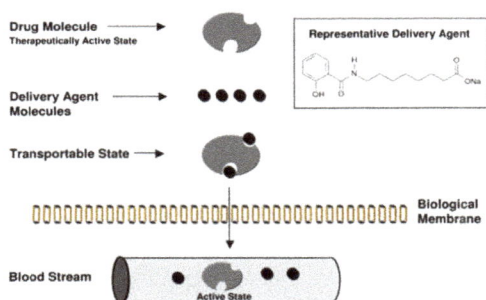

Figure 3. Schematic of Eligen® drug-delivery technology mechanism in intestinal epithelia, as advocated by Emisphere scientists in 2006. "Carrier molecule (delivery agent) associates with drug molecule to create a transportable complex (lipophilic). Because of the weak association, carrier and drug dissociate by simple dilution on entering the blood circulation." Reproduced from Reference [49] under the terms of the Creative Commons Attribution License.

SNAC forms a conjugate base at the pH of the small intestinal lumen, so it can undergo complexation via hydrophobic ion pairing (HIP) with the conjugate acid of basic amino-acid side chains in macromolecules. However, HIP cannot fully account for Eligen®-mediated hydrophobization of anionic payloads including heparin and cromolyn [24]. An alternative interpretation arises from another SNAC study with cromolyn; SNAC increased Caco-2 epithelial cell membrane fluidity as measured by fluorescence anisotropy, consistent with a surfactant-induced membrane perturbation effect, whereas in this study there was no increase in cromolyn's lipophilicity [50]. Still, the overall contribution of transcellular perturbation to the increased flux is not clear since the presence of hydrophilic functional groups in the salicylamide region of SNAC gives rise to inefficient micelle formation (CMC: 56 mM in phosphate-buffered saline (PBS)) [50], and this will not favor membrane insertion. There are a number of other anomalies concerning the original chaperone transcellular mechanism proposed for SNAC (reviewed in Reference [49]). Firstly, since the structure of SNAC comprises MCFA and salicylic-acid moieties, non-specific detergent/surfactant effects on the epithelium should be expected. Secondly, the thermodynamic considerations with respect to the non-covalent linkage between SNAC and payload during epithelial flux are yet to be addressed. Furthermore, there were no calculations on the affinity of SNAC to payloads, except to assert that affinity was weak, now confirmed for exenatide [29]. Thirdly, a transcellular mechanism should account for epithelial endocytosis uptake pathways (e.g., via clathrin- or caveolae-mediated pathways or macropinocytosis), where a template to follow is in place for the other group of transcellular permeability-enhancing agents, the cell-penetrating peptides [51]. Finally, caution must be exercised in making definitive conclusions on mechanism using some of these assays; epithelial TEER values yield information on monolayer integrity, but reveal no direct information about tight junctions. Secondly, the absence of changes in tight-junction-associated antibody imaging for associated proteins is not definitive. Thirdly, fluorescently labeled payloads need to be assessed for their capacity to remain intact during flux. Finally, LDH release from monolayers following exposure to SNAC would not be regarded as a particularly sensitive assay, especially when increased membrane fluidization was observed. In sum, evidence from Caco-2 studies is not yet convincing enough to solely ascribe an exclusive transcellular mechanism for SNAC; moreover, there is little data to directly support the chaperone hypothesis. On the other hand, there are some differences between the mechanism of action of SNAC and those of PEs with mechanisms associated with tight-junction openings (e.g., EDTA).

Recently, Novo Nordisk offered a new mechanism of action for SNAC in its non-enteric coated tablet of the GLP-1 analog, semaglutide ($t_\frac{1}{2}$ = 160 h). Using a ligated dog model, they found that systemic delivery was achieved solely from stomach administration of the tablet [52]. The theory is that SNAC forms a complex around the semaglutide in the stomach and causes a transient increase in local pH around the molecule. It is claimed that semaglutide is protected against pepsin by SNAC and that solubility is increased, resulting in an increased concentration-dependent flux of semaglutide across the gastric mucosa, using a transcellular mechanism as the tablet comes in intimate contact with the epithelium. By shifting the emphasis toward elevation in stomach pH away from conformational changes and increased lipophilicity, the theory takes the focus away from membrane perturbation. Moreover, the authors argue that this mechanism is highly specific for semaglutide, in that similar studies with admixtures of SNAC and liraglutide led to no flux increase across in vitro gastric epithelial models [52]. Part of the role of SNAC seemed to be to convert semaglutide to a more permeable monomeric form and it seems to perform this better when formulated in a stomach-specific tablet. Is this payload-specific and region-specific theory entirely compatible with the previous data from small intestinal studies in which SNAC was paired with many payloads of differing structures? With new cell-imaging tools available, along with advanced biophysical methods to decipher the interaction between SNAC and payloads, it is likely that much of the discrepancy surrounding the mechanism of SNAC will be resolved. Figure 4 is a composite of the possible effects that SNAC has in the stomach when formulated with semaglutide.

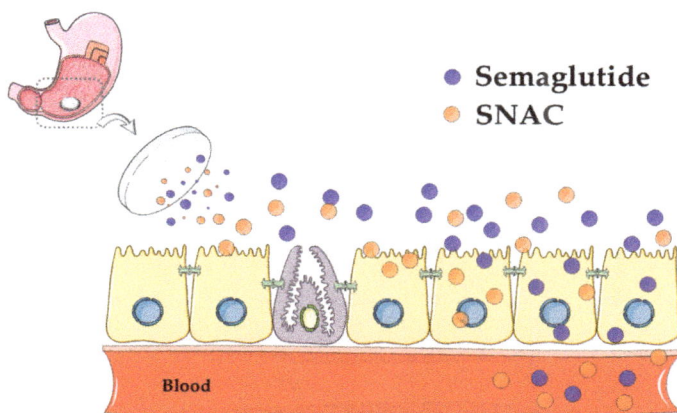

Figure 4. Theory of oral semaglutide absorption, as advocated by Novo Nordisk. Modified from Reference [52]. The diagram represents the proposed mechanism of action of SNAC in inducing transcellular flux of semaglutide across the gastric epithelium of the stomach. The optimum once-daily tablet consists of 14 mg of semaglutide co-formulated with 300 mg of SNAC. After digestion, the tablet erodes rapidly in the stomach, resulting in the release of a highly concentrated amount of SNAC that neutralizes the pH of gastric fluid in the immediate vicinity of the tablet to inactivate pepsin. SNAC is thought to induce semaglutide monomer production and increase gastric epithelial membrane fluidity, but without affecting tight junctions, thereby allowing transcellular passage of semaglutide into systemic circulation. The complex may dissociate at some point in the flux process (Figure 3) due to weak association, but direct evidence for this is scant. Black circles = semaglutide; white circles = SNAC. Image made using a template from Servier Medical Art under a Creative Commons Attribution License.

In sum, the in vitro studies on the mechanism of action of the two agents on cultured intestinal epithelia suggest some common surfactant-based features; however, in contrast to SNAC, there is direct evidence for tight-junction openings induced by C_{10}. The culture models are sub-optimal, however, as they do not discriminate permeation enhancement from perturbation very well, nor do they predict in vivo consequences; the models have difficulty in tolerating both high concentrations of PEs and simulated intestinal fluids.

7. C_{10} and SNAC: Pharmacokinetics and Efficacy in Clinical Trials

7.1. C_{10}

GIPET™ was advanced to clinical testing as enteric-coated tablets containing C_{10} with both peptide and small-molecule payloads [18,42]. Human studies using radiolabeled polyethylene glyol (PEG) revealed that the permeating enhancement effects of GIPET™ were transient and reversible in <1 h [18]. GIPET™ was tested in a range of doses with several poorly absorbed molecules in a total of 16 Phase I studies comprising over 300 subjects [18]. Overall, while oral BA values of >5% were cited for some molecules, the most notable feature was the massive intra-subject variability across all studies, constituting an issue for safety and efficacy.

Pharmacokinetics (PK) analysis of human trials for GIPET™ formulations with low-molecular-weight heparin (LMWH) and desmopressin was described [18]. LMWH–GIPET™ was formulated in tablets containing either 45,000 or 90,000 IU of LMWH at two dose levels of C_{10}. Oral BA was calculated relative to the standard sub-cutaneous (s.c.) dose of 3200 IU following administration to 14–16 subjects. Relative oral BA of 3.9–7.6% was achieved [18]. With a high dose of LMWH combined with a high dose of C_{10}, increased levels of an anti-clotting biomarker were seen in all subjects; the responses were sustained and had a similar time course to the s.c. route. This particular formulation was not progressed clinically (Table 1). When desmopressin was formulated with GIPET™ and administered orally to 18 human subjects, a bioavailability of 2.4% relative to the s.c. route was detected [18], an improvement over the typical 0.2% value for Minirin® tablets. Again, this formulation was not progressed further. The GIPET™ technology was well tolerated even when repeatedly administered in these small Phase I studies [18]. Other clinical trial examples include the gonadotropin-releasing hormone (GnRH) antagonist decapeptide, acyline. In a Phase I study of oral acyline, serum luteinizing hormone (LH), follicle-stimulating hormone (FSH), and testosterone were suppressed within 12 h at the 10-, 20-, and 40-mg single doses tested. However, sustained serum levels of acyline could not be detected, and there was no pharmacokinetic–pharmacodynamic (PK–PD) relationship [53]. The GIPET™ technology was also used to orally deliver the bisphosphonate, zoledronic acid. The rationale was that an oral tablet (Orazol™) administered weekly by patients could compete with a monthly infusion of Zometa® in a hospital setting for cancer patients with bone metastasis. In a Phase I study, urinary excretion of unchanged zoledronic acid suggested equivalent delivery via both routes [54]. The licensing of GIPET™ to Novo Nordisk led to Phase I trials with respect to a proprietary insulin, NN1953, and a GLP-1 analog; however, the resulting data were never published and, ultimately, Merrion's remaining intellectual property (IP) assets were sold to Novo Nordisk, before being liquidated in 2016. Novo Nordisk in turn decided to move away from developing oral insulin to concentrate on its oral GLP-1 analog program. Nonetheless, an important Phase II trial from that time assessing a once-daily long-acting basal insulin (I338) with a $t_\frac{1}{2}$ of 70 h in a GIPET™ formulation was published in 2019 by Novo Nordisk [55]. In this study, a relative oral F versus the long-acting s.c.-administered insulin glargine (Lantus®, Sanofi, Paris) of 1.5–2.0% was achieved without evidence of toxicity over eight weeks. Although similar plasma glucose reduction was achieved by the oral GIPET™-based formulation to the s.c. insulin, the rationale for discontinuation was that the dose of I338 was not commercially viable. The GIPET™ journey with oral peptides and poorly permeable small molecules, therefore, ended without generating a product in 2015. As a post-script, a Phase I study was published in 2018 by Biocon (India) in which a C_{10}-based formulation of their alkylated PEGylated fast-acting meal-time insulin (IN-105; Insulin Tregopil) was shown to have no effect on the PK of oral metformin in fasted conditions and it was well tolerated [56]. Therefore, C_{10} continues to be used in oral peptide formulations both in clinical trials and as a comparator for other PEs in preclinical studies.

The other arm of the original Elan licensing of C_{10}-based matrix tablets in the late 1990s continued in parallel with respect to antisense oligonucleotides. The gene medicine specialty Pharma, Ionis Pharmaceuticals (Carlsbad, CA, USA) (formerly Isis Pharma) developed a number of oral antisense oligonucleotide formulations containing C_{10} for clinical testing against RNA targets. One candidate that progressed to Phase I was ISIS 104838, a tumor necrosis factor (TNF)-α inhibitor. Oral administration of a C_{10}-based tablet to dogs resulted in average absolute oral BA of 1.4% [57]. Tissue histology of the small intestine and large intestine of the dogs indicated no changes following once-daily dosing of tablets containing ~1 g of C_{10} over seven consecutive days. A subsequent Phase I trial examined ISIS 104838 (100 or 140 mg) formulated with C_{10} (660 mg) in immediate-release mini-tablets packaged in enteric-coated gelatin capsules, with or without a second mini-tablet containing only C_{10}. The second group of mini-tablets was coated with different layers of Eudragit® RS30D to allow for subsequent further release of the C_{10} following erosion of the first tablet containing ISIS 104838 [58]. The goal was to create a greater window for absorption by prolonging the time C_{10} was in contact with the epithelium, given that it is rapidly absorbed with a T_{max} of 7 min. All formulations together yielded an average oral BA of 9.5% relative to s.c. injection, with the formulation designed for additional immediate release of C_{10} giving a value of 12%; however, the intra-subject variability ranged from 2–28% [58]. In 2017, Ionis advanced an oral antisense molecule IONIS-JBI1-2.5Rx, aimed at an RNA target associated with a GI autoimmune disorder, to Phase I trials in collaboration with Janssen (Beerse, Belgium) [59]; however, it is unlikely that the formulation contains C_{10} as it is designed for local colonic delivery. Table 1 summarizes the clinical data reported for a range of poorly permeable molecules with C_{10}. Of these, there are only four peer-reviewed original research papers for GIPET™ tablets.

Table 1. Summary of data from selected studies in humans reported for a range of poorly permeable molecules formulated with sodium caprate (C_{10}).

Description	Treatment	Outcome	Reference
Ampicillin with C_{10} in healthy subjects ($n = 12$).	Rectal suppository containing 250 mg of ampicillin and 25 mg of C_{10}.	C_{max} increased 2.6-fold compared to ampicillin alone and BA increased 1.8-fold. Some local tissue damage not ascribed to C_{10}.	[17]
Phenoxymethylpenicillin, antipyrine with C_{10} in healthy subjects ($n = 6$).	Rectal perfusion containing 2 g of phenoxymethylpenicillin, 8 mg of antipyrine, and 0.7 g of C_{10}. Two treatments (T), T1: pH 6 and T2: pH 7.4. Each subject received control (no C_{10}) and treatment.	C_{10} was ineffective at increasing permeability across rectal epithelium.	[60]
GIPET™: oral acyline in healthy subjects ($n = 8$).	3 oral tablet doses of acyline: 10, 20, and 40 mg. Subjects received all doses, 1 week apart, under fasting conditions.	Significant reduction in LH, FSH, and testosterone. No serious treatment related adverse effects.	[53]
GIPET™: oral zoledronic acid in prostate cancer patients with bone metastasis ($n = 30$).	Once-weekly enteric-coated Orazol™ tablets containing 20 mg of zoledronic acid versus weekly Zometa® (4 mg) i.v. infusion over 49 days.	Equivalent urine output biomarkers; claim of 5% bioavailability (BA) in patent.	[54]
Antisense oligonucleotide with C_{10} (ISIS 104838) in healthy subjects ($n = 15$).	Enteric-coated tablets, four formulations, and one after a high-fat meal. Subjects received all treatments.	9.5% bioavailability compared to s.c. No study-related adverse effects.	[58]
Basal insulin in C_{10} formulation versus insulin glargine in Type 2 diabetics (s.c.) ($n = 25$).	Daily tablets of a long-acting insulin (I338) over 8 weeks.	1.5–2.0% bioavailability compared to s.c. Comparable reductions in plasma glucose.	[55]
Insulin tregopil (IN-105) in C_{10} tablets in healthy subjects.	Single treatments of insulin along with metformin over 4 periods of 2 days.	No effects on the pharmacokinetics (PK) of metformin; good safety.	[56]

LH, luteinizing hormone; FSH, follicle-stimulating hormone; s.c., sub-cutaneous; i.v., intravenous. The Phase II study [55] is the most comprehensive of these studies.

7.2. SNAC

SNAC was in a succession of clinical trials in oral formulations with poorly permeable actives since the late 1990s, culminating with approval for cyanocobalamin as a medical food for vitamin B_{12}-deficient anemic subjects in 2014 [20,21]. The initial clinical trials were carried out using unfractionated heparin in 1998 [61]. In the first Phase I study, 2.25 g of taste-masked SNAC was combined with 30,000–150,000 IU of heparin and administered to subjects via gavage; the formulation achieved increases in outputs associated with anti-coagulation efficacy: activated partial thromboplastin time (aPTT) and production of anti-factor Xa. This led to subsequent Phase I and II trials with taste-masked 10–15-mL liquid formulations in patients undergoing total hip replacements; oral heparin was dosed at either 60,000 or 90,000 IU with 1.5 or 2.25 g of SNAC respectively, and results were compared to s.c. administration of 5000 IU of heparin [62]. The oral dosing regimen comprised 12–16 doses over a four-day period after surgery. Data from the second Phase I study showed that the oral heparin liquid formulation induced anti-factor Xa activity similar to s.c. heparin. In the Phase II trial, major bleeding events were similar between oral and s.c. heparin groups, thereby offering encouragement on the safety front. In 2002, the oral liquid heparin formulation ultimately missed its primary efficacy end-point in a Phase III trial (PROTECT) comparing oral heparin (either 60,000 IU/1.5 g SNAC or 90,000 IU/2.25 g SNAC three times a day) to s.c. LMWH (enoxaparin) over a 30-day period with assessment for deep vein thrombosis as the read-out. The study comprised over 2000 patients undergoing elective hip replacement, a study that was associated with poor compliance due to the bitter taste of the solution [49]. Direct leveraging from a taste-masked drink to a solid dosage form was not possible, due to the high quantities of SNAC and heparin. Subsequently, a new Phase I PK–PD study was eventually carried out in 2007 in 16 subjects receiving a 75,000 IU heparin/500 mg

SNAC total dose in soft gel capsules [63]. It confirmed the effect on aPTT and the orally delivered heparin had a C_{max} of 58 min. Ultimately, a solid dose formulation of oral heparin/SNAC never reached Phase III and was abandoned, perhaps in part because of the advantages of LMWH over unfractionated heparin, as well as the advent of alternative oral anti-thrombotics.

In relation to other payloads and Eligen® carriers, a caprylic-acid derivative, possibly SNAC, was also formulated with sCT, and a Phase I study in eight volunteers was published in 2002, with a comprehensive analysis of PK [64]. This benchmark study described tablets of 0.4 mg of sCT with 225 mg of SNAC that were dosed singly, in duplicate, or in triplicate to present individual doses of 0.4, 0.8, and 1.2 mg of sCT. The resulting absolute oral BA values versus an intravenous (i.v.) dose of 10 μg ranged from 0.5–1.4%. An Eligen® formulation of insulin was also assessed in a 2010 trial in 14 Type 2 diabetics (T2D) where the carrier was monosodium *N*-(4-chlorosalicyloyl)-4-aminobutyrate (4-CNAB). An oral BA of $7 \pm 4\%$ was achieved from a 300-IU dose (with 200–400 mg of 4-CNAB) versus an s.c. dose of 15 IU in fasting subjects [65]. Such large variability would not be acceptable for this low-therapeutic-index drug. A third related Eligen® carrier, 8-(*N*-2-hydroxy-5-chloro-benzoyl)-amino-caprylic acid (5-CNAC), was also evaluated by Novartis (Switzerland) and Nordic Biosciences (Herlev, Denmark) in three large Phase III trials for oral sCT: two for osteoarthritis [66] (NCT00486434 and NCT00704847) and one for osteoporosis [67] (NCT00525798). The dosing to several thousand patients across the three trials comprised one tablet (0.8 mg sCT with 200 mg of 5-CNAC) in a tablet administered twice a day with 50 mL of water approximately 30 min ahead of meals. These studies lasted 24 months for the osteoarthritis trials and 36 months for the osteoporosis trial. Although these trials missed their primary efficacy end-points, interesting assessments concerning dosing formats and regimes were published with conclusions that may have relevance for SNAC trials [68]. Differences in sCT absorption and effects on bone biomarkers occurred depending on the volume of water, proximity to a meal, and the time of day (reflecting circadian rhythms in bone turnover). Table 2 summarizes the clinical trial performance of oral SNAC and related Emisphere carrier formulations across a range of poorly permeable molecules.

Table 2. Summary of data from selected studies in humans reported for a range of poorly permeable molecules formulated with either salcaprozate sodium (SNAC), monosodium *N*-(4-chlorosalicyloyl)-4-aminobutyrate (4-CNAB), or 8-(*N*-2-hydroxy-5-chloro-benzoyl)-amino-caprylic acid (5-CNAC). T2D—type 2 diabetes; sCT—salmon calcitonin.

Description	Treatment	Outcome	Reference
Vitamin B_{12} with SNAC in tablets in healthy subjects (n = 20). Medical food clinical study.	(A) Two tablets, each with 5 mg of vitamin B_{12} with 100 mg of SNAC (B) One tablet: 5 mg of vitamin B_{12} with 100 mg of SNAC (C) One commercial tablet: 5 mg of vitamin B_{12} (D) 1 mg of vitamin B_{12} via i.v. injection.	Treatment (B) achieved 3% higher absolute BA compared to the commercial oral formulation. No adverse effects.	[20]
Heparin with SNAC in hip replacement patients, (n = 123). Phase II.	Two studies: one dose every 8 h (max 16 doses), and two doses every 8 h (max 12 doses).	Achieved anti-factor Xa activity comparable to s.c. heparin. No change in major bleeding events compared to s.c.	[62]
Insulin with 4-CNAB in untreated T2D (n = 10). Phase II.	300 mg of insulin with 400 mg of 4-CNAB, or 15 IU of insulin s.c. Performed under fasting conditions.	C_{max} was higher and was reached faster compared to s.c. Shorter duration and high subject variability. No adverse effects.	[65]
sCT with 5-CNAC in osteoarthritic patients over 24 months (n = 1176 and n = 1030) Phase III.	0.8 mg of sCT in tablets twice daily for 24 months.	No significant effect compared to placebo.	[66]
sCT with 5-CNAC in postmenopausal women with osteoporosis (n = 4665). Phase III.	0.8 mg or placebo in tablets daily, together with vitamin D and calcium for 36 months.	No beneficial effect on fractures was observed. No change in quality of life.	[6]

Recent focus, however, shifted entirely to the clinical development of the oral semaglutide/SNAC tablet by Novo Nordisk. Once-daily oral semaglutide with 300 mg of SNAC resulted in improved glycemic control and greater reductions in body weight than placebo in a 26-week Phase II dose-escalation study in doses ranging from 2.5–40 mg of semaglutide per day in over 600 patients with T2D [69]. Daily oral administration of semaglutide (20 mg and 40 mg) with SNAC lowered glycated hemoglobin (HbA1c) by over 1.4% and these data were comparable with that seen with weekly s.c. administration of semaglutide (1 mg). For oral semaglutide with SNAC, the oral BA is likely to be ~1%, although the focus of the publications was on the PD effect and biomarkers. Clues come from Beagle dog studies where tablets containing 300 mg of SNAC with 5–20 mg of semaglutide gave oral BA values of 1.22 ± 0.25% following oral administration [52,70]. Novo Nordisk completed ten Phase IIIa PIONEER trials in 2018. Top-line data from PIONEER 1 achieved significance with respect to a reduction in HbA1c of 1.5% with a 14-mg semaglutide dose in T2D, along with evidence of some weight loss [71]. Recent trials also revealed that renal impairment did not affect PK parameters of 5 mg and 10 mg of semaglutide formulated with 300 mg of SNAC over a short time frame in diabetics [72]. This design was repeated in diabetic patients with hepatic impairment with the same outcome in that PK values were not altered and, therefore, no dose adjustment was needed in these patients [73]. The question of the impact of omeprazole on PK was also assessed, as elevation of bulk stomach pH might have confounded the purported mechanism of SNAC. Using a 5-mg semaglutide dose in patients taking 40 mg of omeprazole over a 10-day period with a follow-up period out to 21 days, overall PK values for both semaglutide and SNAC were unchanged, leading to a conclusion that dose adjustment would be also unnecessary in patients on concomitant omeprazole [74]. The implications of these findings would support the determination that the pH increase created by SNAC in the stomach must be at the semaglutide tablet surface [52] and does not impact bulk stomach pH; otherwise, a large effect of omeprazole on PK would have been expected. The PIONEER 6 Phase III study enrolled diabetics with cardiovascular disease in order to exam oral semaglutide PK and PD in this cohort to see if the daily 14-mg formulation increases cardiovascular risk [75]. Selected oral semaglutide clinical data are summarized in Table 3. It will be interesting to examine patient compliance with the current rather inconvenient dosing regime, especially in post-marketing studies if oral semaglutide is approved, since the daily tablet must be taken at least 30 min before meals in the morning in order to avoid food interference with formulation performance.

Table 3. Selected clinical trial data with an emphasis on peer-reviewed literature from the daily semaglutide/SNAC oral tablet formulation from Novo Nordisk in T2D patients.

Description	Parameters	Comment	Reference
Phase II dose-ranging 26-week study in patients ($n = 632$) (NCT01923181).	0.7–1.9% reduction in glycated hemoglobin (HbA1c); some weight reduction; mild gastro-intestinal (GI) side effects common.	The key trial which supported moving to Phase III.	[69]
PIONEER-1 Phase IIIa 26-week study in patients ($n = 703$) (NCT02906930).	Mean 1.5% reduction in HbA1c confirmed with 14-mg dose; 4.1-kg weight reduction; mild–moderate nausea in 16% versus 6% in placebo.	14 mg established as semaglutide dose with 300 mg of SNAC in all studies.	[71]
PIONEER 5 Phase IIIa in renal-impaired patients ($n = 71$) (NCT02014259).	5 mg of semaglutide for 5 days; 10 mg for 5 days, assessed up to 21 days after; no change in PK overall.	Area under curve (AUC) and half-life ($t_{\frac{1}{2}}$) similar to regular T2D patients, no need to change dose regime.	[72]
Trial in hepatic-impaired patients ($n = 56$) (NCT02016911).	Design as for PIONEER-5.	AUC, C_{max}, and $t_{\frac{1}{2}}$ unchanged, no need to change in dose regime.	[73]

Table 3. *Cont.*

Description	Parameters	Comment	Reference
Trial in healthy subjects [1] taking omeprazole (*n* = 54) (NCT02249871).	5 mg for 5 days, followed by 10 mg for 5 days) ± 40 mg omeprazole.	AUC and stomach pH slightly higher in semaglutide/omeprazole group, but no need to change dose regime.	[74]
PIONEER-6 Phase IIIa assessed cardiovascular (CV) risk in T2D patients (*n* = 3183) (NCT02692716).	Primary end-points: reduction in major CV events over median 16-month period.	Cardiovascular (CV) outcomes not different from placebo, but suggestion of a mortality benefit of oral tablet.	[75]

[1] All studies in T2D patients except for the omeprazole study. [2] PIONEER Phase III 10 study designs are available at https://pharmaintelligence.informa.com/resources/product-content/novos-oral-semaglutide-passes-pioneer-2-but-weight-loss-result-a-bit-disappointing (accessed 12 February 2019). Details of all oral semaglutide trials are available at www.clinicaltrials.gov.

8. Safety of SNAC and C_{10} in Preclinical and Clinical Studies

Although C_{10} was previously marketed in a rectal product, this has limited relevance to the safety of an orally delivered tablet formulation. The approval of SNAC in an oral vitamin-B_{12} medical food product, though encouraging, is also only partially informative. Nonetheless, the clinical trial experience with both PEs in hundreds of subjects over more than 20 years suggest that only very low numbers of subjects experienced side-effects that caused drop out from trials, and the majority of reports were related to mild GI effects including nausea and diarrhea for GIPET™ [18,42] and SNAC [69]. Reversibility studies performed with C_{10} in humans using the lactulose:mannitol urinary excretion ratio (LMER) assay showed that, following intra-jejunal administration to human subjects, the enhancer only increased permeability in a 20-min window [42]. It seems that dilution, spreading, and rapid intestinal absorption of both C_{10} and SNAC prevents prolonged exposure in vivo. There is no direct evidence, even from studies with a duration as long as six months, that stomach or duodenal ulcers are caused by these PEs, nor that pathogens can gain entry across a compromised intestinal epithelium. Still, post-marketing surveillance will provide more safety data in the context of daily administration over several years, at least in the case of SNAC with both vitamin B_{12} and semaglutide in the event of Food and Drug Administration (FDA) approval. Additional safety experience for SNAC will be ascertained from extensive Phase III oral semaglutide trials, which will fully report in 2019.

In terms of preclinical safety data, the experience for both molecules is extensive. Numerous studies reveal little toxicity of high doses of C_{10} in rats, dogs, and pigs following oral administration alone and in combination with payloads [18,42,76]. In a study of the acute effects of a C_{10}-based dosage form (Orasense™) in Beagles, Raoof et al. provided evidence of the safety of oral hydroxypropyl methyl cellulose-coated C_{10}/antisense tablets [57]. Several hundred milligrams of C_{10} were used in each tablet and dogs received treatment three times per day for seven days. Clinical chemistry and blood biochemistry parameters were normal; the dogs tolerated the formulation and there was normal weight gain. Canine intestinal issues were also adjudged normal following macroscopic examination post mortem. Five separate canine daily tolerance studies revealed encouraging safety data for selected components of the GIPET I and II technology [42]. Similar studies were also carried out intra-intestinal catheterized pigs where C_{10} was formulated with antisense oligonucleotides at doses up to 100 mg/kg of the MCFA; it was well tolerated following multiple doses and with little evidence of intestinal epithelial damage post mortem [77].

For SNAC, Riley et al. carried out a sub-chronic oral toxicity test of SNAC in rats and found a no observed adverse effect (NOAEL) level of 1 g/kg/day in rats for up to 13 weeks; it was only a massive dose of 2 g/kg/day that eventually caused significant mortality [78]. It was also examined for gestational toxicity in pregnant rats at oral doses up to 1 g/kg/day where slight weight loss was seen; there was no effect on growth of pups, but some evidence of a small increase in the still-birth rate was noted [79]. Some GI effects including emesis and diarrhea were observed in studies involving monkeys at a dose of ≥ 1.8 g/kg/day [80]. SNAC ultimately achieved provisional GRAS status as a food additive. The safety data from clinical and preclinical studies, therefore, raised no red flags for either agent in oral dosage forms at high concentrations with a wide range of actives tested to date. An important safety consideration is the high inter-subject variability typically associated with the low oral bioavailability values for all payloads tested with both PEs to date; formulation with these PEs will, therefore, not be suitable for molecules with low therapeutic indices.

It is clear that surfactant-based PEs cause a mild degree of reversible perturbation of the intestinal mucosa. The small intestinal epithelium is entirely renewed every 72 h [81]; there is a high rate of cellular turnover and the intestine has a high capacity to replace cells, due to migrating stem cells from the intestinal crypt. There is also a reserve of stem cells that are dormant until epithelial injury occurs, at which point they are recruited to assist with restoration [82]. The capacity of the intestinal mucosa to repair is also associated with secretion of mucus, prostaglandins, and bicarbonate [80]. For a comprehensive review of repair and restoration of the intestinal barrier, see Blikslager et al. [38]. The capacity for epithelial repair following C_{10} exposure was investigated in rat jejunal instillations, where full restitution was seen within 60 min of exposure [83]. These data were similar to that seen in rat models with other PEs including bile salts [84] and sodium dodecyl sulfate (SDS) [85]. Since C_{10} and SNAC are rapidly and completely absorbed, one interpretation is that, following local and transient mucosal perturbation leading to a transient increase in permeability, the epithelium recovers due to gradual dilution of the PE.

Another concern over routine use of PEs is based on their potential capacity to promote microbiome changes and absorption of microorganisms, antigens, and toxins leading to local inflammation, autoimmune disease, and sepsis [86]. Surfactants may impair the protective mucus layer, facilitating the diffusion of luminal bacteria to the intestinal epithelium and ultimately disturbing the host microbiota [87]. In a recent study which generated much debate, evidence was provided that the approved excipient emulsifiers, polysorbate-80 and carboxymethyl cellulose, disturb microbiota composition and induce obesity in mice [88]. Whether these data have any true significance for humans is not known at this point, but it is clear that intestinal microbiome research is going to become more relevant in toxicology profiling of oral formulations. A second concern that is continually raised is the potential increase in permeability of bystander molecules arising from tissue damage induced by PEs [89,90]. Taking into account the precise conditions required for permeation enhancement (high concentrations of payload and PE contemporaneously at the intestinal epithelium), as well as the marked difference in the MW of candidate payloads (<10 kDa) compared to that of typical bacteria, viruses, and bacterial lipopolysaccharide (LPS) (>100 kDa), this concern may be overstated. Nonetheless, clinical pharmacology data from binge-drinking human subjects suggests that alcohol can permit absorption of endotoxins and can promote elevation of type 1 cytokines in plasma, akin to a low-grade infection [91]; thus, together with the study of relevant microbiome changes, more research is needed to filter the true toxicological risks of orally delivered PEs following chronic exposure.

Several studies describe an anti-microbial effect of C_{10} at high concentrations. Cox et al. [92] demonstrated the bactericidal property of C_{10} against *Salmonella typhimurium*, and it also prevented its attachment to intestinal epithelia. Moreover, there was no evidence from the same study that C_{10} promoted permeation of this gut pathogen across isolated rat intestinal mucosa. At low mM concentrations, C_{10} is also bactericidal against *Helicobacter pylori* [93]. In an in vivo study with chickens, incorporation of C_{10} in feed at a level of 3 g/kg protected them from colonization by *Salmonella enterica* [94]. Finally, capric acid has antifungal activities on *Microsporium gypsum* mycelia and spores in vitro [95]. These data are consistent with the well-known anti-microbial actions of MCFAs [96]. Although, to our knowledge, similar data are not reported for SNAC, it would be surprising if, upon examining its structure, it did not have similar anti-microbial actions.

9. Conclusions

In comparing the safety and efficacy of C_{10} and SNAC as PEs in preclinical and clinical studies, examination of 20–30 years of literature would suggest that several of the key parameters are similar. Both can permit oral bioavailability of a range of macromolecular payloads by <5%, with mean values closer to ~1%. The SNAC clinical PK data with semaglutide seem to be on a par with previous performance, for example, with sCT; however, it is due to its formulation with a potent peptide with a long $t_{\frac{1}{2}}$ and high TI that is of particular interest. It is the long $t_{\frac{1}{2}}$ that can compensate for large intra-subject variability [52]. Aspects that tip the balance to SNAC compared to C_{10} include the following: broader clinical experience and an approved vitamin B_{12} product, more extensive toxicology studies and GRAS status, and the lack of requirement for protection against stomach acid. There is still controversy over the mechanism of action of SNAC; techniques including surface plasmon resonance and ITC are now providing data that suggest that the non-covalent interaction of peptides with either SNAC or C_{10} is low affinity and quite similar for each agent. Moreover, while the literature seems to offer a consensus that C_{10} (at low concentrations) acts on tight junctions via intracellular events, and at high concentrations via transcellular perturbation arising from its surfactant effect, there is not the same consensus concerning the mechanism of action of SNAC. The 1990s theory of an exclusive transcellular action arising from increased lipophilicity of a non-covalent complex between SNAC and the payload was not convincing. The new mechanism suggested for SNAC arising from ligated dog studies argues for a local increase in stomach pH around semaglutide, a mechanism that appears to be specific for this molecule. Finally, the main argument advanced for oral peptide delivery is improved convenience over needles leading to better compliance. Patients will, however, be required to wait 30 min before eating and drinking after taking tablets of semaglutide/SNAC each morning; thus, patients will ultimately decide if this is an inconvenience preferable to a once-a-week injection.

Author Contributions: All authors contributed conceptually, to drafting, to figure and table designs, and to the final editing.

Funding: This project received funding from the Science Foundation Ireland Grant 13/RC/2073, the CÚRAM Center for Medical Devices (DB); the EU Horizon 2020 Research and Innovation Program under Marie Skłodowska-Curie Grant agreement No 666010 (SF); and the French National Agency of Research and Technology, CIFRE grant number: 2016/0439, with additional support from Sanofi Pharma (CT).

Conflicts of Interest: In the past two years, D.B. consulted for on oral peptide delivery at Sanofi, AstraZeneca/ MedImmune, and Boehringer-Ingelheim. Sanofi (D.B., E.F.), Gattefosse (D.B.), and Nuritas (D.B.) provided research grant funding. The funding sponsors played no role in the article.

References

1. Fosgerau, K.; Hoffmann, T. Peptide therapeutics: Current status and future directions. *Drug Discov. Today* **2015**, *20*, 122–128. [CrossRef] [PubMed]
2. Usmani, S.S.; Bedi, G.; Samuel, J.S.; Singh, S.; Kalra, S.; Kumar, P.; Ahuja, A.A.; Sharma, M.; Gautam, A.; Raghava, G.P.S. THPdb: Database of FDA-approved peptide and protein therapeutics. *PLoS ONE* **2017**, *12*, e0181748. [CrossRef] [PubMed]
3. Lakkireddy, H.R.; Urmann, M.; Besenius, M.; Werner, U.; Haack, T.; Brun, P.; Alié, J.; Illel, B.; Hortala, L.; Vogel, R.; et al. Oral delivery of diabetes peptides—Comparing standard formulations incorporating functional excipients and nanotechnologies in the translational context. *Adv. Drug Deliv. Rev.* **2016**, *106*, 196–222. [CrossRef] [PubMed]
4. Cowan Report. *Therapeutic Categories Outlook: Comprehensive Study*; Cowan & Co.: New York, NY, USA, 2014.
5. Lewis, A.L.; Richard, J. Challenges in the delivery of peptide drugs: An industry perspective. *Ther. Deliv.* **2015**, *6*, 149–163. [CrossRef]
6. Aguirre, T.A.; Teijeiro-Osorio, D.; Rosa, M.; Coulter, I.S.; Alonso, M.J.; Brayden, D.J. Current status of selected oral peptide technologies in advanced preclinical development and in clinical trials. *Adv. Drug Deliv. Rev.* **2016**, *106*, 223–241. [CrossRef] [PubMed]

7. Benet, L.Z. The drug transporter-metabolism alliance: Uncovering and defining the interplay. *Mol. Pharm.* **2009**, *6*, 631–643. [CrossRef] [PubMed]

8. Eligen® Technology: Summary and Value Proposition. Available online: https://www.emisphere.com/wp-content/uploads/2017/02/Eligen-Technology-Presentation_2.15-Update.pdf (accessed on 12 February 2019).

9. Baluom, M.; Friedman, M.; Assaf, P.; Haj-Yehia, A.I.; Rubinstein, A. Synchronized release of sulpiride and sodium decanoate from HPMC matrices: A rational approach to enhance sulpiride absorption in the rat intestine. *Pharm. Res.* **2000**, *17*, 1071–1076. [CrossRef] [PubMed]

10. Maher, S.; Mrsny, R.J.; Brayden, D.J. Intestinal permeation enhancers for oral peptide delivery. *Adv. Drug Deliv. Rev.* **2016**, *106*, 277–319. [CrossRef] [PubMed]

11. Card, J.W.; Magnuson, B.A. A review of the efficacy and safety of nanoparticle-based oral insulin delivery systems. *Am. J. Physiol. Gastrointest. Liver Physiol.* **2011**, *301*, G956–G967. [CrossRef]

12. Banerjee, A.; Mitragotri, S. Intestinal patch systems for oral drug delivery. *Curr. Opin. Pharmacol.* **2017**, *36*, 58–65. [CrossRef] [PubMed]

13. Whitehead, K.; Karr, N.; Mitragotri, S. Safe and effective permeation enhancers for oral drug delivery. *Pharm. Res.* **2008**, *25*, 1782–1788. [CrossRef] [PubMed]

14. Maher, S.; Ryan, B.; Duffy, A.; Brayden, D.J. Formulation strategies to improve oral peptide delivery. *Pharm. Pat. Anal.* **2014**, *3*, 313–336. [CrossRef] [PubMed]

15. Aungst, B.J. Absorption enhancers: Applications and advances. *AAPS J.* **2012**, *14*, 10–18. [CrossRef] [PubMed]

16. EFSA Panel on Food Additives and Nutrient Sources added to Food (ANS); Younes, M.; Aggett, P.; Aguilar, F.; Crebelli, R.; Dusemund, B.; Filipič, M.; Frutos, M.J.; Galtier, P.; Gott, D.; et al. Re-evaluation of sodium, potassium and calcium salts of fatty acids (E 470a) and magnesium salts of fatty acids (E 470b) as food additives. *EFSA J.* **2018**. [CrossRef]

17. Lindmark, T.; Söderholm, J.D.; Olaison, G.; Alván, G.; Ocklind, G.; Artursson, P. Mechanism of absorption enhancement in humans after rectal administration of ampicillin in suppositories containing sodium caprate. *Pharm. Res.* **1997**, *14*, 930–955. [CrossRef] [PubMed]

18. Walsh, E.; Adamczyk, B.; Chalasani, K.B.; Maher, M.; O'Toole, E.B.; Fox, J.; Leonard, T.W.; Brayden, D.J. Oral delivery of macromolecules: Rationale underpinning Gastrointestinal Permeation Enhancement Technology (GIPET®). *Ther. Deliv.* **2011**, *2*, 1595–1610. [CrossRef]

19. Leone-Bay, A.; Santiago, N.; Achan, D.; Chaudhary, K.; DeMorin, F.; Falzarano, L.; Haas, S.; Kalbag, S.; Kaplan, D.; Leipold, H.; et al. N-acylated alpha amino acids as novel oral delivery agents for proteins. *J. Med. Chem.* **1995**, *38*, 4263–4269. [CrossRef]

20. Castelli, M.C.; Wong, D.F.; Friedman, K.; Riley, M.G. Pharmacokinetics of oral cyanocobalamin formulated with sodium N-[8-(2-hydroxybenzoyl)amino]caprylate (SNAC): An open-label, randomized, single-dose, parallel-group study in healthy male subjects. *Clin. Ther.* **2011**, *33*, 934–945. [CrossRef]

21. Smith, L.; Mosley, J.; Ford, M.; Courtney, J. Cyanocobalamin/Salcaprozate Sodium: A novel way to treat vitamin B_{12} deficiency and anemia. *J. Hematol. Oncol. Pharm.* **2016**, *6*, 42–45.

22. Leone-Bay, A.; Paton, D.R.; Variano, B.; Leipold, H.; Rivera, T.; Miura-Fraboni, J.; Baughman, R.A.; Santiago, N. Acylated non-alpha-amino acids as novel agents for the oral delivery of heparin sodium, USP. *J. Control. Release* **1998**, *50*, 41–49. [CrossRef]

23. Goldberg, M. Gomez-Orellana I. Challenges for the oral delivery of macromolecules. *Nat. Rev. Drug Discov.* **2003**, *2*, 289–295. [CrossRef] [PubMed]

24. Leone-Bay, A.; Leipold, H.; Sarubbi, D.; Variano, B.; Rivera, T.; Baughman, R.A. Oral delivery of sodium cromolyn: Preliminary studies in vivo and in vitro. *Pharm. Res.* **1996**, *13*, 222–226. [CrossRef] [PubMed]

25. Anonymous, Sodium Decanoate, PubChem ID 16211937. Available online: https://pubchem.ncbi.nlm.nih.gov/compound/16211937 (accessed on 12 February 2019).

26. Anonymous, Sodium Caprozate PubChem ID 22669833. Available online: https://pubchem.ncbi.nlm.nih.gov/compound/23669833 (accessed on 12 February 2019).

27. Brayden, D.J.; Gleeson, J.; Walsh, E. A head-to-head multi-parametric high content analysis of a series of medium chain fatty acid intestinal permeation enhancers in Caco-2 cells. *Eur. J. Pharm. Biopharm.* **2014**, *88*, 830–839. [CrossRef] [PubMed]

28. Khafagy, E.S.; Morishita, M.; Takayama, K. The role of intermolecular interactions with penetratin and its analogue on the enhancement of absorption of nasal therapeutic peptides. *Int. J. Pharm.* **2010**, *388*, 209–212. [CrossRef]

29. Twarog, C.; Hillaireau, H.; Taverna, M.; Noiray, M.; Illel, B.; Vogel, R.; Brayden, D.J.; Fattal, E. Oral peptide delivery: Understanding interactions between a peptide and permeation enhancers. In Proceedings of the 11th World Meeting on Pharmaceutics, Biopharmaceutics and Pharmaceutical Technology, Granada, Spain, 19–22 March 2018.

30. Lindmark, T.; Nikkila, T.; Artursson, P. Mechanisms of absorption enhancement by medium chain fatty acids in intestinal epithelial Caco-2 cell monolayers. *J. Pharmacol. Exp. Ther.* **1995**, *275*, 958–964.

31. Sawada, T.; Ogawa, T.; Tomita, M.; Hayashi, M.; Awazu, S. Role of paracellular pathway in nonelectrolyte permeation across rat colon epithelium enhanced by sodium caprate and sodium caprylate. *Pharm. Res.* **1991**, *8*, 1365–1371. [CrossRef]

32. Maher, S.; Kennelly, R.; Bzik, V.A.; Baird, A.W.; Wang, X.; Winter, D.; Brayden, D.J. Evaluation of intestinal absorption enhancement and local mucosal toxicity of two promoters. I. Studies in isolated rat and human colonic mucosae. *Eur. J. Pharm. Sci.* **2009**, *38*, 291–300. [CrossRef]

33. Tomita, M.; Hayashi, M.; Awazu, S. Absorption-enhancing mechanism of EDTA, caprate, and decanoylcarnitine in Caco-2 cells. *J. Pharm. Sci.* **1996**, *85*, 608–611. [CrossRef]

34. Lindmark, T.; Kimura, Y.; Artursson, P. Absorption enhancement through intracellular regulation of tight junction permeability by medium chain fatty acids in Caco-2 cells. *J. Pharmacol. Exp. Ther.* **1998**, *284*, 362–369.

35. Feighery, L.M.; Cochrane, S.W.; Quinn, T.; Baird, A.W.; O'Toole, D.; Owens, S.E.; O'Donoghue, D.; Mrsny, R.J.; Brayden, D.J. Myosin light chain kinase inhibition: Correction of increased intestinal epithelial permeability in vitro. *Pharm. Res.* **2008**, *2*, 1377–1386. [CrossRef]

36. Shimazaki, T.; Tomita, M.; Sadahiro, S.; Hayashi, M.; Awazu, S. Absorption-enhancing effects of sodium caprate and palmitoyl carnitine in rat and human colons. *Dig. Dis. Sci.* **1998**, *43*, 641–645. [CrossRef] [PubMed]

37. Krug, S.M.; Amasheh, M.; Dittmann, I.; Christoffel, I.; Fromm, M.; Amasheh, S. Sodium caprate as an enhancer of macromolecule permeation across tricellular tight junctions of intestinal cells. *Biomaterials* **2013**, *34*, 275–282. [CrossRef] [PubMed]

38. Blikslager, A.T.; Moeser, A.J.; Gookin, J.L.; Jones, S.L.; Odle, J. Restoration of barrier function in injured intestinal mucosa. *Physiol. Rev.* **2007**, *87*, 545–564. [CrossRef]

39. Sugibayashi, K.; Onuki, Y.; Takayama, K. Displacement of tight junction proteins from detergent-resistant membrane domains by treatment with sodium caprate. *Eur. J. Pharm. Sci.* **2009**, *36*, 46–253. [CrossRef]

40. Maher, S.; Heade, J.; McCartney, F.; Waters, S.; Bleiel, S.B.; Brayden, D.J. Effects of surfactant-based permeation enhancers on mannitol permeability, histology, and electrogenic ion transport responses in excised rat colonic mucosae. *Int. J. Pharm.* **2018**, *539*, 11–22. [CrossRef] [PubMed]

41. Brayden, D.J.; Maher, S.; Bahar, B.; Walsh, E. Sodium caprate-induced increases in intestinal permeability and epithelial damage are prevented by misoprostol. *Eur. J. Pharm. Biopharm.* **2015**, *94*, 194–206. [CrossRef]

42. Leonard, T.W.; Lynch, J.; McKenna, M.J.; Brayden, D.J. Promoting absorption of drugs in humans using medium-chain fatty acid-based solid dosage forms: GIPET. *Exp. Opin. Drug Deliv.* **2006**, *3*, 685–692. [CrossRef]

43. Gradauer, K.; Nishiumi, A.; Unrinin, K.; Higashino, H.; Kataoka, M.; Pedersen, B.L.; Buckley, S.T.; Yamashita, S. Interaction with mixed micelles in the intestine attenuates the permeation enhancing potential of alkyl-maltosides. *Mol. Pharm.* **2015**, *12*, 2245–2253. [CrossRef]

44. Brayden, D.; Creed, E.; O'Connell, A.; Leipold, H.; Agarwal, R.; Leone-Bay, A. Heparin absorption across the intestine: Effects of sodium N-[8-(2-hydroxybenzoyl)amino]caprylate in rat in situ intestinal instillations and in Caco-2 monolayers. *Pharm. Res.* **1997**, *14*, 1772–1779. [CrossRef]

45. Malkov, D.; Angelo, R.; Wang, H.Z.; Flanders, E.; Tang, H.; Gomez-Orellana, I. Oral delivery of insulin with the eligen technology: Mechanistic studies. *Curr. Drug Deliv.* **2005**, *2*, 191–197. [CrossRef]

46. Hess, S.; Rotshild, V.; Hoffman, A. Investigation of the enhancing mechanism of sodium N-[8-(2-hydroxybenzoyl)amino]caprylate effect on the intestinal permeability of polar molecules utilizing a voltage clamp method. *Eur. J. Pharm. Sci.* **2005**, *25*, 307–312. [CrossRef] [PubMed]

47. Malkov, D.; Wang, H.Z.; Dinh, S.; Gomez-Orellana, I. Pathway of oral absorption of heparin with sodium N-[8-(2-hydroxybenzoyl)amino] caprylate. *Pharm. Res.* **2002**, *19*, 1180–1184. [CrossRef] [PubMed]

48. Ding, X.; Rath, P.; Angelo, R.; Stringfellow, T.; Flanders, E.; Dinh, S.; Gomez-Orellana, I.; Robinson, J.R. Oral absorption enhancement of cromolyn sodium through noncovalent complexation. *Pharm. Res.* **2004**, *21*, 2196–2206. [CrossRef] [PubMed]

49. Arbit, E.; Goldberg, M.; Gomez-Orellana, I.; Majuru, S. Oral heparin: Status review. *Thromb. J.* **2006**, *4*, 6. [CrossRef] [PubMed]

50. Alani, A.W.; Robinson, J.R. Mechanistic understanding of oral drug absorption enhancement of cromolyn sodium by an amino acid derivative. *Pharm. Res.* **2008**, *25*, 48–54. [CrossRef] [PubMed]

51. Rehmani, S.; Dixon, J.E. Oral delivery of anti-diabetes therapeutics using cell penetrating and transcytosing peptide strategies. *Peptides* **2018**, *100*, 24–35. [CrossRef] [PubMed]

52. Buckley, S.T.; Bækdal, T.A.; Vegge, A.; Maarbjerg, S.J.; Pyke, C.; Ahnfelt-Rønne, J.; Madsen, K.G.; Schéele, S.G.; Alanentalo, T.; Kirk, R.K.; et al. Transcellular stomach absorption of a derivatized glucagon-like peptide-1 receptor agonist. *Sci. Transl. Med.* **2018**, *10*. [CrossRef]

53. Amory, J.K.; Leonard, T.W.; Page, S.T.; O'Toole, E.; McKenna, M.J.; Bremner, W.J. Oral administration of the GnRH antagonist acyline, in a GIPET-enhanced tablet form, acutely suppresses serum testosterone in normal men: Single-dose pharmacokinetics and pharmacodynamics. *Cancer Chemother. Pharmacol.* **2009**, *64*, 641–645. [CrossRef]

54. Leonard, T.W. Composition and Drug Delviery of Bisphosphonates. U.S. Patent 0,215,743 A1, 26 August 2010.

55. Halberg, I.B.; Lyby, K.; Wassermann, K.; Heise, T.; Zijlstra, E.; Plum-Morchel, L. Efficacy and safety of oral basal insulin versus subcutaneous insulin in type 2 diabetes: A randomised, double-blind Phase II trial. *Lancet Diabetes Endocrinol.* **2019**. [CrossRef]

56. Khedkar, A.; Lebovitz, H.; Fleming, A.; Cherrington, A.; Jose, V.; Athalye, S.N.; Vishweswaramurthy, A. Impact of insulin tregopil and its permeation enhancer on pharmacokinetics of metformin in healthy volunteers: Randomized, open-label, placebo-controlled, crossover study. *Clin. Transl. Sci.* **2018**. [CrossRef]

57. Raoof, A.A.; Chiu, P.; Ramtoola, Z.; Cumming, I.K.; Teng, C.; Weinbach, S.P.; Hardee, G.E.; Levin, A.A.; Geary, R.S. Oral bioavailability and multiple dose tolerability of an antisense oligonucleotide tablet formulated with sodium caprate. *J. Pharm. Sci.* **2004**, *93*, 1431–1439. [CrossRef] [PubMed]

58. Tillman, L.G.; Geary, R.S.; Hardee, G.E. Oral delivery of antisense oligonucleotides in man. *J. Pharm. Sci.* **2008**, *97*, 225–236. [CrossRef] [PubMed]

59. Available online: http://ir.ionispharma.com/news-releases/news-release-details/ionis-pharmaceuticals-licenses-first-oral-antisense-drug-acting (accessed on 12 February 2019).

60. Lennernäs, H.; Gjellan, K.; Hallgren, R.; Graffner, C. The influence of caprate on rectal absorption of phenoxymethylpenicillin: Experience from an in-vivo perfusion in humans. *J. Pharm. Pharmacol.* **2002**, *54*, 499–508. [CrossRef] [PubMed]

61. Baughman, R.A.; Kapoor, S.C.; Agarwal, R.K.; Kisicki, J.; Catella-Lawson, F.; FitzGerald, G.A. Oral delivery of anticoagulant doses of heparin. A randomized, double-blind, controlled study in humans. *Circulation* **1998**, *98*, 1610–1615. [CrossRef] [PubMed]

62. Berkowitz, S.D.; Marder, V.J.; Kosutic, G.; Baughman, R.A. Oral heparin administration with a novel drug delivery agent (SNAC) in healthy volunteers and patients undergoing elective total hip arthroplasty. *J. Thromb. Haemost.* **2003**, *1*, 1914–1919. [CrossRef] [PubMed]

63. Mousa, S.A.; Zhang, F.; Aljada, A.; Chaturvedi, S.; Takieddin, M.; Zhang, H.; Chi, L.; Castelli, M.C.; Friedman, K.; Goldberg, M.M.; et al. Pharmacokinetics and pharmacodynamics of oral heparin solid dosage form in healthy human subjects. *J. Clin. Pharmacol.* **2007**, *47*, 1508–1520. [CrossRef] [PubMed]

64. Buclin, T.; Cosma Rochat, M.; Burckhardt, P.; Azria, M.; Attinger, M. Bioavailability and biological efficacy of a new oral formulation of salmon calcitonin in healthy volunteers. *J. Bone Miner. Res.* **2002**, *17*, 1478–1485. [CrossRef] [PubMed]

65. Kapitza, C.; Zijlstra, E.; Heinemann, L.; Castelli, M.C.; Riley, G.; Heise, T. Oral insulin: A comparison with subcutaneous regular human insulin in patients with type 2 diabetes. *Diabetes Care* **2010**, *33*, 1288–1290. [CrossRef] [PubMed]

66. Karsdal, M.A.; Byrjalsen, I.; Alexandersen, P.; Bihlet, A.; Andersen, J.R.; Riis, B.J.; Bay-Jensen, A.C.; Christiansen, C.; CSMC021C2301/2 investigators. Treatment of symptomatic knee osteoarthritis with oral salmon calcitonin: Results from two phase 3 trials. *Osteoarthr. Cartil.* **2015**, *23*, 532–543. [CrossRef]

67. Henriksen, K.; Byrjalsen, I.; Andersen, J.R.; Bihlet, A.R.; Russo, L.A.; Alexandersen, P.; Valter, I.; Qvist, P.; Lau, E.; Riis, B.J.; et al. SMC021 investigators., A randomized, double-blind, multicenter, placebo-controlled study to evaluate the efficacy and safety of oral salmon calcitonin in the treatment of osteoporosis in postmenopausal women taking calcium and vitamin D. *Bone* **2016**, *91*, 122–129. [CrossRef]

68. Karsdal, M.A.; Henriksen, K.; Bay-Jensen, A.C.; Molloy, B.; Arnold, M.; John, M.R.; Byrjalsen, I.; Azria, M.; Riis, B.J.; Qvist, P.; et al. Lessons learned from the development of oral calcitonin: The first tablet formulation of a protein in phase III clinical trials. *J. Clin. Pharmacol.* **2011**, *51*, 460–471. [CrossRef] [PubMed]

69. Davies, M.; Pieber, T.R.; Hartoft-Nielsen, M.L.; Hansen, O.K.H.; Jabbour, S.; Rosenstock, J. Effect of oral semaglutide compared with placebo and subcutaneous semaglutide on glycemic control in patients with Type 2 diabetes: A Randomized Clinical Trial. *JAMA* **2017**, *318*, 1460–1470. [CrossRef] [PubMed]

70. Bjerregaard, S.; Nielsen, F.S.; Sauerberg, P. Solid Compositions Comprising a GLP-1 Agonist and a Salt of n-(8-(2-Hydroxybenzoyl)Amino)Caprylic Acid. U.S. Patent WO2012080471A1, 8 March 2016.

71. Available online: https://globenewswire.com/news-release/2018/02/22/1379640/0/en/Novo-Nordisk-successfully-completes-the-first-phase-3a-trial-PIONEER-1-with-oral-semaglutide.html (accessed on 28 November 2018).

72. Granhall, C.; Søndergaard, F.L.; Thomsen, M.; Anderson, T.W. Pharmacokinetics, safety and tolerability of oral semaglutide in subjects with renal impairment. *Clin. Pharm.* **2018**, *57*, 1571–1580. [CrossRef] [PubMed]

73. Baekdal, T.A.; Thomsen, M.; Kupčová, V.; Hansen, C.W.; Anderson, T.W. Pharmacokinetics, safety, and tolerability of oral semaglutide in subjects with hepatic impairment. *J. Clin. Pharmacol.* **2018**, *58*, 1314–1323. [CrossRef] [PubMed]

74. Bækdal, T.A.; Breitschaft, A.; Navarria, A.; Hansen, C.W. A randomized study investigating the effect of omeprazole on the pharmacokinetics of oral semaglutide. *Expert Opin. Drug Metab. Toxicol.* **2018**, *14*, 869–877. [CrossRef] [PubMed]

75. Bain, S.C.; Mosenzon, O.; Arechavaleta, R.; Bogdański, P.; Comlekci, A.; Consoli, A.; Deerochanawong, C.; Dungan, K.; Faingold, M.C.; Farkouh, M.E.; et al. Cardiovascular safety of oral semaglutide in patients with type 2 diabetes: Rationale, design and patient baseline characteristics for the PIONEER 6 trial. *Diabetes Obes. Metab.* **2018**. [CrossRef]

76. Maher, S.; Leonard, T.W.; Jacobsen, J.; Brayden, D.J. Safety and efficacy of sodium caprate in promoting oral drug absorption: From in vitro to the clinic. *Adv. Drug Deliv. Rev.* **2009**, *61*, 1427–1449. [CrossRef]

77. Raoof, A.A.; Ramtoola, Z.; McKenna, B.; Yu, R.Z.; Hardee, G.; Geary, R.S. Effect of sodium caprate on the intestinal absorption of two modified antisense oligonucleotides in pigs. *Eur. J. Pharm. Sci.* **2002**, *17*, 131–138. [CrossRef]

78. Riley, M.G.; Castelli, M.C.; Paehler, E.A. Subchronic oral toxicity of salcaprozate sodium (SNAC) in Sprague-Dawley and Wistar rats. *Int. J. Toxicol.* **2009**, *28*, 278–293. [CrossRef]

79. Riley, M.G.; York, R.G. Peri-and postnatal developmental toxicity of salcaprozate sodium (SNAC) in Sprague-Dawley rats. *Int. J. Toxicol.* **2009**, *28*, 266–277. [CrossRef]

80. McCartney FGleeson, J.; Brayden, D.J. Safety concerns over the use of intestinal permeation enhancers: A mini-review. *Tissue Barriers* **2016**, *4*, e1176822. [CrossRef] [PubMed]

81. Van der Flier, L.G.; Clevers, H. Stem cells, self-renewal, and differentiation in the intestinal epithelium. *Annu. Rev. Physiol.* **2009**, *71*, 241–260. [CrossRef]

82. Laine, L.; Takeuchi, K.; Tarnawski, A. Gastric mucosal defense and cytoprotection: Bench to bedside. *Gastroenterology* **2008**, *135*, 41–60. [CrossRef] [PubMed]

83. Wang, X.; Maher, S.; Brayden, D.J. Restoration of rat colonic epithelium after in situ intestinal instillation of the absorption promoter, sodium caprate. *Ther. Deliv.* **2010**, *1*, 75–82. [CrossRef]

84. Gookin, J.L.; Galanko, J.A.; Blikslager, A.T.; Argenzio, R.A. PG-mediated closure of paracellular pathway and not restitution is the primary determinant of barrier recovery in acutely injured porcine ileum. *Am. J. Physiol.* **2003**, *285*, G967–G979. [CrossRef] [PubMed]

85. Narkar, Y.; Burnette, R.; Bleher, R.; Albrecht, R.; Kandela, A.; Robinson, J.R. Evaluation of mucosal damage and recovery in the gastrointestinal tract of rats by a penetration enhancer. *Pharm. Res.* **2008**, *25*, 25–38. [CrossRef] [PubMed]

86. König, J.; Wells, J.; Cani, P.D.; García-Ródenas, C.L.; MacDonald, T.; Mercenier, A.; Whyte, J.; Troost, F.; Brummer, R.J. Human intestinal barrier function in health and disease. *Clin. Transl. Gastroenterol.* **2016**, *7*, e196. [CrossRef]

87. Cani, P.D. Human gut microbiome: Hopes, threats and promises. *Gut* **2018**, *67*, 1716–1725. [CrossRef]
88. Chassaing, B.; Koren, O.; Goodrich, J.K.; Poole, A.C.; Srinivasan, S.; Ley, R.E.; Gewirtz, A.T. Dietary emulsifiers impact the mouse gut microbiota promoting colitis and metabolic syndrome. *Nature* **2015**, *519*, 92–96. [CrossRef]
89. Choonara, B.F.; Choonara, Y.E.; Kumar, P.; Bijukumar, D.; du Toit, L.C.; Pillay, V. A review of advanced oral drug delivery technologies facilitating the protection and absorption of protein and peptide molecules. *Biotechnol. Adv.* **2014**, *32*, 1269–1282. [CrossRef]
90. Tscheik, C.; Blasig, I.E.; Winkler, L. Trends in drug delivery through tissue barriers containing tight junctions. *Tissue Barriers* **2013**, *1*, e24565. [CrossRef] [PubMed]
91. Bala, S.; Marcos, M.; Gattu, A.; Catalano, D.; Szabo, G. Acute binge drinking increases serum endotoxin and bacterial DNA levels in healthy individuals. *PLoS ONE* **2014**, *9*, e96864. [CrossRef] [PubMed]
92. Cox, A.B.; Rawlinson, L.; Baird, A.W.; Bzik, V.; Brayden, D.J. In vitro interactions between the oral absorption promoter, sodium caprate (C10) and S. typhimurium in rat intestinal ileal mucosae. *Pharm. Res.* **2008**, *25*, 114–122. [CrossRef] [PubMed]
93. Petschow, B.W.; Batema, R.P.; Ford, L.L. Susceptibility of *Helicobacter pylori* to bactericidal properties of medium-chain monoglycerides and free fatty acids. *Antimicrob. Agents Chemother.* **1996**, *40*, 302–306. [CrossRef]
94. Van Immerseel, F.; De Buck, J.; Boyen, F.; Bohez, L.; Pasmans, F.; Volf, J.; Sevcik, M.; Rychlik, I.; Haesebrouck, F.; Ducatelle, R. Medium-chain fatty acids decrease colonization and invasion through hilA suppression shortly after infection of chickens with *Salmonella enterica* serovar *Enteritidis. Appl. Environ. Microbiol.* **2004**, *70*, 3582–3587. [CrossRef] [PubMed]
95. Chadeganipour, M.; Haims, A. Antifungal activities of pelargonic and capric acid on *Microsporum gypseum. Mycoses* **2001**, *44*, 109–112. [CrossRef] [PubMed]
96. Huang, C.B.; Alimova, Y.; Myers, T.M.; Ebersole, J.L. Short and medium-chain fatty acids exhibit antimicrobial activity for oral microorganisms. *Arch. Oral Biol.* **2011**, *56*, 650–654. [CrossRef]

pharmaceutics

MDPI

Article

Synthesis, Structure–Activity Relationships and In Vitro Toxicity Profile of Lactose-Based Fatty Acid Monoesters as Possible Drug Permeability Enhancers

Simone Lucarini [1], Laura Fagioli [1], Robert Cavanagh [2], Wanling Liang [3], Diego Romano Perinelli [4], Mario Campana [5], Snjezana Stolnik [2], Jenny K. W. Lam [3], Luca Casettari [1,*] and Andrea Duranti [1]

[1]   Department of Biomolecular Sciences, School of Pharmacy, University of Urbino, 61029 Urbino (PU), Italy; simone.lucarini@uniurb.it (S.L.); laura.fagioli@uniurb.it (L.F.); andrea.duranti@uniurb.it (A.D.)
[2]   Drug Delivery and Tissue Engineering Division, School of Pharmacy, University of Nottingham, Nottingham NG7 2RD, UK; robert.cavanagh@nottingham.ac.uk (R.C.); Snow.Stolnik@nottingham.ac.uk (S.S.)
[3]   Department of Pharmacology & Pharmacy, The University of Hong Kong, 21 Sassoon Road, Pokfulam, Hong Kong, China; sophiawlliang@gmail.com (W.L.); jkwlam@hku.hk (J.K.W.L.)
[4]   School of Pharmacy, University of Camerino, 62032 Camerino (MC), Italy; diego.perinelli@unicam.it
[5]   Science and Technology Facilities Council (STFC), ISIS Neutron and Muon Source, Rutherford Appleton Laboratory, Didcot OX11 0QX, UK; mario.campana@stfc.ac.uk
*   Correspondence: luca.casettari@uniurb.it; Tel.: +39-0722-303332

Received: 30 May 2018; Accepted: 2 July 2018; Published: 3 July 2018

Abstract: Permeability enhancers are receiving increased attention arising from their ability to increase transepithelial permeability and thus, bioavailability of orally or pulmonary administered biopharmaceutics. Here we present the synthesis and the in vitro assaying of a series of lactose-based non-ionic surfactants, highlighting the relationship between their structure and biological effect. Using tensiometric measurements the critical micelle concentrations (CMCs) of the surfactants were determined and demonstrate that increasing hydrophobic chain length reduces surfactant CMC. In vitro testing on Caco-2 intestinal and Calu-3 airway epithelia revealed that cytotoxicity, assessed by 3-(4,5-dimethylthiazol-2-yl)-2,5-diphenyltetrazolium bromide (MTT) and lactate dehydrogenase (LDH) release assays, is presented for most of the surfactants at concentrations greater than their CMCs. Further biological study demonstrates that application of cytotoxic concentrations of the surfactants is associated with depolarizing mitochondrial membrane potential, increasing nuclear membrane permeability and activation of effector caspases. It is, therefore, proposed that when applied at cytotoxic levels, the surfactants are inducing apoptosis in both cell lines tested. Importantly, through the culture of epithelial monolayers on Transwell® supports, the surfactants demonstrate the ability to reversibly modulate transepithelial electrical resistance (TEER), and thus open tight junctions, at non-toxic concentrations, emphasizing their potential application as safe permeability enhancers in vivo.

Keywords: absorption enhancers; sugar-based surfactants; biocompatibility studies; transmucosal drug delivery

1. Introduction

Sugar-based fatty acid esters usually belong to the class of non-ionic surfactants and possess desirable characteristics suitable for different applications in food, cosmetic and pharmaceutical fields. They are constituted by a sugar moiety as hydrophilic head (polar) linked via an ester bond to a fatty acid chain as hydrophobic tail (non-polar). Various modifications, both on polar head or non-polar tail, have been rationally designed to obtain a broad class of sugar esters with different properties. Particularly, sugar-based fatty acid esters made up of carbohydrate moieties, including mono-, di- or tri-saccharides condensed with saturated or unsaturated fatty acids with different chain lengths have been synthesized to give products with various degree of esterification [1]. Constituted of natural substrates, easily available and therefore inexpensive and renewable, these products are considered ideal raw materials to be employed for a large variety of technological applications such as emulsification, stabilization of disperse systems, solubility or drug permeation enhancement [2–5].

Sugar-based fatty acid esters are receiving a growing attention due to the large demand for non-toxic, non-irritant and highly biocompatible and biodegradable amphiphilic compounds in different fields [6]. Many studies have recently reported the synthesis and possible applications of selective 6-*O*-sugar fatty acid monoesters, generally referred as sugar monoesters [7–9]. Several physico-chemical and biological properties have been studied [10,11], to develop advanced drug delivery systems, including skin penetration enhancing effect or transmucosal permeability enhancement [12–15]. The use of amphiphilic compounds as permeability enhancers (PEs) for transmucosal drug delivery represents one of the most promising application of surfactants in biopharmaceutics, able to provide a valid alternative (e.g., oral or pulmonary administration) to the conventional (e.g., injection) route of administrations of many therapeutic peptides [16–20].

Among the class of sugar monoesters, sorbitan and sucrose derivatives are those most easily available on the market. However, sugar-based surfactants bearing a different sugar moiety can also represent a valid alternative to the currently available amphiphilic compounds; particularly when industrial waste can be easily transformed in valued-added products. In this respect, the lactose monoester derivatives have been recently brought back into the spotlight, as promising eco-friendly emulsifier and antimicrobial compounds for pharmaceutical, food and cosmetic fields. These surfactants were synthesized for the first time in the 1970s [21], and, over the last decades, they have been proposed, including as excipients in drug formations, additives in the food industry and are being explored for their potential anticancer activity [22]. Despite being well-characterized in term of surface activity [23,24], and emulsifying properties [25], no detailed studies have been performed aimed at defining cytotoxicity profiles of these surfactants. Such information is required to broaden the potential applications of this class of sugar-based amphiphiles for pharmaceutical and cosmetic applications.

The aim of this work was to investigate the relationship between the structure and cytotoxicity of a series of lactose esters derivatives, enzymatically synthesized using saturated fatty acids with different chain lengths (C10; C12; C14; C16). The critical micelle concentration (CMC) was compared with cytotoxicity (IC_{50}) evaluated on two selected cell lines as models for the intestinal (Caco-2) and respiratory (Calu-3) epithelia, which are common route of drug administration. In addition, mitochondrial membrane potential, nuclear membrane permeability and effector caspase activation were studied on the same cell lines to deeper understand the mechanism upon cellular toxicity. Finally, transepithelial electrical resistance (TEER) measurements were performed to investigate the effect of saturated acyl chain lactose monoesters on the integrity of the cellular barrier and to provide a preliminary evidence of their transmucosal perturbance action, which is commonly exerted by surfactants acting as permeability enhancers across mucosa.

2. Materials and Methods

2.1. Materials

Decanoic, lauric, myristic and palmitic acids were purchased from TCI (Zwijndrecht, Belgium), lactose monohydrate from Carlo Erba (Milan, Italy), while Lipozyme® (immobilized from Mucor miehei), *p*-toluenesulfonic acid, 2,2-dimethoxypropane, tetrafluoroboric acid diethyl ether complex, carbonyl cyanide 4-(trifluoromethoxy) phenylhydrazone (FCCP) and all organic solvents used in this study were purchased from Sigma-Aldrich (Milan, Italy). Prior to use, acetonitrile was dried with molecular sieves with an effective pore diameter of 4 Å and toluene was saturated with water. CellEvent™ caspase-3/7 green detection reagent was purchased from Thermo Fisher Scientific (Waltham, MA, USA) and the CellTox™ green cytotoxicity assay acquired from Promega (Madison, WI, USA). The JC-1 probe (5,5′,6,6′-Tetrachloro-1,1′,3,3′-tetraethylbenzimidazolylcarbocyanine, iodide) was purchased from Biotium (Fremont, CA, USA).

2.2. Cell Culture Conditions

Caco-2 and Calu-3 cells were obtained from American Type Culture Collection. Caco-2 cells were cultured in advanced Dulbecco Modified Eagle Medium (DMEM) supplemented with 10% v/v Fetal Bovine Serum (FBS) and 1% v/v antibiotics-antimycotic. Calu-3 cells were cultured in DMEM F-12 supplemented with 10% v/v FBS and 1% v/v antibiotics-antimycotic. All cell lines were maintained at a 5% CO_2 in a humidified incubator at 37 °C. Caco-2 cells were used between passages 30–45 and Calu-3 cells between 25–40.

2.3. Synthesis of Lactose-Based Surfactants

The structures of compounds were unambiguously assessed by ^{1}H NMR and ^{13}C NMR recorded on a Bruker AC 400 or 100 (Milan, Italy), respectively, spectrometer and analyzed using the TopSpin software package (version 2.1). Chemical shifts were measured using the central peak of the solvent. Column chromatography purifications were performed under "flash" conditions using Merck 230–400 mesh silica gel. TLC was carried out on Merck silica gel 60 F254 plates, which were visualized by exposure to an aqueous solution of ceric ammonium molibdate.

2.3.1. General Procedure for the Synthesis of Lactose Tetra Acetal Monoesters

Lipozyme® (0.078 g) was added to a solution of the fatty acid (**1a–d**) (0.79 mmol) and 4-O-(3′,4′-O-isopropylidene-β-D-galactopyranosyl)-2,3:5,6-di-O-isopropylidene-1,1-di-O-methyl-D-glucopyranose (lactose tetra acetate, LTA) [26] (**2**) (0.402 g, 0.79 mmol) in water-saturated toluene at 25 °C [12,27]. The mixture was stirred at 75 °C for 12 h, cooled and diluted with acetone, then the enzyme was filtered, and the filtrate was concentrated. The purification of the residue by column chromatography (cyclohexane/EtOAc 8:2) gave **3a–d** as pale yellow oils. (Scheme 1).

[6′-O-Decanoyl-4-O-(3′,4′-O-isopropylidene-β-D-galactopyranosyl)-2,3:5,6-di-O-isopropylidene-1,1-di-O-methyl-D-glucopyranose] (**3a**) [27]. Yield: 53% (0.275 g). ^{1}H NMR (400 MHz, MeOD) δ: 0.92 (t, 3H, J = 6.7 Hz, CH$_3$), 1.32 (s, 6H, 2CH$_3$), 1.33–1.37 [m, 12H, (CH$_2$)$_n$], 1.39 (s, 3H, CH$_3$), 1.41 (s, 3H, CH$_3$), 1.44 (s, 3H, CH$_3$), 1.49 (s, 3H, CH$_3$), 1.61–1.67 (m, 2H, CH$_2$CH$_2$COOR), 2.40 (t, 2H, J = 7.0 Hz, CH$_2$COOR), 3.46 (s, 6H, 2OCH$_3$), 3.47 (dd, 1H, J_{8-9} = 7.0 Hz, J_{8-7} = 8.0 Hz, H^8), 3.91 (dd, 1H, J_{4-3} = 1.2 Hz, J_{4-5} = 5.0 Hz, H^4), 4.04 (ddd, 1H, J_{11-12a} = 1.5 Hz, J_{11-10} = 2.1 Hz, J_{11-12b} = 6.8 Hz, H^{11}), 4.05 (dd, 1H, J_{6b-5} = 6.0 Hz, J_{6b-6a} = 8.7 Hz, H^{6b}), 4.08 (dd, 1H, J_{9-10} = 5.5 Hz, J_{9-8} = 7.0 Hz, H^9), 4.14 (dd, 1H, J_{3-4} = 1.2 Hz, J_{3-2} = 7.5 Hz, H^3), 4.17 (dd, 1H, J_{6a-5} = 6.0 Hz, J_{6a-6b} = 8.7 Hz, H^{6a}), 4.22 (dd, 1H, J_{10-11} = 2.1 Hz, J_{10-9} = 5.5 Hz, H^{10}), 4.27 (dd, 1H, J_{12b-11} = 6.8 Hz, $J_{12b-12a}$ = 11.5 Hz, H^{12b}), 4.30 (dd, 1H, J_{12a-11} = 1.5 Hz, $J_{12a-12b}$ = 11.5 Hz, H^{12a}), 4.31 (ddd, 1H, J_{5-4} = 5.0 Hz, J_{5-6a} ≅ J_{5-6b} = 6.0 Hz, H^5), 4.41 (d, 1H, J_{1-2} = 6.2 Hz, H^1), 4.51 (d, 1H, J_{7-8} = 8.0 Hz, H^7), 4.51 (dd, 1H, J_{2-1} = 6.2 Hz, J_{2-3} = 7.5 Hz, H^2) ppm. ^{13}C NMR (100 MHz, MeOD) δ: 13.0, 22.3, 24.2, 24.6, 25.1, 25.5, 25.6, 26.2, 27.0, 28.8, 29.00, 29.02, 29.2, 31.6, 33.5, 53.0, 55.1, 63.0, 65.5, 70.8, 73.3, 73.5, 75.4, 76.4, 76.8, 77.6, 79.4, 103.1, 105.7, 108.5, 109.7, 109.9, 173.8 ppm.

[6′-O-Dodecanoyl-4-O-(3′,4′-O-isopropylidene-β-D-galactopyranosyl)-2,3:5,6-di-O-isopropylidene-1,1-di-O-methyl-D-glucopyranose] (**3b**) [27]. Yield: 50% (0.274 g). ^{1}H NMR (400 MHz, MeOD) δ: 0.92 (t, 3H, J = 6.7 Hz, CH$_3$), 1.32 (s, 6H, 2CH$_3$), 1.33–1.37 [m, 16H, (CH$_2$)$_n$], 1.39 (s, 3H, CH$_3$), 1.41 (s, 3H, CH$_3$), 1.44 (s, 3H, CH$_3$), 1.49 (s, 3H, CH$_3$), 1.62–1.67 (m, 2H, CH$_2$CH$_2$COOR), 2.40 (t, 2H, J = 7.0 Hz, CH$_2$COOR), 3.46 (s, 6H, 2OCH$_3$), 3.47 (dd, 1H, J_{8-9} = 7.1 Hz, J_{8-7} = 8.0 Hz, H^8), 3.91 (dd, 1H, J_{4-3} = 1.2 Hz, J_{4-5} = 5.0 Hz, H^4), 4.05 (ddd, 1H, J_{11-12a} = 1.2 Hz, J_{11-10} = 2.1 Hz, J_{11-12b} = 6.8 Hz, H^{11}),

4.05 (dd, 1H, J_{6b-5} = 6.0 Hz, J_{6b-6a} = 8.7 Hz, H^{6b}), 4.08 (dd, 1H, J_{9-10} = 5.6 Hz, J_{9-8} = 7.1 Hz, H^9), 4.14 (dd, 1H, J_{3-4} = 1.2 Hz, J_{3-2} = 7.5 Hz, H^3), 4.17 (dd, 1H, J_{6a-5} = 6.0 Hz, J_{6a-6b} = 8.7 Hz, H^{6a}), 4.22 (dd, 1H, J_{10-11} = 2.1 Hz, J_{10-9} = 5.6 Hz, H^{10}), 4.27 (dd, 1H, J_{12b-11} = 6.8 Hz, $J_{12b-12a}$ = 11.5 Hz, H^{12b}), 4.30 (dd, 1H, J_{12a-11} = 1.2 Hz, $J_{12a-12b}$ = 11.5 Hz, H^{12a}), 4.31 (ddd, 1H, J_{5-4} = 5.0 Hz, J_{5-6a} ≅ J_{5-6b} = 6.0 Hz, H^5), 4.41 (d, 1H, J_{1-2} = 6.2 Hz, H^1), 4.51 (d, 1H, J_{7-8} = 8.0 Hz, H^7), 4.51 (dd, 1H, J_{2-1} = 6.2 Hz, J_{2-3} = 7.5 Hz, H^2) ppm. ^{13}C NMR (100 MHz, MeOD) δ: 13.0, 22.3, 24.2, 24.6, 25.1, 25.5, 25.7, 26.2, 27.0, 28.8, 29.0, 29.1, 29.2, 29.3, 31.7, 33.5, 53.0, 55.1, 63.1, 65.5, 70.8, 73.3, 73.5, 75.4, 76.4, 76.8, 77.6, 79.4, 103.1, 105.7, 108.5, 109.7, 109.9, 173.8 ppm.

[6′-O-Tetradecanoyl-4-O-(3′,4′-O-isopropylidene-β-D-galactopyranosyl)-2,3:5,6-di-O-isopropylidene-1,1-di-O-methyl-D-glucopyranose] (**3c**) [27]. Yield: 44% (0.248 g). ^{1}H NMR (400 MHz, MeOD) δ: 0.92 (t, 3H, *J* = 6.7 Hz, CH$_3$), 1.30–1.33 [m, 20H, (CH$_2$)$_n$], 1.35 (s, 6H, 2CH$_3$), 1.39 (s, 3H, CH$_3$), 1.41 (s, 3H, CH$_3$), 1.44 (s, 3H, CH$_3$), 1.49 (s, 3H, CH$_3$), 1.61–1.67 (m, 2H, CH$_2$CH$_2$COOR), 2.40 (t, 2H, *J* = 7.0 Hz, CH$_2$COOR), 3.46 (s, 6H, 2OCH$_3$), 3.47 (dd, 1H, J_{8-9} = 7.1 Hz, J_{8-7} = 8.0 Hz, H^8), 3.91 (dd, 1H, J_{4-3} = 1.2 Hz, J_{4-5} = 5.0 Hz, H^4), 4.04 (ddd, 1H, J_{11-12a} = 1.0 Hz, J_{11-10} = 2.2 Hz, J_{11-12b} = 6.8 Hz, H^{11}), 4.05 (dd, 1H, J_{6b-5} = 6.0 Hz, J_{6b-6a} = 8.7 Hz, H^{6b}), 4.08 (dd, 1H, J_{9-10} = 5.6 Hz, J_{9-8} = 7.1 Hz, H^9), 4.15 (dd, 1H, J_{3-4} = 1.2 Hz, J_{3-2} = 7.5 Hz, H^3), 4.17 (dd, 1H, J_{6a-5} = 6.0 Hz, J_{6a-6b} = 8.7 Hz, H^{6a}), 4.22 (dd, 1H, J_{10-11} = 2.2 Hz, J_{10-9} = 5.6 Hz, H^{10}), 4.27 (dd, 1H, J_{12b-11} = 6.8 Hz, $J_{12b-12a}$ = 11.5 Hz, H^{12b}), 4.30 (dd, 1H, J_{12a-11} = 1.0 Hz, $J_{12a-12b}$ = 11.5 Hz, H^{12a}), 4.31 (ddd, J_{5-4} = 5.0 Hz, J_{5-6a} ≅ J_{5-6b} = 6.0 Hz, H^5), 4.41 (d, 1H, J_{1-2} = 6.2 Hz, H^1), 4.51 (d, 1H, J_{7-8} = 8.0 Hz, H^7), 4.51 (dd, 1H, J_{2-1} = 6.2 Hz, J_{2-3} = 7.5 Hz, H^2) ppm. ^{13}C NMR (100 MHz, MeOD) δ: 13.0, 22.3, 24.2, 24.6, 25.1, 25.5, 25.6, 26.2, 27.0, 28.8, 29.0, 29.1, 29.2, 29.31, 29.34, 29.4, 31.7, 33.5, 53.0, 55.1, 63.1, 65.5, 70.8, 73.3, 73.6, 75.4, 76.4, 76.8, 77.6, 79.4, 103.1, 105.7, 108.5, 109.7, 109.9, 173.8 ppm.

[6′-O-Esadecanoyl-4-O-(3′,4′-O-isopropylidene-β-D-galactopyranosyl)-2,3:5,6-di-O-isopropylidene-1,1-di-O-methyl-D-glucopyranose] (**3d**) [27]. Yield: 34% (0.200 g). ^{1}H NMR (400 MHz, MeOD) δ: 0.92 (t, 3H, *J* = 6.7 Hz, CH$_3$), 1.30–1.33 [m, 24H, (CH$_2$)$_n$], 1.35 (s, 6H, 2CH$_3$), 1.39 (s, 3H, CH$_3$), 1.41 (s, 3H, CH$_3$), 1.44 (s, 3H, CH$_3$), 1.49 (s, 3H, CH$_3$), 1.60–1.67 (m, 2H, CH$_2$CH$_2$COOR), 2.40 (t, 2H, *J* = 7.4 Hz, CH$_2$COOR), 3.46 (s, 6H, 2OCH$_3$), 3.47 (dd, 1H, J_{8-9} = 7.1 Hz, J_{8-7} = 8.0 Hz, H^8), 3.91 (dd, 1H, J_{4-3} = 1.2 Hz, J_{4-5} = 5.0 Hz, H^4), 4.04 (ddd, 1H, J_{11-12a} = 1.5 Hz, J_{11-10} = 2.2 Hz, J_{11-12b} = 6.8 Hz, H^{11}), 4.05 (dd, 1H, J_{6b-5} = 6.0 Hz, J_{6b-6a} = 8.7 Hz, H^{6b}), 4.08 (dd, 1H, J_{9-10} = 5.5 Hz, J_{9-8} = 7.1 Hz, H^9), 4.14 (dd, 1H, J_{3-4} = 1.2 Hz, J_{3-2} = 7.5 Hz, H^3), 4.17 (dd, 1H, J_{6a-5} = 6.0 Hz, J_{6a-6b} = 8.7 Hz, H^{6a}), 4.22 (dd, 1H, J_{10-11} = 2.2 Hz, J_{10-9} = 5.5 Hz, H^{10}), 4.27 (dd, 1H, J_{12b-11} = 6.8 Hz, $J_{12b-12a}$ = 11.5 Hz, H^{12b}), 4.30 (dd, 1H, J_{12a-11} = 1.5 Hz, $J_{12a-12b}$ = 11.5 Hz, H^{12a}), 4.31 (ddd, 1H, J_{5-4} = 5.0 Hz, J_{5-6a} ≅ J_{5-6b} = 6.0 Hz, H^5), 4.41 (d, 1H, J_{1-2} = 6.2 Hz, H^1), 4.51 (d, 1H, J_{7-8} = 8.0 Hz, H^7), 4.51 (dd, 1H, J_{2-1} = 6.2 Hz, J_{2-3} = 7.5 Hz, H^2) ppm. ^{13}C NMR (100 MHz, MeOD) δ: 13.0, 22.3, 24.2, 24.6, 25.1, 25.7, 26.2, 27.0, 28.8, 29.1, 29.2, 29.4, 31.7, 33.5, 53.0, 55.1, 63.1, 65.5, 70.8, 73.3, 73.6, 75.4, 76.4, 76.9, 77.6, 79.4, 103.1, 105.7, 108.5, 109.7, 109.9, 173.8 ppm.

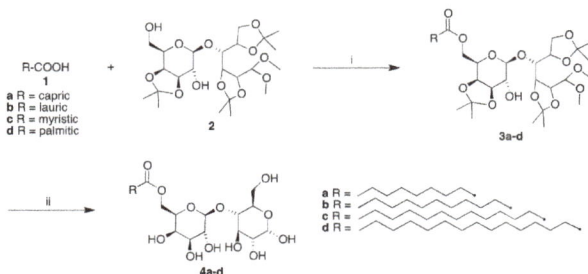

Scheme 1. Reagents and conditions: (**a**) toluene, 75 °C, 12 h; (**b**) HBF$_4$ Et$_2$O, CH$_3$CN, 30 °C, 3 h.

2.3.2. General Procedure for the Synthesis of Lactose Fatty Acid Monoesters

Compounds **3a–d** (0.25 mmol) were dissolved in tetrafluoroboric acid diethyl ether complex/water/acetonitrile (2.1 mL, 1:5:500) and the mixture was stirred at 30 °C for 3 h [12,27]. The white solids precipitated were then filtered, washed with acetonitrile and dried. The purification by recrystallization from methanol gave **4a–d** as white solids. (Scheme 1).

[6′-O-Decanoyl-4-O-(β-D-galactopyranosyl)-D-glucopyranose, lactose caprate] (**4a**) [27]. Yield: 75% (0.093 g). ^{1}H NMR (400 MHz, DMSO) δ: 0.86 (t, 3H, J = 6.6 Hz, CH$_3$), 1.20–1.32 [m, 12H, (CH$_2$)$_n$], 1.48–1.57 (m, 2H, CH$_2$CH$_2$COOR), 2.31 (t, 2H, J = 7.3 Hz, CH$_2$COOR), 3.17 (ddd, 1H, J_{2-1} = 4.0 Hz, J_{2-OH2} = 7.0 Hz, J_{2-3} = 9.5 Hz, H^2), 3.27 (dd, 1H, $J_{4-3} \cong J_{4-5}$ = 9.5 Hz, H^4), 3.33–3.37 (m, 2H, H^8, H^9), 3.57 (dd, 1H, $J_{3-2} \cong J_{3-4}$ = 9.5 Hz, H^3), 3.60–3.67 (m, 3H, H^{6a}, H^{6b}, H^{10}), 3.68–3.76 (m, 2H, H^5, H^{11}), 4.09 (dd, 1H, J_{12b-11} = 4.5 Hz, $J_{12b-12a}$ = 11.5 Hz, H^{12b}), 4.17 (dd, 1H, J_{12a-11} = 8.5 Hz, $J_{12a-12b}$ = 11.5 Hz, H^{12a}), 4.20–4.25 (m, 2H, H^7, OH^3), 4.43 (dd, 1H, $J_{OH6-6a} \cong J_{OH6-6b}$ = 6.0 Hz, OH^6), 4.55 (d, 1H, J_{OH2-2} = 7.0 Hz, OH^2), 4.78 (d, 1H, $J_{OH10-10}$ = 5.0 Hz, OH^{10}), 4.86 (d, 1H, J = 3.0 Hz, OH), 4.90 (dd, 1H, $J_{1-OH1} \cong J_{1-2}$ = 4.0 Hz, H^1), 5.15 (d, 1H, J = 3.0 Hz, OH), 6.33 (d, 1H, J_{OH1-1} = 4.0 Hz, OH^1) ppm. ^{13}C NMR (100 MHz, DMSO) δ: 14.4, 22.6, 24.8, 28.9, 29.1, 29.2, 29.3, 31.7, 33.8, 60.9, 63.8, 68.7, 70.2, 70.8, 71.7, 72.7, 72.9, 73.3, 81.6, 92.5, 104.0, 173.4 ppm.

[6′-O-Dodecanoyl-4-O-(β-D-galactopyranosyl)-D-glucopyranose, lactose laurate] (**4b**) [27]. Yield: 44% (0.058 g). ^{1}H NMR (400 MHz, DMSO) δ: 0.86 (t, 3H, J = 6.6 Hz, CH$_3$), 1.19–1.30 [m, 16H, (CH$_2$)$_n$], 1.48–1.57 (m, 2H, CH$_2$CH$_2$COOR), 2.31 (t, 2H, J = 7.3 Hz, CH$_2$COOR), 3.17 (ddd, 1H, J_{2-1} = 4.0 Hz, J_{2-OH2} = 7.0 Hz, J_{2-3} = 9.5 Hz, H^2), 3.27 (dd, 1H, $J_{4-3} \cong J_{4-5}$ = 9.5 Hz, H^4), 3.33–3.38 (m, 2H, H^8, H^9), 3.56 (dd, 1H, $J_{3-2} \cong J_{3-4}$ = 9.5 Hz, H^3), 3.60–3.67 (m, 3H, H^{6a}, H^{6b}, H^{10}), 3.68–3.76 (m, 2H, H^5, H^{11}), 4.09 (dd, 1H, J_{12b-11} = 4.5 Hz, $J_{12b-12a}$ = 11.5 Hz, H^{6a}), 4.17 (dd, 1H, J_{12a-11} = 8.5 Hz, $J_{12a-12b}$ = 11.5 Hz, H^{6b}), 4.20–4.24 (m, 2H, H^7, OH^3), 4.43 (dd, 1H, $J_{OH6-6a} \cong J_{OH6-6b}$ = 6.0 Hz, OH^6), 4.56 (d, 1H, J_{OH2-2} = 7.0 Hz, OH^2), 4.79 (d, 1H, $J_{OH10-10}$ = 5.0 Hz, OH^{10}), 4.86 (d, 1H, J = 5.0 Hz, OH), 4.90 (dd, 1H, $J_{1-OH1} \cong J_{1-2}$ = 4.0 Hz, H^1), 5.16 (d, 1H, J = 4.0 Hz, OH), 6.34 (d, 1H, J_{OH1-1} = 4.0 Hz, OH^1) ppm. ^{13}C NMR (100 MHz, DMSO) δ: 14.4, 22.6, 24.8, 28.9, 29.2, 29.4, 29.46, 29.48, 31.8, 33.8, 60.9, 63.8, 68.7, 70.2, 70.7, 71.7, 72.7, 72.9, 73.3, 81.6, 92.5, 104.0, 173.4 ppm.

[6′-O-Tetradecanoyl-4-O-(β-D-galactopyranosyl)-D-glucopyranose, lactose myristate] (**4c**) [27]. Yield: 65% (0.090 g). ^{1}H NMR (400 MHz, DMSO) δ: 0.86 (t, 3H, J = 6.6 Hz, CH$_3$), 1.17–1.32 [m, 20H, (CH$_2$)$_n$], 1.48–1.57 (m, 2H, CH$_2$CH$_2$COOR), 2.30 (t, 2H, J = 7.4 Hz, CH$_2$COOR), 3.16 (ddd, 1H, J_{2-1} = 4.0 Hz, J_{2-OH2} = 7.0 Hz, J_{2-3} = 9.5 Hz, H^2), 3.27 (dd, 1H, $J_{4-3} \cong J_{4-5}$ = 9.5 Hz, H^4), 3.31–3.37 (m, 2H, H^8, H^9), 3.56 (dd, 1H, $J_{3-2} \cong J_{3-4}$ = 9.5 Hz, H^3), 3.60–3.66 (m, 3H, H^{6a}, H^{6b}, H^{10}), 3.67–3.76 (m, 2H, H^5, H^{11}), 4.08 (dd, 1H, J_{12b-11} = 4.5 Hz, $J_{12b-12a}$ = 11.5 Hz, H^{12b}), 4.16 (dd, 1H, J_{12a-11} = 8.5 Hz, $J_{12a-12b}$ = 11.5 Hz, H^{12a}), 4.20–4.25 (m, 2H, H^7, OH^3), 4.47 (dd, 1H, $J_{OH6-6a} \cong J_{OH6-6b}$ = 6.0 Hz, OH^6), 4.60 (d, 1H, J_{OH2-2} = 7.0 Hz, OH^2), 4.82 (d, 1H, $J_{OH10-10}$ = 5.0 Hz, OH^{10}), 4.89 (d, 1H, J = 4.0 Hz, OH), 4.90 (dd, 1H, $J_{1-OH1} \cong J_{1-2}$ = 4.0 Hz, H^1), 5.19 (d, 1H, J = 4.0 Hz, OH), 6.37 (d, 1H, J_{OH1-1} = 4.0 Hz, OH^1) ppm. ^{13}C NMR (100 MHz, DMSO) δ: 14.4, 22.6, 24.8, 29.0, 29.18, 29.19, 29.4, 29.48, 29.51, 29.53, 31.8, 33.8, 60.9, 63.8, 68.7, 70.2, 70.7, 71.7, 72.7, 72.9, 73.3, 81.6, 92.5, 104.0, 173.4 ppm.

[6′-O-Esadecanoyl-4-O-(β-D-galactopyranosyl)-D-glucopyranose, lactose palmitate] (**4d**) [27]. Yield: 80% (0.116 g). ^{1}H NMR (400 MHz, DMSO) δ: 0.86 (t, 3H, J = 6.6 Hz, CH$_3$), 1.18–1.32 [m, 24H, (CH$_2$)$_n$], 1.47–1.58 (m, 2H, CH$_2$CH$_2$COOR), 2.31 (t, 2H, J = 7.4 Hz, CH$_2$COOR), 3.18 (ddd, 1H, J_{2-1} = 4.0 Hz, J_{2-OH2} = 7.0 Hz, J_{2-3} = 9.5 Hz, H^2), 3.27 (dd, 1H, $J_{4-3} \cong J_{4-5}$ = 9.5 Hz, H^4), 3.32–3.38 (m, 2H, H^8, H^9), 3.57 (dd, 1H, $J_{3-2} \cong J_{3-4}$ = 9.5 Hz, H^3), 3.61–3.67 (m, 3H, H^{6a}, H^{6b}, H^{10}), 3.68–3.76 (m, 2H, H^5, H^{11}), 4.09 (dd, 1H, J_{12b-11} = 4.5 Hz, $J_{12b-12a}$ = 11.5 Hz, H^{12b}), 4.17 (dd, 1H, J_{12a-11} = 8.5 Hz, $J_{12a-12b}$ = 11.5 Hz, H^{12a}), 4.20–4.28 (m, 2H, H^7, OH^3), 4.39 (dd, 1H, $J_{OH6-6a} \cong J_{OH6-6b}$ = 6.0 Hz, OH^6), 4.51 (d, 1H, J_{OH2-2} = 7.0 Hz, OH^2), 4.75 (d, 1H, $J_{OH10-10}$ = 5.0 Hz, OH^{10}), 4.82 (br s, 1H, OH), 4.90 (dd, 1H, $J_{1-OH1} \cong J_{1-2}$ = 4.0 Hz, H^1), 5.12 (br s, 1H, OH), 6.31 (d, 1H, J_{OH1-1} = 4.0 Hz, OH^1) ppm. ^{13}C NMR (100 MHz, DMSO) δ: 14.4,

22.5, 24.8, 29.0, 29.1, 29.2, 29.4, 29.46, 29.50, 31.7, 33.8, 61.0, 63.7, 68.7, 70.2, 70.8, 71.7, 72.7, 72.9, 73.3, 81.6, 92.5, 104.0, 173.4 ppm.

2.4. Surface Tension Measurements

Surface tension of different concentrations of surfactant solutions in water was measured using a platinum cylindrical rod probe with wetted length of 1.6 mm (K100-Krüss force tensiometer, Hamburg, Germany) at room temperature. Approximately 1 mL of each surfactant solution was placed onto a Teflon plate and the surface of the liquid was aspirated to remove any remaining impurities. Then, the rod probe was immersed 2 mm into the liquid. Data are expressed as the mean of three repeated measurements performed at room temperature. The critical micelle concentration and the surface tension at the CMC (γCMC) were calculated through the straight-line interception method, while the Gibbs surface excess (Γ_{max}) was calculated from the following equation:

$$\Gamma_{max} = \frac{1}{2.303 \times n \times R \times T} \left(\frac{\delta_\gamma}{\delta logC} \right) \tag{1}$$

where T is the absolute temperature, R is the gas constant (8.314 J/mol K), C is the surfactant concentration, n = 1 for a non-ionic candidate. $\delta_\gamma / \delta logC$ was calculated from the maximum slope of the plot surface tension vs. surfactant concentration in the linear region before CMC.

The minimum area per surfactant molecule at the air-water interface (A_{min}) was determined as follow:

$$A_{min} = \frac{10^{18}}{N \times \Gamma_{max}} \tag{2}$$

where N is the Avogadro number.

2.5. MTT Cell Viability Assays

Caco-2 and Calu-3 cells were seeded in sterile 96-well culture plates at a density of 3×10^4 cells per well. The cells were incubated to attain at least 80% confluence before the experiment. Stock solutions of surfactants were prepared in phosphate buffered saline (PBS). They were diluted at various concentrations (from 0.0078 to 1 mg/mL) in cell culture medium before added to the cells. Complete culture media were used as control. The cytotoxic effect of each surfactant was evaluated using the MTT cell viability assay. After 24 h of incubation, surfactant solution was discarded and replaced by MTT solution (0.8 mg/mL). The cells were subjected to MTT treatment for 2 h. Formazan crystals formed were then dissolved in absolute isopropanol and incubated with gentle shaking at room temperature for 15 min. Absorbance was measured at 570 nm using a microplate reader (Multiskan™ GO Microplate Spectrophotometer Thermo Scientific, Waltham, MA, USA). Percentage of viable cells was calculated using untreated cells as control with 100% cell viability. The percentage of viable cells was plotted against log concentration of the surfactants. IC_{50} (mg/mL), the concentration of surfactant that caused a 50% reduction in cell viability was calculated by fitting the experimental data with dose–response model (Prism 6, Version 6.0b, GraphPad Software).

2.6. Lactate Dehydrogenase (LDH) Release Assay

LDH assay was used to evaluate the membrane disruption effect exhibited by the surfactants. Caco-2 and Calu-3 cells were seeded in sterile 96-well culture plates at a density of 3×10^4 cells per well. Surfactant solutions (at the same concentration as in MTT assay described above) were added to the cells and incubated at 37 °C for 24 h. Triton X-100 at 1% v/v was used as positive control. LDH release assay was conducted according to the manufacturer's protocol. The percentage of released LDH was calculated relative to the controls by taking samples treated with Triton X-100 as complete LDH release and untreated cells as nil LDH release.

The concentration of surfactant that caused a 50% release of LDH (IC_{50}, mM), was calculated by fitting the experimental data with dose–response model (Prism 6, Version 6.0b, GraphPad Software).

2.7. Mitochondrial Membrane Potential (JC-1 Assay)

Caco-2 and Calu-3 cells were seeded in sterile 96 well plates at a density of 1×10^4 cells per well and cultured for 24 h. As above, surfactant solutions were applied in Hank's balanced salt solution (HBSS) for 24 h. One millimolar FCCP was employed as the positive, mitochondrial depolarizing control. Following exposure, treatments were removed and cells were washed twice with PBS prior to the addition of 50 µL (5 µg/mL) JC-1 dye diluted in complete DMEM (without antibiotics) per well for 15 min at 37 °C. Dye solution was then removed and wells washed with PBS followed by addition of 50 µL/well PBS prior to measuring fluorescence at 550/600 nm ($\lambda_{ex}/\lambda_{em}$) for detection of JC-1 J-aggregates and 485/535 nm ($\lambda_{ex}/\lambda_{em}$) for detection of JC-1 monomers. A ratio between JC-1 aggregates and JC-1 monomer signals was then taken, and data normalized by setting the untreated control as a value of 1.0 and the positive control (1.0 mM FCCP) as a value of 0.0.

2.8. Caspase 3/7 Activation (CellEvent™ Assay)

Caco-2 and Calu-3 cells were seeded in sterile 96 well plates at a density of 1×10^4 cells per well and cultured for 24 h. Following 24 h exposure on cells, surfactant solutions were removed, and cells washed twice with PBS followed by the addition of 100 µL 1.0% CellEvent™ Caspase-3/7 detection reagent diluted in HBSS buffer per well for 60 min. Fluorescence was then analyzed at 490/540 nm ($\lambda_{ex}/\lambda_{em}$), and data presented normalized to the untreated control set as a value of 1.0.

2.9. Nuclear Membrane Permeability (CellTox™ Green Cytotoxicity Assay)

Caco-2 and Calu-3 cells were seeded at a density of 1×10^4 cells per well in sterile 96 well plates for 24 h prior to assaying. Cells were exposed to treatments for 24 h, followed by the addition of 100 µL (2×) CellTox™ Green reagent (1:500 dilution of CellTox™ Green Dye in Assay Buffer) per well. The resulting solution was incubated at room temperature for 15 min and fluorescence then measured at 495/519 nm ($\lambda_{ex}/\lambda_{em}$). CellTox™ green signals were normalized by setting the untreated control as 0% and the positive control (1% Triton X-100) as 100% permeabilization of cell nuclei.

2.10. Measurement of Trans-Epithelial Electrical Resistance (TEER)

Caco-2 and Calu-3 cells were seeded at a density of 2×10^5 cells per well on filter inserts (Transwell® Permeable Support 12 mm Insert, Corning Life Sciences, Tewksbury, MA, USA) and cultured to confluence under air-liquid interface conditions. Culture media on the baso-lateral sides of the cells were changed every 24 h. For TEER measurements, culture medium was discarded from the cell layer and replaced with Kreb's Balanced Saline Solutions (KBSS) on both the apical and baso-lateral sides of the monolayers. Cell layers were allowed equilibrating in KBSS at 37 °C, 5% CO_2 for 45 min prior to sample application. Baseline TEER was measured before the treatment with surfactants. For each surfactant, concentrations that caused 50% cell viability, and the highest concentration that maintained 100% cell viability (according to the MTT assay) were added to the apical sides of the cell layers and incubated for 2 h. TEER was then measured at 5, 30, 60, 90 and 120 min after surfactant addition. Between TEER measurements, cells were incubated at normal cell culture conditions. After 120 min, surfactant was removed, and culture media were added to both sides of the filter inserts. TEER measurement was conducted again after 24 h to evaluate the recovery of cell monolayers. A volt-ohmmeter (Millcell® ERS-2 Voltohmmeter, Millipore, Burlington, MA, USA) equipped with a pair of electrodes was used for TEER measurement. Baseline TEER measured from cell layers incubated in KBSS was used as control and the change in TEER was presented as a percentage relative to baseline value. Three independent experiments were performed in duplicate.

3. Results and Discussion

3.1. Surface Tension and CMC Determination

Figure 1 shows the variation of surface tension over concentrations for each lactose fatty acid monoester. From the plotted curves, it is possible to observe the relevant influence of the carbon chain length on the surface properties of the amphiphiles.

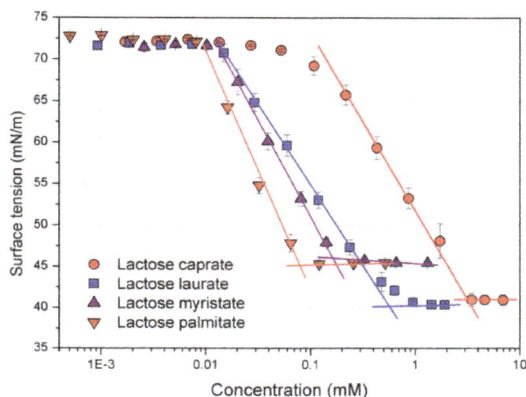

Figure 1. Surface tension (mN/m) vs. concentration (mM) plot for the lactose fatty acid monoester surfactants. Surface tension data are the mean of three repeated measurements (n = 3) performed at room temperature. The CMC (critical micelle concentration) is calculated from the straight-line interception method [28].

A clear relationship between the calculated CMC values (Table 1) and the carbon chain length can be established.

Table 1. Air-water surface parameters (critical micelle concentration (CMC), surface tension at CMC (γCMC), maximum surface excess (Γ_{max}) and minimum area per surfactant molecule (A_{min})) of the synthetized lactose fatty acid monoesters determined by tensiometry.

Entry	CMC (mM)	γCMC (mN/m)	$\Gamma_{max} \times 10^{-6}$ (mol/m^2)	A_{min} (Å^2)
Lactose caprate	2.58 ± 0.32	40.6 ± 0.04	9.52 ± 0.11	17.46 ± 0.25
Lactose laurate	0.55 ± 0.02	40.4 ± 0.02	9.52 ± 0.05	17.45 ± 0.09
Lactose myristate	0.14 ± 0.05	45.6 ± 0.19	8.37 ± 0.46	19.86 ± 0.80
Lactose palmitate	0.08 ± 0.03	45.1 ± 0.33	6.46 ± 0.11	25.69 ± 0.43

Indeed, lactose esters with longer carbon chains show a lower CMC because of the higher hydrophobicity. This translates in a lower water solubility and micellization reasonably occurs at lower concentrations. These results agree with those previously reported by Becerra et al. and Garofalakis et al. [24,29].

The surface tension at the CMC (γCMC) was calculated to be around 40 mN/m for lactose caprate and lactose laurate, while it was around 45 mN/m for derivatives with a longer hydrocarbon chain (C14 and C16), demonstrating the potential application of these compounds as surface-active agents (Table 1).

The absorption of the surfactants at the interface is described by the maximum surface excess concentration (Γ_{max}), according to the Gibbs isotherm.

The packing ability of surfactants at the interface is influenced by both the hydrocarbon chain length and polar head group. Surfactants with the bulkiest organization are generally characterized by a higher area per surfactants (A_{min}). In fact, as previously reported, A_{min} depends not only on the hydrophilic head group dimensions (number of hydroxyl group), but also on packing and stereochemistry of the whole structure [29].

According to Becerra et al., the surface excess is inversely dependent on the hydrocarbon chain length, therefore as the carbon chain length increase, the Γ_{max} decreases. Conversely, the area occupied by each molecule of surfactant increases as the carbon chain length increases [24]. Lactose caprate and lactose laurate, characterized by short hydrocarbon chain lengths, showed the highest Γ_{max}, suggesting the organization in a more packed monolayer as indicated by the lower area per molecule.

3.2. Biocompatibility Studies

3.2.1. MTT and LDH Assays on Calu-3 and Caco-2 Cells

MTT and LDH assays were carried out to assess the cytotoxicity of various concentration of lactose esters on Calu-3 and Caco-2 cells after 24 h exposure.

Results from the MTT assay (Figure 2) clearly suggest that cell viability of Calu-3 and Caco-2 cells is influenced by both carbon chain length and surfactant concentration. It is interesting to notice how, by increasing the carbon chain length of the synthetized surfactants, cell viability decreases at lower concentrations.

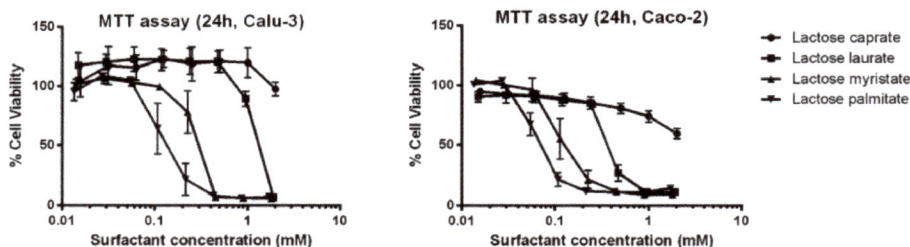

Figure 2. MTT assay of the lactose ester surfactants on Calu-3 and Caco-2 cell lines. The graph plots cell viability (%) as a function of different surfactant concentrations. Data are expressed as mean $\pm$ SD ($n = 3$).

A similar toxicological profile of lactose surfactants was observed when tested on both Caco-2 and Calu-3 cell lines.

Besides the MTT assay, another commonly employed in vitro cytotoxicity assay (LDH assay) was performed. The LDH assay highlights the effect of lactose esters on the cell membrane integrity, confirming the influence of the carbon chain length on the surfactant cytotoxicity on both cell lines (Figure 3).

A comparison on the cytotoxicity of lactose surfactants can be performed by calculation IC_{50} values, which is the concentration of surfactant that causes 50% maximum effect, in terms of 50% reduction of viable cells (MTT assay) or 50% release of LDH (LDH assay) (Table 2).

IC_{50} values decrease from lactose caprate to lactose palmitate independently from the cytotoxicity tests (MTT or LDH assay) or cell lines (Calu-3 and Caco-2). Indeed, for lactose caprate surfactant an IC_{50} value cannot be calculated since it is higher than the tested concentration range, confirming it has the lowest cytotoxicity. For the other lactose surfactants, it is noted that comparable IC_{50} values were calculated from the LDH assay between the two cell lines, while slightly higher IC_{50} values were found in Calu-3 with respect to Caco-2 from the MTT assay.

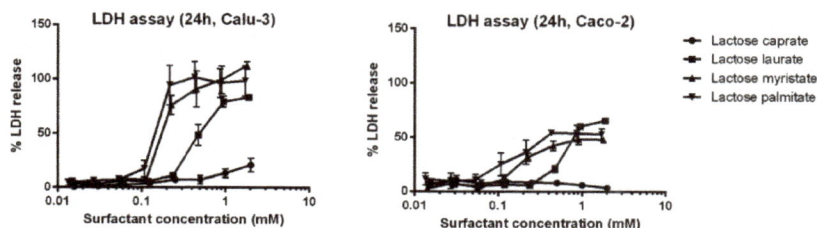

Figure 3. LDH assay of the series of lactose surfactants. The graph plots LDH release (%) from Calu-3 and Caco-2 cell lines as a function of different surfactant concentrations. Data are expressed as mean $\pm$ SD ($n = 3$).

Table 2. MTT and LDH cytotoxicity studies of the lactose ester surfactants on Calu-3 and Caco-2 cells. IC_{50} is the concentration of surfactant that causes 50% maximum effect, thus 50% reduction of viable cells (MTT assay) or 50% release of LDH (LDH assay).

Entry	MTT Assay IC_{50} (mM)		LDH Assay IC_{50} (mM)	
	Calu-3	Caco-2	Calu-3	Caco-2
Lactose caprate	>2	>2	>2	>2
Lactose laurate	1.069	0.376	0.452	0.597
Lactose myristate	0.261	0.112	0.189	0.194
Lactose palmitate	0.122	0.060	0.142	0.163

Interestingly, previous studies demonstrate the relationship between the hydrocarbon chain length and the cytotoxicity of sugar-based surfactants. The cytotoxic effect results from the interplay of different factors such as the ability of the hydrocarbon chain to insert into the lipid bilayer and to perturb membrane as well as the availability of free surfactant molecules, as indicated by CMC value [30,31]. Perinelli et al. recently investigated the correlation between the CMC and the cytotoxicity of *N*-decanoyl amino acid-based surfactants with different polar head groups. The authors demonstrated that toxicity is affected by both the polar head and the hydrocarbon chain length, with the latter parameter causing the main effect [32,33].

Lactose palmitate, which is characterized by the lowest CMC (0.08 mM), demonstrated the highest cytotoxicity in both cell lines. The calculated IC_{50} values for lactose palmitate, were 0.122 mM (Calu-3) and 0.060 mM (Caco-2) for the MTT assay and 0.142 mM (Calu-3) and 0.194 mM (Caco-2) for the LDH assay, respectively.

Moreover, IC_{50} values were compared to the CMC values, since it has already been demonstrated that surfactants with high cytotoxicity, show IC_{50} values lower than the CMC [33,34]. All the surfactants demonstrated IC_{50} values higher or comparable to the CMC in both cell lines (MTT and LDH assays), showing a low toxicity potential of the investigated lactose ester series on the two selected cell lines under defined conditions. This result obtained on cell-based methods in vitro is a preliminary evaluation of the toxicological profile of these surfactants, which should be confirmed by in vivo studies to assess the safety of these amphiphiles for pharmaceutical applications.

3.2.2. JC-1 Assay to Monitor Mitochondrial Health on Caco-2 and Calu-3

To examine the effect of lactose surfactants on the variation of mitochondrial membrane potential ($\Delta\Psi_m$), the ratiometric dye JC-1 assay was employed. The JC-1 dye readily permeates across the cell plasma membrane where it specifically accumulates in active mitochondria, in a potential dependent way. When present in the mitochondria, the dye forms J-aggregates, emitting fluorescence at red 595 nm wavelength, distinct from the dye presents in the cytoplasm which remains in monomeric form emitting fluorescence at green 530 nm wavelength [34]. Mitochondrial depolarization, due to the dissipation of negative charges across the mitochondrial membrane because of mitochondrial disruption, is consequently indicated by a decrease in the J-aggegrate:monomer intensity ratio, thus representing an arbitrary value for $\Delta\Psi_m$.

The effect of different concentration of lactose surfactants on the mitochondrial membrane potential is reported in Figure 4.

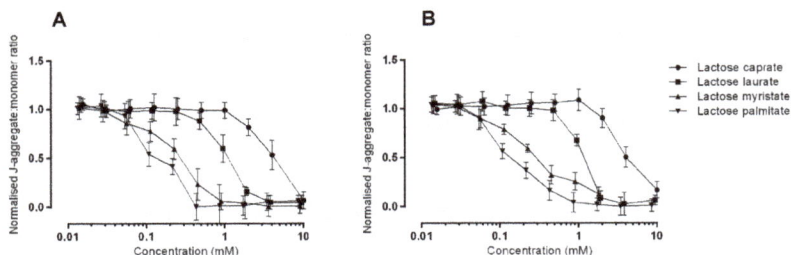

Figure 4. Mitochondrial membrane potential as measured by JC-1 assay in (**A**) Caco-2 and (**B**) Calu-3 cells. Responses are relative to those induced by untreated (HBSS buffer) which were set to a value of 1.0 and to 1.0 mM FCCP (carbonyl cyanide 4-(trifluoromethoxy) phenylhydrazone), known to induce total depolarization of mitochondrial membrane which were set to a value of 0.0. Data represents mean ± SD of triplicates from three independent experiments except for data for Caco-2 dosing of lactose myristate 3.6 mM and 9.0 mM, which comes from one repeat.

Loss of mitochondrial membrane potential is influenced by both concentration and hydrocarbon chain length of the tested surfactants, thus reflecting the results obtained from the MTT and LDH assays. In general, all the surfactants exert a similar toxicological profile in the two cell lines. When applied at the same concentrations, the highest cytotoxic effect is observed with lactose palmitate, as indicated by the lower J-aggretates:J-monomers ratio.

It is likely that the decline in metabolic activity measured by the MTT assay, observed above (Figure 2), is related to the interruption of mitochondrial respiration that would occur because of mitochondrial membrane potential disruption.

A common cause of mitochondrial depolarization is the induction of apoptosis. Both intrinsic and extrinsic apoptosis cause depolarization, which induces the release of key pro-apoptotic proteins/messengers from the mitochondria.

Depolarization of the mitochondrial membrane potential is commonly caused by the formation of pores or channels across the inner mitochondrial membrane, such as the permeability transition pore that is activated by the pro-apoptotic Bcl-2 family members [35]. Various accounts demonstrate that the dissipation of mitochondrial membrane potential occurs shortly after the permeabilization of the outer mitochondrial membrane [36]. Once the outer membrane is permeabilized, the soluble proteins present in the inner mitochondrial space are released [37,38], many of which play crucial roles in the induction of apoptosis. Therefore, the results gathered suggest the potentially involvement of apoptosis in surfactant toxicity and is explored further in the next section.

3.2.3. Caspase 3/7 Detection

Detection of activated effector caspases 3/7 is a well-recognized marker of programmed cell death. CellEvent™ Caspase-3/7 detection reagent is a four-amino acid peptide (DEVD) conjugated to a specific dye, thus inhibiting its ability to bind to DNA. The conjugated dye is non-fluorescent until the DEVD peptide sequence is recognized and cleaved by activated caspase-3/7, which in turn enables the dye to bind to DNA.

Figure 5 shows the detection of activated caspase 3/7 induced by the tested lactose surfactants as a function of the applied concentration, in Caco-2 and Calu-3 cells. Based on these results, it is reasonable to assume that the compounds induce caspase 3/7 activation, indicating that apoptosis is occurring. Furthermore, the induction of activated caspases occurs in a compound-dependent manner; therefore, as carbon chain length is increased, the potency to elicit apoptosis increases also since caspase 3/7 activation occurs at lower concentrations. Nevertheless, starting from a certain concentration, the normalized level of caspase 3/7 activation decreases, returning to the baseline values (or lower as is the case for lactose palmitate).

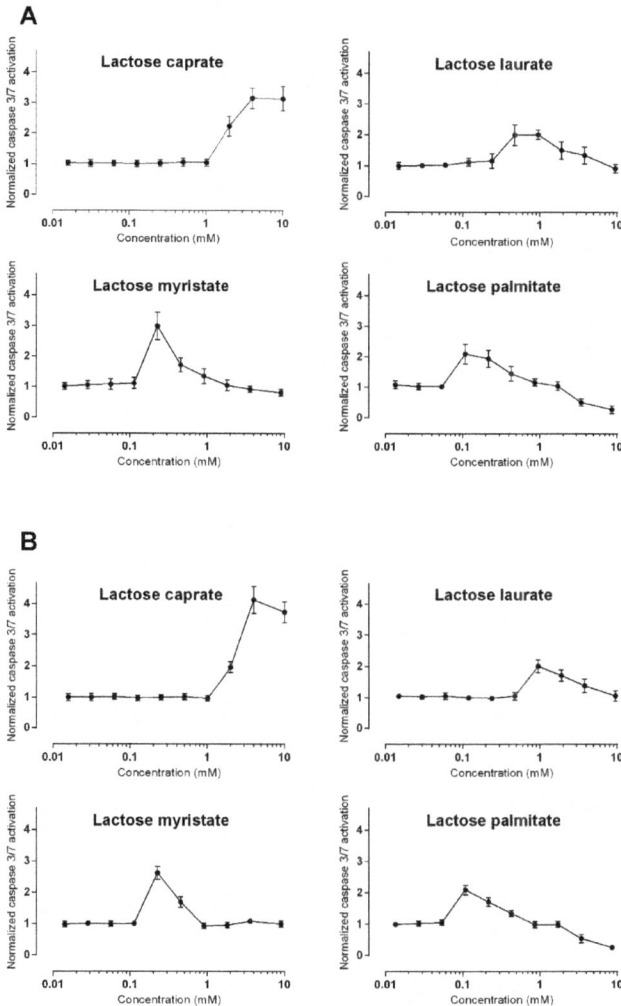

Figure 5. Detection of activated caspase 3/7 in (**A**) Caco-2 and (**B**) Calu-3 cells. Responses are displayed normalized to those induced by vehicle control (HBSS buffer). Data is presented as mean ± SD and represents triplicates from three experiments except for data for dosing of lactose myristate 3.6 mM and 9.0 mM in both Caco-2 and Calu-3 cells, which comes from one repeat.

These unusual profiles (Figure 5) observable for all the lactose surfactants may be explained by the dynamic and transient nature of caspase expression. Once cellular death has occurred, indicated by total loss of metabolic activity, the apoptotic process is likely over, therefore cellular expression of effector caspases is no longer necessary. When a cell population undergoes apoptosis, however, caspase levels significantly increase, and the breakdown of the cellular components occurs.

An alternative interpretation to the obtained results that should not be overlooked, is the induction of necrosis at higher concentrations rather than apoptosis, as was observed with quaternary ammonium surfactants [39]. This data set could therefore benefit from the inclusion of an intermediate exposure point (6 or 12 h) which could test the theory based on dynamic caspase expression discussed above. Additional approaches, such as the detection of apoptotic DNA fragmentation, would also aid in deciphering if apoptosis is occurring at higher surfactant concentrations or indeed if necrosis was prevalent.

3.2.4. CellTox^{TM} Green Cytotoxicity Assay

CellTox^{TM} green is a DNA binding dye that measures changes in membrane integrity that occurs because of cell death [40]. Signal generation occurs when the cell-impermeable dye binds DNA, and this can occur when DNA is released from cells. Thus, this assay detects for both loss of cellular and nuclear membrane integrity. Alternatively, compounds that enhance membrane permeability can also facilitate dye entry via permeabilization of the cell and nuclear membrane, thus binding to intracellular DNA. Figure 6 shows the results obtained from CellTox^{TM} green assay in Caco-2 and Calu-3 cells treated with different concentration of lactose surfactants. It is possible to observe a concentration and compound dependent increase in nuclear permeability.

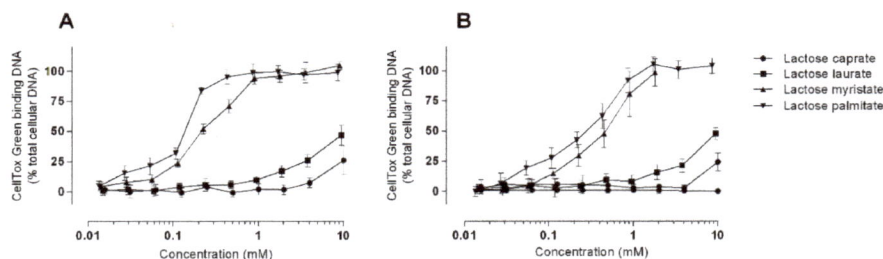

Figure 6. Nuclear membrane permeability as measured using the CellTox^{TM} green assay in (**A**) Caco-2 and (**B**) Calu-3 cells. Responses are relative to those caused by 1.0% Triton X-100, which were set to 100%. Data is presented as mean ± SD and represents triplicates from three independent experiments except for data for Caco-2 dosing of lactose myristate 3.6 mM and 9.0 mM, which comes from one repeat.

Permeabilization of the plasma membrane that may enable the CellTox^{TM} green dye to enter the cell is likely an effect of direct surfactant interaction and incorporation into phospholipid bilayer resulting in altered membrane fluidity, a commonly observed surfactant effect [41]. The increases in nuclear membrane permeability could then subsequently occur as a direct consequence of surfactant incorporation into the nuclear membranes. Additionally, increased permeability in nuclear membranes may be induced because of cellular apoptosis—a late event in apoptosis, mediating the formation of apoptotic bodies. Thus, taken together with the activation of caspase-3/7, increased nuclear membrane permeability at low surfactant concentrations may be occurring in an apoptotic manner. However, at higher concentrations the presence of LDH release alongside increased nuclear membrane permeabilization is likely indicative of surfactant-mediated perturbation of cellular membranes.

3.3. Trans-Epithelial Electrical Resistance (TEER) Studies in Calu-3 and Caco-2 Cells

TEER studies were performed in Calu-3 and Caco-2 cells to evaluate the ability of lactose surfactants to act as absorption enhancers, through transmucosal perturbation possibly by transiently opening tight junctions (Figure 7). Results obtained from TEER measurements should be interpreted carefully with the toxicological profile of the tested compounds to ensure that the changes in TEER was not due to the permeant damage of the membrane integrity. In fact, a transient modulation of tight junction opening commonly translates in a reversible effect on the TEER, while a permanent perturbation of the membrane integrity, on the other hand, is evidenced by a non-reversible effect on the TEER. However, it should also be noted that reversible effect on TEER could be a consequence of mechanisms other than tight junction opening.

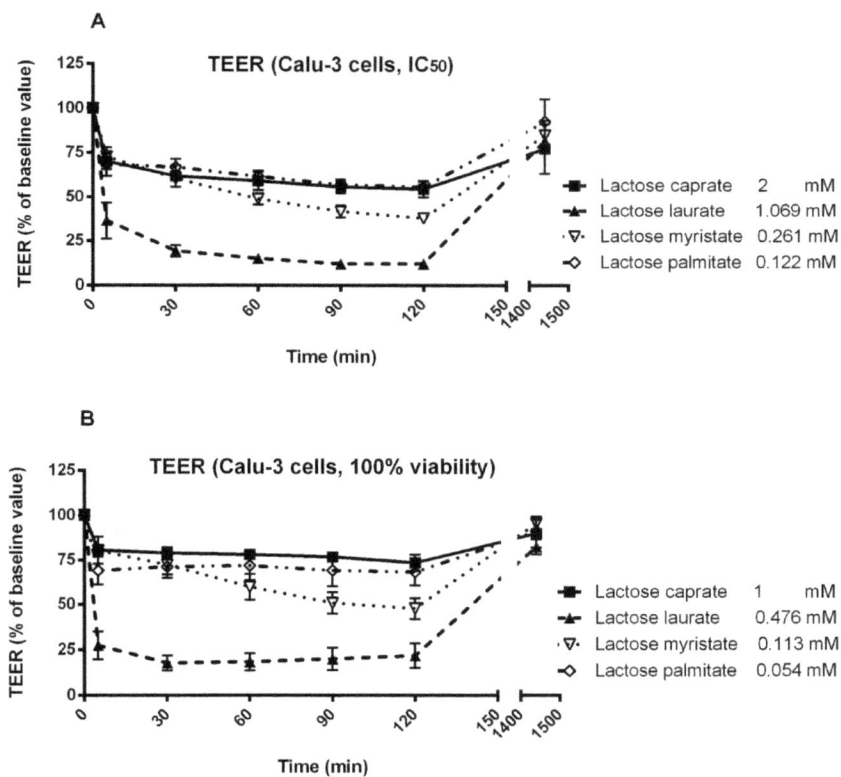

Figure 7. Effect of two different concentrations of lactose surfactants on Calu-3 cell monolayer TEER. (A) IC_{50} calculated from MTT assay and (B) the highest concentration that shows 100% viability from MTT assay. Data are presented as the mean of three independent experiments.

In the present study, two concentrations of each lactose surfactant were selected for TEER studies, specifically the IC_{50} calculated from MTT assay and the highest concentration that shows 100% viability in MTT assay, to evaluate the potential application of lactose surfactants within this range of concentrations. Hence, the effect observed on TEER for each surfactant must be correlated with the specific applied concentration, in addition to the structure of the compound (hydrocarbon chain length).

Regarding Calu-3 cells, lactose laurate was found to be the most effective surfactant in decreasing the TEER at both tested concentrations, while all the other surfactants showed only a moderate decrease in the TEER. Lactose laurate was effective in decreasing the TEER at the lowest applied concentration (0.476 mM; 0.025% w/v), with an effect comparable to the highest applied concentration (1.069 mM; 0.056% w/v). On the other hand, lactose caprate, applied at a similar concentration (1 mM), only slightly affected the TEER. It is noted that the surfactants were tested at different concentrations according to their toxicity profile. The ability of lactose laurate to lower the TEER significantly at the tested concentrations indicated that this surfactant exhibits a good balance between safety and efficacy.

Interestingly, TEER reversed to the initial value after 25 h with all the tested surfactants and concentrations, suggesting a transient effect on the membrane permeability, possibly by tight junction opening. To elucidate the mechanism and to confirm whether the surfactants could be serve as permeation enhancers, a macromolecule permeability assay could be performed in future study.

Regarding Caco-2 cells, different concentrations of surfactants were selected for TEER experiments, based on the IC_{50} calculated from the MTT assay (Figure 8). Due to the higher cytotoxicity displayed on Caco-2 cells, surfactants were tested at lower concentrations.

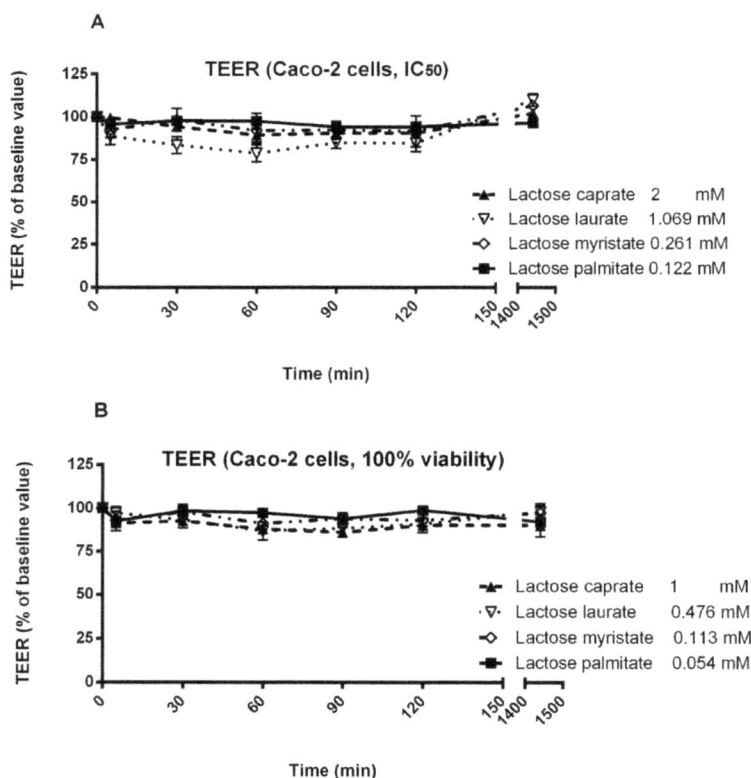

Figure 8. Effect of two different concentrations of lactose surfactants on Caco-2 cell monolayer TEER. (**A**) IC_{50} calculated from MTT assay and (**B**) the highest concentration that shows 100% viability from MTT assay. Data are presented as the mean of three independent experiments.

Caco-2 cells were significantly less sensitive than Calu-3 cells. This was mainly because Caco-2 cells were more prone to the cytotoxic effect of the surfactants, hence a much lower concentrations were used in the TEER study than on Calu-3 cells, rendering the rather poor response on this cell line. Lactose caprate tested at 2 mM, induced a more significant decrease in TEER in Calu-3 cells compared to Caco-2 cells. All the surfactants, tested at their IC_{50} concentration, only poorly affected the TEER, suggesting a reduced efficacy in tight junction opening or other membrane perturbation mechanisms. Nevertheless, lactose laurate showed a more significant effect, with a moderate reduction of TEER. On the other hand, all the surfactants tested at the lowest concentration (100% cell viability from MTT assay) did not induced a significant decrease of TEER.

4. Conclusions

This work reports an extensive and comprehensive study of the cytotoxicity profile of selected lactose-based surfactants, as function of their structure (different hydrocarbon chain length) and concentration. Cytotoxicity of the tested surfactants was found to be closely related to their hydrocarbon tail for this specific homologues series in cell cultures tested, thus increasing the hydrocarbon chain length also increased the cytotoxicity. Hence, higher IC_{50} values were observed in presence of more hydrophilic compounds (shorter hydrocarbon chain length). Moreover, comparing CMC and IC_{50} values reveals that the CMCs of the surfactants are lower or similar, thus showing a low toxicity potential on the selected cell lines. Furthermore, the compounds tested showed a comparable cytotoxicity in Caco-2 colonic epithelium and Calu-3 airway epithelium according to both MTT and LDH assay. When applied for 24 h the compounds induced, in a dose-dependent manner, depolarization of the mitochondrial membrane potential and permeabilization of plasma and nuclear membranes, as shown by JC-1 assay and CellTox^{TM} green assay, respectively. The activation of caspase-3/7 suggests apoptosis may play a role in surfactant-induced cell death, particularly at lower surfactant concentrations; however, at higher concentrations, surfactant-mediated membrane perturbation may possibly result in necrotic-like cell death. The initiating factor behind induction of apoptosis remains unknown but is likely associated to alterations in membrane fluidity and the subsequent effect on ion gradient homeostasis and intracellular redox environment. Interestingly, lactose laurate showed a good ability to decrease the TEER at a concentration close to IC_{50} value, while all the other surfactants showed only a moderate effect on membrane perturbation across cell monolayer.

Overall, results from cytotoxicity assays suggest a possible "mild behavior" of lactose monoester surfactants in term of toxicological profile, providing a preliminary evidence regarding one of the possible advantages of using these amphiphiles in different fields.

Author Contributions: Conceptualization, L.C., S.L., A.D., J.W.K.L. and S.S.; Methodology, S.L., R.C., M.C. and D.R.P.; Formal Analysis, S.L., M.C., R.C., D.R.P. and W.L.; Investigation, L.F., R.C., W.L. and D.R.P.; Resources, L.C., A.D., J.W.K.L. and S.S.; Writing-Original Draft Preparation, L.F. R.C., D.R.P., S.L. and L.C.; Writing-Review and Editing, L.C., A.D., S.L., D.R.P. and R.C.; Supervision, L.C., A.D., S.S. and J.W.K.L.

Funding: This research received no external funding.

Acknowledgments: The authors wish to thank Fabio De Belvis for the design and realization of the graphical abstract.

Conflicts of Interest: The authors declare no conflict of interest.

References

1. Plou, F.J.; Cruces, M.A.; Ferrer, M.; Fuentes, G.; Pastor, E.; Bernabé, M.; Christensen, M.; Comelles, F.; Parra, J.L.; Ballesteros, A. Enzymatic acylation of di- and trisaccharides with fatty acids: Choosing the appropriate enzyme, support and solvent. *J. Biotechnol.* **2002**, *96*, 55–66. [CrossRef]
2. Hill, K.; Rhode, O. Sugar-based surfactants for consumer products and technical applications. *Lipid* **1999**, *101*, 25–33. [CrossRef]

3. Neta, N.S.; Teixeira, J.A.; Rodrigues, L.R. Sugar Ester Surfactants: Enzymatic Synthesis and Applications in Food Industry. *Crit. Rev. Food Sci. Nutr.* **2015**, *55*, 595–610. [CrossRef] [PubMed]
4. Plat, T.; Linhardt, R.J. Syntheses and applications of sucrose-based esters. *J. Surfactants Deterg.* **2001**, *4*, 415–421. [CrossRef]
5. Szuts, A.; Szabó-Révész, P. Sucrose esters as natural surfactants in drug delivery systems—A mini-review. *Int. J. Pharm.* **2012**, *433*, 1–9. [CrossRef] [PubMed]
6. De, S.; Malik, S.; Ghosh, A.; Saha, R.; Saha, B. A review on natural surfactants. *RSC Adv.* **2015**, *5*, 65757–65767. [CrossRef]
7. Zhang, X.; Wei, W.; Cao, X.; Feng, F. Characterization of enzymatically prepared sugar medium-chain fatty acid monoesters. *J. Sci. Food Agric.* **2015**, *95*, 1631–1637. [CrossRef] [PubMed]
8. Zhao, K.-H.; Cai, Y.-Z.; Lin, X.-S.; Xiong, J.; Halling, P.; Yang, Z. Enzymatic Synthesis of Glucose-Based Fatty Acid Esters in Bisolvent Systems Containing Ionic Liquids or Deep Eutectic Solvents. *Molecules* **2016**, *21*, 1294. [CrossRef] [PubMed]
9. Cruces, M.A.; Plou, F.J.; Ferrer, M.; Bernabé, M.; Ballesteros, A. Improved synthesis of sucrose fatty acid monoesters. *J. Am. Oil Chem. Soc.* **2001**, *78*, 541–546. [CrossRef]
10. Zhang, X.; Song, F.; Taxipalati, M.; Wei, W.; Feng, F. Comparative Study of Surface-Active Properties and Antimicrobial Activities of Disaccharide Monoesters. *PLoS ONE* **2014**, *9*, e114845. [CrossRef] [PubMed]
11. Ferrer, M.; Comelles, F.; Plou, F.J.; Cruces, M.A.; Fuentes, G.; Parra, J.L.; Ballesteros, A. Comparative Surface Activities of Di- and Trisaccharide Fatty Acid Esters. *Langmuir* **2002**, *18*, 667–673. [CrossRef]
12. Lucarini, S.; Fagioli, L.; Campana, R.; Cole, H.; Duranti, A.; Baffone, W.; Vllasaliu, D.; Casettari, L. Unsaturated fatty acids lactose esters: Cytotoxicity, permeability enhancement and antimicrobial activity. *Eur. J. Pharm. Biopharm.* **2016**, *107*, 88–96. [CrossRef] [PubMed]
13. Perinelli, D.R.; Lucarini, S.; Fagioli, L.; Campana, R.; Vllasaliu, D.; Duranti, A.; Casettari, L. Lactose oleate as new biocompatible surfactant for pharmaceutical applications. *Eur. J. Pharm. Biopharm.* **2018**, *124*, 55–62. [CrossRef] [PubMed]
14. Kiss, L.; Hellinger, É.; Pilbat, A.-M.; Kittel, Á.; Török, Z.; Füredi, A.; Szakács, G.; Veszelka, S.; Sipos, P.; Ózsvári, B.; et al. Sucrose esters increase drug penetration, but do not inhibit p-glycoprotein in caco-2 intestinal epithelial cells. *J. Pharm. Sci.* **2014**, *103*, 3107–3119. [CrossRef] [PubMed]
15. Maher, S.; Heade, J.; McCartney, F.; Waters, S.; Bleiel, S.B.; Brayden, D.J. Effects of surfactant-based permeation enhancers on mannitol permeability, histology, and electrogenic ion transport responses in excised rat colonic mucosae. *Int. J. Pharm.* **2018**, *539*, 11–22. [CrossRef] [PubMed]
16. Aguirre, T.A.S.; Rosa, M.; Guterres, S.S.; Pohlmann, A.R.; Coulter, I.; Brayden, D.J. Investigation of coco-glucoside as a novel intestinal permeation enhancer in rat models. *Eur. J. Pharm. Biopharm.* **2014**, *88*, 856–865. [CrossRef] [PubMed]
17. Maher, S.; Mrsny, R.J.; Brayden, D.J. Intestinal permeation enhancers for oral peptide delivery. *Adv. Drug Deliv. Rev.* **2016**, *106*, 277–319. [CrossRef] [PubMed]
18. McCartney, F.; Gleeson, J.P.; Brayden, D.J. Safety concerns over the use of intestinal permeation enhancers: A mini-review. *Tissue Barriers* **2016**, *4*, e1176822. [CrossRef] [PubMed]
19. Touitou, E. Enhancement of intestinal peptide absorption. *J. Control. Release* **1992**, *21*, 139–144. [CrossRef]
20. Ghadiri, M.; Canney, F.; Pacciana, C.; Colombo, G.; Young, P.M.; Traini, D. The use of fatty acids as absorption enhancer for pulmonary drug delivery. *Int. J. Pharm.* **2018**, *541*, 93–100. [CrossRef] [PubMed]
21. Scholnick, F.; Sucharski, M.K.; Linfield, W.M. Lactose-derived surfactants (I) fatty esters of lactose. *J. Am. Oil Chem. Soc.* **1974**, *51*, 8–11. [CrossRef]
22. Staroń, J.; Dąbrowski, J.M.; Cichoń, E.; Guzik, M. Lactose esters: Synthesis and biotechnological applications. *Crit. Rev. Biotechnol.* **2018**, *38*, 245–258. [CrossRef] [PubMed]
23. Drummond, C.J.; Wells, D. Nonionic lactose and lactitol based surfactants: Comparison of some physico-chemical properties. *Colloids Surf. A Physicochem. Eng. Asp.* **1998**, *141*, 131–142. [CrossRef]
24. Becerra, N.; Toro, C.; Zanocco, A.L.; Lemp, E.; Günther, G. Characterization of micelles formed by sucrose 6-O-monoesters. *Colloids Surf. A Physicochem. Eng. Asp.* **2008**, *327*, 134–139. [CrossRef]
25. Neta, N.D.A.S.; dos Santos, J.C.S.; de Oliveira Sancho, S.; Rodrigues, S.; Gonçalves, L.R.B.; Rodrigues, L.R.; Teixeira, J.A. Enzymatic synthesis of sugar esters and their potential as surface-active stabilizers of coconut milk emulsions. *Food Hydrocoll.* **2012**, *27*, 324–331. [CrossRef]

26. Thelwall, L.A.W.; Hough, L.; Richardson, A.C. Sugar Acetals, Their Preparation and Use. U.S. Patent 4,284,763, 2 April 1980.
27. Sarney, D.B.; Kapeller, H.; Fregapane, G.; Vulfson, E.N. Chemo-enzymatic synthesis of disaccharide fatty acid esters. *J. Am. Oil Chem. Soc.* **1994**, *71*, 711–714. [CrossRef]
28. Mukherjee, I.; Moulik, S.P.; Rakshit, A.K. Tensiometric determination of Gibbs surface excess and micelle point: A critical revisit. *J. Colloid Interface Sci.* **2013**, *394*, 329–336. [CrossRef] [PubMed]
29. Garofalakis, G.; Murray, B.S.; Sarney, D.B. Surface Activity and Critical Aggregation Concentration of Pure Sugar Esters with Different Sugar Headgroups. *J. Colloid Interface Sci.* **2000**, *229*, 391–398. [CrossRef] [PubMed]
30. Lu, B.; Vayssade, M.; Miao, Y.; Chagnault, V.; Grand, E.; Wadouachi, A.; Postel, D.; Drelich, A.; Egles, C.; Pezron, I. Physico-chemical properties and cytotoxic effects of sugar-based surfactants: Impact of structural variations. *Colloids Surf. B. Biointerfaces* **2016**, *145*, 79–86. [CrossRef] [PubMed]
31. Li, X.; Turánek, J.; Knötigová, P.; Kudláčková, H.; Mašek, J.; Parkin, S.; Rankin, S.E.; Knutson, B.L.; Lehmler, H.-J. Hydrophobic tail length, degree of fluorination and headgroup stereochemistry are determinants of the biocompatibility of (fluorinated) carbohydrate surfactants. *Colloids Surf. B Biointerfaces* **2009**, *73*, 65–74. [CrossRef] [PubMed]
32. Perinelli, D.R.; Casettari, L.; Cespi, M.; Fini, F.; Man, D.K.W.; Giorgioni, G.; Canala, S.; Lam, J.K.W.; Bonacucina, G.; Palmieri, G.F. Chemical–physical properties and cytotoxicity of *N*-decanoyl amino acid-based surfactants: Effect of polar heads. *Colloids Surf. A Physicochem. Eng. Asp.* **2016**, *492*, 38–46. [CrossRef]
33. Perinelli, D.R.; Cespi, M.; Casettari, L.; Vllasaliu, D.; Cangiotti, M.; Ottaviani, M.F.; Giorgioni, G.; Bonacucina, G.; Palmieri, G.F. Correlation among chemical structure, surface properties and cytotoxicity of *N*-acyl alanine and serine surfactants. *Eur. J. Pharm. Biopharm.* **2016**, *109*, 93–102. [CrossRef] [PubMed]
34. Sakamuru, S.; Li, X.; Attene-Ramos, M.S.; Huang, R.; Lu, J.; Shou, L.; Shen, M.; Tice, R.R.; Austin, C.P.; Xia, M. Application of a homogenous membrane potential assay to assess mitochondrial function. *Physiol. Genom.* **2012**, *44*, 495–503. [CrossRef] [PubMed]
35. Marzo, I.; Brenner, C.; Zamzami, N.; Jürgensmeier, J.M.; Susin, S.A.; Vieira, H.L.; Prévost, M.C.; Xie, Z.; Matsuyama, S.; et al. Bax and adenine nucleotide translocator cooperate in the mitochondrial control of apoptosis. *Science* **1998**, *281*, 2027–2031. [CrossRef] [PubMed]
36. Kroemer, G.; Galluzzi, L.; Brenner, C. Mitochondrial Membrane Permeabilization in Cell Death. *Physiol. Rev.* **2007**, *87*, 99–163. [CrossRef] [PubMed]
37. Patterson, S.D.; Spahr, C.S.; Daugas, E.; Susin, S.A.; Irinopoulou, T.; Koehler, C.; Kroemer, G. Mass spectrometric identification of proteins released from mitochondria undergoing permeability transition. *Cell Death Differ.* **2000**, *7*, 137–144. [CrossRef] [PubMed]
38. Van Loo, G.; Demol, H.; van Gurp, M.; Hoorelbeke, B.; Schotte, P.; Beyaert, R.; Zhivotovsky, B.; Gevaert, K.; Declercq, W.; Vandekerckhove, J.; et al. A matrix-assisted laser desorption ionization post-source decay (MALDI-PSD) analysis of proteins released from isolated liver mitochondria treated with recombinant truncated Bid. *Cell Death Differ.* **2002**, *9*, 301–308. [CrossRef] [PubMed]
39. Inácio, Â.S.; Costa, G.N.; Domingues, N.S.; Santos, M.S.; Moreno, A.J.M.; Vaz, W.L.C.; Vieira, O.V. Mitochondrial dysfunction is the focus of quaternary ammonium surfactant toxicity to mammalian epithelial cells. *Antimicrob. Agents Chemother.* **2013**, *57*, 2631–2639. [CrossRef] [PubMed]
40. McDougall, M.; Dwight, S. Nucleic Acid Binding Dyes and Uses Therefor. U.S. Patent 8,598,198 B2, 3 December 2013.
41. Heerklotz, H. Interactions of surfactants with lipid membranes. *Q. Rev. Biophys.* **2008**, *41*, 205–264. [CrossRef] [PubMed]

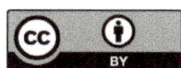

pharmaceutics

MDPI

Article

Hydrophobic Amino Acid Tryptophan Shows Promise as a Potential Absorption Enhancer for Oral Delivery of Biopharmaceuticals

Noriyasu Kamei, Hideyuki Tamiwa, Mari Miyata, Yuta Haruna, Koyo Matsumura, Hideyuki Ogino, Serena Hirano, Kazuhiro Higashiyama and Mariko Takeda-Morishita *

Laboratory of Drug Delivery Systems, Faculty of Pharmaceutical Sciences, Kobe Gakuin University, 1-1-3 Minatojima, Chuo-ku, Kobe, Hyogo 650-8586, Japan; noriyasu@pharm.kobegakuin.ac.jp (N.K.); hideyuki.ko192@gmail.com (H.T.); poffc263@s.kobegakuin.ac.jp (M.M.); pphgl074@s.kobegakuin.ac.jp (Y.H.); pohje089@s.kobegakuin.ac.jp (K.M.); pooww214@s.kobegakuin.ac.jp (H.O.); pofip292@s.kobegakuin.ac.jp (S.H.); podtk272@s.kobegakuin.ac.jp (K.H.)
* Correspondence: mmtakeda@pharm.kobegakuin.ac.jp; Tel.: +81-78-974-4816; Fax: +81-78-974-4820

Received: 24 August 2018; Accepted: 8 October 2018; Published: 10 October 2018

Abstract: Cell-penetrating peptides (CPPs) have great potential to efficiently deliver drug cargos across cell membranes without cytotoxicity. Cationic arginine and hydrophobic tryptophan have been reported to be key component amino acids for cellular internalization of CPPs. We recently found that L-arginine could increase the oral delivery of insulin in its single amino acid form. Therefore, in the present study, we evaluated the ability of another key amino acid, tryptophan, to enhance the intestinal absorption of biopharmaceuticals. We demonstrated that co-administration with L-tryptophan significantly facilitated the oral and intestinal absorption of the peptide drug insulin administered to rats. Furthermore, L-tryptophan exhibited the ability to greatly enhance the intestinal absorption of other peptide drugs such as glucagon-like peptide-1 (GLP-1), its analog Exendin-4 and macromolecular hydrophilic dextrans with molecular weights ranging from 4000 to 70,000 g/mol. However, no intermolecular interaction between insulin and L-tryptophan was observed and no toxic alterations to epithelial cellular integrity—such as changes to cell membranes, cell viability, or paracellular tight junctions—were found. This suggests that yet to be discovered inherent biological mechanisms are involved in the stimulation of insulin absorption by co-administration with L-tryptophan. These results are the first to demonstrate the significant potential of using the single amino acid L-tryptophan as an effective and versatile bioavailability enhancer for the oral delivery of biopharmaceuticals.

Keywords: tryptophan; oral delivery; insulin; GLP-1; intestinal absorption; amino acid; cell-penetrating peptide

---

1. Introduction

During the past few decades, cell-penetrating peptides (CPPs) have been established as potential tools for delivering bioactive macromolecules and lipidic or polymeric particulate carriers into cells via mainly covalent conjugation [1,2]. Conversely, our recent studies demonstrate that CPPs can dramatically accelerate the intestinal and nasal absorption of therapeutic peptides and proteins including insulin and the GLP-1 receptor agonist, Exendin-4, by the means of noncovalent co-administration [3–5]. In particular, we found that artificial cationic peptides such as octaarginine (R8) and the amphipathic sequence derived from antennapedia homeoprotein—penetratin—are CPPs that have shown the greatest potential to act as bioavailability enhancers for facilitating mucosal absorption of poorly absorbable peptides and proteins [3,6]. Several reports suggested that CPPs may enter into cells by multiple internalization mechanisms including endocytosis, mainly macropinocytosis and energy-independent direct translocation into the cytoplasm compartment [7–10].

Alternatively, in an earlier study examining the effects of arginine peptides with different chain lengths (4–16 residues), Futaki and coworkers found that the cationic amino acid arginine is a key common amino acid in arginine-rich CPPs, including the human immunodeficiency virus (HIV)-1 Tat peptide and identified an optimal arginine chain length that maximized cellular internalization efficiency [11]. We also examined the relationship between chain length of arginine peptides and their ability to enhance the intestinal absorption of insulin and confirmed that the effect of R8 was stronger than that of shorter or longer peptides [12]. Apart from the discussion regarding the effects of peptides with different numbers of amino acids, we recently found that the L-form of the amino acid arginine (L-arginine) could strongly enhance the intestinal absorption of insulin in its single amino acid form, although its effectiveness was relatively less than peptide forms of arginine [13]. Other studies suggest that when hydrophobic moieties such as stearyl groups or hydrophobic amino acids such as tryptophan are found within the peptide structure they synergistically enhance the potential of the original arginine-rich peptides [14–17]. R8 modified with a stearyl group and penetratin containing tryptophan residues are typical examples of CPPs with both cationic and amphipathic properties [18–20]. In fact, we demonstrated the stronger effect of penetratin over R8 on the intestinal and nasal absorption of various peptide and protein drugs [3,6,21,22]. These findings have shown the importance of the hydrophobic amino acid tryptophan for boosting the action of arginine-rich peptides in the facilitation of the intestinal absorption of insulin. It was expected that single amino acid tryptophan would affect the modulation of intestinal absorption of insulin similar to L-arginine. However, little is known about the ability of tryptophan to enhance the absorption of insulin.

Therefore, in the present study, we examined the effects of single amino acid tryptophan on the intestinal absorption of insulin and compared its effectiveness to other useful and conventional absorption enhancers including CPP (penetratin), tight junction-modulator (sodium caprate, C10) [23–25] and lipid membrane-disrupting bile acid (sodium taurodeoxycholate) [26,27]. Among the diversity of biopharmaceuticals currently available, the majority include peptides and proteins that must be administered as injectable forms [28]. Therefore, we further evaluated the applicability of tryptophan to enhance intestinal absorption of other biopharmaceuticals including peptide drugs (GLP-1 and Exendin-4) and different sizes of model hydrophilic macromolecules (dextrans, FD-4, FD-20 and FD-70; with molecular weights of 4000, 20,000 and 70,000 g/mol, respectively). Regarding the safe use of tryptophan as a potential absorption enhancer, we evaluated the irreversibility of action and possible cytotoxic effects on the intestinal mucosa. Furthermore, to better understand the mechanism of action, the structural isomeric difference and its specificity among hydrophobic amino acids on the ability of tryptophan and the possibility of intermolecular interaction between insulin and tryptophan in absorption enhancement were examined. As the possible transepithelial pathway utilized by tryptophan, the involvement of paracellular transport via tight junction opening effect of tryptophan itself or its major metabolite serotonin was examined. In addition, the ability of tryptophan to protect the peptide drugs from intestinal enzymatic degradation was tested.

2. Materials and Methods

2.1. Materials

Recombinant human insulin (27.5 IU/mg) and amino acids (L-tryptophan, D-tryptophan, L-phenylalanine, L-isoleucine and L-proline) were purchased from Wako Pure Chemical Industries, Ltd. (Osaka, Japan). Exendin-4 was synthesized by Sigma Genosys, Life Science Division of Sigma-Aldrich Japan Co. (Hokkaido, Japan). L-Penetratin (RQIKIWFQNRRMKWKK; capital letters indicate the L-form of amino acids) and GLP-1 were synthesized by Toray Research Center, Inc. (Tokyo, Japan). D-R8 (rrrrrrrr; lowercase letters indicate the D-form of amino acids) was synthesized by Scrum Inc. (Tokyo, Japan). Fluorescein isothiocyanate-labeled dextran with average molecular weights 4400,

20,000 and 70,000 g/mol (FD-4, FD-20 and FD-70, respectively), sodium taurodeoxycholate and Triton X-100 were purchased from Sigma-Aldrich Co. (Darmstadt, Germany). C10 was purchased from Tokyo Chemical Industry, Co. Ltd. (Tokyo, Japan). Methylcellulose (MC, METOLOSE) was purchased from Shin-Etsu Chemical Co., Ltd. (Tokyo, Japan). Human colon adenocarcinoma-derived Caco-2 cell line was purchased form the American Type Culture Collection (Rockville, MD, USA) at passage 18. Dulbecco's modified Eagle's medium (DMEM) with 4.5 g/L glucose, nonessential amino acids (NEAA), antibiotic mixture (10,000 U/mL penicillin, 10,000 µg/mL streptomycin and 29.2 mg/mL L-glutamine in 10 mM citric acid-buffered saline), 0.05% trypsin-ethylenediaminetetraacetic acid (EDTA) and Hanks' balanced salt solution (HBSS) were purchased from Gibco Laboratories (Lenexa, KS, USA). Fetal bovine serum (FBS) was purchased from Biowest (Nuaillé, France). Carboxymethyl dextran (CM5)-coated sensor chips were purchased from GE Healthcare (Little Chalfont, Buckinghamshire, UK). All other chemicals were of analytical grade and are commercially available.

2.2. Preparation of Mixed Solutions of Peptide Drugs and Amino Acids or CPPs

To prepare the insulin solution, specific amounts of recombinant human insulin were dissolved in 100 µL of 0.1 M HCl. The insulin solution was diluted with 0.8 mL of phosphate buffered saline (PBS, pH 7.4) (137 mM NaCl, 2.7 mM KCl, 8.1 mM Na_2HPO_4 and 1.47 KH_2PO_4 without calcium and magnesium) containing 0.001% MC, which prevents the adsorption of insulin and penetratin to the tube surface and was then normalized with 100 µL of 0.1 M NaOH. The final insulin concentration of the stock solution was 40 IU/mL. Stock solutions of other peptide drugs (GLP-1 and Exendin-4) and macromolecular compounds (FD-4, FD-20 and FD-70) were created by dissolving in PBS (pH 7.4) containing 0.001% MC (1.0 mg/mL and 8.0 mg/mL, respectively). Two times concentrations of amino acids (L-arginine, L- or D-tryptophan, L-phenylalanine, L-isoleucine and L-proline) were prepared using PBS (pH 7.4) containing 0.001% MC. To aid in the dissolution of high concentrations of hydrophobic amino acids such as L- or D-tryptophan and L-phenylalanine, the solutions were immersed in a water bath at 60 °C resulting in a clear solution. To create the solution used for the intestinal absorption study, two times concentrations of peptide drugs or macromolecular compounds and amino acid stock solutions were mixed together in equal volumes.

In the comparison study, specific amounts of L-penetratin, D-R8, C10, or sodium taurodeoxycholate were dissolved in PBS (pH 6.0 or 7.4) containing 0.001% MC at appropriate concentrations. For the in vitro study with Caco-2 cells, HBSS (LDH assay and transepithelial electrical resistance [TEER] measurement) or completed DMEM (WST-8 assay) were used instead of PBS to produce the test solution.

2.3. Animal Study

Animal experiments were performed at Kobe Gakuin University and complied with the regulations of the Committee on Ethics in the Care and Use of Laboratory Animals (approved as A16-15 and A17-4). Male Sprague Dawley rats weighing 180–220 g and male ddY mice weighing 30–40 g were purchased from Japan SLC, Inc. (Shizuoka, Japan), housed in temperature controlled rooms (23 ± 1 °C) with a relative humidity of 55 ± 5% and had free access to water and food during acclimatization. Animals were fasted for 18 h (rats) and 24 h (mice) before the experiments; however, they were allowed to drink water ad libitum.

2.4. In Situ Closed Ileum Loop Administration Study

Following anesthetization by intraperitoneal (i.p.) injection of sodium pentobarbital (50 mg/kg, Somnopentyl®, Kyoritsu Seiyaku Corp., Tokyo, Japan), which has been conventionally used in our insulin delivery study as confirmed to have a minimal effect on the blood glucose levels, rats were restrained in a supine position on a thermostatically controlled board at 37 °C. Additional i.p. injections of sodium pentobarbital (12.5 mg/kg) were administered every 1 h to maintain anesthesia. The ileum was exposed following a small midline incision made carefully in the abdomen. Its proximal to ileocecal junction segments (length = 10 cm) were cannulated at both ends using polypropylene tubing and ligated securely to prevent fluid loss. To wash out the intestinal contents, PBS warmed to 37 °C was circulated through the cannula at 5.0 mL/min for 4 min using an infusion pump. The cannulation tubing was removed, the segments were closed tightly and returned carefully to their original location inside the peritoneal cavity. Rats were kept on the board at 37 °C for an additional 30 min to calm biological reactions such as elevated blood glucose levels resulting from the stress imposed by surgery. After 30 min rest period, 0.5 mL of test insulin or other drug solution with or without amino acids and/or L-penetratin was administered directly into a 6 cm ileal loop created from the 10 cm pretreated segment. The insulin dose was administered at 50 IU/kg body weight (20 IU/mL) for all animal experiments. To examine dose dependency, the final concentrations of tryptophan were adjusted to 4, 8, 16 and 32 mM. In the comparison study with three hydrophobic amino acids or metabolite of L-tryptophan, the final concentrations of L-isoleucine, L-proline, L-phenylalanine and serotonin were 32 mM. In the study examining the synergistic effect of L-arginine and L-tryptophan, the final concentration of L-arginine was fixed at 40 mM. The doses of GLP-1 and Exendin-4 were both 1.25 mg/kg (0.5 mg/mL) and the doses of FDs were all 10 mg/kg (4 mg/mL). In the study examining the effect of pretreatment with L-tryptophan, D-R8, L-penetratin and other positive controls, ileal loop was exposed to these solutions during 30 min rest period after surgery and before the administration of insulin solution. For a part of above experiments involving pretreatment with L-tryptophan, C10 and sodium taurodeoxycholate for 30 min, an additional rest period of 30 min was added before the administration of insulin.

During the experiment, 0.25 mL blood aliquots were taken from the jugular vein at 0, 5, 10, 15, 30, 60, 120 and 180 min after dosing. The tuberculin syringes (1 mL, Terumo Corp., Tokyo, Japan) were heparinized by the standard procedure of coating the syringe wall with aspirated heparin and then expelling all the heparin. Plasma was separated by centrifugation at $13,400 \times g$ for 1 min and stored at -80 °C until analysis. The plasma concentrations of insulin, GLP-1 and Exendin-4 were determined using a human insulin ELISA kit (Mercodia AB, Uppsala, Sweden), GLP-1 ELISA kit (Wako Pure Chemical Industries, Ltd.) and Exendin-4 EIA kit (Phoenix Pharmaceuticals, Inc., Burlingame, CA, USA), respectively. The plasma concentrations of FDs were measured with a microplate fluorimeter (Synergy HT, BioTek Instruments Inc., Winooski, VT, USA) at excitation and emission wavelengths of 485 and 528 nm, respectively. The total area under the drug concentration time curve (AUC) from 0–3 h was estimated using the sum of successive trapezoids fitted between each set of data points in the time profiles of the plasma drug concentration.

2.5. Pharmacokinetic Analysis

The bioavailability of intestinal administered insulin was calculated relative to the subcutaneous (s.c.) route. Briefly, an insulin solution was prepared by dissolving an appropriate amount of insulin in PBS for s.c. injection (1 IU/kg). The peak plasma concentration (C_{max}) and time to reach C_{max} (T_{max}) were determined directly from the plasma insulin concentration–time curves. The total area under the insulin concentration–time curve (AUC) for 0–3 h was estimated from the sum of successive trapezoids between each data point. The relative bioavailability (BA) of insulin was calculated relative to the s.c. injection as follows:

$$BA (\%) = ([AUC]/dose)/([AUC]_{s.c.}/dose_{s.c.}) \times 100$$

2.6. In Vivo Oral Administration Study

After 24 h fasting, mice were dosed with insulin (50 IU/kg) with or without L-tryptophan (32 mM) (100 µL) by using oral gavage tube (i.d. $0.9 \times$ length 50 mm) (Natsume Seisakusho Co., Ltd., Tokyo, Japan). Blood glucose levels were measured (One Touch Ultra View, Johnson & Johnson K.K., Tokyo, Japan) by collection of blood (one drop) from a small cut in the tail vein at t = 0 (prior to dosing), 15, 30, 60, 120, 180, 240, 300 and 360 min after administration. Blood glucose levels are depicted as percentage of the initial value in same mouse. Mice were trained with oral dosing and tail cutting at 24 h and

60 min prior to actual drug administration to avoid the unexpected elevation of blood glucose levels during experiments.

2.7. Insulin Degradation in Intestinal Enzymatic Fluid

Intestinal fluid was collected from male Sprague-Dawley rats by inserting a Sonde needle into the upper portion of the small intestine and the intestine was then cannulated on the lower side (length = 20 cm) to remove the intestinal fluid. The contents of the small intestine were washed out with 30 mL of PBS. Because intestinal fluid contains a high lipid content, the efflux solution was treated with equal volume of methylene chloride to remove any lipids that might interfere with the analysis of insulin by HPLC. This removal of lipid contents was repeated five times. L- or D-tryptophan (8–32 mM as final concentration) was mixed with insulin (10 IU/mL final concentration) and incubated in the intestinal fluid at 37 °C. At 5, 15, 30, 45 and 60 min, 50 μL was collected and added to 50 μL of ice-cold mobile phase solution to terminate the reaction. L- or D-penetratin (0.25 mM as final concentration) and STI (1.25 mg/mL final concentration) were used as a CPP and positive conventional inhibitor, respectively. Insulin concentration was measured by HPLC (LaChrom Elite System, Hitachi High-Technologies Corporation, Tokyo, Japan) using the following conditions: mobile phase, acetonitrile, trifluoroacetic acid (0.1%) and sodium chloride (31:69:0.58, $v/v/w$); 20 μL injection volume; 1.0 mL/min flow rate; 220 nm wave length; analytical column (4.6 × 150 mm; 5 μm) with guard column (4.6 × 150 mm; 5 μm) (ChemcoPak Nucleosil 5C18, Chemco Plus Scientific Co., Ltd., Osaka, Japan).

2.8. Cell Culture

Caco-2 cells were cultured in 75 cm^2 culture dishes (Nippon Becton Dickinson, Tokyo, Japan) with 10 mL of culture medium. The culture medium consisted of DMEM containing 10% FBS, 0.1 mM NEAA, 2 mM glutamine, 100 U/mL penicillin and 100 μg/mL streptomycin (completed DMEM). The seeding density for cultivation was 8.0×10^5 cells/dish. The cells were maintained in an incubator at 37 °C, 95% relative humidity and 5% CO$_2$. The culture medium was replaced with fresh medium every second day for approximately 7 days until the cells reached 80% confluence, at which time they were subcultured. For the subculture procedure, the cells were detached from the culture dishes by trypsinization with 0.05% trypsin–EDTA, counted with a hemocytometer and transferred at the desired seeding density to new culture dishes or experimental wells. We used cells between passages 25 and 35.

2.9. In Vitro and In Situ the Lactate Dehydrogenase (LDH) Leakage

To assess the cytotoxic effects of L-tryptophan, the integrity of the cell membrane after treatment with the CPPs was examined by measuring the lactate dehydrogenase (LDH) released from the cytoplasm under both in vitro and in situ conditions.

In the in vitro assay, the Caco-2 cells were grown in 24-well plates with a 1.88 cm^2 culture area (Nippon Becton Dickinson) at the density of 1.0×10^5 cells/cm^2 and then grown in completed DMEM for 3 or 4 days. Before the addition of L-tryptophan, cell membranes were allowed to equilibrate in 0.5 mL of assay buffer for 30 min. HBSS containing 0.001% MC (pH 7.4) was added to the wells as the transport buffer. After a 30 min pre-incubation with transport buffer, the assay was initiated by replacing 50 μL of transport buffer with 50 μL of L-tryptophan stock solution (ten times concentration) or transport buffer. Various concentrations (300–2400 μM) of L-tryptophan were incubated in Caco-2-seeded wells for 120 min at 37 °C. The incubation buffer was collected and LDH released from the cytoplasm into the incubation buffer was determined using a CytoTox 96 Non-Radioactive Cytotoxicity Assay kit (Promega Corp., Madison, WI, USA). Cytotoxicity was expressed as the percentage calculated by dividing the absorbance of the vehicle (HBSS) or the L-tryptophan-treated sample by that of a sample treated with 0.8% Triton X-100, according to the instructions of assay kit.

In the in situ assay, various concentrations of L-tryptophan solution (16, 32 or 50 mM) with 50 IU/kg insulin were administered into rat ileal segments in the same manner as the closed loop administration study described above. For the trial with the highest concentration of L-tryptophan (50 mM), L-arginine (40 mM) was added as a solubilizing agent. For this test, 5% sodium taurodeoxycholate was used as a positive control. At 60 min after administration, the ileal loop was washed with 5.0 mL of PBS and then intestinal fluid was collected. After adjusting the collected intestinal fluid to a total volume of 6.0 mL with PBS, the activity of LDH (Unit) leaked into the intestinal fluid was determined using an LDH kit (Promega Corp.).

2.10. Cell Viability Assay

To examine the cellular viability of Caco-2 cells exposed to L-tryptophan, a WST-8 assay was performed with Cell Counting Kit-8 (CCK-8, Dojindo Laboratories, Kumamoto, Japan). The Caco-2 cells were grown in 96-well plates with a $0.33\ cm^2$ culture area (Nippon Becton Dickinson) to a density of $3.0 \times 10^4\ cells/cm^2$ and then grown in 100 μL of completed DMEM for 3 or 4 days. In this assay, the completed DMEM was used in place of the incubation buffer to prevent the possible loss of cell viability during total 5 h incubation in HBSS. First, 10 μL of L-tryptophan stock solution (eleven times concentration) or transport buffer was added to 100 μL of completed DMEM and the cells were incubated with various concentrations of L-tryptophan (600–2400 μM) for 2 h. Then, 10 μL of CCK-8 reagent was added to the wells and the cells were incubated for an additional 3 h to allow for the reductive reaction of WST-8. The resulting absorbances of the incubated solution in the wells were read with a microplate reader (Synergy HT, BioTek Instruments Inc.) at a wavelength of 450 nm. In this assay, 0.8% of Triton X-100 was used as a positive control, same as the LDH assay.

2.11. Transcellular Transport Assay

For TEER measurement, Caco-2 cells were grown in 12-well transwell plates with a $1.13\ cm^2$ culture area (collagen-coated polytetrafluoroethylene (PTFE) membrane with 0.4 μm pore size, Corning Inc., Corning, NY, USA). The cells were cultured to a density of $1.0 \times 10^5\ cells/cm^2$. The cells were grown in completed DMEM for 21 days until they achieved a constant TEER reading of $>500\ \Omega\ cm^2$, which indicated that tight junctions had formed in the monolayer. The culture medium was changed every second day and the electrical resistance was monitored by the method described below. Each well consisted of apical (top) and basal (bottom) chambers, which were separated by a collagen-coated polytetrafluoroethylene membrane with a pore size of 0.4 μm and a filter area of $1.12\ cm^2$.

In preparation for the assays, the cell membranes were allowed to equilibrate for 30 min in transport buffer; HBSS (pH 7.4) with 0.001% MC was added to the apical (0.5 mL) and basal (1.5 mL) chambers of the transwell. After a 30 min pre-incubation for equilibration, an initial TEER measurement was taken of the monolayer in each well and then 100 μL of transport buffer was removed from the apical chamber and replaced with 50 μL of insulin and 50 μL of L-tryptophan or serotonin stock solutions (ten times concentration) or transport buffer. L-tryptophan (600, 1200 or 16,000 μM) or serotonin (2.4 or 16 mM) was incubated with insulin (15 μM) in the apical chamber of the Caco-2-seeded transwell for 2 h. During the incubation, the Caco-2 monolayer was kept at physiological temperature (37 °C).

2.12. TEER Measurement

The TEER of the Caco-2 monolayer was measured to confirm cell growth and differentiation on the insert filter of the transwell using a Millicell ERS-2 (Millipore Corp., Bedford, MA, USA). Before seeding the Caco-2 cells, the electrical resistance of the insert filter in the medium was measured and subtracted from the total electrical resistance determined for the monolayer to calculate the intrinsic TEER of the monolayer. The TEER of the monolayer was measured at the end of the 2 h incubation to detect any negative effects of the applied L-tryptophan on the intercellular tight junctions. The TEER is expressed as a percentage calculated by dividing the TEER value ($\Omega\ cm^2$) at 2 h by the initial value.

2.13. Surface Plasmon Resonance (SPR)-Based Binding Assay

The intermolecular interactions between insulin and L-tryptophan or L-penetratin were analyzed by SPR (Biacore X-100, GE Healthcare). To measure the binding of L-tryptophan or L-penetratin to insulin, insulin was immobilized at the carboxymethyl dextran surface of a CM5 sensor chip by using an amine coupling method. For the immobilization procedure, insulin was diluted to a concentration of 50 μg/mL using acetate buffer at pH 4.5 and immobilized on the chip surface in separate flow cells at 5 μL/min for 7 min. Reference surfaces were prepared by amine coupling activation followed by immediate deactivation. For binding measurements, different concentrations of L-tryptophan or L-penetratin (2–200 μM) were injected for 90 s followed by an additional 90 s dissociation phase. At the end of each cycle, the surface was regenerated by a 30 s injection of 1 M NaCl. Measurements were carried out in HBSS (pH 7.4) supplied with 0.001% MC at 20 μL/min at 25 °C. Each sensorgram was determined by subtracting nonspecific binding on the surface of the reference flow cell from total binding on the immobilized-insulin surface.

2.14. Statistical Analysis

Each value is expressed as the mean and standard error of the mean (SEM) of multiple determinations. The significance of the differences in the mean values of multiple groups was evaluated using analysis of variance with Dunnett's test. IBM SPSS Statistics (version 24; IBM Corp., Armonk, NY, USA) was used for statistical analysis. Differences were considered significant when the *p* value was less than 0.05.

3. Results

3.1. Stimulatory Effect of L-Tryptophan on the Intestinal Absorption of Insulin

It was reported that tryptophan residues at position 6 and 14 in the penetratin amino acid sequence aid in lipid interaction in cell membranes and are therefore an important moiety involved in the cellular internalization of penetratin [18]. To test the ability of hydrophobic amino acid tryptophan as an absorption enhancer for insulin, we first conducted an in situ absorption study in which insulin was administered with various concentrations of the L-form of tryptophan (8–32 mM) into rat ileal closed loops. As shown in Figure 1A, the plasma insulin concentration increased after administration of insulin with L-tryptophan in a concentration dependent manner and with a late onset of action 30–60 min after administration. This result suggests that L-tryptophan has the potential to strongly enhance the intestinal absorption of insulin as single amino acid form. On the other hand, we confirmed the effect of the amphipathic CPP penetratin on the intestinal absorption of insulin. The effect of L-penetraitn shown in Figure 1A was consistent with our previous publication using L-penetratin [3,6], in which insulin co-administered with L-penetratin was absorbed immediately at 15 min post administration. The difference of action onset between L-tryptophan and L-penetratin suggested that L-tryptophan as single amino acid played a role in increasing absorption of insulin in a different way from tryptophan residues as a component of the peptide structure of L-penetratin. We further compared the effect of other hydrophobic amino acids such as phenylalanine, proline and isoleucine on the absorption of insulin. The results in Figure 1B show that there was no stimulatory effect on insulin absorption by these three hydrophobic amino acids suggesting that the bioenhancing effect is unique to tryptophan among the hydrophobic amino acids. The pharmacokinetic parameters are summarized in Table 1.

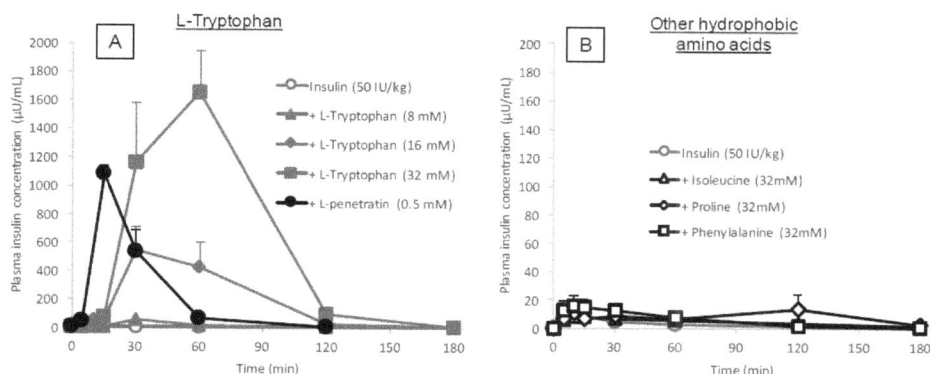

Figure 1. Time profiles of plasma insulin concentration after in situ administration of insulin (50 IU/kg) with or without L-tryptophan, L-penetratin or other hydrophobic amino acid additives into rat ileal loop. Panel (**A**), L-tryptophan (8–32 mM) or L-penetratin (0.5 mM); panel (**B**), hydrophobic amino acids (L-isoleucine, L-proline and L-phenylalanine, 32 mM). Each data point represents the mean ± SEM of *N* = 3–8, except for the group with L-tryptophan (8 mM, *N* = 2).

Table 1. Pharmacokinetic parameters following in situ administration of insulin with various amino acid additives, L-penetratin, or after pretreatment of amino acids or control reagents.

		Experiment	C_{max} (µU/mL)	T_{max} (min)	AUC (µU·h/mL)	BA (%)
Insulin (50 IU/kg)		8	10.6 ± 2.4	9.4 ± 1.1	8.5 ± 2.5	0.1 ± 0.0
+L-Tryptophan	(8 mM)	2	52.9	30	35.8	0.4
	(16 mM)	4	563.0 ± 162.4	45.0 ± 8.7	558.4 ± 195.2 **	5.8 ± 2.0 **
	(32 mM)	4	2008.2 ± 196.9	52.5 ± 7.5	1785.7 ± 153.5 **	18.7 ± 1.6 **
+D-Tryptophan	(16 mM)	3	84.7 ± 35.8	60.0 ± 0.0	75.4 ± 30.2	0.8 ± 0.3
	(32 mM)	3	723.5 ± 153.0	60.0 ± 0.0	606.3 ± 132.8 **	6.3 ± 1.4 **
+L-penetratin (0.5 mM)		4	1079.0 ± 54.4	15.0 ± 0.0	481.8 ± 85.0 **	5.0 ± 0.9 **
+Serotonin (32 mM)		3	258.3 ± 124.7	60.0 ± 0.0	304.8 ± 174.1	3.2 ± 1.8
Pretreatment study						
+PBS		4	1.7 ± 0.3	7.5 ± 2.5	2.0 ± 0.2	0.0 ± 0.0
+L-Tryptophan (32 mM)		4	1040.5 ± 455.9	18.8 ± 3.8	582.1 ± 229.2	6.1 ± 2.4
+D-R8 (0.5 mM)		3	22.7 ± 5.2	8.3 ± 3.3	22.5 ± 6.7	0.2 ± 0.1
+L-penetratin (0.5 mM)		3	356.3 ± 241.3	5.0 ± 0.0	141.0 ± 73.8	1.5 ± 0.8
+C10 (100 mM)		3	1574.8 ± 772.9	20.0 ± 5.0	1235.9 ± 686.2	12.9 ± 7.2
+Sodium taurodeoxycholate (5%)		3	4038.0 ± 1685.4	8.3 ± 3.3	2386.2 ± 1114.6 *	25.0 ± 11.7 *
Pretreatment with 30 min rest						
+L-Tryptophan (32 mM)		3	41.2 ± 11.2	11.7 ± 3.3	25.8 ± 5.4	0.3 ± 0.1
+C10 (100 mM)		3	165.1 ± 22.7	11.7 ± 3.3	128.3 ± 35.6	1.3 ± 0.4
+ Sodium taurodeoxycholate (5%)		3	393.7 ± 225.2	8.3 ± 3.3	203.3 ± 121.3	2.1 ± 1.3
Insulin s.c. (1 IU/kg)		3	133.8 ± 3.4	25.0 ± 5.0	191.2 ± 5.2	100

C_{max}, the maximum concentration; T_{max}, the time to reach the C_{max}; AUC, the area under the curve; BA, relative bioavailability compared to subcutaneous injection. Each data point represents the mean ± SEM of *N* =3–8, except for the group with L-tryptophan (8 mM, *N* = 2). * $p < 0.05$, ** $p < 0.01$, significantly different with corresponding control insulin (50 IU/kg).

3.2. Identification of the Ability of L-Tryptophan as the Oral Absorption Enhancer for Insulin

The above-mentioned results suggested that L-tryptophan has the ability to effectively increase the intestinal absorption of insulin. Therefore, the potential of L-tryptophan as oral absorption enhancer was further tested after in vivo oral administration of insulin to mice. As shown in Figure 2, the hypoglycemic reaction elevated after oral administration of insulin (50 IU/kg) with L-tryptophan (32 mM) suggested that L-tryptophan could enhance the oral absorption of insulin. The elevation in the blood glucose levels just after oral administration in all groups might be because of the stress by oral gavage, even though mice were trained before administration.

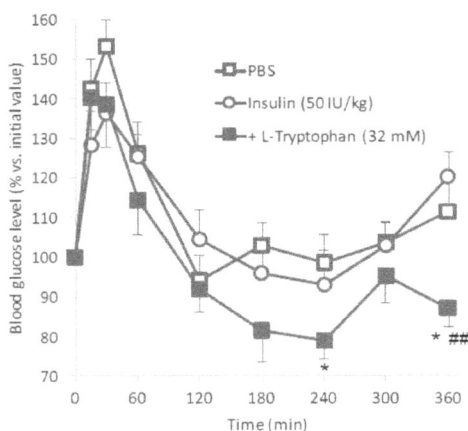

Figure 2. Blood glucose levels in mice following oral administration of insulin (50 IU/kg) with or without L-tryptophan (32 mM). Each data point represents the mean ± SEM of N = 6–8. * $p < 0.05$, ## $p < 0.01$, significantly different with PBS and insulin (50 IU/kg), respectively.

3.3. Applicability of L-Tryptophan to Enhance the Intestinal Absorption of Various Biopharmaceuticals

Although the mechanism involved in the absorption-stimulatory effect of L-tryptophan is still unclear, our results strongly suggest that L-tryptophan has potential as an effective absorption enhancer for the oral delivery of insulin. We additionally researched the ability of L-tryptophan to aid in the delivery of other biopharmaceuticals.

To examine the ability of L-tryptophan to assist in the transport of a range of differently sized potential drug cargo, we evaluated the effect of L-tryptophan co-administered with fluorescently labeled hydrophilic dextrans of various molecular weights (4400, 20,000 and 70,000 g/mol). As shown in Figure 3A–C, the intestinal absorption of all dextrans (FD-4, FD-20 and FD-70) was effectively enhanced by co-administration with L-tryptophan (32 mM), although the effectiveness of enhancement tended to decrease with increase in the molecular weight of the cargo compounds. Furthermore, the effect of L-tryptophan on the intestinal absorption of other peptide drugs, GLP-1 and Exendin-4, was examined. As shown in Figure 4A,B, these peptide drugs were efficiently absorbed in the presence of L-tryptophan (32 mM). Thus, L-tryptophan has the potential to enhance the intestinal absorption of a wide variety of biopharmaceuticals in a safe manner. The AUC values of dextrans and peptide drugs are summarized in Table 2.

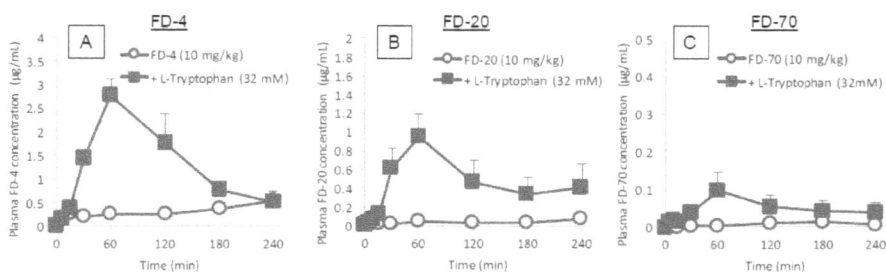

Figure 3. Time profiles of plasma concentrations of model hydrophilic macromolecules (FD-4, FD-20 and FD-70) after their in situ administration with or without L-tryptophan (32 mM) into rat ileal loop. Panels (**A**–**C**) show the absorption of FD-4, FD-20 and FD-70, respectively. Each data point represents the mean ± SEM of N = 3–8.

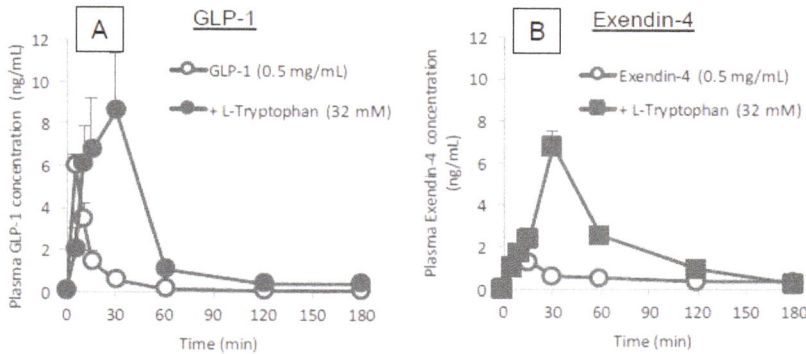

Figure 4. Time profiles of plasma concentrations of peptide drugs (GLP-1 and Exendin-4) after their in situ administration with or without L-tryptophan (32 mM) into rat ileal loop. Panels (**A**) and (**B**) show the absorption of GLP-1 and Exendin-4, respectively. Each data point represents the mean ± SEM of $N = 4$.

Table 2. AUCs following in situ administration of dextrans (FD-4, FD-20 and FD-70) with L-tryptophan into rat ileal loop.

	AUC (ng·h/mL)	
	−L-Tryptophan	+L-Tryptophan (32 mM)
FD-4 (10 mg/kg)	1194.2 ± 463.2	5512.7 ± 1034.9**
FD-20 (10 mg/kg)	146.0 ± 44.8	1973.2 ± 801.8*
FD-70 (10 mg/kg)	25.4 ± 24.6	205.6 ± 115.0
GLP-1 (0.5 mg/mL)	1.35 ± 0.27	6.35 ± 2.06*
Exendin-4 (0.5 mg/mL)	1.54 ± 0.62	6.17 ± 0.67**

AUC, the area under the curve. Each data point represents the mean ± SEM of $N = 3$–8. * $p < 0.05$, ** $p < 0.01$, significantly different with corresponding control without L-tryptophan.

3.4. Mucosal Cytotoxic Examinations for Intestinal Administration of L-Tryptophan

3.4.1. Effect of L-Tryptophan on the Membrane Integrity and Cell Viability in the Intestinal Epithelium

The intestinal absorption of insulin accelerated by co-administration with L-tryptophan might be attributed to the modulation of biological structures and functions in the intestinal mucosa. To establish the safety of L-tryptophan as a potential absorption enhancer for biopharmaceuticals, changes in the integrity of epithelial cell membranes, cellular viability and the tightness of the paracellular junctions after administration of L-tryptophan were examined.

Figure 5A,B shows the leakage of an intracellular protein, LDH, from intestinal epithelial cells after in situ administration into rat ileal loop (A) and in vitro exposure onto the epithelial model Caco-2 cells (B). In Figure 5A, the leakage of LDH was negligible after in situ administration of insulin with L-tryptophan at all tested concentrations (16 and 32 mM) and these measurements were significantly low when compared to the positive control (the administration of 5% sodium taurodeoxycholate). Similarly, in the in vitro assay (Figure 5B), no release of LDH into the media was observed after the exposure of Caco-2 cells to L-tryptophan at all concentrations (300–2400 μM). Figure 5C shows the viability of Caco-2 cells after applying L-tryptophan to culture media. The results indicate no decrease in cell viability after addition of L-tryptophan at all concentrations (600–2400 μM). The toxicity examinations suggest that L-tryptophan has no adverse effect on the intestinal mucosa and may therefore become a potentially safe absorption enhancer.

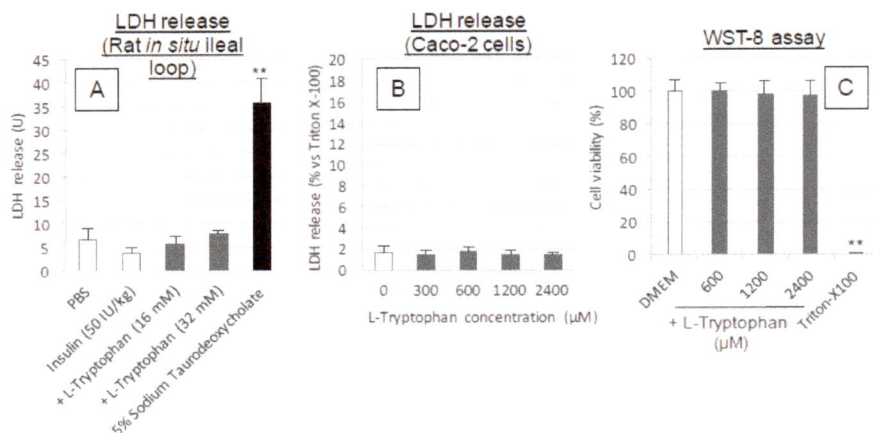

Figure 5. Cytotoxicity examinations after the exposure of intestinal epithelium to L-tryptophan. Panel (**A**), the LDH release in the intestinal fluid collected at 60 min after ileal administration of PBS, insulin (50 IU/kg) with or without L-tryptophan (16–50 mM) and sodium taurodeoxycholate (5%). Panel (**B**), LDH released from the cytoplasm into the incubation medium (HBSS) after incubation with various concentrations of L-tryptophan (200–2400 μM). The value is expressed as a percentage calculated by dividing the absorbance of the L-tryptophan treated medium sample by that of the sample treated with Triton X-100 (0.8%). Panel C, cell viability after incubation with various concentrations of L-tryptophan (600–2400 μM). Each data point represents the mean ± SEM of $N = 3$, 3 and 6–11 for panels (**A**–**C**), respectively. * $p < 0.05$, ** $p < 0.01$, significantly different with corresponding control PBS- (panel (**A**)), or DMEM- (panel (**C**)) treatment group.

3.4.2. Effect of Intestinal Pretreatment with L-Tryptophan on the Intestinal Absorption of Insulin

The results from the previous section suggest that L-tryptophan can enhance the intestinal absorption of insulin via functional and structural modification of the intestinal mucosa, while not exhibiting cytotoxicity (Figure 5). When further considering the safe use of absorption enhancers, it is important that these agents exhibit either no effect or only a temporal effect on the functions of the mucosal membrane since this membrane is an integral component of the defense system protecting against exogenous pathogens. To assess the reversibility of L-tryptophan activity, an insulin solution was administered to rat ileal loop after pretreatment with L-tryptophan (32 mM), CPPs (D-R8 and L-penetratin), or conventional enhancers (C10 and sodium taurodeoxycholate) for 30 min and then washing the pretreated ileal segment with fresh PBS.

As shown in Figure 6A, an increase in plasma insulin concentration was observed after the administration of insulin to the ileal loop pretreated with L-tryptophan and L-penetratin, however, the extent of insulin absorption was lower than the effect of co-administration with these enhancers (Figure 1A). In addition, the onset of insulin absorption could be shifted to an early time point, (5 min after administration of insulin), by pretreating withL-tryptophan. In contrast, pretreatment with C10 and sodium taurodeoxycholate had a stronger stimulatory response on intestinal absorption of insulin than L-tryptophan and L-penetratin (Figure 6B). When insulin was administered into the ileal loop after 30 min of pretreatment with L-tryptophan followed by washing and further rest for 30 min, the increase in the plasma insulin concentration was almost completely eliminated (Figure 6C), suggesting that the action of L-tryptophan was temporal and reversible. The pharmacokinetic parameters are summarized in Table 1.

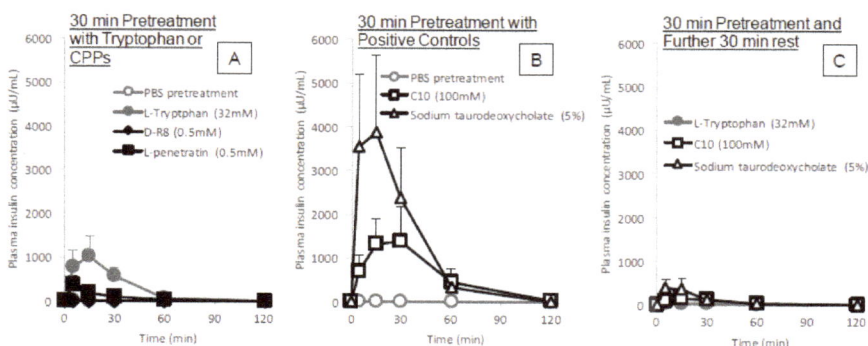

Figure 6. Time profiles of plasma insulin concentration after in situ administration of insulin (50 IU/kg) into rat ileal loop pretreated with L-tryptophan (32 mM), D-R8 (0.5 mM), L-penetratin (0.5 mM), C10 (100 mM), or sodium taurodeoxycholate (5%). In the results shown in Panels (**A**,**B**), insulin solution was administered immediately after washing the pretreatment solution from the ileal loop. For the results shown in Panel (**C**), insulin solution was administered at 30 min after washing out the pretreatment solution. Each data point represents the mean $\pm$ SEM of $N = 3$–4.

3.5. Mechanistic Analysis for the Intestinal Absorption of Insulin Facilitated by L-Tryptophan

3.5.1. Possibility of the Intermolecular Interaction between Insulin and L-Tryptophan

The above-mentioned results suggest that single amino acid L-tryptophan is unique in its ability to enhance the intestinal absorption of insulin. The binding affinity of L-tryptophan with insulin and/or possible activity of L-tryptophan in the modulation of biological functions and structures may explain its specificity for absorption enhancement. In this section, we analyzed the intermolecular interaction between insulin and L-tryptophan using a SPR-based assay.

Figure 7 shows the binding sensorgrams obtained from the assay. Various concentrations of L-tryptophan (2–200 µM) or L-penetratin (2–200 µM) were injected into the flow cells containing immobilized insulin. The resulting sensorgrams do not show an increase after the injection of L-tryptophan at any concentration (Figure 7A). For comparison, L-penetratin was bound to the insulin-immobilized flow cells depending on the applied insulin concentration (Figure 7B) in a manner consistent with our previous publications [29]. These results suggest that L-tryptophan can enhance the absorption of insulin without intermolecular interaction and that the modulation of mucosal epithelial structure might be important for the enhancement of intestinal insulin absorption mediated by L-tryptophan.

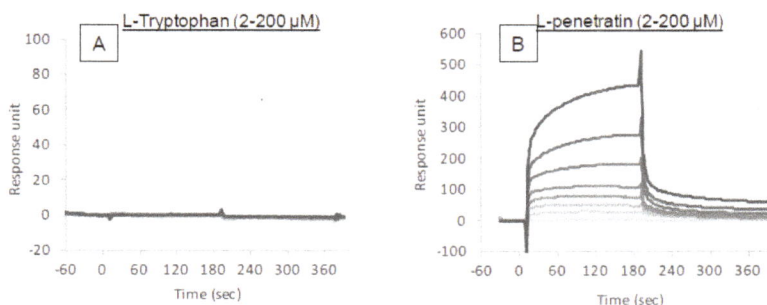

Figure 7. Binding sensorgrams obtained by SPR analysis. Various concentrations of L-tryptophan (**A**) or L-penetratin (**B**) solutions (pH 7.4) were injected into insulin-immobilized flow cells.

3.5.2. Possible Ability of Tryptophan to Protect Insulin from Enzymatic Degradation

The formation of the complex via intermolecular interaction between insulin and L-tryptophan or L-penetratin might be related to the protection of insulin from the intestinal enzymatic degradation. Therefore, we further evaluated the protective effect of L-tryptophan and L-penetratin on the degradation of insulin in the intestinal enzymatic fluid. As shown in Figure 8B, the positive control STI (1.25 mg/mL) completely abolished the activity of proteases in the intestinal fluid and the co-incubation with L-penetratin partially protected insulin from the enzymatic degradation. This was consistent with the result in our previous work [6]. This suggested that the stabilization of insulin in the presence of L-penetratin could be probably explained by steric hindrance via their intermolecular interaction (Figure 7B). In contrast, L-tryptophan did not have the ability to protect insulin from intestinal enzymatic degradation (Figure 8A). This may be attributed to the lack of intermolecular interaction between insulin and L-tryptophan (Figure 7A).

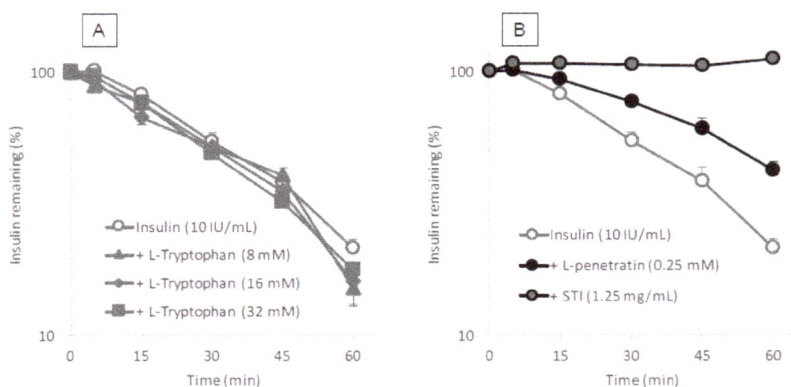

Figure 8. Degradation profiles of insulin in the presence of tryptophan or positive controls (penetratin and STI) in rat intestinal enzymatic fluid. Panel (**A**), various concentrations of L-tryptophan (8–32 mM); panel (**B**), L-penetratin (0.25 mM) or STI (positive control, 1.25 mg/mL). Each data point represents the mean ± SEM of $N = 3$.

3.5.3. Possibility of Paracellular Transport via Tight Junction Opening Effect Induced by L-Tryptophan and Its Metabolite

The temporal effect of pretreatment with L-tryptophan on the intestinal absorption of insulin (Figure 6A,C) suggested that L-tryptophan could possibly modify the structure of the lipid membrane or tight junctions in the intestinal epithelium, resulting in enhanced transcellular or paracellular transport of insulin. Therefore, the epithelial transport of insulin in the in vitro Caco-2 cell monolayer model was then examined in the absence or presence of L-tryptophan. Figure 9A shows the TEER values which reflect the integrity of paracellular tight junctions after the application of L-tryptophan into Caco-2 cells grown in transwells. No change in the TEER values was observed after addition of L-tryptophan at all concentrations examined (600–16,000 μM), although a significant reduction in TEER was observed after addition of typical enhancer C10. The maintained TEER confirmed that the cellular lipid membrane was retained after addition of L-tryptophan, consistent with the LDH release assays (Figure 5A,B). Consistent with the result in TEER measurement, Figure 9B showed no change in the in vitro epithelial permeation of insulin after co-incubation with various concentrations of L-tryptophan.

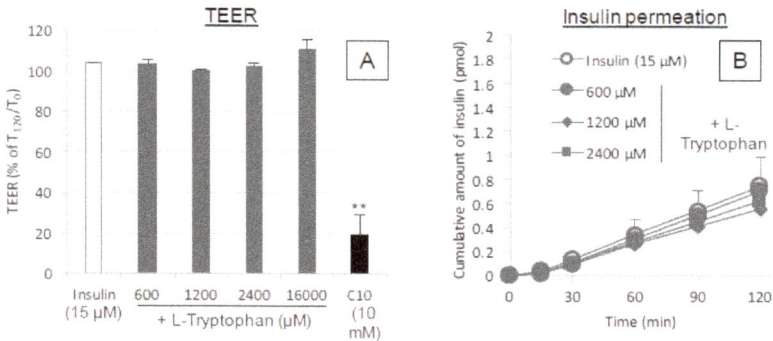

Figure 9. Cytotoxicity examinations after the exposure of intestinal epithelium to L-tryptophan. Panel (**A**), changes in the TEER of Caco-2 cell monolayers after the incubation with insulin (15 μM) and various concentrations of L-tryptophan (600–16,000 μM). The values are expressed as a percentage calculated by dividing the TEER measurement (Ω cm^2) at 120 min by the initial value. Panel (**B**), time courses of permeation of insulin through Caco-2 monolayer in the presence or absence of L-Tryptophan (600–2400 μM). Each data point represents the mean $\pm$ SEM of $N = 3$. * $p < 0.05$, ** $p < 0.01$, significantly different with corresponding insulin control group.

3.5.4. Isomeric Dependent Effect of Tryptophan Co-Administration on the Intestinal Absorption of Insulin

The lack of L-tryptophan effect in the in vitro transport assay (Figure 9B) contradicted the in situ and in vivo effect of L-tryptophan on the absorption of insulin (Figures 1A and 2), suggesting that inherent active transport systems might potentially be associated with the action of L-tryptophan but that these transport systems might be diminished or deficient in Caco-2 cells. In our recent work, we found that only the L-form of arginine in its amino acid form can facilitate the intestinal absorption of insulin [13]. As it is possible that the effect of tryptophan may also vary between L- and D-forms, we conducted an in situ absorption study of insulin with D-tryptophan (16 and 32 mM) and compared its effectiveness to that of L-tryptophan (Figure 1A). The results in Figure 10 show that the effect of D-tryptophan appears much weaker than that of L-tryptophan but the onset of action by D-tryptophan (60 min after administration) was similar to that of L-tryptophan.

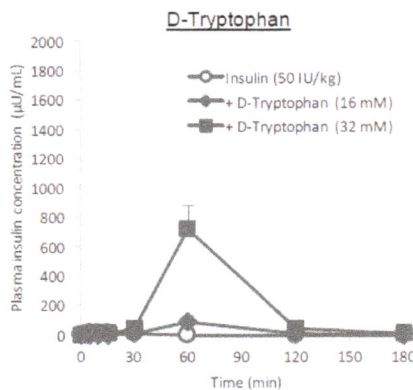

Figure 10. Time profiles of plasma insulin concentration after in situ administration of insulin (50 IU/kg) with or without D-tryptophan (16 or 32 mM) into rat ileal loop. Each data point represents the mean $\pm$ SEM of $N = 3$.

3.5.5. Possible Involvement of Serotonin as Active Metabolite of L-Tryptophan to Enhance the Intestinal Absorption of Insulin

On the other hand, it is possible that the metabolite of L-tryptophan, serotonin, has the potential to enhance the epithelial permeability of insulin and other macromolecular drugs [30] and the delayed action of L-tryptophan might be attributed to the time required for conversion from tryptophan to serotonin after administration to the intestine. Therefore, we then tested the effect of serotonin on the permeation and absorption of insulin under the in vitro and in situ conditions. The result of the permeation study with Caco-2 cell monolayer (Figure 11A,B) showed that serotonin had no stimulatory effect on the permeation of insulin, in fact, serotonin increased the TEER as shown in Figure 11C, suggesting that paracellular space was tightened by addition of serotonin. Consistent with the increase in TEER, the permeability of insulin through the Caco-2 cell monolayer decreased by co-incubation with serotonin (Figure 11B). On the other hand, serotonin (32 mM) could enhance the intestinal absorption of insulin after administration to a rat ileal loop but it was less effective than L-tryptophan (Figure 11D). The pharmacokinetic parameters are summarized in Table 1. The relationship between results in the in vitro and in vivo conditions is unknown.

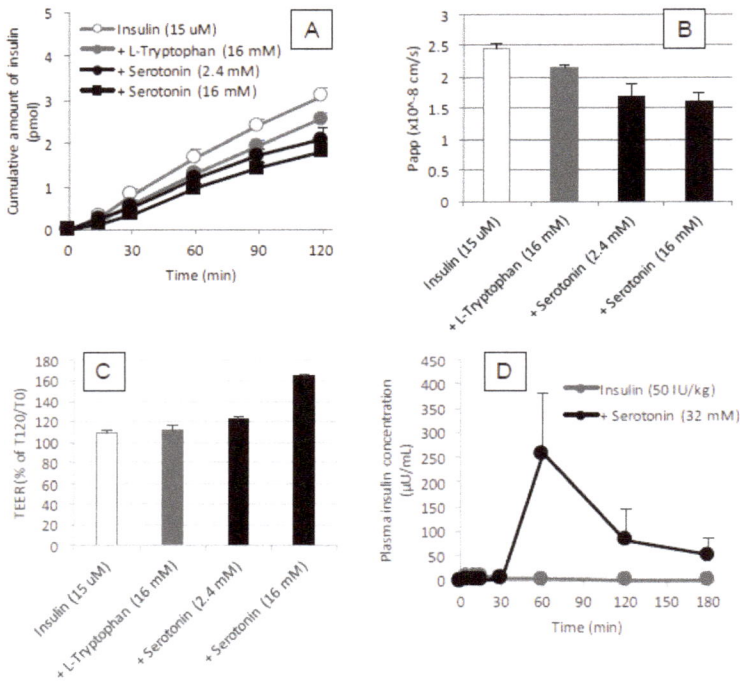

Figure 11. Permeation of insulin through the Caco-2 cell monolayer panels (**A**,**B**) and TEER values panel (**C**) during coincubation with L-tryptophan (16 mM) or serotonin (2.4 or 16 mM) and the absorption of insulin after its in situ administration of insulin (50 IU/kg) with or without serotonin (32 mM) into rat ileal loop panel (**D**). Each data point represents the mean ± SEM of $N = 3$.

3.5.6. Combined Effect of Co-Administration of L-Tryptophan with L-Penetratin on the Intestinal Absorption of Macromolecules

The difference in the action onset between L-tryptophan (slow) and L-penetratin (rapid) shown in Figure 1A suggested that these two enhancers used different pathways to enhance the intestinal absorption of insulin and other macromolecular drugs. No intermolecular interaction between insulin and L-tryptophan (Figure 7A,B) confirmed that L-tryptophan uses a different mechanism than L-penetratin. Therefore, we then examined the additive or synergistic potential of the combination of L-tryptophan and L-penetratin to increase the intestinal absorption of macromolecular dextran (FD-4) in the in situ ileal loop administration study.

As shown in Figure 12, the individual effect of L-tryptophan (16 mM) and L-penetratin (0.5 mM) on the absorption of FD-4 was confirmed as being delayed and rapid onset, respectively, consistent with the above-mentioned results with insulin (Figure 1). Contrary to our expectation, the effect of the combined co-administration with L-tryptophan (16 mM) and L-penetratin (0.5 mM) on the absorption of FD-4 was almost equal to that co-administered with only L-penetratin (0.5 mM). As L-penetratin had the capacity to interact with FD-4 similar to insulin, L-tryptophan might be deprived of a chance to facilitate the absorption of FD-4. Possibly, a large part of FD-4 administered to the intestine could be systemically and quickly absorbed by complexing with L-penetratin, while FD-4 which could be delivered by L-tryptophan was scarce due to the slow mechanism of action. The results suggested that the action mechanism of L-tryptophan to facilitate the intestinal absorption of macromolecular drugs was different from that of L-penetratin.

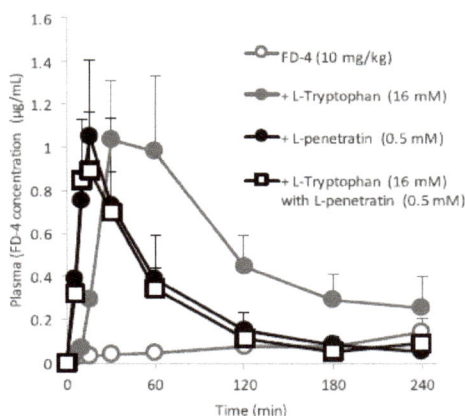

Figure 12. Time profiles of plasma concentrations of FD-4 after its in situ administration with or without L-tryptophan (16 mM) and/or L-penetratin (0.5 mM) into rat ileal loop. Each data point represents the mean $\pm$ SEM of N = 3–4.

4. Discussion

We recently discovered that single amino acid arginine, particularly the L-form of arginine, an important component in cationic CPPs, has the potential to facilitate the intestinal absorption of insulin without being part of a peptide structure such as arginine-rich CPPs [13]. Another amino acid, the hydrophobic amino acid tryptophan, is known to play an important role in the cellular association and internalization of the amphipathic CPP, penetratin [16,18]. In fact, our previous study demonstrated that the amphipathic CPP enhanced the intestinal absorption of insulin to a greater degree than cationic CPPs such as R8 and Tat peptide [3]. Therefore, we hypothesized that addition of tryptophan to insulin might potentially improve the intestinal absorption of insulin.

The data showed that the intestinal absorption of insulin was significantly enhanced by co-administration with L-tryptophan (16 or 32 mM, Figure 1A and Table 1), comparable to the effect of L-penetratin (0.5 mM). Interestingly, the onset patterns of insulin absorption after co-administration were quite different between L-arginine (T_{max} 12.8 $\pm$ 0.9 min at 40 mM) and L-tryptophan (T_{max} 52.5 $\pm$ 7.5 min at 32 mM), as shown in Figure 1A, Table 1 and our previous publication [13], suggesting that different mechanisms might be associated with the absorption enhancement by cationic arginine versus hydrophobic tryptophan. On the other hand, we showed in our previous publications that the simple cationic CPP (R8) generated a relatively slow enhancing effect, whereas the typical amphipathic CPP (penetratin), containing two tryptophan residues, rapidly enhanced the absorption of insulin [3,21], contradicting the effect of amino acids, L-arginine and L-tryptophan, observed in the present and current studies [13]. This suggests that L-tryptophan and L-arginine could enhance intestinal absorption via mechanisms distinctly different from that involving CPPs.

The binding analysis showed no intermolecular interaction between insulin and L-tryptophan (Figure 7), implying that L-tryptophan has no capacity to bring the noncovalently mixed drugs as a delivery carrier. L-arginine also showed no binding with insulin (data not shown). This observation is quite different from the mechanism of penetratin and R8 in which intermolecular interaction is essential to their ability as absorption enhancers. There was no protective effect of L-tryptophan on the enzymatic degradation of insulin (Figure 8A), confirming no possible interaction between insulin and L-tryptophan. With respect to the opening of tight junctions as a possible mechanism, the examination in our recent report suggested that no opening of tight junctions was observed after adding the effective concentrations of L-arginine (9.6 mM equivalent to 4.2 mg/kg in the animal study) to the transwell with Caco-2 cell monolayers [13]. In regard to tryptophan, while there is an earlier report suggesting that mucosal exposure of L-tryptophan (1 mM or more) increases the paracellular permeability of macromolecules in an energy- and sodium-dependent manner [31], more recent study suggests that indole-containing molecules like tryptophan strengthen the epithelial barrier function via the increased expression of tight junction-related proteins such as claudins and occludins [32,33]. No change in the TEER values of Caco-2 cell monolayers was observed after addition of various concentrations of L-tryptophan (600–16,000 μM) (Figure 9A). Therefore, it is expected that the mechanism resulting in the enhancement of the mucosal absorption by both amino acids does not occur via opening of tight junctions.

Interestingly, it was suggested that the enteric nervous system was associated with the intestinal transport of low molecular weight compounds and hydrophilic macromolecules [34,35]. While the adrenergic stimulation has been known to decrease the intestinal absorption of dextran with molecular weights of 20,000 and 40,000 g/mol [35], vascular perfusion with the cholinergic agonist bethanechol can contribute to the increase in intestinal drug transport [34]. Furthermore, serotonin, a major metabolite of tryptophan, is known to promote the secretion of acetylcholine via the stimulation of the serotonin 5-HT$_4$ receptor, possibly contributing to the increased intestinal absorption of macromolecules [30]. No enhancement of the epithelial permeation of insulin in the presence of L-tryptophan (Figure 9B) may strengthen the hypothesis that L-tryptophan needs to be metabolized for enhancing the epithelial permeation of drugs. However, our in vivo data (Figure 11D) in the present study was inconsistent with such a hypothesis, as the effect of serotonin (32 mM) on the intestinal absorption of insulin was weaker than that of L-tryptophan (32 mM) and the action onset of serotonin was delayed compared to L-tryptophan. Furthermore, our in vitro data partially negated the possible cholinergic contribution, as serotonin appeared to tighten the paracellular space and decrease the epithelial transport of insulin through a Caco-2 cell monolayer (Figure 11A–C). In the present study regarding the ability of tryptophan to enhance intestinal absorption, the L-form is more effective than the D-form (Figure 10), similar to arginine. Considering the differences between how L- and D-amino acids affect insulin absorption, endogenous systems such as the enteric nervous system, the transporter-mediated influx, or receptor-mediated influx mechanisms might be involved either directly or indirectly. Although some effects of D-tryptophan remained at the higher dose (32 mM), it was considerably small compared to that of L-tryptophan (Figure 10 and Table 1), suggesting that stereospecificity might be partially involved in their absorption enhancing mechanisms.

The in situ administration study conducted after pretreatment with L-tryptophan indicated its reversibility in the enhancement of the intestinal absorption of insulin. As shown in Figure 6C, the absorption stimulatory effect of L-tryptophan greatly diminishes at 30 min after pretreatment with L-tryptophan followed by washing, like the effect of conventional positive controls such as C10 and sodium taurodeoxycholate. These results along with the cytotoxic analysis (Figure 5A–C and Figure 9A) suggest L-tryptophan has no irreversible effect on the mucosal structure, which means that L-tryptophan does not induce permanent functional change to the intestinal membrane. Future studies are needed to clarify the mechanism.

Based on the results of the in situ intestinal insulin absorption study, we examined the potential of L-tryptophan as an oral absorption enhancer for insulin in vivo. Figure 2 clearly showed the hypoglycemic effects after oral administration of insulin (50 IU/kg) with L-tryptophan (32 mM). In this study, insulin and L-tryptophan were administered just as a solution, therefore, the development of an appropriate formulation could be expected to increase the biological effect of insulin. Figures 3 and 4 clearly demonstrates the wide applicability of L-tryptophan as an absorption enhancer for macromolecules having peptide- to protein-sized molecular weights. In contrast, L-arginine had no effect on the intestinal absorption of such peptide drugs (data not shown). The effectiveness of absorption enhancement by L-tryptophan was comparable to that by L-penetratin, although L-tryptophan required relatively higher concentrations (16 mM or more) than L-penetratin (0.5 mM). Since L-tryptophan is currently used as an oral supplement and it appears to facilitate the intestinal absorption of a wide variety of biopharmaceuticals, its potential as an intestinal absorption enhancer is meritorious and quite unique.

As mentioned above, tryptophan is first metabolized into serotonin which stimulates the cholinergic nervous system, balancing neural activity. Therefore, although L-tryptophan is one of the essential amino acids, its excess use has to be carefully considered for safe pharmacotherapy. In addition, another metabolite from tryptophan, melatonin, is used as a sleep-inducing agent and therefore may affect circadian rhythm. The required dose of L-tryptophan for inducing sleepiness is roughly to 1500–3000 mg·day^{-1}·human^{-1}, which is comparable to the maximum dose used to enhance the intestinal absorption of biopharmaceuticals (32 mM equivalent to 16.3 mg/kg) in this study. However, the dose of L-tryptophan used as an absorption enhancer could be further optimized by precisely evaluating the relation between its co-administered concentration and the efficiency of the resultant absorption enhancement. Considering the effective plasma concentration of insulin (<100 μU/mL), it is expected that the dose of L-tryptophan can be reduced to 10 mM, the equivalent to 5.1 mg/kg (300 mg/human). Further examination will be essential to establish the potential of L-tryptophan as a safe and effective absorption enhancer for the oral delivery of biopharmaceuticals.

5. Conclusions

In the process of studying the role of the hydrophobic amino acid tryptophan, which was widely known as a key amino acid in the function of CPPs, we discovered that tryptophan singly improves the intestinal absorption of various biopharmaceuticals having peptide to protein molecular sizes. When examining the absorption of insulin in particular, the bioavailability enhancement effect of L-tryptophan was far stronger than that of L-arginine [13], another key cationic amino acid component of CPPs and comparable to the potent CPP, L-penetratin. However, the mechanism of action remains unclear. In the present study, the cell integrity of the intestinal epithelium (demonstrated by assessing cell viability, cell membrane integrity and the tightness of paracellular junctions) was not changed in the presence of L-tryptophan. Furthermore, no intermolecular interaction between insulin and L-tryptophan was observed and insulin was not protected from enzymatic degradation when in the presence of L-tryptophan. Tryptophan is the precursor of a wide array of bioactive compounds, such as serotonin, melatonin and so forth. [36]. Considering the stronger action of L-tryptophan as an absorption enhancer relative to the D-form, inherent biological functions might be involved in its action mechanisms. To utilize L-tryptophan as a safe absorption enhancer, further studies are required to identify the complete mechanism of action.

Author Contributions: M.T.-M. conceived the study and acquired research grants. N.K. and M.T.-M. designed the study. H.T. and M.M. conducted in situ loop absorption experiments. H.T., M.M. and K.H. conducted in vivo oral absorption experiments. H.T conducted in situ intestinal toxicity examinations (LDH assay). H.O. and S.H.

conducted in vitro cytotoxicity examinations (LDH and WST-8 assays) and transcellular transport assays. M.M. conducted SPR-binding assays. Y.H. and K.M. conducted enzymatic degradation assays. N.K. prepared the manuscript. All authors analyzed and discussed the results and reviewed the manuscript.

Funding: This research was funded by JSPS KAKENHI Scientific Research (C) (grant number 16K08211) and a Kobe Gakuin University Research Grants (A and C). The APC was also funded by JSPS KAKENHI Scientific Research (C) (grant number 16K08211).

Acknowledgments: The authors are grateful to Matthew Miller (Laboratory of Biomaterials, Drug Delivery, and Bionanotechnology, McKetta Department of Chemical Engineering, Cockrell School of Engineering, The University of Texas at Austin) for his assistance in improving English in the manuscript.

Conflicts of Interest: Authors declare no conflict of interest. The funders had no role in the design of the study; in the collection, analyses, or interpretation of data; in the writing of the manuscript, and in the decision to publish the results.

References

1. Komin, A.; Russell, L.M.; Hristova, K.A.; Searson, P.C. Peptide-based strategies for enhanced cell uptake, transcellular transport, and circulation: Mechanisms and challenges. *Adv. Drug Deliv. Rev.* **2017**, *110–111*, 52–64. [CrossRef] [PubMed]

2. Salzano, G.; Torchilin, V.P. Intracellular delivery of nanoparticles with cell penetrating peptides. *Methods Mol. Biol.* **2015**, *1324*, 357–368. [PubMed]

3. Kamei, N.; Morishita, M.; Eda, Y.; Ida, N.; Nishio, R.; Takayama, K. Usefulness of cell-penetrating peptides to improve intestinal insulin absorption. *J. Control. Release* **2008**, *132*, 21–25. [CrossRef] [PubMed]

4. Kamei, N.; Morishita, M.; Takayama, K. Importance of intermolecular interaction on the improvement of intestinal therapeutic peptide/protein absorption using cell-penetrating peptides. *J. Control. Release* **2009**, *136*, 179–186. [CrossRef] [PubMed]

5. Khafagy, E.-S.; Morishita, M.; Kamei, N.; Eda, Y.; Ikeno, Y.; Takayama, K. Efficiency of cell-penetrating peptides on the nasal and intestinal absorption of therapeutic peptides and proteins. *Int. J. Pharm.* **2009**, *381*, 49–55. [CrossRef] [PubMed]

6. Khafagy, E.S.; Iwamae, R.; Kamei, N.; Takeda-Morishita, M. Region-dependent role of cell-penetrating peptides in insulin absorption across the rat small intestinal membrane. *AAPS J.* **2015**, *17*, 1427–1437. [CrossRef] [PubMed]

7. Brock, R. The uptake of arginine-rich cell-penetrating peptides: Putting the puzzle together. *Bioconjug. Chem.* **2014**, *25*, 863–868. [CrossRef] [PubMed]

8. Copolovici, D.M.; Langel, K.; Eriste, E.; Langel, U. Cell-penetrating peptides: Design, synthesis, and applications. *ACS Nano* **2014**, *8*, 1972–1994. [CrossRef] [PubMed]

9. Bechara, C.; Sagan, S. Cell-penetrating peptides: 20 years later, where do we stand? *FEBS Lett.* **2013**, *587*, 1693–1702. [CrossRef] [PubMed]

10. Kamei, N.; Onuki, Y.; Takayama, K.; Takeda-Morishita, M. Mechanistic study of the uptake/permeation of cell-penetrating peptides across a caco-2 monolayer and their stimulatory effect on epithelial insulin transport. *J. Pharm. Sci.* **2013**, *102*, 3998–4008. [CrossRef] [PubMed]

11. Futaki, S.; Suzuki, T.; Ohashi, W.; Yagami, T.; Tanaka, S.; Ueda, K.; Sugiura, Y. Arginine-rich peptides. An abundant source of membrane-permeable peptides having potential as carriers for intracellular protein delivery. *J. Biol. Chem.* **2001**, *276*, 5836–5840. [CrossRef] [PubMed]

12. Morishita, M.; Kamei, N.; Ehara, J.; Isowa, K.; Takayama, K. A novel approach using functional peptides for efficient intestinal absorption of insulin. *J. Control. Release* **2007**, *118*, 177–184. [CrossRef] [PubMed]

13. Kamei, N.; Khafagy, E.S.; Hirose, J.; Takeda-Morishita, M. Potential of single cationic amino acid molecule "arginine" for stimulating oral absorption of insulin. *Int. J. Pharm.* **2017**, *521*, 176–183. [CrossRef] [PubMed]

14. Bechara, C.; Pallerla, M.; Zaltsman, Y.; Burlina, F.; Alves, I.D.; Lequin, O.; Sagan, S. Tryptophan within basic peptide sequences triggers glycosaminoglycan-dependent endocytosis. *FASEB J.* **2013**, *27*, 738–749. [CrossRef] [PubMed]

15. Jobin, M.L.; Bonnafous, P.; Temsamani, H.; Dole, F.; Grelard, A.; Dufourc, E.J.; Alves, I.D. The enhanced membrane interaction and perturbation of a cell penetrating peptide in the presence of anionic lipids: Toward an understanding of its selectivity for cancer cells. *Biochim. Biophys. Acta* **2013**, *1828*, 1457–1470. [CrossRef] [PubMed]

16. Jobin, M.L.; Blanchet, M.; Henry, S.; Chaignepain, S.; Manigand, C.; Castano, S.; Lecomte, S.; Burlina, F.; Sagan, S.; Alves, I.D. The role of tryptophans on the cellular uptake and membrane interaction of arginine-rich cell penetrating peptides. *Biochim. Biophys. Acta* **2015**, *1848*, 593–602. [CrossRef] [PubMed]

17. Crombez, L.; Aldrian-Herrada, G.; Konate, K.; Nguyen, Q.N.; McMaster, G.K.; Brasseur, R.; Heitz, F.; Divita, G. A new potent secondary amphipathic cell-penetrating peptide for sirna delivery into mammalian cells. *Mol. Ther.* **2009**, *17*, 95–103. [CrossRef] [PubMed]

18. Christiaens, B.; Grooten, J.; Reusens, M.; Joliot, A.; Goethals, M.; Vandekerckhove, J.; Prochiantz, A.; Rosseneu, M. Membrane interaction and cellular internalization of penetratin peptides. *Eur. J. Biochem.* **2004**, *271*, 1187–1197. [CrossRef] [PubMed]

19. Futaki, S.; Ohashi, W.; Suzuki, T.; Niwa, M.; Tanaka, S.; Ueda, K.; Harashima, H.; Sugiura, Y. Stearylated arginine-rich peptides: A new class of transfection systems. *Bioconjug. Chem.* **2001**, *12*, 1005–1011. [CrossRef] [PubMed]

20. Khalil, I.A.; Futaki, S.; Niwa, M.; Baba, Y.; Kaji, N.; Kamiya, H.; Harashima, H. Mechanism of improved gene transfer by the n-terminal stearylation of octaarginine: Enhanced cellular association by hydrophobic core formation. *Gene Ther.* **2004**, *11*, 636–644. [CrossRef] [PubMed]

21. Kamei, N.; Morishita, M.; Kanayama, Y.; Hasegawa, K.; Nishimura, M.; Hayashinaka, E.; Wada, Y.; Watanabe, Y.; Takayama, K. Molecular imaging analysis of intestinal insulin absorption boosted by cell-penetrating peptides by using positron emission tomography. *J. Control. Release* **2010**, *146*, 16–22. [CrossRef] [PubMed]

22. Khafagy, E.-S.; Morishita, M.; Isowa, K.; Imai, J.; Takayama, K. Effect of cell-penetrating peptides on the nasal absorption of insulin. *J. Control. Release* **2009**, *133*, 103–108. [CrossRef] [PubMed]

23. Maher, S.; Leonard, T.W.; Jacobsen, J.; Brayden, D.J. Safety and efficacy of sodium caprate in promoting oral drug absorption: From in vitro to the clinic. *Adv. Drug Deliv. Rev.* **2009**, *61*, 1427–1449. [CrossRef] [PubMed]

24. Krug, S.M.; Amasheh, M.; Dittmann, I.; Christoffel, I.; Fromm, M.; Amasheh, S. Sodium caprate as an enhancer of macromolecule permeation across tricellular tight junctions of intestinal cells. *Biomaterials* **2013**, *34*, 275–282. [CrossRef] [PubMed]

25. Brayden, D.J.; Maher, S.; Bahar, B.; Walsh, E. Sodium caprate-induced increases in intestinal permeability and epithelial damage are prevented by misoprostol. *Eur. J. Pharm. Biopharm.* **2015**, *94*, 194–206. [CrossRef] [PubMed]

26. Swenson, E.S.; Milisen, W.B.; Curatolo, W. Intestinal permeability enhancement: Efficacy, acute local toxicity, and reversibility. *Pharm. Res.* **1994**, *11*, 1132–1142. [CrossRef] [PubMed]

27. Whitehead, K.; Karr, N.; Mitragotri, S. Safe and effective permeation enhancers for oral drug delivery. *Pharm. Res.* **2008**, *25*, 1782–1788. [CrossRef] [PubMed]

28. Karsdal, M.A.; Riis, B.J.; Mehta, N.; Stern, W.; Arbit, E.; Christiansen, C.; Henriksen, K. Lessons learned from the clinical development of oral peptides. *Br. J. Clin. Pharmacol.* **2015**, *79*, 720–732. [CrossRef] [PubMed]

29. Kamei, N.; Aoyama, Y.; Khafagy, E.-S.; Henmi, M.; Takeda-Morishita, M. Effect of different intestinal conditions on the intermolecular interaction between insulin and cell-penetrating peptide penetratin and on its contribution to stimulation of permeation through intestinal epithelium. *Eur. J. Pharm. Biopharm.* **2015**, *94*, 42–51. [CrossRef] [PubMed]

30. Hiraoka, H.; Kimura, N.; Furukawa, Y.; Ogawara, K.; Kimura, T.; Higaki, K. Up-regulation of p-glycoprotein expression in small intestine under chronic serotonin-depleted conditions in rats. *J. Pharmacol. Exp. Ther.* **2005**, *312*, 248–255. [CrossRef] [PubMed]

31. Madara, J.L.; Carlson, S. Supraphysiologic l-tryptophan elicits cytoskeletal and macromolecular permeability alterations in hamster small intestinal epithelium in vitro. *J. Clin. Investig.* **1991**, *87*, 454–462. [CrossRef] [PubMed]

32. Bansal, T.; Alaniz, R.C.; Wood, T.K.; Jayaraman, A. The bacterial signal indole increases epithelial-cell tight-junction resistance and attenuates indicators of inflammation. *Proc. Natl. Acad. Sci. USA* **2010**, *107*, 228–233. [CrossRef] [PubMed]

33. Shimada, Y.; Kinoshita, M.; Harada, K.; Mizutani, M.; Masahata, K.; Kayama, H.; Takeda, K. Commensal bacteria-dependent indole production enhances epithelial barrier function in the colon. *PLoS ONE* **2013**, *8*, e80604. [CrossRef] [PubMed]

34. Higaki, K.; Sone, M.; Ogawara, K.; Kimura, T. Regulation of drug absorption from small intestine by enteric nervous system i: A poorly absorbable drug via passive diffusion. *Drug Metab. Pharmacokinet.* **2004**, *19*, 198–205. [CrossRef] [PubMed]
35. Kimoto, T.; Takanashi, M.; Mukai, H.; Ogawara, K.; Kimura, T.; Higaki, K. Effect of adrenergic stimulation on drug absorption via passive diffusion in caco-2 cells. *Int. J. Pharm.* **2009**, *368*, 31–36. [CrossRef] [PubMed]
36. Kaluzna-Czaplinska, J.; Gatarek, P.; Chirumbolo, S.; Chartrand, M.S.; Bjorklund, G. How important is tryptophan in human health? *Crit. Rev. Food Sci. Nutr.* **2017**, 1–17. [CrossRef] [PubMed]

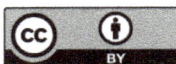

pharmaceutics

MDPI

Article

Delivery of Nanoparticles across the Intestinal Epithelium via the Transferrin Transport Pathway

Jing M. Yong, Julia Mantaj, Yiyi Cheng and Driton Vllasaliu *

School of Cancer and Pharmaceutical Sciences, Faculty of Life Sciences & Medicine, King's College London, London SE1 9NH, UK
* Correspondence: driton.vllasaliu@kcl.ac.uk; Tel.: +207-848-1728

Received: 17 May 2019; Accepted: 25 June 2019; Published: 26 June 2019

Abstract: The aim of this study was to probe whether the transferrin (Tf) transport pathway can be exploited for intestinal delivery of nanoparticles. Tf was adsorbed on 100 nm model polystyrene nanoparticles (NP), followed by size characterisation of these systems. Cell uptake of Tf and Tf-adsorbed NP was investigated in intestinal epithelial Caco-2 cells cultured on multi-well plates and as differentiated polarised monolayers. Tf-NP demonstrated a remarkably higher cell uptake compared to unmodified NP in both non-polarised (5-fold) and polarised cell monolayers (16-fold difference). Application of soluble Tf significantly attenuated the uptake of Tf-NP. Notably, Tf-NP displayed remarkably higher rate (23-fold) of epithelial transport across Caco-2 monolayers compared to unmodified NP. This study therefore strongly suggests that the Tf transport pathway should be considered as a candidate biological transport route for orally-administered nanomedicines and drugs with poor oral bioavailability.

Keywords: Caco-2; intestinal absorption; nanomedicine; nanoparticle; oral delivery; transferrin

1. Introduction

The oral drug administration route offers the ultimate patient convenience, preference and therefore adherence to drug therapy. However, with a few exceptions, oral administration is currently an option only for small drug molecules that show acceptable intestinal absorption. As a rapidly expanding class of drugs, biologics are presently predominantly given by injection. Significant research efforts over a number of decades have explored technologies to enable oral delivery of biologics, but progress has been relatively poor. Drug delivery strategies in this area mostly utilise absorption or permeation enhancers and focus on smaller biologics, such as glucagon-like peptide 1 (GLP-1) analogues [1]. However, safety concerns, including those related to many surfactants [2], have hindered the clinical translation of these approaches. Recent progress in this area seeks to utilise advances in materials, engineering and electronics, leading to swallowable "devices", such as mucoadhesive patches [3] and the microneedle "robotic pill" [4].

The key challenge in the field of oral delivery of macromolecular biologics concerns the difficulty in overcoming the formidable intestinal epithelial barrier, rather than additional barriers such as the stomach acid and mucosal enzymes, which can be addressed via relatively established technologies. A key requirement for technologies enabling therapeutically-relevant oral delivery of biologics is safety. Rather than disrupting and increasing the permeability of the intestinal epithelium non-selectively (i.e., an effect that a classical permeation enhancer would display), it is desirable to engineer delivery systems that selectively permeate the intestinal mucosa. This can be achieved by targeting and hijacking the natural, physiological transport processes present in the intestinal epithelium. This approach usually requires a ligand or transport-enabling entity capable of intestinal translocation, which is linked (e.g., conjugated or fused) to the biotherapeutic. Alternatively, the ligand can be presented on the surface of drug carriers, particularly nanocarriers [5–7], which may also serve to protect the drug against mucosal enzymatic degradation or enable targeted delivery post absorption.

Transferrin (Tf) has been explored as a potential ligand to enable drug targeting and delivery across biological barriers, particularly the blood-brain barrier (BBB) [8,9], because of its high expression in BBB endothelium [10]. The transferrin receptor (TfR) is expressed in the human gastrointestinal epithelial cells [11]. Furthermore, TfR is overexpressed in colon cancer (similarly to other types of cancer) [12] and the inflamed colon; it was detected in both basolateral and apical sides of enterocytes from the colon tissue biopsies of inflammatory bowel disease (IBD) patients and rats with colitis [13]. Therefore, TfR and TfR-mediated transcytosis could be exploited as a biological system for systemic delivery of biologics, in addition to its potential as a targeting receptor for local delivery in intestinal cancer or IBD.

However, it must be noted that it is currently unclear whether TfR-mediated transcytosis offers opportunity for improving intestinal delivery of biologics in the context of systemic delivery, or local, targeted delivery to the intestinal diseased tissue. This is because of predominant distribution of TfR on the basolateral surface in polarised cells, which presents an obvious obstacle for receptor-mediated mucosal delivery [14]. There are however reports of TfR-mediated transcytosis being explored for oral delivery of biologics via a Tf recombinant fusion protein approach [15] or Tf conjugation to therapeutic macromolecule [16]—both these approaches have shown evidence and potential for the use of TfR-mediated transport as a strategy to enhance the intestinal absorption (i.e., in the apical-to-basolateral direction) of biologics. Importantly, a recent landmark study clearly showed a complete and enhanced apical-to-basolateral transcytosis of Tf-functionalised nanogranules in Caco-2 cells, with Tf modification upregulating the expression of trafficking-related (endocytosis and transcytosis) proteins [17].

This study probed the possibility of improving the intestinal epithelial delivery of nanoparticles (NP), as potentially useful carriers of biologics, by targeting TfR-mediated transcytosis. A fundamental study of this nature is imperative to assess the possibility that TfR-mediated transcytosis may be utilised to facilitate intestinal translocation of nanomedicines. This is important as, with the exception of two studies [17,18], TfR-mediated transcytosis has not been investigated for intestinal delivery of nanosystems. We show here that TfR targeting of NP significantly improves their uptake into intestinal epithelial cells (Caco-2), as well as translocation across cell monolayers serving as an in vitro intestinal model.

2. Materials and Methods

2.1. Materials

Hank's balanced salt solution (HBSS; with sodium bicarbonate, without phenol red), Dulbecco's Modified Eagle's Medium (DMEM) and all other reagents (including cell culture media supplements, antibiotic-antimycotic solution and foetal bovine serum), unless otherwise stated, were purchased from Sigma-Aldrich (Poole, UK). Fluorescently-labelled ("fluospheres"), carboxylate-modified polystyrene microspheres of 0.1 μm diameter (referred to as "NP") and multiwell cell culture plates were purchased from Thermo Fisher Scientific (Waltham, MA, USA). Human holotransferrin (Tf) was purchased from LEE biosolutions (Maryland Heights, MO, USA), while fluorescently-labelled human Tf-CF®488A dye conjugate was purchased from Biotium (Fremont, CA, USA). Transwell permeable inserts of 12 mm diameter and polycarbonate filters and 0.4μm pore size were obtained from Corning (Corning, NY, USA).

2.2. Adsorption of Tf to Nanoparticles

Tf-adsorbed nanoparticles (Tf-NP) were prepared based on a procedure that was previously reported [19]. A 1:2 Tf to NP mass ratio (1.1 mg/mL Tf and 2.2 mg/mL carboxylic-modified NPs) was used, with adsorption achieved by incubation in 50mM 2-(*N*-morpholino)ethanesulfonic acid (MES) buffer at pH 5.9 for 2 h at 20 °C. A previous study characterising Tf adsorption to latex NP reported the

1:1 mass ratio to produce full surface coverage on the same NP systems [19]. Given that we used a lower amount of Tf (below adsorption saturation), the presence of unadsorbed Tf was assumed to be very low and dialysis was not carried out.

2.3. Nanoparticle Characterisation

Average hydrodynamic size (dynamic light scattering, DLS), polydispersity and zeta potential of NP before and post Tf adsorption were measured by using a Malvern zetasizer (Malvern Instruments Ltd., Malvern, UK). Unmodified and Tf-NP were diluted in HBSS (biological buffer used in cell experiments). Measurements were conducted at a scattering angle $\theta = 173$ and at a temperature of 25 °C. For DLS, each measurement was an average of 12 repetitions of 10 s each. Both DLS and zeta potential measurements were repeated three times.

2.4. Cell Culture

Caco-2 cells were cultured on 24-well plates for two days as undifferentiated system and Transwell inserts as differentiated monolayers, following plating at 10^5 cells/cm^2 using DMEM. Cells were cultured on inserts for at least 21 days prior to the experiments, with culture medium replaced every other day. For differentiated Caco-2 system, transepithelial electrical resistance (TEER) was measured periodically and before uptake and transport experiments to ensure integrity of the monolayer and tight junction formation (polarisation). Prior to cell uptake and transport experiments, both undifferentiated and differentiated Caco-2 cells were equilibrated in HBSS for 45 min to minimise the potential impact of media change on cell uptake and transport studies.

2.5. Cell Uptake of Tf

Human Tf CF488A conjugate was applied to Caco-2 cells (cultured on 24-well plates) at 50 μg/mL and cells incubated at 37 °C for two hours. This was followed by removing the applied sample and repeated cell washing using HBSS. Triton X-100 (1% *v/v*) was applied to cells for 10 min to permeabilise and detach the cells. Permeabilised cells were then centrifuged and the supernatant harvested. Tf CF488A conjugate was quantified by measuring the fluorescence of supernatant using a Tecan Fluorescence Plate Reader (Tecan Trading AG, Männedorf, Switzerland) at 515 nm emission/490 nm excitation. Quantitation of samples was carried out via a calibration curve.

2.6. Cell Uptake of Tf-NP

Tf-NPs (1:2 mass ratio) were applied to Caco-2 cells cultured on 24-well plates at 40 μg/mL. Cells were incubated with the samples at 37 °C for two hours, following washing with HBSS. Cells were then permeabilised via the application of Triton X-100 (1% *v/v* in HBSS). Cells were then harvested and transferred to 1 mL vials for centrifugation. Tf-NPs were quantified by measuring NP fluorescence following centrifugation of permeabilised cells and measurement of fluorescence of the supernatant using a Tecan fluorescence plate reader at 590 nm/645 nm (excitation/emission).

2.6.1. Competition Studies

For competition studies, cells were pre-treated with 10 μg/mL of Tf, shortly followed by application of Tf-NP. Cell uptake was examined as above.

2.6.2. Uptake in Differentiated Monolayers

In addition to examining uptake of Tf-NP in multiwell plate-grown Caco-2 cells, we also tested cell internalisation of these systems in differentiated Caco-2 cells (i.e., following culture on Transwell inserts). Only cell monolayers displaying TEER ≥ 500 Ωcm^2 were used in the experiments (given the typical range observed in our work of 700–1400 Ωcm^2). Application of Tf-NP and cell monolayer permeabilisation was conducted in the same manner as above.

2.7. Transport of Tf-NP across Differentiated Caco-2 Monolayers

Caco-2 cells were cultured as polarised monolayers on Transwell inserts as described above. Prior to the transport study, cells were equilibrated in HBSS. Tf-NP (1:2 ratio) were then applied to the apical side of Caco-2 cells at 40 µg/mL for two hours. Unmodified NPs were also applied at equivalent concentration. Cells were incubated with the samples at 37 °C for two hours, with periodic sampling of the basolateral solution every 20 min (this was replaced with fresh HBSS). Samples were transferred onto a black 96-well plate for NP fluorescence quantitation as above.

2.8. Statistical Analysis

Unpaired, unequal variance t test (or Welch t test) was performed for comparisons of two group means, while one-way analysis of variance (ANOVA) was utilised for comparison of three or more group means. p value of <0.05 was considered statistically significant. ***, ** and * indicate $p < 0.001$, $p < 0.01$ and $p < 0.05$, respectively, whereas "ns" denotes nonsignificant. Statistical analysis was conducted using GraphPad Prism® Software.

3. Results

This study examined whether TfR-mediated transcytosis may be utilised as a biological transport route to facilitate intestinal delivery of nanomedicines (Figure 1).

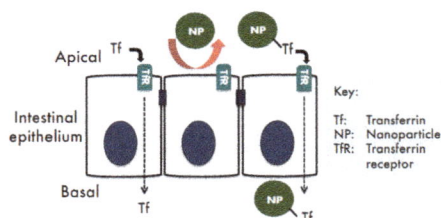

Figure 1. Transferrin transcytosis pathway as a potential route for intestinal delivery of nanomedicines.

3.1. Nanoparticle Characterisation

To assess the effect of physical adsorption of Tf to NP on their size, we conducted size characterisation of bare NP and Tf-NP. Data shown in Figure 2 highlight that adsorption of Tf on model polystyrene NP produced an increase in the hydrodynamic diameter of the NP (measured by DLS) from approximately 130 nm to 176 nm, indicating the formation of an adsorbed Tf surface layer of about 23 nm.

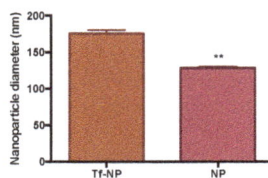

Figure 2. Hydrodynamic size of bare nanoparticles (NP) and transferrin-adsorbed systems (Tf-NP). Size was characterised by dynamic light scattering (DLS), with systems suspended in Hank's Balanced Salt Solution (HBSS). Measurements were done at scattering angle θ = 173 and at a temperature of 25 °C. Data shown as mean ± SD. Each measurement was an average of 12 repetitions of 10 s each and repeated three times. ** denotes $p < 0.01$.

In terms of surface charge, the zeta potential of unmodified NP was −35.7 (± 1.57), whereas for Tf-NP this amounted to −14.3 (± 1.03), resulting in a statistically significant reduction of negative surface charge post Tf adsorption ($p = 0.0001$).

3.2. Cell Uptake of Tf

Uptake of Tf by multiwell-cultured (undifferentiated) Caco-2 cells following application at 50 µg/mL (at 37 °C for two hours) was 0.18 µg/well (24-well plate).

3.3. Cell Uptake of Tf-NP

The internalisation of Tf-NP by intestinal Caco-2 cells was tested under different conditions in non-polarised, multiwell-cultured cells (Figure 3), prior to subsequent examination in differentiated cell monolayers (Figure 4). Considering the multiwell-cultured cells, Figure 2 shows the internalisation of Tf-NP after application alone, or following treatment with soluble Tf ('+Tf'). The figure also depicts the uptake of bare NP. The data highlight more than five-fold higher cell uptake of Tf-NP compared to bare NP. Importantly, following cell treatment of Tf-NP in conjunction with excess free Tf, cell internalisation of the former was attenuated by more than three-fold.

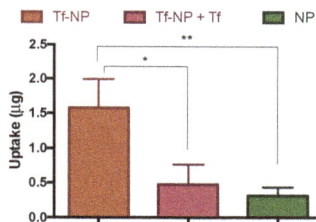

Figure 3. Uptake of transferrin-adsorbed nanoparticles ('Tf-NP') and bare nanoparticles (NP) by Caco-2 cells cultured on multiwell plates. Tf-NP were applied to cells at 40 µg/mL alone or just after application of 10 µg/mL soluble Tf ('Tf-NP + Tf'). Cells were incubated with the samples at 37 °C for two hours. Cell internalisation was measured following permeabilization with Triton X-100 (1% *v/v* in Hank's Balanced Salt Solution), centrifugation and measurement of nanoparticle fluorescence. Data shown as the mean ± SD ($n = 3$). ** and * denote $p < 0.01$ and $p < 0.05$, respectively.

3.4. NP-Tf Uptake in, and Transport across, Differentiated Monolayers

Cell uptake of Tf-NP in differentiated Caco-2 monolayers is depicted in Figure 4. The data demonstrate more than 16-fold higher cell uptake of Tf-NP compared to bare NP.

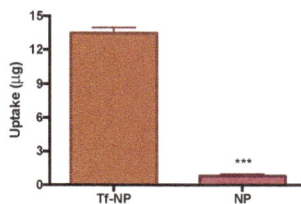

Figure 4. Uptake of transferrin-adsorbed nanoparticles ('Tf-NP') and bare nanoparticles (NP) by Caco-2 cells cultured as differentiated monolayers. Tf-NP were applied to the apical side of Caco-2 monolayers at 40 µg/mL in Hank's Balanced Salt Solution (HBSS) as biological buffer. Cells were incubated with the samples at 37 °C for two hours. Cells were permeabilised via the application of 100 µL of Triton X-100 (1% *v/v* in HBSS). Nanoparticles were quantified by fluorescence. Data presented as the mean ± SD ($n = 3$). *** denotes $p < 0.001$

Following the demonstration of Tf-NP uptake by intestinal Caco-2 cells, the final set of experiments looked into the transepithelial transport. In this regard, Figure 5 shows that Tf-NP traversed differentiated Caco-2 monolayers remarkably more efficiently; specifically a 23-fold higher rate of NP translocation was observed with Tf-NP compared to bare counterparts.

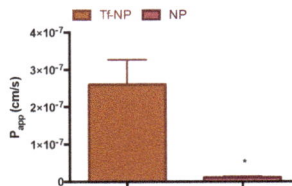

Figure 5. Transport of transferrin-adsorbed nanoparticles ('Tf-NP') and bare nanoparticles (NP) across differentiated Caco-2 cells (cultured on inserts for three weeks). Tf-NP were applied to the apical side of Caco-2 monolayers at 40 µg/mL in Hank's Balanced Salt Solution (HBSS) as biological buffer. Cells were incubated with the samples at 37 °C for two hours, during which sampling from the basolateral compartment was carried out periodically. Data presented as the mean ± SD ($n = 3$). * denotes $p < 0.05$.

4. Discussion

The intestinal mucosa acts as a selective barrier to systemic absorption of material present in the lumen. Large and complex biologics are usually not capable of crossing the intestinal epithelium, therefore displaying very low bioavailabilities following oral administration. One way to improve the oral bioavailability of such drugs is to enhance epithelial absorption by targeting the transcytosis pathways as physiological routes of transport in the intestinal epithelium. This strategy has been made possible by advances in biotechnology and nanotechnology, which have facilitated the production of fusion proteins and drug nanocarriers, respectively. We and other groups have demonstrated that a number of physiological transcytosis processes functioning in the intestinal epithelium can potentially be used to shuttle material (nanoparticles and macromolecules) across the intestinal epithelium, including the transport system for IgG [20,21], neurotensin [22] and albumin [23,24]. This study provides further progress in this arena, by demonstrating that the biological machinery for Tf transport can also be considered as a potential pathway for intestinal delivery of nanomedicines.

Tf is an abundant human plasma glycoprotein responsible for transport of iron, binding to TfR when bound to iron, activating receptor mediated endocytosis [25]. As tumour cells generally overexpress the TfR because of high demand for iron, Tf-mediated drug delivery strategy has been predominantly used for its potential to target cancer cells, usually as a ligand to guide NP to these cells.

Transferrin receptor (TfR)-mediated endocytosis and transcytosis in intestinal Caco-2 cells was previously investigated using Tf-fusion proteins. It was shown that apically-endocytosed Tf in Caco-2 cells is transported to a Rab11-positive compartment, which may control its release to follow either slow recycling to apical membrane or progress to transcytotic compartments [26]. Shah and Shen studied the transport of Tf-conjugated insulin across Caco-2 cell monolayers and reported that transport of the complex, which was mediated via the TfR, was increased by 5- to 15-fold compared to free insulin [16]. In another study, Tf recombinant fusion protein approach was explored for oral delivery for human growth hormone (hGH) [15]. Fusion proteins of 100 kDa, which retained bioactivity of both hGH and Tf, were tested in hGH-deficient hypophysectomised rats for in vivo biological activity. It was shown that one of the tested fusion proteins—containing a helical linker as spacer between hGH and Tf domain—induced a statistically significant weight gain after oral dosing.

We utilised fluorescently-labelled model polystyrene NP systems and achieved ligand (Tf) presentation on NP via physical adsorption. This produced Tf-NP of approximately 180 nm (Figure 2), which fall within the optimal size range for intestinal epithelial transport [6,20,27,28]. Furthermore, it was previously shown that following presentation as coating on the surface of NP via physical adsorption, Tf retains the ability to target and interact with TfR [29].

We first probed the internalisation of Tf by Caco-2 cells, demonstrating that the extent of Tf uptake by Caco-2 cells ($0.18 \, \mu g/1.9 \, cm^2$) is likely to be comparable with a previous study [16] showing that cell internalization of insulin-Tf conjugate was around 1.9 pmoles per $3.5 \, cm^2$ monolayer (Caco-2), equivalent to around $0.15 \, \mu g$ (the final insulin:Tf ratio in the conjugate was 3:1).

Cell internalisation of Tf-NP was tested both in multiwell-cultured cells and differentiated cell monolayers. This was done to determine any potential difference in cell uptake capacity between undifferentiated and differentiated cells (cultured on inserts), given the difference in surface area available for uptake and potential differential receptor expression between undifferentiated and differentiated cells. In undifferentiated cells (multiwell culture) cell uptake of Tf-NP was over five-fold higher relative to bare NP. Furthermore, excess free Tf reduced cell uptake of Tf-NP by more than three-fold (Figure 3). With regards to cell uptake of Tf-NP in differentiated cells, data revealed more than 16-fold higher cell uptake of Tf-NP compared to bare NP (Figure 4), with the latter displaying a similar uptake level to that previously reported by us (around $2 \, \mu g$ here versus $5 \, \mu g$ in previously published work [30]), confirming the pattern observed in undifferentiated cells. The notably larger magnitude of effect (enhanced cell uptake following Tf presentation on NP) may be related to differential TfR expression in undifferentiated *versus* differentiated cells. The implications of these findings are important, pointing to significant enhancement of cell uptake of NP following presentation of Tf on their surface.

It is noted that the definitive biological pathway of Tf-NP uptake in Caco-2 cells cannot be ascertained from this work. However, suppression of internalisation by excess free Tf does point to a TfR-dependent uptake, similarly to the study by Shah and Shen [16] who demonstrated that the binding and uptake of the radiolabelled insulin-Tf conjugate in Caco-2 cells were inhibited by 70% and 80%, respectively, with excess unlabeled Tf.

We finally considered the transport of Tf-NP across differentiated Caco-2 monolayers. The data concerning this showed remarkably higher (23-fold) transport of Tf-NP across cells compared to bare NP (Figure 5). It must be pointed out that this remarkable enhancement in the permeation of NP across intestinal epithelium in vitro is much higher than that previously seen with other transcytosis receptor systems exploited in a similar manner (i.e., for intestinal NP delivery). This includes the neonatal Fc receptor (FcRn), whereby the uptake into Caco-2 cells of polyethylene glycol-poly(lactic-*co*-glycolic acid) (PEG-PLGA) NP modified with Fc was improved (compared to non Fc-modified NP) by a maximum three-fold [20]. Similarly, a different study showed that the translocation of 63 nm Fc-targeted poly(lactic acid)-*b*-poly(ethylene glycol) (PLA-PEG) across Caco-2 monolayers was increased by approximately a factor of two (compared to non-modified NP) [21].

Overall, this work highlights that the TfR transport system shows potential as a pathway for cell entry and transepithelial permeation of NP in the intestinal epithelium. Therefore, this system should be given consideration as a potential pathway for intestinal delivery of nanomedicines intended for systemic effect or local action. The latter is particularly applicable to colon cancer and IBD, given TfR overexpression in the intestinal mucosa in these diseases [12,13]. Therefore, TfR-mediated delivery should be probed further for its potential usefulness in the area of oral or intestinal delivery of nanomedicines.

Author Contributions: Conceptualization, D.V.; Methodology, D.V., J.M. and J.M.Y.; Software, D.V., J.M.Y.; Validation, J.M.Y. and J.M.; Formal Analysis, D.V., J.M.Y. and J.M.; Investigation, J.M.Y., Y.C. and J.M.; Resources, D.V.; Data Curation, J.M.Y., Y.C. and J.M.; Writing-Original Draft Preparation, D.V. and J.M.Y.; Writing-Review & Editing, D.V.; Supervision, D.V.

Funding: This research was partially funded by the Engineering and Physical Sciences Research Council (EPSRC); grant reference number EP/P002544/2.

Conflicts of Interest: The authors declare no conflict of interest.

References

1. Nordisk, N. Available online: https://www.novonordisk.com/content/Denmark/HQ/www-novonordisk-com/en_gb/home/media/news-details.2226662.html (accessed on 17 December 2018).
2. Vllasaliu, D.; Shubber, S.; Fowler, R.; Garnett, M.; Alexander, C.; Stolnik, S. Epithelial toxicity of alkylglycoside surfactants. *J. Pharm. Sci.* **2013**, *102*, 114–125. [CrossRef] [PubMed]
3. Anselmo, A.C.; Gokarn, Y.; Mitragotri, S. Non-invasive delivery strategies for biologics. *Nat. Rev. Drug Discov.* **2018**, *18*, 19–40. [CrossRef] [PubMed]
4. Therapeutics, R. Available online: https://www.ranitherapeutics.com (accessed on 17 December 2018).
5. Vllasaliu, D.; Alexander, C.; Garnett, M.; Eaton, M.; Stolnik, S. Fc-mediated transport of nanoparticles across airway epithelial cell layers. *J. Control. Release* **2012**, *158*, 479–486. [CrossRef] [PubMed]
6. Kim, K.S.; Suzuki, K.; Cho, H.; Youn, Y.S.; Bae, Y.H. Oral Nanoparticles Exhibit Specific High-Efficiency Intestinal Uptake and Lymphatic Transport. *ACS Nano* **2018**, *12*, 8893–8900. [CrossRef] [PubMed]
7. Pridgen, E.M.; Alexis, F.; Farokhzad, O.C. Polymeric nanoparticle drug delivery technologies for oral delivery applications. *Expert. Opin. Drug Deliv.* **2015**, *12*, 1459–1473. [CrossRef] [PubMed]
8. Lajoie, J.M.; Shusta, E.V. Targeting receptor-mediated transport for delivery of biologics across the blood-brain barrier. *Annu. Rev. Pharmacol. Toxicol.* **2015**, *55*, 613–631. [CrossRef]
9. Lam, F.C.; Morton, S.W.; Wyckoff, J.; Han, T.L.; Hwang, M.K.; Maffa, A.; Balkanska-Sinclair, E.; Yaffe, M.B.; Floyd, S.R.; Hammond, R.T. Enhanced efficacy of combined temozolomide and bromodomain inhibitor therapy for gliomas using targeted nanoparticles. *Nat. Commun.* **2018**, *9*, 1991. [CrossRef]
10. Uchida, Y.; Ohtsuki, S.; Katsukura, Y.; Ikeda, C.; Suzuki, T.; Kamiie, J.; Terasaki, T. Quantitative targeted absolute proteomics of human blood-brain barrier transporters and receptors. *J. Neurochem.* **2011**, *117*, 333–345. [CrossRef]
11. Banerjee, D.; Flanagan, P.R.; Cluett, J.; Valberg, L.S. Transferrin receptors in the human gastrointestinal tract. Relationship to body iron stores. *Gastroenterology* **1986**, *91*, 861–869. [CrossRef]
12. Shen, Y.; Li, X.; Dong, D.; Zhang, B.; Xue, Y.; Shang, P. Transferrin receptor 1 in cancer: A new sight for cancer therapy. *Am. J. Cancer Res.* **2018**, *8*, 916–931.
13. Tirosh, B.; Khatib, N.; Barenholz, Y.; Nissan, A.; Rubinstein, A. Transferrin as a luminal target for negatively charged liposomes in the inflamed colonic mucosa. *Mol. Pharm.* **2009**, *6*, 1083–1091. [CrossRef] [PubMed]
14. Du, W.; Fan, Y.; Zheng, N.; He, B.; Yuan, L.; Zhang, H.; Wang, X.; Wang, J.; Zhang, X.; Zhang, Q. Transferrin receptor specific nanocarriers conjugated with functional 7peptide for oral drug delivery. *Biomaterials* **2013**, *34*, 794–806. [CrossRef] [PubMed]
15. Amet, N.; Wang, W.; Shen, W.C. Human growth hormone-transferrin fusion protein for oral delivery in hypophysectomized rats. *J. Control. Release* **2010**, *141*, 177–182. [CrossRef] [PubMed]
16. Shah, D.; Shen, W.C. Transcellular delivery of an insulin-transferrin conjugate in enterocyte-like Caco-2 cells. *J. Pharm. Sci.* **1996**, *85*, 1306–1311. [CrossRef] [PubMed]
17. Yang, D.; Liu, D.; Deng, H.; Zhang, J.; Qin, M.; Yuan, L.; Zou, X.; Shao, B.; Li, H.; Dai, W.; et al. Transferrin Functionization Elevates Transcytosis of Nanogranules across Epithelium by Triggering Polarity-Associated Transport Flow and Positive Cellular Feedback Loop. *ACS Nano* **2019**, *13*, 5058–5076. [CrossRef] [PubMed]
18. Ganugula, R.; Arora, M.; Guada, M.; Saini, P.; Kumar, M.N.R. Noncompetitive Active Transport Exploiting Intestinal Transferrin Receptors for Oral Delivery of Proteins by Tunable Nanoplatform. *ACS Macro Lett.* **2017**, *6*, 161–164. [CrossRef]
19. Pitek, A.S.; O'Connell, D.; Mahon, E.; Monopoli, M.P.; Bombelli, F.B.; Dawson, K.A. Transferrin coated nanoparticles: Study of the bionano interface in human plasma. *PLoS ONE* **2012**, *7*, e40685. [CrossRef]
20. Shi, Y.; Sun, X.; Zhang, L.; Sun, K.; Li, K.; Li, Y.; Zhang, Q. Fc-modified exenatide-loaded nanoparticles for oral delivery to improve hypoglycemic effects in mice. *Sci. Rep.* **2018**, *8*, 726. [CrossRef]
21. Pridgen, E.M.; Alexis, F.; Kuo, T.T.; Levy-Nissenbaum, E.; Karnik, R.; Blumberg, R.S.; Langer, L.; Farokhzad, O.C. Transepithelial transport of Fc-targeted nanoparticles by the neonatal fc receptor for oral delivery. *Sci. Transl. Med.* **2013**, *5*, 213ra167. [CrossRef]
22. Bird, J.L.; Simpson, R.; Vllasaliu, D.; Goddard, A.D. Neurotensin receptor 1 facilitates intracellular and transepithelial delivery of macromolecules. *Eur. J. Pharm. Biopharm.* **2017**, *119*, 300–309. [CrossRef]
23. Hashem, L.; Swedrowska, M.; Vllasaliu, D. Intestinal uptake and transport of albumin nanoparticles: Potential for oral delivery. *Nanomedicine (Lond.)* **2018**, *13*, 1255–1265. [CrossRef] [PubMed]

24. Martins, J.P.; D'Auria, R.; Liu, D.; Fontana, F.; Ferreira, M.P.; Correia, A.; Kemell, M.; Moslova, K.; Makila, K.; Salonen, J.; et al. Engineered Multifunctional Albumin-Decorated Porous Silicon Nanoparticles for FcRn Translocation of Insulin. *Small* **2018**, *14*, e1800462. [CrossRef] [PubMed]
25. Qian, Z.M.; Li, H.; Sun, H.; Ho, K. Targeted drug delivery via the transferrin receptor-mediated endocytosis pathway. *Pharmacol. Rev.* **2002**, *54*, 561–587. [CrossRef] [PubMed]
26. Lim, C.J.; Norouziyan, F.; Shen, W.C. Accumulation of transferrin in Caco-2 cells: A possible mechanism of intestinal transferrin absorption. *J. Control. Release* **2007**, *122*, 393–398. [CrossRef] [PubMed]
27. Fowler, R.; Vllasaliu, D.; Falcone, F.H.; Garnett, M.; Smith, B.; Horsley, H.; Alexander, C.; Stolnik, S. Uptake and transport of B12-conjugated nanoparticles in airway epithelium. *J. Control. Release* **2013**, *172*, 374–381. [CrossRef]
28. Song, Y.; Shi, Y.; Zhang, L.; Hu, H.; Zhang, C.; Yin, M.; Chu, L.; Yan, X.; Zhao, M.; Zhang, X.; et al. Synthesis of CSK-DEX-PLGA Nanoparticles for the Oral Delivery of Exenatide to Improve Its Mucus Penetration and Intestinal Absorption. *Mol. Pharm.* **2019**, *16*, 518–532. [CrossRef] [PubMed]
29. Chang, J.; Paillard, A.; Passirani, C.; Morille, M.; Benoit, J.P.; Betbeder, D.; Garcion, E. Transferrin adsorption onto PLGA nanoparticles governs their interaction with biological systems from blood circulation to brain cancer cells. *Pharm. Res.* **2012**, *29*, 1495–1505. [CrossRef]
30. Bannunah, A.M.; Vllasaliu, D.; Lord, J.; Stolnik, S. Mechanisms of nanoparticle internalization and transport across an intestinal epithelial cell model: Effect of size and surface charge. *Mol. Pharm.* **2014**, *11*, 4363–4373. [CrossRef]

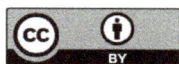

pharmaceutics

MDPI

Article

N-(2-Hydroxy)-propyl-3-trimethylammonium, O-Mysristoyl Chitosan Enhances the Solubility and Intestinal Permeability of Anticancer Curcumin

Daniella S. Silva [1], Danilo M. dos Santos [2], Andreia Almeida [3,4,5], Leonardo Marchiori [1], Sérgio P. Campana-Filho [6], Sidney J. L. Ribeiro [1] and Bruno Sarmento [3,4,5,*]

[1]   Institute of Chemistry, São Paulo State University—UNESP, Araraquara 4800-900, Brazil; danyss8@hotmail.com (D.S.S.); leonardo.marchiori.lm@gmail.com (L.M.); sidney.jl.ribeiro@unesp.br (S.J.L.R.)
[2]   Embrapa Instrumentação, Rua XV de Novembro 1452, São Carlos 13560-970, Brazil; danilomartins_1@hotmail.com
[3]   Institute for Research and Innovation in Health (i3S), Rua Alfredo Allen, 208, 4200-393 Porto, Portugal; andreia.almeida@ineb.up.pt
[4]   ICBAS—Institute of Biomedical Sciences Abel Salazar, University of Porto, Rua de Jorge Viterbo Ferreira, 228, 4050-313 Porto, Portugal
[5]   CESPU—Institute for Research and Advanced Training in Health Sciences and Technologies, Rua Central de Gandra, 1317, 4585-116 Gandra, Portugal
[6]   Sao Carlos Institute of Chemistry, University of Sao Paulo—USP, Av. Trabalhador São-Carlense, 400, São Carlos 13566-590, Brazil; scampana@iqsc.usp.br
*   Correspondence: bruno.sarmento@ineb.up.pt; Tel.: +351-226-074-949

Received: 30 September 2018; Accepted: 16 November 2018; Published: 20 November 2018

Abstract: An amphiphilic derivative of chitosan containing quaternary ammonium and myristoyl groups, herein named as ammonium myristoyl chitosan (DMCat), was synthesized by reacting glycidyltrimethylammonium chloride (GTMAC) and myristoyl chitosan (DMCh). The success of the modification was confirmed using Fourier-transform infrared spectroscopy (FTIR) and ^{1}H nuclear magnetic resonance (NMR) spectroscopy. The average degrees of alkylation and quaternization ($\overline{DQ}$) were determined by using ^{1}H NMR and conductometric titration. The zeta potential of the micelles was higher than 28 mV while its average size and encapsulation efficiency ranged from 280 nm to 375 nm and 68% to 100%, respectively. The in vitro cytotoxicity of the unloaded and curcumin (CUR)-loaded micelles was tested against Caco-2 and HT29-MTX intestinal epithelial cell lines. The results showed no cytotoxic effect from loaded and unloaded micelles as compared to free CUR. In the permeability test, it was observed that both types of micelles, i.e., DMCh and DMCat, improved CUR permeability. Additionally, higher permeability was verified for both systems in Caco-2/HT29-MTX:Raji B because of the mucoadhesive character of chitosan and its ability to open tight junctions. The results indicated that DMCat micelles, due to the physico-chemical, improved characteristics may be a promising carrier to encapsulate CUR aiming cancer therapy.

Keywords: chitosan derivatives; amphiphilic polymers; polymeric micelles; quaternization; curcumin; intestinal delivery

---

1. Introduction

Polymeric micelles have attracted considerable interest for controlled drug delivery over the last few years, due to their unique properties and behaviors resulting from their small size and high load capacity [1]. These nanostructured materials show potential to deliver chemotherapeutics to tumor cells maintaining their concentration at the desired site for a sufficient time to have a therapeutic effect, increasing the efficacy of treatment and reducing the toxicity [2].

Curcumin (CUR) is a naturally occurring phytochemical that has been widely used as a therapeutic agent against a variety of cancers [3–8]. In particular, CUR is a cheap compound (especially when compared with popular anticancer agents like paclitaxel and camptothecin) and has properties in antioxidant, anti-inflammatory, antimicrobial, anticancer, anticarcinogenic, chemopreventive, chemotherapeutic, and chemosensitizing activities [9,10]. Although CUR possesses remarkable medicinal properties, its bioavailability during cancer treatments is limited due to its low solubility and poor stability in aqueous solution. Other than its rapid degradation in physiological conditions, however, there is a wide interest in the development of systems to solve problems related to the limitations of the applicability of CUR as a therapeutic agent [4–7,11]. To enhance solubility, stability, pharmacokinetics profile of curcumin and thus its therapeutic efficiency, various drug delivery systems have been investigated, including nanoemulsions, nanosuspensions, and polymeric micelles [11,12].

In recent years, drug delivery systems based on polymeric micelles have been the subject of research. Several formulations are undergoing clinical trials due to the ability of the micelles to encapsulate hydrophobic and hydrophilic drugs [13–15]. In addition, these systems have shown greater physical stability and encapsulation efficiency, when compared to liposomes [16–20]. Shell/core polymeric micelles, in particular, exhibit advantages regarding encapsulation and controlled release of drugs since their hydrophobic nuclei promote the solubilization of hydrophobic actives, avoiding drug degradation. On the other hand, hydrophilic outer shells avoid recognition by the immune system, prolonging the circulation time of the drug in the body [21,22].

Lately, micelles formulations based on chitosan have presented promising results in the drug delivery field [23–28]. This cationic biopolymer exhibits biological activities, such as biocompatibility, biodegradability, mucoadhesiveness, and antimicrobial activity, in addition to presenting antioxidant properties [29–31]. Chitosan has present in its backbone reactive groups (–OH and –NH$_2$) that make it susceptible to chemical modifications. Various derivatives of chitosan are obtained via the addition of hydrophobic groups with different degrees of substitution (DS). In particular, chitosan modified with stearic acid (DS = 4.96%) [32] and linoleic acid (DS = 1.8%) [33] exhibit self-assembly and loading abilities, which improve the solubility of hydrophobic drugs [34,35]. However, the addition of a small portion of hydrophobic units makes chitosan extremely insoluble in neutral medium, leading to a low loading capacity of the micelles for non-ionic hydrophobic drugs [34,36].

Previous studies with the structural modification of chitosan via an *O*-acylation reaction with myristoyl chloride showed excellent capacity for encapsulation and solubilization of hydrophobic drugs, such as paclitaxel [37]. This is due to the affinity of the acyl chains within the drug. However, because such a derivative exhibited a low degree of substitution (DS = 6.8%), the characteristics of the starting chitosan have been maintained, and its limited solubility at a neutral pH has hindered its application. Thus, the limitations resulting from the modification of chitosan with myristoyl chloride via an *O*-substitution reaction can be solved by carrying out a further chemical modification.

The introduction of hydrophilic and hydrophobic groups has shown excellent results in the encapsulation of hydrophobic drugs, such as paclitaxel and doxorubicin. In this sense, different amphiphilic derivatives of chitosan have been synthesized, such as *N*-octyl-*N*, *O*-carboxymethylchitosan [18], colic acid grafted *N*-(2,3-(dihydroxypropyl) chitosan [38], chitosan-*g*-polylactic [39], *N*-octyl-*N*-trimethylchitosan [40], *N*-propyl-*N*-methylenephosphonic chitosan [41], *N*-naphthyl-*N*, *O*-succinylchitosan [42]. In all of these studies, amphiphilic derivatives of chitosan are suggested to be promising efficient carriers for hydrophobic drugs, especially when compared to hydrophobically modified chitosan.

This work aims to develop a new amphiphilic derivative of chitosan via *O*-acylation and quaternization reactions in chitosan (Scheme 1), since the first step (*O*-acylation) has already been conducted with excellent results for anticancer drug delivery [37]. Studies showed that the synthesis of quaternized chitosan via *N*-substitution by reacting it with *N*-(2-hydroxyl) propyl-3-trimethyl ammonium chloride presented properties of interest, such as water solubility, antibacterial activity, mucoadhesiveness, increased permeability to hydration, and strong stereochemical hindrance of quaternary amine groups [43–45].

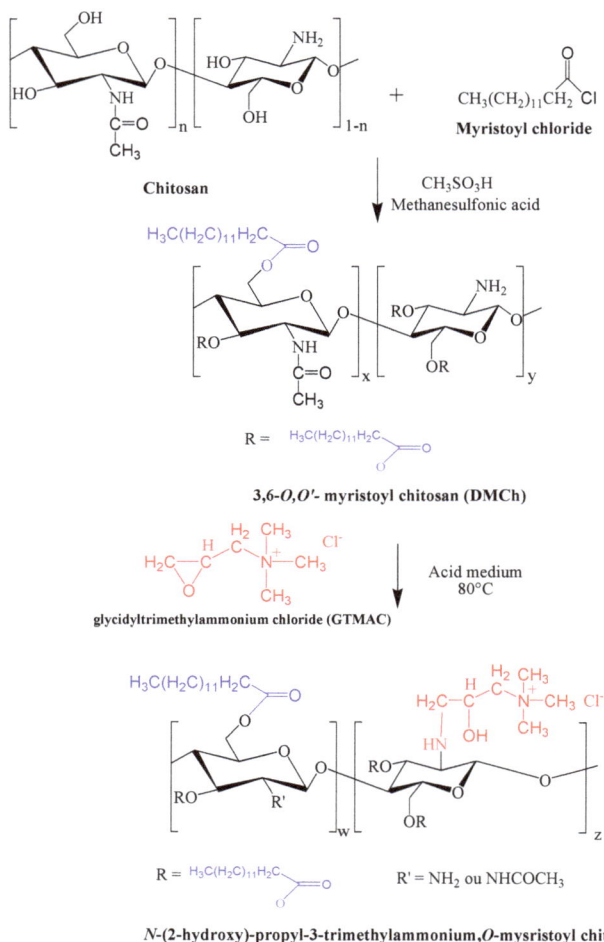

Scheme 1. The synthesis of *N*-(2-hydroxy)-propyl-3-trimethylammonium,*O*-mysristoyl chitosan.

In this study, an amphiphilic derivative of chitosan containing quaternary ammonium and myristoyl goups was prepared and its ability to form self-assembled micelles with ability to encapsulate curcumin was explored. The efficiency of the structural modification was evaluated by FTIR and ^{1}H nuclear magnetic resonance (NMR) spectroscopy and conductometric titration. The physical-chemical characteristics such as average size, zeta potential, drug loading efficiency, and critical aggregation concentration (CAC) were determined. The in vitro cytotoxicity was evaluated using Caco-2 (clone C2BBe1) and HT29-MTX cell lines, as well as the in vitro intestinal permeability.

2. Materials and Methods

2.1. Materials

Chitosan acquired from a commercial supplier (Cheng Yue Plating Co. Ltd.; Pequim, China) was purified according to Santos et al. [46], and then dried at 30 °C. The average degree of acetylation ($\overline{DA}$) of chitosan was 5%, as determined by the ^{1}H NMR analysis. The viscosity average molecular weight ($\overline{Mv}$) of chitosan was calculated from its intrinsic viscosity, which was determined in 0.3 mol L^{-1} acetic acid/0.2 mol L^{-1} sodium acetate buffer (pH 4.5) at 25.00 ± 0.01 °C, by using the Mark-Houwink-Sakurada equation, resulting in $\overline{Mv} \approx 87.000$ g mol^{-1} [46,47]. Glycidyltrimethylammonium chloride (GTMAC) was acquired from Sigma-Aldrich (Saint Louis, MO, USA). All other reagents and solvents were used as acquired, i.e., without any purification.

2.2. Synthesis of 3,6-O,O'-Myristoyl Chitosan

The synthesis of 3,6-*O,O'*-myristoyl chitosan (DMCh) was realized by adding 1 g of chitosan in 25 mL of methanesulfonic acid (MeSO$_3$H). In addition, an amount of myristoyl chloride was added in order to generate an excess of chitosan ($\approx$13.3). After 1 h of reaction, the product was (i) neutralized with 5% (*w/v*) aqueous sodium bicarbonate solution, (ii) centrifugated, (iii) extensively washed with distilled water, (iv) purified in Soxhlet, and finally, (v) dried in a vacuum oven at room temperature. This procedure can be found in detail in a previous work [37].

2.3. Synthesis of N-(2-Hydroxy)-Propyl-3-Trimethylammonium Chitosan Chloride

The reaction of glycidyltrimethylammonium chloride (GTMAC) and DMCh in an acid medium was carried out as described in the literature [46] to result in *N*-(2-hydroxy)-propyl-3-trimethylammonium,*O*-mysristoyl chitosan chloride. Briefly, 1 g of DMCh was dissolved in 60 mL of acetic acid 1% (*v/v*), until complete dissolution. An aqueous solution of GTMAC was added dropwise to the DMCh solubilized; the reaction mixture was then stirred in a glycerin bath for 8 h, under constant stirring at 80 °C. Following, excess acetone was added to the reaction medium to result in the precipitation of the product, which was filtered. Finally, the solid was purified by extraction with acetone in Soxhlet during 6 h and dried in a vacuum oven (30 °C), obtaining as final product the DMCat polymer.

2.4. Preparation of CUR-Loaded DMCh and DMCat Micelles

Both CUR-loaded DMCh and DMCat micelles were prepared by following the steps described in earlier works [37,48,49]. In essence, DMCh is dissolved in acetic acid 0.1% while DMCat is dissolved in deionized water. CUR was dissolved in acetone (1 mg/mL). Next, aliquots containing 50, 100 and 150 µg of CUR were added in the different polymer solutions (DMCh and DMCat). Then, the solutions are magnetically stirred at 300 rpm for 2 h (room temperature) and freeze-dried. Finally, the CUR-loaded micelles are resuspended and separated by centrifugation at 5000 rpm for 10 min.

2.5. Characterization

2.5.1. Fourier-Transform Infrared Spectroscopy (FTIR)

FTIR was performed on an IRAffinity Shimadzu spectrometer (Shimadzu Scientific Instruments, Columbia, MD, USA) in a 4000–400 cm^{-1} wavelength range, with an accumulation of 32 scans and resolution of 4 cm^{-1}. In order to prepare the pellets, the sample and KBr were dried at 60 °C for 8 h and mixed in a ratio of 1:100 (sample:KBr).

2.5.2. ¹H NMR Spectroscopy

A Bruker AVANCE III spectrophotometer 400 MHz (Bruker, Billerica, MA, EUA) was used to obtain ¹H NMR spectra, aiming the samples' characterization. Basically, the Equations (1)–(3) are used to determine the average degree of acetylation of chitosan ($\overline{DA}$) ([50,51]), degree of substitution ($\overline{DS}$) of the derivative 3,6-O,O'-myristoyl chitosan ([37]) and degree of quaternization ($\overline{DQ}$) of the derivative N-(2-hydroxy)-propyl-3-trimethylammonium, O-mysristoyl chitosan ([46]), respectively. In other words, $\overline{DA}$, $\overline{DS}$, and $\overline{DQ}$ refers to the amount of acetylated units present in chitosan, as well as both the myristoyl groups added to chitosan and the quaternary groups present in derivative N-(2-hydroxy)-propyl-3-trimethylammonium,O-mysristoyl chitosan.

$$\overline{DA}(\%) = \left(\frac{A_{CH_3}/3}{A_{H_2-H_6}/6} \right) * 100 \tag{1}$$

A_{CH3} = area of the methyl hydrogens of the acetamido group (of GlcNAc units);
A_{H2-H6} = area of hydrogens bonded to the C (2–6) carbon of the glycopyranose ring.

$$\overline{DS}(\%) = \left(\frac{A_{Me}/3}{A_{H_2-H_6}/6} \right) * 100 \tag{2}$$

A_{Me} = area of the methyl hydrogens of the myristoyl group;
A_{H2-H6} = area of hydrogens bonded to the C (2–6) carbon of the glycopyranose ring.

$$\overline{DQ}(\%) = \frac{IH1'}{IH1' + IH1} \cdot 100 \tag{3}$$

$I_{H1'}$= the integral of the signal due to the anomeric hydrogen bonded to N-substituted GlcN (units);
I_{H1} = is the integral of the signal due to the anomeric units hydrogen bonded to unsubstituted GlcN (units).

2.5.3. Conductometric Titration

The $\overline{DQ}$ of DMcat samples were also determined by dosing the counter-ions Cl^- through titration with standardized 0.017 mol L^{-1} aqueous $AgNO_3$ solution. Thus, the quaternized derivative (0.1 g) was dissolved in deionized water (100 mL) and the conductivity of the solution was measured at 25.00 ± 0.01 °C as a function of the added volume of aqueous $AgNO_3$ by using a Handylab LF1 conductivimeter (SI Analytics, Mainz, Germany). The value of $\overline{DQ}$ of samples was calculated from the titration curves according to [46].

2.5.4. Critical Aggregation Concentration (CAC)

The conductivity method was performed to determine the CAC by using a Consort C863 conductivity meter. In order to prepare the samples, different polymer concentrations were utilized (1×10^{-6} mg/mL $\leq$ Cp $\leq$ 1 mg/mL). The DMCh sample was solubilized in acid medium due to its limited solubility in neutral medium, while deionized water was used to dissolve DMCat.

2.5.5. Particle Size and Surface Charge

The average size, polydispersity, and zeta potential of DMCh (in acid medium) and DMCat (in water) micelles were determined using dynamic light scattering (DLS) measurements (ZetaSizer Nano ZS, Malvern, UK). Three replicates of each formulation were produced and analyzed.

2.5.6. Drug Encapsulation Efficiency

The drug encapsulation efficiency (EE%) was quantified by measuring the absorbance of the CUR solution at 340 nm using a UV-Vis spectrophotometer [3,7]. The measurements were performed by an indirect method in triplicate, in which the unencapsulated drug was solubilized in acetone and quantified. The amount of CUR loaded into the DMCh and DMCat micelles was determined according to Equation (4):

$$EE\% = \frac{(CUR_{total} - CUR_{free})}{CUR_{total}} \times 100 \qquad (4)$$

2.6. In Vitro Studies

2.6.1. Cell Culturing Reagents

Caco-2 cells (clone C2BBe1) were obtained from American Type Culture Collection (ATCC, Manassas, VA, USA) and HT29-MTX cell line was kindly provided by Dr. T. Lesuffleur (INSERMU178, Villejuif, France). Dulbecco's Modified Eagle Medium (DMEM, Lonza, Basel, Switzerland), supplemented with 10% (*v/v*) fetal bovine serum (FBS, Merck Millipore, USA), 1% (*v/v*) penicillin (100 UI/mL, Merck Millipore), streptomycin (100 µg/mL, Merck Millipore), and 1% (*v/v*) nonessential amino acids (NEAA, Merck Millipore). 3-(4,5-dimethylthiazol-2-yl)-2,5-diphenyltetrazolium bromide (MTT), dimethyl sulfoxide (DMSO) and Triton X-100 were obtained from Sigma Aldrich.

2.6.2. Cytotoxicity Assay

The cytotoxicity of CUR-loaded micelles and free CUR was assessed in Caco-2 and HT29-MTX cell lines, using the MTT reagent. Cells were seeded (200 µL) into 96-well plates at a density of 1×10^4 cells/well for HT29-MTX cell line and 2×10^4 cells/well for Caco-2 and then incubated during 24 h in a Binder® incubator at 37 °C with a humidified atmosphere and 5% CO_2 to reach exponential growth prior to the assay test. On the following day, the medium was removed and the cells were washed twice with 200 µL of phosphate buffered saline (PBS). Next, the cells were treated with free CUR and CUR-loaded and unloaded micelles at the concentrations of 5, 10, 20, and 50 µg/mL. The negative control, which were cells treated with cell culture medium and positive control and treated with 1% (*w/v*) Triton X-100 in DMEM [52]. The cultured cells were incubated for 4 h in the presence of different concentrations of the referred samples. After this period, the wells were washed twice with PBS at 37 °C and 200 µL of the MTT reagent (0.5 mg/mL in cell culture medium) was added to each well, followed by an incubation period of 4 h. After, the MTT was removed and 200 µL of DMSO was added to each well to dissolve the formazan crystals. The plates were shaken for 10 min inside the microplate reader before the relative color intensity has been measured at 570 nm and taking the absorbance at 630 nm as a reference, by using a microplate reader (Synergy 2, Biotek Instruments Ltd., Winooski, VT, USA). The percentage of cell viability was calculated according to the Equation (5):

$$Cell\ viability\ (\%) = \frac{experimental\ value - negative\ control}{positive\ control - negative\ control} \times 100 \qquad (5)$$

2.6.3. Permeability Studies

Monoculture model of Caco-2 cells and triple co-culture model of Caco-2/HT29-MTX:Raji B cells were seeded on 6-well Transwell™ cell culture inserts (transparent PET, 3 µm pore size, 4.67 cm², Corning Life Sciences, New York, NY, USA), according to Araújo. F [53,54]. The cell lines were seeded on the apical compartment at a density of 1×10^5 cells/cm². In the case of the triple co-culture model, Caco-2 and HT29-MTX were seeded at the proportion 90:10 and at the 14th day of culture, Raji B cells were added to the basolateral compartment in a density of 1×10^5 cells/cm². Cells were grown for 21 days until reaching confluency and the medium was changed every 2 days.

Before permeability experiments, cells were washed twice with pre-warmed Hank's buffered salt solution (HBSS) and then replaced with new HBSS and allowed to equilibrate for 30 min at 37 °C at 100 rpm. Permeability studies of CUR-loaded micelles and free CUR (20 µg/mL) were run at similar conditions during 3 h and samples were collected at different time (15, 30, 60, 90, 120, and

180 min). Each sample was taken from the basolateral side of the Transwell^{TM} cell culture insert, which contained 1% (v/v) DMSO in HBSS in order to maintain the sink conditions. The same volume of pre-warmed 1% (v/v) DMSO in HBSS was added to replace the withdrawn volume. The cell monolayers integrity was measured at the during 21 days of growth and during the experiment, using an epithelial voltohmmeter EVOM$^{2®}$ with chopstick electrodes (World Precision Instruments, Sarasota, FL, USA). The transepithelial electrical resistance (TEER) values, expressed in percentage, were normalized in function of the TEER value after equilibrium. All experiments were performed in triplicate and the CUR was quantified by measuring the absorbance at 340 nm as referred previously.

2.7. Statistical Analysis

The experiments were performed in triplicate and are represented as mean ± standard deviation (SD). A two-way ANOVA with Bonferroni multiple/post hoc group comparisons was used to analyze the cytotoxicity and permeability data. GraphPadPrism software (GraphPad Software, San Diego, CA, USA) was used and the level of significance was set at probabilities of * $p < 0.05$, ** $p < 0.01$, *** $p < 0.001$ and **** $p < 0.0001$.

3. Results and Discussion

3.1. Spectroscopic Characterizatio

The infrared spectra of chitosan, DMCh, and DMCat derivatives (Figure 1) were characterized by an intense and broad band centered at 3434 cm^{-1}, associated to the axial stretching of hydroxyl and amine groups; a band at 2915 cm^{-1} corresponding to stretching vibration of CH; the bands at 1654 and 1600 cm^{-1} assigned to the C=O stretching and N–H bending, respectively [55]. The spectrum of DMCh (Figure 1B) also exhibits a weak band centered at 1732 cm^{-1}, due to axial deformation of carbonyl ester that is related to the O-acylation of chitosan [37]. In the spectrum of DMCat, a new band is observed at 1483 cm^{-1}, which is attributed to the CH bending of $^{+}N(CH_3)_3$ group [56]. Additionally, the band corresponding to the primary amine observed at 1600 cm^{-1} in the spectrum of chitosan and DMCh is less intense in the spectrum of DMCat and it is shifted to lower wavenumber while that band observed at 1654 cm^{-1} is more intense in the spectra of DMCat, which confirms that the primary amine group of GlcN units of DMCh has been modified to secondary amine group as a consequence of the reaction with GTMAC [46,57].

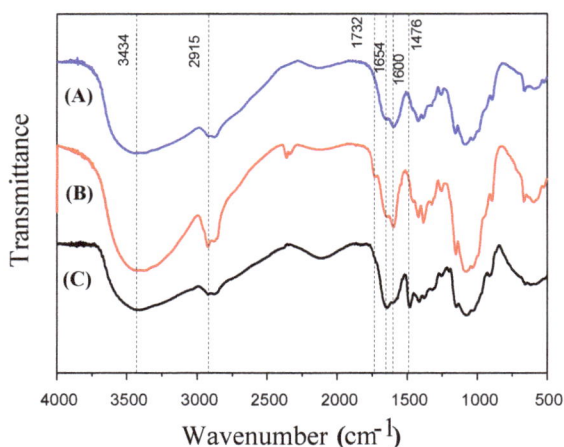

Figure 1. (**A**) Infrared spectra of chitosan, (**B**) DMCh, and (**C**) DMCat.

The comparison of the ^{1}H NMR of chitosan (Figure 2A), DMCh (Figure 2B), and DMCat (Figure 2C) provide additional evidences for the structural modifications resulting of *O*-acylation of chitosan and the quaternization of DMCh. The ^{1}H NMR spectrum of chitosan exhibited singlets at 2.0 ppm and 3.2 ppm characteristics of methyl hydrogens of GlcNAc units and to the hydrogen bonded to C2 of GlcN units, respectively. The set of signals in the range of 3.3–4.0 ppm is attributed to the hydrogens H3–H6 from GlcN unit and the hydrogen bonded to C2 of GlcNAc unit, while that signal occurring at 4.80 ppm is due to the hydrogen (H1) bonded to the anomeric carbon (C1) [46]. The average degree of deacetylation of chitosan was calculated from its ^{1}H NMR spectrum by taking into account the intensity of the signals due to methyl hydrogens from acetamido groups (2.0 ppm) and due to H2–H6 of GlcN/GlcNAc units (3.3–4.0 ppm) and resulted in $\overline{DA}$ = 5%.

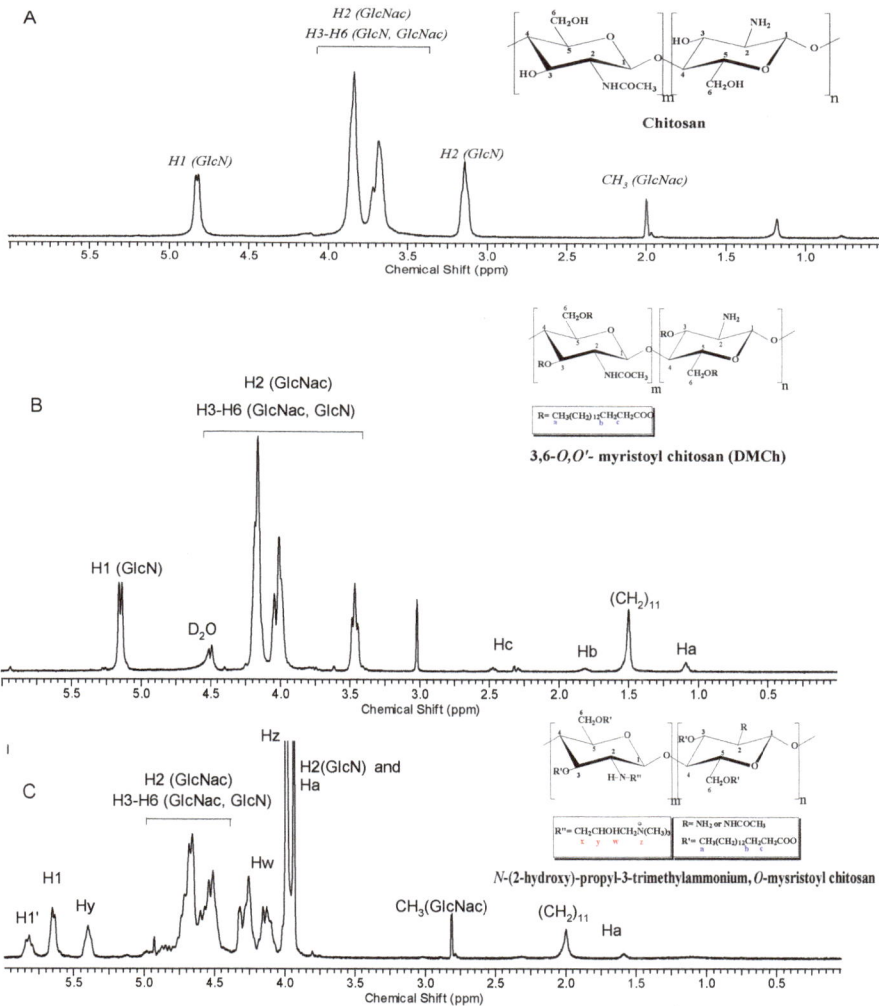

Figure 2. (A) ^{1}H nuclear magnetic resonance (NMR) spectra of chitosan, (B) DMCh, and (C) DMCat in solution D_2O/HCl 1% (*v/v*) acquired at 80 °C.

The ^{1}H NMR spectrum of DMCh (Figure 2B) exhibits additional signals at 1.1, 1.5, 1.8, 2.5, and 3.1 ppm corresponding to the hydrogen atoms of CH3, CH2, CH2 (β), and CH2 (α) moieties of myristoyl group. The peaks at 3.2–4.2 ppm refer to the hydrogens H3–H6 from the GlcN unit and the hydrogen bonded to C2 of the GlcNAc unit [37]. The $\overline{DS}$ of DMCh was calculated from ^{1}H NMR spectrum, as described in the Section 2.5.2, and resulted in $\overline{DS}$ = 6%. As a consequence of quaternization of DMCh, the ^{1}H NMR spectrum of DMCat (Figure 2B) showed signals at 4.0 ppm and 4.2 ppm assigned to the methyl hydrogens of $N^+(CH_3)_3$ and methylene hydrogens of $NHCH_2$, respectively, which were due to the introduction of the substituent on the chitosan chains. Additionally, the signals of the hydrogens H3–H6 from GlcN unit and the hydrogen bonded to C2 of GlcNAc unit shifted from 3.2–4.2 ppm to 4.4–4.9 ppm upon the chemical modification of DMCh. The signals at 5.6 ppm and 5.7 ppm are ascribed to the hydrogen bonded to the anomeric carbon of unsubstituted and substituted GlcN units, respectively. The $\overline{DQ}$ was calculated from the corresponding ^{1}H NMR spectrum by using Equation (2) and resulted in $\overline{DQ}$ = 34.7%. The average degree of quaternization of DMcat was also determined from conductometric titration and resulted in $\overline{DQ}$ = 36%, thus demonstrating a good agreement with that calculated from the ^{1}H NMR spectra.

3.2. Critical Aggregation Concentration

The critical aggregation concentration (CAC) was evaluated with the conductivity measurements of sample aqueous solutions of DMCh and DMCat at different concentrations, resulting in CAC values of 8.9×10^{-3} mg/mL [37] and 9.38×10^{-6} mg/mL, respectively. The CAC result of the DMCat sample was calculated from the data shown in Figure 3; the result related to the DMCh sample is presented in a previous work [37]. It is also important to note that each polymer was solubilized in a different aqueous medium, according to its solubility, because the aggregation behavior of the polymers was evaluated depending on their solubility as a function of the polymer concentration, thus enabling quantification of the dilution limit that each system presents until its aggregation occurs. When it came to evaluating the stability of micellar systems, the CAC of the polymer was extremely important, as it was possible to know the minimum concentration required of the amphiphilic polymer to obtain stable micelles [18]. Therefore, the ability of the micelles to withstand the dilution is described in terms of their thermodynamic stability and micelles with low CAC values can be maintained in a more dilute solution, and therefore, thermodynamically more stable [58]. A previous study [37] on the physical chemical properties of DMCh evidenced its lower CAC as compared to non-polymeric surfactants, showing that the former was thermodynamically more stable as the micelles are formed and kept stable in more dilute solutions [58]. In the same sense, taking into account that the CAC value of DMCat was much lower as compared to that of DMCh, the former system was able to form micelles at more dilute solutions, evidencing its higher stability as compared to DMCh [59,60]. DMCat derivative was more stable than the DMCh, a fact that can be explained by the permanent positive charges present in the DMCat, as these charges prevent agglomeration of the micelles by the effect of electrostatic repulsion [37,49].

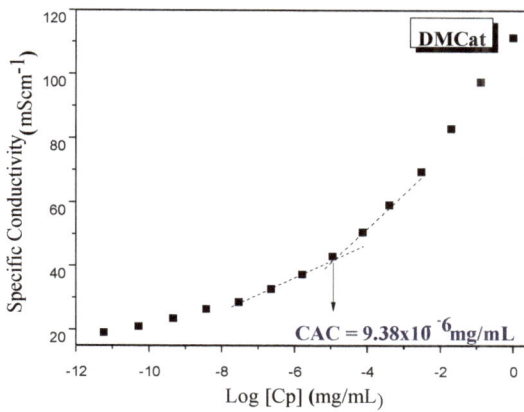

Figure 3. Graphic of specific conductivity versus function of logarithm concentration of DMCat of 1 mg/mL to 1×10^{-6} mg/mL. DMCat sample solubilized in water.

3.3. Drug Encapsulation Efficiency

The encapsulation efficiency (EE) of curcumin in the micellar systems of the DMCh and DMCat derivatives was evaluated through UV spectroscopy. The quantification was performed through the indirect method, from the no-encapsulated CUR contained in the supernatant. The EE values were calculated from the equation of the line obtained from the analytical curve and the results are presented in Table 1. According to the data in Table 1, both micellar systems presented high EE values. However, DMCh micelles had higher EE values when compared to DMCat. This difference may have occurred due to the difficulty of CUR crossing the barrier of positive charges as a consequence of the electronsteric effect. In addition, it was observed that all systems remained stable, with no formation of larger particles and/or particles precipitation.

Table 1. Size, polydispersity index, zeta potential, and encapsulation efficiency of DMCh and DMCat micelles.

Drug (µg)	Micelles–CUR							
	Sample DMCh				Sample DMCat			
	Size (nm) [1]	PDI [2]	Zeta (mV) [3]	EE (%) [4]	Size (nm) [1]	PDI [2]	Zeta (mV) [3]	EE (%) [4]
0	356 ± 21	0.53 ± 0.03	32.1 ± 4.4	-	343 ± 19	0.21 ± 0.02	34.0 ± 0.8	-
50	289 ± 17	0.49 ± 0.04	42.5 ± 2.1	92.7 ± 0.8	268 ± 43	0.62 ± 0.01	30.5 ± 1.2	100 ± 0.5
100	281 ± 38	0.44 ± 0.04	49.1 ± 0.2	81.8 ± 1.0	231 ± 15	0.66 ± 0.02	28.8 ± 1.0	73.8 ± 1.0
150	386 ± 168	0.44 ± 0.16	46.6 ± 4.12	80.9 ± 0.9	372 ± 23	0.49 ± 0.03	33.0 ± 1.5	68.6 ± 0.9

Size [1], polydispersity index [2], and zeta potential [3] were determined by carrying out dynamic light scattering measurements. Encapsulation efficiency [4] of curcumin (CUR) in percentage. Values were reported as mean ± SD (*n* = 3).

3.4. Particle Size and Surface Charge

In case of DMCh micelles, the mean diameter of the micelles varied from 281 nm to 386 nm and from 231 to 372 nm, in case of DMCat micelles (Table 1). CUR-loaded micelles presented lower values than empty micelles (Figure 4), probably due to a contraction of the micelles in the presence of the drug, caused by the greater interaction between the hydrophobic groups pertaining to the core of the micelles and the drug [37]. However, the micelles with higher CUR encapsulation reached a limit, which in turn resulted in the expansion of the volume of the micelles to accommodate a larger amount of CUR and hydrophobic groups inside. The same behavior was observed for the micelles of DMCat, showing that the hydrophobic groups present in both micellar systems have a direct influence on the size of the micelles. Therefore, from the mean diameter results it can be stated that such micelles were promising for delivery of hydrophobic drugs via oral administration.

Zeta potential of the micelles were also evaluated and according to the data presented in Table 1, loaded and empty micelles had high positive zeta potential values (> +28 mV), regardless of whether they were made up of DMCh or DMCat. In the case of DMCh micelles, the net positive charge at the micelles surface was due to the high content of amine groups pertaining to GlcN units, which were converted to ammonium groups when the polymer was dissolved in acid medium [48]. In contrast, the surface of DMCat micelles had permanent positive charges regardless of the pH of the medium because of the presence of quaternized nitrogen atoms pertaining to the substituent groups N-(2-hydroxy)-propyl-3-trimethylammonium.

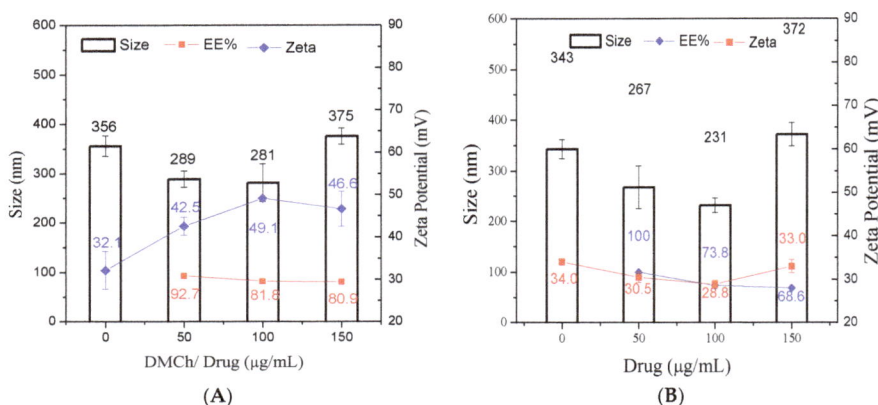

Figure 4. (**A**) the particle size, zeta potential, and encapsulation efficiency of micelles DMCh-CUR and (**B**) DMCat-CUR with different drug concentrations.

The zeta potential values of the empty and loaded micelles were slightly different. It was observed that the DMCh micelles showed an increase of the zeta potential with increase of the CUR loading. This behavior can be attributed to the fact that the formation of the micelles occurred by association of the hydrophobic moieties of the polymer chain to constitute the micelle core, while the hydrophilic portions of the positively charged polymer were exposed to the aqueous medium, i.e., the latter was predominantly located on the surface of the micelles. On the other hand, it was observed for DMCat micelles a small decrease on zeta potential values, which may be justified by the micelles surface, probably containing hydrophobic moieties, as well as a certain fraction of hydrophilic groups may be located in the micelles nuclei, varying the zeta potential in a narrow range. Thus, the high density of permanent positive charge in the hydrophilic shell of the micelles contributes strongly to stabilize them and also favors the interactions of the micelles with the negatively charged cell wall, resulting in the greater absorption and penetration of CUR.

According to the literature, formulations with PdI values ≤0.3 are representative of monodisperse systems [61,62]. From the PdI results of both micelles, it was possible to observe values ranging from 0.21 to 0.66 (Table 1), indicating that the systems did not present a monodisperse distribution. This fact can be justified by the non-uniform distribution of the acyl groups added to the chitosan chains, because it was a derivative from a heterogeneous reaction, which lead to the block distribution of the substituent groups. However, the values obtained were in agreement with the results obtained in the literature for chitosan derivatives [48,63–65].

3.5. Cytotoxicity Assay

The in vitro cell viability studies were carried out with Caco-2 and HT29-MTX intestinal cell lines to evaluate the biocompatibility and safety for the oral administration of the empty micelles, DMCh and DMCat, the micelles loaded with CUR, DMCh-CUR and DMCat-CUR, and free CUR. Loaded micelles were incubated during 4 h with different concentrations of drug (5 to 50 µg/mL) and the correspondent amount of empty micelles was also incubated in the same conditions. The cell viability was assessed using an MTT assay (Figure 5). According to the results shown in the Figure 4, it was observed that all the tested samples had no cytotoxic effect on both cell lines for the concentrations 5, 10, and 20 µg/mL. However, at the concentration of 50 µg/mL, it was possible to note a slight decrease on cell viability for unloaded and loaded micelles. This was more evident in the case of HT29-MTX cell line, which dropped very close to 70%. This 70% of cell viability is a threshold that was considered as the cytotoxic level, according to the ISO 10993-5 guideline [52].

It is important to notice that CUR presented a cytotoxic effect for the highest concentration tested with statistical significance when compared with the unloaded and loaded micelles. This means that both micelles systems had the ability to maintain and protect the drug inside of the core, at least during 4 h, showing their potential to be used in the micelles for the release of the drug in the intestine, avoiding the apparent cytotoxicity of CUR. It was assumed based on our previous published studies, where similar chitosan micelles were able to retain and protect the drug, providing a hydrophobic drug release less than 20% after 4 h in the gastric and intestinal fluids [49]. The absence of cytotoxicity from the polymers was also expected taking into account our previous work [37,49]. HT29-MTX cell line showed greater sensitivity to the tested samples. However, it is known that the intestine is constituted by a small portion of these mucus-producing cells, being the majority constituted by Caco-2 cells, which presented higher cell viability levels. Taking into account these cytotoxicity results, the concentration chosen to proceed for the in vitro intestinal permeability was 20 µg/mL, since no cytotoxic effect was observed either for the free drug or for the unloaded or loaded micelles in both cell lines.

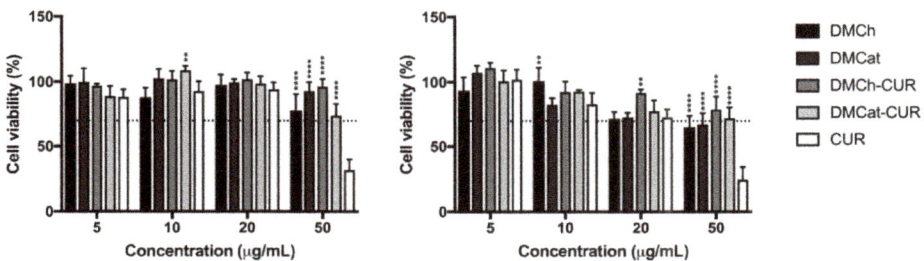

Figure 5. Cell viability of DMCh, DMCat, DMCh-CUR, DMCat-CUR, and free CUR against Caco-2 (**left**) and HT29-MTX (**right**) cell lines, respectively, at CUR concentrations between 5 and 50 µg/mL after 4 h of incubation. Values were reported as mean ± SD (*n* = 4). ** $p < 0.01$ and **** $p < 0.0001$ denotes a significant difference when compared with free CUR.

3.6. Permeability Studies

In order to evaluate the in vitro permeability estudies, non-toxic concentrations of free CUR and DMCh/DMCat loaded with CUR were selected based on cell viability results. Tests were carried out uni-directionally from the apical to the basolateral compartment. Therefore, a monoculture model consisting of Caco-2 cells was used, which represents the standard model that mimics human enterocytes. In addition, the triple co-culture model, Caco-2/HT29-MTX:Raji B was used due to be a model that better mimic the human intestine when compared to isolated Caco-2 cells, since HT29-MTX are secretory cells of mucus and Raji B cells can induce differentiation of the Caco-2 cell phenotype into M cells.

The monolayer's integrity and growth were carefully verified before the day of the experiment by measuring the TEER regularly during 21 days in order to make sure that a confluent monolayer was formed (Figure 6). As can be seen in Figure 6, Caco-2 model presented much higher TEER values compared to the triple model. These higher values were expected due to the tight junctions presented in Caco-2 cells [66]. On the other hand, the triple model presented lower TEER values due to the presence of HT29-MTX. Both models presented TEER values after 21 days that supported those monolayers to be used in the permeability experiment.

TEER values before starting the experiment were about 1600 Ω/cm^2 in the case of Caco-2 model and up to 450 Ω/cm^2 in the case of the triple model (Figure 6). The TEER values were normalized in percentage by the value at the beginning of the experiment (time zero). The permeability profile of CUR permeated through both models was plotted as a function of time expressed in percentage and is shown in Figure 7. It is possible to observe the permeability of CUR across Caco-2 monoculture model ranged from around 15% in the case of free CUR to around 18% and 24% for DMCh-CUR and DMCat-CUR, respectively, showing that both polymers are capable of carrying CUR. However, the micellar system constituted by DMCat-CUR presented no statistical difference in terms of permeability through monoculture compared to DMCh-CUR, as the first one appeared to have a faster CUR release over time, reaching almost the same permeability after 60 min compared to the CUR permeability at 180 min. The triple co-culture model presented a permeability value in the range of 10% in case of free CUR to 16% and 19% in the case of DMCat-CUR and DMCh-CUR, respectively.

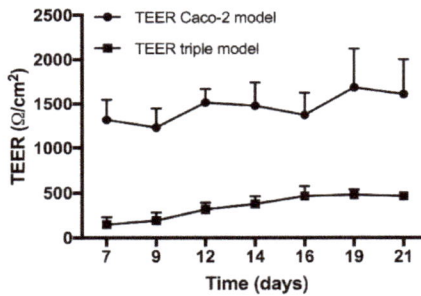

Figure 6. Transepithelial electrical resistance (TEER) values (Ω/cm^2) monitored in function of time during the 21 days of culture on Transwell™ membranes for Caco-2 monoculture model and Caco-2/HT29-MTX:Raji B triple co-culture model.

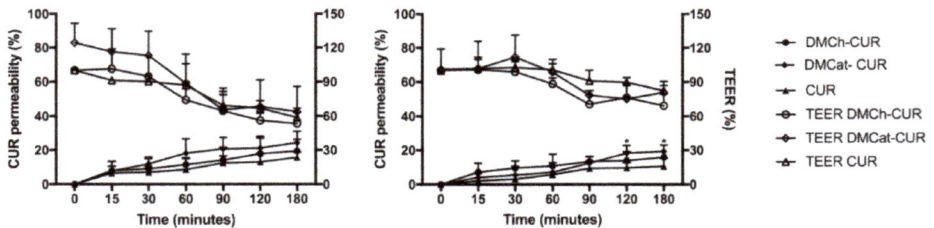

Figure 7. In vitro permeability profile of DMCh-CUR, DMCat-CUR, and free CUR across Caco-2 monoculture model (**left**) and across Caco-2/HT29-MTX:Raji B triple co-culture model (**right**) expressed in percentage. All experiments were conducted from the apical to basolateral compartment in 1% (v/v) DMSO in HBSS at 37 °C. Error bars represent mean $\pm$ SD ($n = 3$) and * $p < 0.05$ denotes a significant difference between DMCat-CUR and CUR.

In this model, a more controlled permeability of CUR was observed over time possibly due to the presence of mucus, which may delay the transport of CUR through the intestinal barrier. In addition, and as can be concluded, there is no significative difference in CUR permeability between both micellar systems. However, for the triple model, DMCat-CUR presented a statistical significance compared with free CUR, evidencing that this system presents a greater capacity to permeate in a more controlled way through the biological barriers and to do the release of the drug.

The decrease on TEER values in Caco-2 monoculture model were in agreement with the higher permeability observed in this mode. The triple co-culture model presented lower CUR permeability values for all the samples tested and this may be due to two important factors to consider due to the complexity of evaluating different biological systems. First, TEER values presented at the end of the 21 days for the triple model presented a lower value (below 500 Ω/cm^2) than that observed in the co-culture (above 1500 Ω/cm^2), making it impossible to compare between the two models. Second, the presence of mucus that entrapes the free CUR avoiding their passage through the monolayer. The lower ability of the micellar systems to permeate through the biological barriers is explained by the high capacity of mucoadhesion that the polymer presents. Preliminary studies show that the DMCat sample had a mucoadhesion capacity greater than the chitosan [67–69], due to the permanent charges present in the polymer chain (DMCat), emphasizing the importance of electrostatic forces for the establishment of interaction with the biological substrate. The effect of mucoadhesion is responsible for maintaining the DMCat-CUR system on the surface of the biological barrier, allowing the release of the sustained release of the drug over time, and in this case, the release of the drug occurs through degradation of the carrier or by diffusion through the polymeric wall. In the process of degradation are involved lysozyme and/or *N*-acetyl-beta-D-glucosaminidase (NAGase), which are enzymes present in the human body, capable of performing the hydrolysis of 1,4-beta-linkages between *N*-acetyl-D-glucosamine, a constituent of polymer chains of chitosan derivatives [67,70,71]. Perhaps, a longer experiment would be necessary to verify if CUR release from DMCat-CUR and subsequent CUR permeation would increase with time. Still, DMCat-CUR presented a more sustained and higher CUR intestinal permeability, which according to the previous results, demonstrate this system as a potential CUR intestinal delivery system.

4. Conclusions

Modification of the derivative 3,6-*O*,*O'*-dimyristoyl chitosan by the addition of quaternary groups was conducted to improve the solubility of the promising system to carry hydrophobic drugs; it was successfully performed. The presence of the permanent positive charges in the DMCat derivative allowed the solubilization of the polymer over a wide pH range. In addition, the characteristics of this polymer allowed the recognition thereof by the immunological system, thus facilitating its passage through the biological barriers, allowing the circulation of the polymer charged with a hydrophobic drug of interest.

Author Contributions: D.S.S., D.M.d.S., A.A., L.M. conceived, designed, and performed the experiments; S.P.C.-F., S.J.L.R. and B.S. contributed reagents/materials/analysis tools; the manuscript was jointly written by all authors. The manuscript has been reviewed by S.P.C.-F., S.J.L.R. and B.S.

Funding: The authors gratefully acknowledge the support from the Brazillian agency Conselho Nacional de Desenvolvimento Tecnológico (CNPQ 150964/2017-0). This article is a result of the project NORTE-01-0145-FEDER-000012, supported by Norte Portugal Regional Operational Programme (NORTE 2020), under the PORTUGAL 2020 Partnership Agreement, through the European Regional Development Fund (ERDF). This work was also financed by FEDER (Fundo Europeu de Desenvolvimento Regional) funds through the COMPETE 2020 Operacional Programme for Competitiveness and Internationalisation (POCI), Portugal 2020, and by Portuguese funds through Fundação para a Ciência e a Tecnologia (FCT)/Ministério da Ciência, Tecnologia e Ensino Superior in the framework of the project "Institute for Research and Innovation in Health Sciences" (POCI-01-0145-FEDER-007274). Andreia Almeida (grant SFRH/BD/118721/2016) would like to thank Fundação para a Ciência e a Tecnologia (FCT), Portugal for financial support.

Conflicts of Interest: The authors declare no conflict of interest. The funders had no role in the design of the study; in the collection, analyses, or interpretation of data; in the writing of the manuscript, and in the decision to publish the results.

References

1. Crucho, C.I.C.; Barros, M.T. Polymeric nanoparticles: A study on the preparation variables and characterization methods. *Mater. Sci. Eng. C* **2017**, *80*, 771–784. [CrossRef] [PubMed]
2. Lu, Z.R.; Qiao, P. Drug Delivery in Cancer Therapy, Quo Vadis? *Mol. Pharm.* **2018**, *15*, 3603–3616. [CrossRef] [PubMed]
3. Anitha, A.; Maya, S.; Deepa, N.; Chennazhi, K.P.; Nair, S.V.; Tamura, H.; Jayakumar, R. Efficient water soluble O-carboxymethyl chitosan nanocarrier for the delivery of curcumin to cancer cells. *Carbohydr. Polym.* **2011**, *83*, 452–461. [CrossRef]
4. Sajomsang, W.; Gonil, P.; Saesoo, S.; Ruktanonchai, U.R.; Srinuanchai, W.; Puttipipatkhachorn, S. Synthesis and anticervical cancer activity of novel pH responsive micelles for oral curcumin delivery. *Int. J. Pharm.* **2014**, *477*, 261–272. [CrossRef] [PubMed]
5. Ghalandarlaki, N.; Alizadeh, A.M.; Ashkani-Esfahani, S. Nanotechnology-applied curcumin for different diseases therapy. *Biomed. Res. Int.* **2014**, *2014*, 39426. [CrossRef] [PubMed]
6. Sarisozen, C.; Abouzeid, A.H.; Torchilin, V.P. The effect of co-delivery of paclitaxel and curcumin by transferrin-targeted PEG-PE-based mixed micelles on resistant ovarian cancer in 3-D spheroids and in vivo tumors. *Eur. J. Pharm. Biopharm.* **2014**, *88*, 539–550. [CrossRef] [PubMed]
7. Popat, A.; Karmaka, S.R.; Jambhrunkar, S.; Xu, C.; Yu, C. Curcumin-cyclodextrin encapsulated chitosan nanoconjugates with enhanced solubility and cell cytotoxicity. *Colloids Surf. B Biointerfaces* **2014**, *117*, 520–527. [CrossRef] [PubMed]
8. Aggarwal, B.B.; Gupta, S.C.; Sung, B. Curcumin: An orally bioavailable blocker of TNF and other pro-inflammatory biomarkers. *Br. J. Pharmacol.* **2013**, *169*, 1672–1692. [CrossRef] [PubMed]
9. Khan, S.; Imran, M.; Butt, T.T.; Ali Shah, S.W.; Sohail, M.; Malik, A.; Das, S.; Thu, H.E.; Adam, A.; Hussain, Z. Curcumin based nanomedicines as efficient Nanoplatform for treatment of cancer: New developments in reversing cancer drug resistance, rapid internalization, and improved anticancer efficacy. *Trends Food Sci. Technol.* **2018**, *80*, 8–22. [CrossRef]
10. Rauf, A.; Imran, M.; Orhan, I.E.; Bawazeer, S. Health perspectives of a bioactive compound curcumin: A review. *Trends Food Sci. Technol.* **2018**, *74*, 33–45. [CrossRef]
11. Nelson, K.M.; Dahlin, J.L.; Bisson, J.; Graham, J.; Pauli, G.F.; Walters, M.A. The Essential Medicinal Chemistry of Curcumin. *J. Med. Chem.* **2017**, *60*, 1620–1637. [CrossRef] [PubMed]
12. Anand, P.; Kunnumakkara, A.B.; Newman, R.A.; Aggarwal, B.B. Bioavailability of Curcumin: Problems and Promises. *Mol. Pharm.* **2007**, *4*, 807–818. [CrossRef] [PubMed]
13. Angeles, L.; Angeles, L.; Haven, N. Phase 1 study of PSMA-targeted docetaxel-containing nanoparticle BIND-014 in patients with advanced solid tumors. *Clin. Cancer Res.* **2016**, *22*, 3157–3163. [CrossRef]
14. Kyung, H.; Minkyu, A.; Sun, J.; Sym, J. A phase II trial of Cremorphor EL-free paclitaxel (Genexol-PM) and gemcitabine in patients with advanced non-small cell lung cancer. *Cancer Chemother. Pharmacol.* **2014**, *74*, 277–282. [CrossRef]
15. Cortez, A.J.; Tudre, P.J.; Kujawa, K.A.; Lisowska, K.M. Advances in ovarian cancer therapy. *Cancer Chemother. Pharmacol.* **2018**, *81*, 17–38. [CrossRef] [PubMed]
16. Tien, C.L.; Lacroix, M.; Ispas-Szabo, P.; Mateescu, M.A. N-acylated chitosan: Hydrophobic matrices for controlled drug release. *J. Control. Release* **2003**, *93*, 1–13. [CrossRef]
17. Ishihar, M.A.; Kishimoto, M.; Fujita, S.; Hattori, H.; Kanatani, Y. Biological, Chemical and Physical Compatibility of Chitosan and Biopharmaceuticals. *Chitosan-Based Syst. Biopharm. Deliv. Target. Polym. Ther.* **2012**, 93–106. [CrossRef]
18. Huo, M.; Zhang, Y.; Zhou, J.; Zou, A.; Li, J. Formation, microstructure, biodistribution and absence of toxicity of polymeric micelles formed by N-octyl-N,O-carboxymethyl chitosan. *Carbohydr. Polym.* **2011**, *83*, 1959–1969. [CrossRef]
19. Matsumura, Y.; Kataoka, K. Preclinical and clinical studies of anticancer agent-incorporating polymer micelles. *Cancer Sci.* **2009**, *100*, 572–579. [CrossRef] [PubMed]
20. Nishiyama, N.; Kataoka, K. Current state, achievements, and future prospects of polymeric micelles as nanocarriers for drug and gene delivery. *Pharmacol. Ther.* **2006**, *112*, 630–648. [CrossRef] [PubMed]
21. Gao, J.; Ming, J.; He, B.; Fan, Y.; Gu, Z.; Zhang, X. Preparation and characterization of novel polymeric micelles for 9-nitro-20(S)-camptothecin delivery. *Eur. J. Pharm. Sci.* **2008**, *34*, 85–93. [CrossRef] [PubMed]

22. Muley, P.; Kumar, S.; El Kourati, F.; Kesharwani, S.S.; Tummala, H. Hydrophobically modified inulin as an amphiphilic carbohydrate polymer for micellar delivery of paclitaxel for intravenous route. *Int. J. Pharm.* **2016**, *500*, 32–41. [CrossRef] [PubMed]

23. Ito, T.; Yoshida, C.; Murakami, Y. Design of novel sheet-shaped chitosan hydrogel for wound healing: A hybrid biomaterial consisting of both PEG-grafted chitosan and crosslinkable polymeric micelles acting as drug containers. *Mater. Sci. Eng. C* **2013**, *33*, 3697–3703. [CrossRef] [PubMed]

24. Du, Y.; Cai, L.; Liu, P.; You, J.; Yuan, H.; Hu, F. Biomaterials Tumor cells-speci fi c targeting delivery achieved by A54 peptide functionalized polymeric micelles. *Biomaterials* **2012**, *33*, 8858–8867. [CrossRef] [PubMed]

25. Jiao, J.; Li, X.; Zhang, S.; Liu, J.; Di, D.; Zhang, Y.; Zhao, Q.; Wang, S. Redox and pH dual-responsive PEG and chitosan-conjugated hollow mesoporous silica for controlled drug release. *Mater. Sci. Eng. C* **2016**, *67*, 26–33. [CrossRef] [PubMed]

26. Elsaid, Z.; Taylor, K.M.G.; Puri, S.; Cath, A.; Al-jamal, K.; Bai, J.; Klippstein, R.; Wang, T.; Forbes, B.; Chana, J. Mixed micelles of lipoic acid-chitosan-poly(ethylene glycol) and distearoylphosphatidylethanolamine-poly(ethylene glycol) for tumor delivery. *Eur. J. Pharm. Sci.* **2017**, *101*, 228–242. [CrossRef] [PubMed]

27. Jin, X.; Li, N.; Ju, C.; Sun, M.; Zhang, C.; Pin, Q.G. Biomaterials The mechanism of enhancement on oral absorption of paclitaxel by N-octyl-O-sulfate chitosan micelles. *Biomaterials* **2011**, *32*, 4609–4620. [CrossRef]

28. Huo, M.; Liu, Y.; Wang, L.; Yin, T.; Qin, C.; Xiao, Y.; Yin, L.; Liu, J.; Zhou, J. Redox-sensitive micelles based on O,N-hydroxyethyl chitosan-octylamine conjugates for triggered intracellular delivery of paclitaxel Redox-sensitive micelles based on O,N-hydroxyethyl chitosan-octylamine conjugates for triggered intracellular deliver. *Mol. Pharm.* **2016**, *13*, 1750–1762. [CrossRef] [PubMed]

29. Attia, E.A.B.; Ong, Z.Y.; Hedrick, J.L.; Lee, P.P.; Lee, P.L.R.; Hammond, P.T.; Yang, Y.-Y. Mixed micelles self-assembled from block copolymers for drug delivery. *Curr. Opin. Colloid Interface Sci.* **2011**, *16*, 182–194. [CrossRef]

30. Jiang, G.B.B.; Quan, D.; Liao, K.; Wang, H. Novel polymer micelles prepared from chitosan grafted hydrophobic palmitoyl groups for drug delivery. *Mol. Pharm.* **2006**, *3*, 152–160. [CrossRef] [PubMed]

31. Zhang, C.; Qu, G.; Sun, Y.; Wu, X.; Yao, Z.; Guo, Q.; Ding, Q.; Yuan, S.; Shen, Z.; Ping, Q.; et al. Pharmacokinetics, biodistribution, efficacy and safety of N-octyl-O-sulfate chitosan micelles loaded with paclitaxel. *Biomaterials* **2008**, *29*, 1233–1241. [CrossRef] [PubMed]

32. Hu, F.Q.Q.; Zhao, M.D.D.; Yuan, H.; You, J.; Du, Y.Z.Z.; Zeng, S. A novel chitosan oligosaccharide-stearic acid micelles for gene delivery: Properties and in vitro transfection studies. *Int. J. Pharm.* **2006**, *315*, 158–166. [CrossRef] [PubMed]

33. Chenguang, L.I.U.; Desai, K.G.; Xiguang, C.; Hyun-jin, P. Preparation and Charaterization of Self-assembled Nanoparticles Based on Linolenic-acid Modified Chitosan. *J. Ocean Univ. China* **2005**, *4*, 234–239. [CrossRef]

34. Hu, F.Q.; Ren, G.F.; Yuan, H.; Du, Y.Z.; Zeng, S. Shell cross-linked stearic acid grafted chitosan oligosaccharide self-aggregated micelles for controlled release of paclitaxel. *Colloids Surf. B Biointerfaces* **2006**, *50*, 97–103. [CrossRef] [PubMed]

35. Huo, M.; Zhang, Y.; Zhou, J.; Zou, A.; Yu, D.; Wu, Y.; Li, J.; Li, H. Synthesis and characterization of low-toxic amphiphilic chitosan derivatives and their application as micelle carrier for antitumor drug. *Int. J. Pharm.* **2010**, *394*, 162–173. [CrossRef] [PubMed]

36. Du, Y.Z.Z.; Wang, L.; Yuan, H.; Wei, X.H.H.; Hu, F.Q.Q. Preparation and characteristics of linoleic acid-grafted chitosan oligosaccharide micelles as a carrier for doxorubicin. *Colloids Surf. B Biointerfaces* **2009**, *69*, 257–263. [CrossRef] [PubMed]

37. Silva, D.S.; Almeida, A.; Prezotti, F.; Cury, B.; Campana-Filho, S.P.; Sarmento, B. Synthesis and characterization of 3,6-O,O'-dimyristoyl chitosan micelles for oral delivery of paclitaxel. *Colloids Surf. B Biointerfaces* **2017**, *152*, 220–228. [CrossRef] [PubMed]

38. Pan, Z.; Gao, Y.; Heng, L.; Liu, Y.; Yao, G.; Wang, Y.; Liu, Y. Amphiphilic N-(2,3-dihydroxypropyl)-chitosan-cholic acid micelles for paclitaxel delivery. *Carbohydr. Polym.* **2013**, *94*, 394–399. [CrossRef] [PubMed]

39. Di Martino, A.; Sedlarik, V. Amphiphilic chitosan-grafted-functionalized polylactic acid based nanoparticles as a delivery system for doxorubicin and temozolomide co-therapy. *Int. J. Pharm.* **2014**, *474*, 134–145. [CrossRef] [PubMed]

40. Zhang, C.; Ding, Y.; Lucy, L.; Ping, Q. Polymeric micelle systems of hydroxycamptothecin based on amphiphilic *N*-alkyl-*N*-trimethyl chitosan derivatives. *Colloids Surf. B Biointerfaces* **2007**, *55*, 192–199. [CrossRef] [PubMed]
41. Zuñiga, A.; Debbaudt, A.; Albertengo, L.; Rodríguez, M.S. Synthesis and characterization of *N*-propyl-*N*-methylene phosphonic chitosan derivative. *Carbohydr. Polym.* **2010**, *79*, 475–480. [CrossRef]
42. Woraphatphadung, T.; Sajomsang, W.; Gonil, P.; Treetong, A.; Akkaramongkolporn, P.; Ngawhirunpat, T.; Opanasopit, P. pH-Responsive polymeric micelles based on amphiphilic chitosan derivatives: Effect of hydrophobic cores on oral meloxicam delivery. *Int. J. Pharm.* **2016**, *497*, 150–160. [CrossRef] [PubMed]
43. Wu, J.; Wei, W.; Wang, L.Y.; Su, Z.G.; Ma, G.H. A thermosensitive hydrogel based on quaternized chitosan and poly(ethylene glycol) for nasal drug delivery system. *Biomaterials* **2007**, *28*, 2220–2232. [CrossRef] [PubMed]
44. Sonia, T.A.; Sharma, C.P. In vitro evaluation of *N*-(2-hydroxy) propyl-3-trimethyl ammonium chitosan for oral insulin delivery. *Carbohydr. Polym.* **2011**, *84*, 103–109. [CrossRef]
45. Ruihua, H.; Bingchao, Y.; Zheng, D.; Wang, B. Preparation and characterization of a quaternized chitosan. *J. Mater. Sci.* **2012**, *47*, 845–851. [CrossRef]
46. Santos, D.M.; Bukzem, A.L.; Campana-Filho, S.P. Response surface methodology applied to the study of the microwave-assisted synthesis of quaternized chitosan. *Carbohydr. Polym.* **2016**, *138*, 317–326. [CrossRef] [PubMed]
47. Rinaudo, M.; Milas, M.; Le Dung, P. Characterization of chitosan. Influence of ionic strength and degree of acetylation on chain expansion. *Int. J. Biol. Macromol.* **1993**, *15*, 281–285. [CrossRef]
48. Almeida, A.; Silva, D.S.; Gonçalves, V.; Sarmento, B. Synthesis and characterization of chitosan-grafted-polycaprolactone micelles for modulate intestinal paclitaxel delivery. *Drug Deliv. Transl. Res.* **2017**, *7*, 1–11. [CrossRef] [PubMed]
49. Silva, D.S.; Almeida, A.; Prezotti, F.G.; Facchinatto, W.M.; Colnago, L.A.; Campana-Filho, S.P.; Sarmento, B. Self-aggregates of 3,6-*O*,*O'*-dimyristoylchitosan derivative are effective in enhancing the solubility and intestinal permeability of camptothecin. *Carbohydr. Polym.* **2017**, *177*, 178–186. [CrossRef] [PubMed]
50. Hirai, A.; Odani, H.; Nakajim, A.A. Determination of degree of deacetylation of chitosan by ^{1}H NMR spectroscopy. *Polym. Bull.* **1991**, *94*, 87–94. [CrossRef]
51. Fiamingo, A.; Delezuk, J.A.D.M.; Trombotto, S.; David, L.; Campana-Filho, S.P. Extensively deacetylated high molecular weight chitosan from the multistep ultrasound-assisted deacetylation of beta-chitin. *Ultrason. Sonochem.* **2016**, *32*, 79–85. [CrossRef] [PubMed]
52. ISO/EN10993-5. *International Standard ISO 10993-5 Biological Evaluation of Medical Devices—Part 5: Tests for Cytotoxicity: In Vitro Methods*; International Organization for Standardization: Geneva, Switzerland, 2009; Volume 42.
53. Araújo, F.; Sarmento, B. Towards the characterization of an in vitro triple co-culture intestine cell model for permeability studies. *Int. J. Pharm.* **2013**, *458*, 128–134. [CrossRef] [PubMed]
54. Antunes, F.; Andrade, F.; Araújo, F.; Ferreira, D.; Sarmento, B. Establishment of a triple co-culture in vitro cell models to study intestinal absorption of peptide drugs. *Eur. J. Pharm. Biopharm.* **2013**, *83*, 427–435. [CrossRef] [PubMed]
55. Brugnerotto, J.; Lizardi, J.; Goycoolea, F.M.; Argüelles-Monal, W.; Desbrières, J.; Rinaudo, M. An infrared investigation in relation with chitin and chitosan characterization. *Polymer* **2001**, *42*, 3569–3580. [CrossRef]
56. Cho, J.; Grant, J.; Piquette-miller, M.; Allen, C. Synthesis and Physicochemical and Dynamic Mechanical Properties of a Water-Soluble Chitosan Derivative as a Biomaterial. *Biomacromolecules* **2006**, *10*, 2845–2855. [CrossRef] [PubMed]
57. Xiao, B.; Wan, Y.; Wang, X.; Zha, Q.; Liu, H.; Qiu, Z.; Zhang, S. Synthesis and characterization of *N*-(2-hydroxy)propyl-3-trimethyl ammonium chitosan chloride for potential application in gene delivery. *Colloids Surf. B Biointerfaces* **2012**, *91*, 168–174. [CrossRef] [PubMed]
58. Croy, S.R.; Kwon, G.S. Polymeric micelles for drug delivery. *Curr. Pharm. Des.* **2006**, *12*, 4669–4684. [CrossRef] [PubMed]
59. Li, Y.; Li, L.; Dong, H.; Cai, X.; Ren, T. Pluronic F127 nanomicelles engineered with nuclear localized functionality for targeted drug delivery. *Mater. Sci. Eng. C* **2013**, *33*, 2698–2707. [CrossRef] [PubMed]
60. Li, X.; Yu, Y.; Ji, Q.; Qiu, L. Targeted delivery of anticancer drugs by aptamer AS1411 mediated Pluronic F127/cyclodextrin-linked polymer composite micelles. *Nanomedicine* **2014**, *1*, 175–184. [CrossRef] [PubMed]

61. Rao, J.P.; Geckeler, K.E. Polymer nanoparticles: Preparation techniques and size-control parameters. *Prog. Polym. Sci.* **2011**, *36*, 887–913. [CrossRef]
62. Hickey, J.W.; Santos, J.L.; Williford, J.M.; Mao, H.Q. Control of polymeric nanoparticle size to improve therapeutic delivery. *J. Control. Release* **2015**, *219*, 535–547. [CrossRef] [PubMed]
63. Yuan, H.; Lu, L.; Du, Y.; Hu, F. Stearic acid-g-chitosan polymeric micelle for oral drug delivery: In intro transport and in vivo absorption. *Mol. Pharm.* **2010**, *8*, 225–238. [CrossRef] [PubMed]
64. Zhang, C.; Ping, Q.; Zhang, H.; Shen, J. Preparation of N-alkyl-O-sulfate chitosan derivatives and micellar solubilization of taxol. *Carbohydr. Polym.* **2003**, *54*, 137–141. [CrossRef]
65. Zhang, C.; Qineng, P.; Zhang, H. Self-assembly and characterization of paclitaxel-loaded N-octyl-O-sulfate chitosan micellar system. *Colloids Surf. B Biointerfaces* **2004**, *39*, 69–75. [CrossRef] [PubMed]
66. Lechanteur, A.; Almeida, A.; Sarmento, B. Elucidation of the impact of cell culture conditions of Caco-2 cell monolayer on barrier integrity and intestinal permeability. *Eur. J. Pharm. Biopharm.* **2017**, *119*, 137–141. [CrossRef] [PubMed]
67. Park, J.H.; Saravanakumar, G.; Kim, K.; Kwon, I.C. Targeted delivery of low molecular drugs using chitosan and its derivatives. *Adv. Drug Deliv. Rev.* **2010**, *62*, 28–41. [CrossRef] [PubMed]
68. Hejazi, R.; Amiji, M. Chitosan-based gastrointestinal delivery systems. *J. Control. Release* **2003**, *89*, 151–165. [CrossRef]
69. Tozaki, H.; Komoike, J.; Tada, C.; Maruyama, T.; Terabe, A.; Suzuki, T.; Yamamoto, A.; Muranishi, S. Chitosan capsules for colon-specific drug delivery: Improvement of insulin absorption from the rat colon. *J. Pharm. Sci.* **1997**, *86*, 1016–1021. [CrossRef] [PubMed]
70. Bernkop-Schnürch, A.; Dünnhaupt, S. Chitosan-based drug delivery systems. *Eur. J. Pharm. Biopharm.* **2012**, *81*, 463–469. [CrossRef] [PubMed]
71. Chauvierre, C.; Leclerc, L.; Labarre, D.; Appel, M.; Marden, M.C.; Couvreur, P.; Vauthier, C. Enhancing the tolerance of poly(isobutylcyanoacrylate) nanoparticles with a modular surface design. *Int. J. Pharm.* **2007**, *338*, 327–332. [CrossRef] [PubMed]

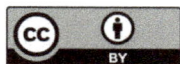

pharmaceutics

MDPI

Article

Intestinal Drug Absorption Enhancement by *Aloe vera* Gel and Whole Leaf Extract: In Vitro Investigations into the Mechanisms of Action

Anja Haasbroek [1], Clarissa Willers [1], Matthew Glyn [2], Lissinda du Plessis [1] and Josias Hamman [1,*]

1   Centre of Excellence for Pharmaceutical Sciences (Pharmacen™), Potchefstroom Campus, North West University, Potchefstroom 2520, South Africa; 22692592@nwu.ac.za or anjahaasbroek11@gmail.com (A.H.); 20672322@nwu.ac.za (C.W.); Lissinda.duPlessis@nwu.ac.za (L.d.P.)
2   Preclinical Drug Development Platform (PCDDP), Potchefstroom Campus, North West University, Potchefstroom 2520, South Africa; mglynmglyn@live.co.uk
*   Correspondence: sias.hamman@nwu.ac.za; Tel.: +27-18-299-4035

Received: 27 November 2018; Accepted: 13 December 2018; Published: 18 January 2019

Abstract: The co-administration of absorption enhancing agents with macromolecular drugs (e.g., protein and peptide drugs) has been identified as a means to improve the oral bioavailability of these drugs. Absorption-enhancing agents of natural origins have received a great deal of attention due to their sustainable production, in support of green chemistry. In previous studies, certain parts of the *Aloe vera* leaf (e.g., gel and whole leaf extract) have shown a potential to enhance drug permeation across the intestinal epithelial barrier. The mechanism of the drug-absorption-enhancement action and the capacity for absorption-enhancement of the *A. vera* gel and whole leaf, were investigated in this study. A clear decrease in transepithelial electrical resistance (TEER) of Caco-2 cell monolayers exposed to *A. vera* gel and wholeleaf extract, in various concentrations, indicated the opening of tight junctions between the epithelial cells. The transport of Fluorescein isothiocyanate (FITC)-dextran, with a molecular weight of 4 kDa (FD-4), could be enhanced across the Caco-2 cell monolayers, by the *A. vera* gel and whole-leaf extract, but not the FITC-dextran with larger molecular weights (i.e., 10, 20, and 40 kDa), which indicated a limited drug absorption enhancement capacity, in terms of the molecular size. Accumulation of FD-4 between the Caco-2 cells (and not within the cells), after treatment with the *A. vera* gel and whole-leaf extract was shown with a confocal laser scanning microscopy (CLSM) imaging, indicating that the paracellular transport of FD-4 occurred after the interaction of the *A. vera* gel and whole-leaf extract, with the epithelial cell monolayers. Furthermore, changes in the F-actin distribution in the cytoskeleton of the Caco-2 cell monolayers was observed by means of a fluorescence staining, which confirmed tight junction modulation as the mechanism of action for the absorption enhancement effect of the *A. vera* gel and whole-leaf extract.

Keywords: *Aloe vera*; gel; whole leaf; absorption enhancement; Caco-2; confocal laser scanning microscopy; F-actin; FITC-dextran; tight junctions; transepithelial electrical resistance

1. Introduction

The oral route of drug administration is associated with relatively high patient compliance and is more affordable, when compared to the injection therapies [1]. Reasons for a high patient compliance with the oral route of administration, include self-treatment, ease of use, and its non-invasive nature [2]. On the other hand, oral drug administration is challenged by the low bioavailability of certain drugs, such as macromolecular drugs [1]. The general low-membrane permeability and oral bioavailability of large compounds (molecular weight > 500 Da) can be ascribed to their unfavorable physico-chemical properties [3], as well as the harsh gastrointestinal environment where enzymatic and chemical activity cause extensive degradation, especially, of protein and peptide drugs [4].

For an orally administered drug to have its desired pharmacological effect, the drug must reach the systemic circulation via absorption, through the intestinal epithelial layer [5], which can occur via the paracellular or transcellular pathways [6,7]. The paracellular pathway is the transport of drug molecules between epithelial cells and occurs by means of size-limited passive diffusion, through the tight junctions and intercellular spaces. Hydrophilic macromolecules, such as peptide and protein drugs are mainly transported via the paracellular route, since they cannot penetrate cell membranes [7,8], however, their paracellular movement is severely restricted by the tight junctions between the adjacent epithelial cells [9]. A promising approach to improve the oral absorption of these hydrophilic macromolecules is the co-administration of absorption enhancers [7].

Tight junctions (zonula occludens) are one of three intercellular complexes, with adherence junctions (zonula adherens) and desmosomes (macula adherens), which link epithelial cells together. Tight junctions can be described as dynamic multi-protein complex structures consisting of various transmembrane proteins, with the main proteins being occludin, tricellulin, and the claudin family. These proteins are connected to the cell actin cytoskeleton, via the scaffolding protein zonula occludens-1 (ZO-1). Thus, a change in the actin distribution can be linked to a modulation of one or more tight junction proteins [10,11]. The dynamic nature of the tight junction ensures that it can be modulated by different stimuli, resulting in an increased paracellular absorption, in a reversible and potentially safe manner [12]. Tight junction modulation can be experimentally confirmed by transepithelial electrical resistance (TEER) measurements, as well as the permeability of paracellular markers. In addition, microscopic examination after staining of cell components and intercellular accumulation of fluorescent probes, can be used to indicate the opening of tight junctions as a mechanism of paracellular drug-absorption enhancement [13,14].

Oral drug-absorption enhancement of protein and peptide drugs can be defined as the process of improving the movement of the drug molecules across the intestinal epithelium, which can be accomplished by the incorporation of functional excipients, in dosage forms. This improved membrane permeation should be accomplished without damaging the cells or causing toxic effects [15,16]. Absorption enhancers are chemical adjuvants that are co-administered with peptides and proteins, to increase their bioavailability, by reversibly removing or disrupting the intestinal barrier, with minimal tissue damage [17]. The mechanisms through which this can be achieved include decreasing mucus viscosity, changing membrane fluidity, disrupting the structural integrity of the intestinal wall or modulating the tight junctions [17,18].

Many compounds have already been investigated for their potential drug-absorption enhancing abilities, including various chemicals of natural origin that are derived from plants (capsaicin, piperine, quercetin, and *Aloe vera*) and from animals (chitosan and zonula occludens toxin). Different mechanisms of absorption enhancement have been suggested for these chemical absorption-enhancing agents, such as regulation of gastrointestinal function, enzyme inhibition, P-gp efflux inhibition, mucoadhesion, and tight junction modulation [12,19–24].

Aloe vera is a succulent perennial xerophyte that displays the water-storage mechanisms in leaves, such as the formation of a viscous mucilage to survive in arid regions with little or irregular rainfall [25,26]. The innermost part of the leaf is made up of clear, moist, soft, and slippery tissue that consists of thin-walled parenchyma cells [27]. As a result, the thick fleshy leaves contain amongst other compounds, storage carbohydrates, such as acetylated mannan (acemannan or aloverose) and cell wall carbohydrates, such as cellulose and hemicellulose [28].

Aloe vera has long been used in traditional medicine, where the latex has been used for its laxative effects and the gel was mainly used for the treatment of wounds and skin ailments, such as psoriasis and genital herpes [29]. Other uses that have also been ascribed to *A. vera* components include anti-bacterial, anti-cancer, anti-diabetic, anti-fungal, anti-obesity, anti-viral effects, and gastric protection against ulcers [25,29,30].

A study was conducted to evaluate the effect of *A. vera* liquid preparations on the absorption of vitamin C and E, in human subjects, and it was found that *A. vera* markedly improved the oral bioavailability of both these vitamins [31]. It was shown in an in vitro study that the *A. vera* gel and whole-leaf extract had the ability to markedly enhance the transport of insulin across the Caco-2 cell monolayers [32]. Thereafter, several in vitro studies were conducted on the effect of the *A. vera* gel and whole-leaf extract on macromolecular and other hydrophilic compounds, across intestinal epithelial cell monolayers, excised intestinal tissues [32–35], excised skin [36,37], and across excised buccal mucosa [38]. The P-gp-modulating effects of the *A. vera* juice was investigated by Djuv and Nilsen [39], but they found that the *A. vera* juice did not inhibit the P-gp mediated transport of digoxin, in a statistically significant way in any of the concentrations that were tested.

The aim of this study was to identify the mechanism of action by which the *A. vera* gel and the whole leaf extract, enhance the gastrointestinal absorption of macromolecules, as well as to establish the capacity of these materials in terms of the size of the molecules, which can be moved across the intestinal epithelium. This was done by determining the transport of the FITC-dextran with different molecular weights across the Caco-2 cell monolayers, after treatment with the *A. vera* gel and whole-leaf extract, by TEER studies, by visualization of the accumulation of the FITC-dextran (4 kDa) between the Caco-2 cells, on the monolayers grown on membrane inserts, and by fluorescence staining and visualization of the F-actin structure of the Caco-2 cells, after incubation with the *A. vera* gel and the whole-leaf extract.

2. Materials and Methods

2.1. Materials

Dehydrated *Aloe vera* gel powder 200X (Dalton Max 700® gel) and whole leaf, decolourised, spray-dried *Aloe vera* powder 100X (whole-leaf extract) were kindly donated by Improve USA. Inc. (De Soto, TX, USA). Chitosan (ChitoClear® with a degree of deacetylation of 96% and viscosity of 8 cP for a 1% solution) was purchased from Primex (Siglufjordur, Iceland). Fluorescein isothiocyanate (FITC)-dextran with molecular weight (MW) of 4 kDa (FD-4), 10 kDa (FD-10), 20 kDa (FD-20), and 40 kDa (FD-40), as well as Lucifer Yellow, were purchased from Sigma-Aldrich/Merck (Darmstadt, Germany). CytoPainter® Phalloidin iFluor 488 and Fluoroshield® mounting medium, with propidium iodide, were purchased from Abcam (Cambridge, MA, USA).

2.2. Chemical Characterisation of the A. vera Gel and the Whole-Leaf Extract

Quantitative proton nuclear magnetic resonance (^{1}H-NMR) analysis was used to chemically characterise the *A. vera* gel and the whole-leaf extract, by determining the content of certain marker molecules, including aloverose, glucose, malic acid, and iso-citric acid (whole-leaf marker), as previously described [40].

2.3. Chemical Characterisation of N-Trimethyl Chitosan Chloride

N-trimethyl chitosan chloride (TMC) was synthesised from chitosan (ChitoClear®, degree of deacetylation of 96% and viscosity of 8 cP, for a 1% solution), as previously described [41], and characterized by the means of ^{1}H-NMR spectroscopy, using an Avance III 600 Hz NMR spectrometer (Bruker BioSpin Corporation, Rheinstetlen, Germany). A sample of the TMC (100 mg) was dissolved in 2 mL D_2O and analyzed in the NMR spectrometer, at 80 °C, with a suppression of the water peak. The degree of quaternization of the TMC was calculated from the ^{1}H-NMR spectra, by using Equation (1), as previously described [42]:

$$DQ\ (\%) = \left[\left(\frac{\int TM}{\int H} \right) \times \frac{1}{9} \right] \times 100 \tag{1}$$

where DQ (%) is the percentage of the degree of quaternization, $\int$TM is the integral of the trimethyl amino group (quaternary amino) peak at 3.7–4.0 ppm, on the ^{1}H-NMR spectra, and $\int$H is the integral of the ^{1}H peaks from 4.7–6.2 ppm, on the ^{1}H-NMR spectra.

2.4. Caco-2 Cell Culturing

The Caco-2 cells were procured from the European Collection of Authenticated Cell Cultures (ECACC). Caco-2 cells were cultured in a growth medium that consisted of high-glucose Dulbecco's Modified Eagles Medium (DMEM), supplemented with 10% v/v fetal bovine serum (FBS), 1% v/v non-essential amino-acid solution (NEAA), 1% v/v penicillin/streptomycin (10,000 U/mL penicillin and 10,000 U/mL streptomycin), 1% v/v amphotericin B (250 µg/mL), and 2 mM L-glutamine. The cells were incubated at 37 °C and exposed to 95% humidified air and 5% CO_2. The Caco-2 cells were used between passages 51–56.

2.5. Cell Monolayer Integrity

The integrity of the cell monolayers was confirmed by measuring the TEER, as well as determining the permeation of the exclusion marker, Lucifer yellow [43,44].

Prior to each permeation experiment, the TEER of the Caco-2 cell monolayers was measured to confirm the formation of a confluent cell monolayer on the insert membrane. The minimum TEER values, as indicated in Table 1, were required and considered as indicative of the presence of intact cell monolayers, in the different Transwell® plates (Corning Costar®, Corning, NY, USA) [45–47].

Table 1. Required transepithelial electrical resistance (TEER) values, as indicative of the intact Caco-2 cell monolayers, on different Transwell®plate insert membranes.

Type of Transwell® Plate	TEER Value Measured (Ω)	TEER Value Normalized for Surface Area (Ω·cm^2)
Transwell® 6-well plates (surface area = 4.67 cm^2) [45]	150	700.5
Transwell® 24-well plates (surface area = 0.33 cm^2) [46]	750	247.5
Snapwell® 6-well plates (surface area = 1.12 cm^2) [47]	179	200.0

Lucifer yellow was used as an exclusion transport marker molecule, to confirm the formation of confluent Caco-2 cell monolayers on the inserts of each Transwell® plate. The growth medium was aspirated from the basolateral chambers of the 6-well Transwell® plate and replaced with the appropriate volume of pre-heated serum-free DMEM, buffered with N-(2-hydroxyethyl) piperazine-N-(2-ethanesulfonic acid) (HEPES) (pH = 7.4), and incubated for 30 min, at 37 °C. After 30 min, the Transwell® plates were removed from the incubator, the growth medium was aspirated from the apical chambers and replaced with an appropriate volume of a pre-heated Lucifer yellow solution (i.e., 50 µg/mL in serum-free DMEM) [44]. The Transwell® plates were incubated with the Lucifer yellow solution and samples (200 µL) were withdrawn from the basolateral chamber, every 20 min, for 120 min, and replaced with equal volumes of pre-heated serum-free DMEM buffered with HEPES. The Lucifer yellow concentration in the samples was quantified by means of fluorescence spectroscopy, at excitation, and at emission wavelengths of 485 nm and 535 nm, respectively [48]. The percentage transport of Lucifer yellow across the Caco-2 cell monolayer should be less than 2% for the two-hour transport period, to indicate intact cell monolayers [48]. Furthermore, apparent permeability coefficient (P_{app}) values of the Lucifer yellow $\leq 0.2 \times 10^{-6}$ cm/s [43] or 0.66–0.75×10^{-6} cm/s [44], were considered indicative of the formation of intact Caco-2 cell monolayers.

2.6. In Vitro Transepithelial Electrical Resistance (TEER) Study

Caco-2 cells were cultured in Transwell® 24-well plates (Corning Costar®) on insert membranes, with a surface area of 0.33 cm² and pore size of 0.4 μm, to form confluent monolayers. The positive control consisted of 0.5% *w/v* TMC (a known tight junction modulator), while the test solutions consisted of *A. vera* gel and whole-leaf extract, each in four different concentrations ranging from 0.1 % *w/v* to 1.5% *w/v*. Serum-free DMEM alone was used as the negative control.

The TEER measurements of the Caco-2 cell monolayers on insert membranes in 24-well Transwell® plates commenced one hour prior to addition of the test solutions, to obtain the TEER values, at a baseline level. DMEM buffered with HEPES (pH = 7.4) (1 mL) was added to the basolateral chamber and incubated for 30 min, prior to the addition of the test solutions (200 μL) to the apical chamber on top of the cell monolayers, on the filter membranes. The TEER (T_0) was measured directly, after application of the test solutions to the apical chamber. TEER measurements were then taken at 20 min intervals up to 120 min, after addition of test solutions. TEER was measured with a Millicell ERS meter (Millipore, Billerica, MA, USA) that was connected to a set of chopstick electrodes.

2.7. In Vitro Permeation Studies

Caco-2 cells were cultured in Transwell® 6-well plates (Corning Costar®) on insert membranes, with a surface area of 4.67 cm² and a pore size of 0.4 μm, to form confluent monolayers. For the in vitro permeation study, four different FITC-dextran (i.e., FD-4, FD-10, FD-20 and FD-40) solutions were prepared, each in a concentration of 125 μg/mL, in serum-free DMEM. Four different concentrations of each of the *A. vera* gel and whole leaf extract (ranging from 0.1 % *w/v* to 1.5% *w/v*) were added to each of the FITC-dextran solutions, to prepare the experimental solutions. Control groups consisted of each FITC-dextran in serum-free DMEM, without *A. vera* gel and the whole-leaf extract.

The in vitro permeation of each of the FITC-dextran molecules, in the absence and presence of the different *A. vera* gel and the whole-leaf extract solutions, was determined in the apical to basolateral (AP-BL, absorptive) direction, across the Caco-2 cell monolayers. First, the growth medium was aspirated from the basolateral chamber and replaced with 2.5 mL pre-heated serum-free DMEM buffered with HEPES (pH = 7.4) and placed back in the incubator (37 °C), to equilibrate for 30 min. After 30 min, the Transwell® plates were removed from the incubator and the growth medium from the apical chamber was aspirated and replaced with 2.5 mL of each of the experimental solutions pre-heated to 37 °C. Samples (200 μL) were extracted from the basolateral chamber at 20 min intervals for a total period of 120 min and replaced with 200 μL pre-heated DMEM buffered with HEPES. The quantification of the FITC-dextran concentrations, in the samples, was done by means of fluorescence spectroscopy, at excitation and at emission wavelengths of 494 and 518 nm, respectively.

The percentage transport was calculated from the concentration of each FITC-dextran (i.e., FD-4, FD-10, FD-20, and FD-40) measured in the samples withdrawn from the basolateral chamber, at each time interval. The percentage transport was calculated with the following equation:

$$\%\text{Transport} = \frac{\text{Drug concentration at specific time interval}}{\text{Initial FITC} - \text{dextran dose}} \times 100 \qquad (2)$$

The apparent permeability coefficient (P_{app}) values were calculated from the percentage transport data across the Caco-2 cell monolayers, for each of the FITC-dextran molecules. P_{app} is defined as the permeability rate that is normalized by the surface area, across which the permeation occurs, as well as the concentration, assuming the starting concentration in the acceptor (basolateral) chamber is zero [49]. The P_{app} was calculated by using the following equation [50,51]:

$$P_{app} = \text{dc/dt} \frac{1}{(A \cdot 60 \cdot C_0)}, \qquad (3)$$

where P_{app} is the apparent permeability coefficient $(cm \cdot s^{-1})$, (dc/dt) represents the permeability rate (concentration/min, represented by the slope of the transport curve), A is the permeation surface area (cm^2), and C_0 is the starting concentration of the permeant.

From the P_{app} values, the permeation-enhancement ratio (R) values were calculated by the following equation [32]:

$$R = \frac{P_{app} \text{ experiment}}{P_{app} \text{ control}} \tag{4}$$

where R is the permeation-enhancement ratio, P_{app} experiment is the apparent permeability coefficient for the test solution, and P_{app} control is the apparent permeability coefficient for the control group.

2.8. Caco-2 Cell Monolayers for the Confocal Laser Scanning Microscopy (CLSM) Study

For the CLSM visualisation studies (for both the transport pathway and the F-actin filament studies), the Caco-2 cells were cultured in Snapwell® 6-well plates (Corning Costar®), with removable filter-rings, which had a surface area of 1.12 cm² and a pore size of 0.4 µm, to form confluent cell monolayers. Stock solutions of the FITC-dextran 4 kDa (FD-4, 1 mg/mL), the *A. vera* gel, the *A. vera* whole-leaf extract (2.0% *w/v*), and TMC (1.0% *w/v*), were each prepared, separately, in a serum-free DMEM. These stock solutions were used to prepare the experimental solutions, which consisted of combinations of the FITC-dextran and each of the permeation enhancers solutions (i.e., *A. vera* gel, *A. vera* whole leaf, and TMC) in a 1:1 ratio that were applied to the Caco-2 cell monolayers. The final concentrations of the test solutions were, therefore, 1.0% *w/v A. vera* gel, 1.0% *w/v A. vera* whole-leaf extract and 0.5% *w/v* TMC, while the final concentration of FITC-dextran (FD-4) in the mixture, applied to the cell monolayers, was 0.5 mg/mL. The negative control group consisted of serum-free DMEM, without any of the chemical permeation enhancers.

For the fluorescence staining, a 10× CytoPainter® Phalloidin iFluor 488 solution was prepared by diluting 5 µL of a 1000× phalloidin conjugate in dimethyl sulfoxide (DMSO) stock solution with 500 µL PBS, containing 1.1% *v/v* foetal bovine serum (FBS). The 0.1% *v/v* Triton X100 solution was prepared by diluting 3 µL of the 100× Triton X-100 solution to 300 µL with phosphate buffer saline (PBS).

2.8.1. Fluorescence Staining

Visualisation of the Transport Pathway

After 21 days of culturing, in the Snapwell® 6-well plates, and confirmation of the cell monolayer formation, the cell monolayers were incubated with the above-mentioned experimental solutions for 2 h at 37°C, 5% CO_2, and 95% air (i.e., the same conditions as for the in vitro permeation study).

After the 2 h incubation period, the cells were fixed with 4% formaldehyde for 10 min [52,53] and gently rinsed, once, with ice-cold PBS [54]. After fixation, the cell monolayers were prepared on the microscope slides, as described below in Section 2.8.2, and confocal images were taken with a Nikon Eclipse TE-3000 inverted microscope (Nikon Instruments, Melville, NY, USA), equipped with 60× and 100× ApoPlanar oil immersion objectives and a DSRi1 Nikon digital camera, for real-time imaging. The microscope was linked to a Nikon D-Eclipse C1 confocal system. The images were taken at room temperature, under light exclusion. All experiments were done in triplicates.

Visualization of the F-Actin Filaments in the Cytoskeleton

Staining of the F-actin in the cytoskeleton of the Caco-2 cells was used to identify if opening of tight junctions was the mechanism of action of the *A. vera* gel and the whole-leaf extract, in terms of drug-absorption enhancement [55,56]. The cell monolayers in the Snapwell® 6-well plates were incubated with the experimental permeation enhancer solutions (*A. vera* gel and whole-leaf extract without FD-4) for 2 h, at 37 °C, 5% CO_2, and 95% air. The cell monolayers were then fixed with 4% formaldehyde, for 10 min, and gently rinsed, once, with ice-cold PBS. Fixation was followed by permeabilization (to increase the accessibility of the F-actin to the CytoPainter® Phalloidin iFluor probe) with 0.1% Triton X-100 for, 3 min, after which the cell monolayers were gently rinsed with PBS. Thereafter, F-actin staining was done with 10X CytoPainter® Phalloidin iFluor 488 for 60 min and gently rinsed for 5 min, with PBS. The cell monolayers were prepared on the microscope slides, as described below in Section 2.8.2, and images were taken with CLSM, as described above. All experiments were done in triplicates.

2.8.2. Preparation of the Microscope Slides for the Confocal Laser Scanning Microscopy (CLSM)

The filter-ring was removed from the Snapwell® insert and placed onto a glass plate, to add support before the filter membrane was cut loose with a scalpel. The filter membrane was cut into smaller sections and a section with a size of, approximately, 1.12 cm × 0.3 cm was transferred to a microscope slide. Three to four drops of the Fluoroshield® mounting medium, containing propidium iodide [57], were added and spread-out, evenly. Care was taken not to touch the cell monolayer on the filter membrane. The propidium iodide, contained in the mounting media was used to visualize the cell nuclei. Finally, the excess Fluoroshield® mounting medium was removed by gently touching the slide with a piece of paper towel, and then a coverslip was added.

2.8.3. Imaging with Confocal Laser Scanning Microscopy

The CLSM was equipped with an Argon Ion laser (emission wavelength of 488 nm or 515 nm), a Helium Neon polarised laser (emission wavelength of 543 nm), and a blue Diode laser (emission wavelength of 409 nm). The excitation and emission wavelengths used for the imaging of the FITC-dextran, Phalloidin iFluor, and the propidium iodide are shown in Table 2.

Table 2. Excitation and emission wavelengths of the dyes and transport marker used in the confocal imaging experiments [51,54,57].

Compound	Excitation Wavelength (nm)	Emission Wavelength (nm)
FITC-dextran	494	518
Phalloidin iFluor	493	517
Propidium Iodide	535	615

2.9. Data Analysis

Data analyses on the in vitro permeation results were performed with STATISTICA Version 12 (Statsoft, Tulsa, OK, USA, 2013). All data sets were subjected to the Brown-Forsythe test to establish the normality and homogeneity of the data distribution. Normally distributed data were analyzed by analysis of variance (ANOVA) with Dunnet's post-hoc tests (two-sided). For data sets that were not normally distributed, non-parametric Kruskal-Wallis testing was applied. Statistically significant differences were accepted when $p < 0.05$.

3. Results and Discussion

3.1. Characterisation of the A. vera Gel and the Whole-Leaf Extract

The quantitative ^{1}H-NMR analysis indicated that the *A. vera* gel contained 15.2% aloverose; 9.8% glucose; 2.0% citric acid, and 20.7% malic acid, while the *A. vera* whole-leaf extract contained 4.9% aloverose; 8.6% glucose, 8.9% citric acid, 24.7% malic acid, and 14.6% iso-citric acid, or whole-leaf marker [33].

3.2. Characterization of the N-trimethyl Chitosan (TMC)

The degree of quaternization (DQ) of the TMC was calculated to be 45.995%, from the ^{1}H-NMR spectrum of the TMC (Figure 1), using Equation (1).

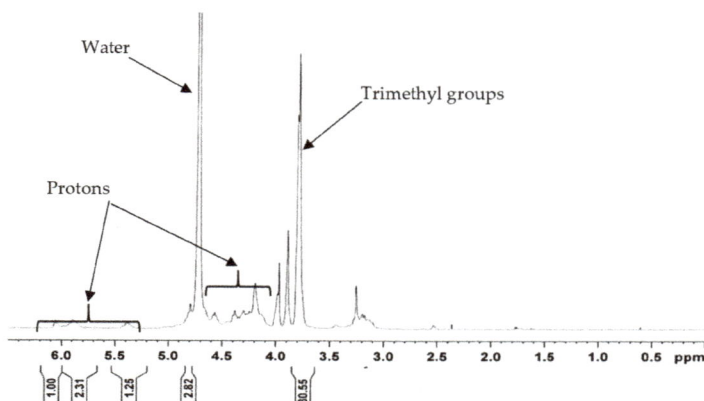

Figure 1. Proton nuclear magnetic resonance (^{1}H-NMR) spectrum for the *N*-trimethyl chitosan chloride (TMC).

3.3. Cell Monolayer Integrity Using Lucifer Yellow

The cumulative percentage transport of Lucifer yellow, across the Caco-2 cell monolayers was below 2%, over a period of 120 min, which indicated an acceptable integrity of the Caco-2 cell monolayers, as suggested by Wahlang et al. [48]. The apparent permeability coefficient (P_{app}) value for the Lucifer yellow was calculated to be 0.346×10^{-6} cm/s, from the transport curve, which was also within the range of the suggested P_{app} values for the Lucifer yellow, when transported across the Caco-2 cell monolayers, with an acceptable integrity, namely 0.2–0.75×10^{-6} cm/s [43,44].

3.4. In Vitro Transepithelial Electrical Resistance (TEER) Study

The TEER value of a cell monolayer is indicative of the tight junction integrity and a decrease in TEER has been related to the opening of tight junctions and, therefore, also to an increase in the paracellular permeability [56]. The TEER studies were performed to indicate the capability of the *A. vera* gel and the whole-leaf extract, to open tight junctions. From the results it was clear that maximum TEER reduction was already evident at 20 min, after application of the test solutions, and the TEER started to recover over the 120 min period, towards the initial value. The percentage TEER of the Caco-2 cell monolayers, after application of the test solutions and the positive control (i.e., TMC) plotted as a function of time, are shown in Figure 2, for four different concentrations of the *A. vera* gel, and in Figure 3, for the four different concentrations of the *A. vera* whole-leaf extract.

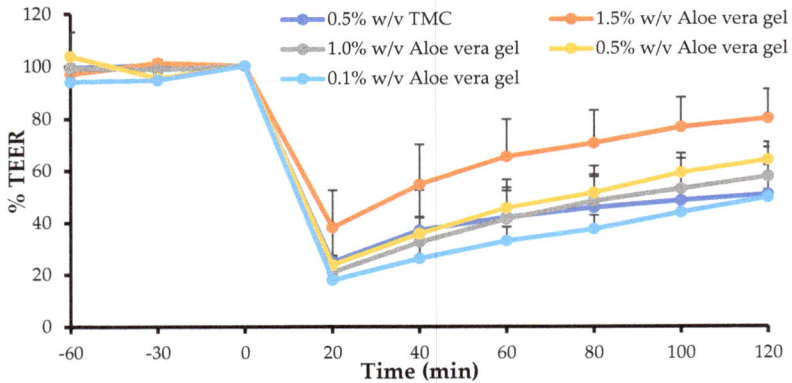

Figure 2. Percentage transepithelial electrical resistance (TEER) of the Caco-2 cell monolayers, after application of the *A. vera* gel, at different concentrations, and N-trimethyl chitosan chloride (TMC) (0.5% *w/v*, positive control), plotted as a function of time (*n* = 3) (Error bars represent standard deviation (SD)).

From Figure 2, it is clear that a rapid (within 20 min) and relatively large decrease in the percentage TEER of Caco-2 cell monolayers occurred after the application of the *A. vera* gel solutions, which was similar in extent to that of the positive control (TMC at 0.5% *w/v*), except for the 1.5% *w/v* *A. vera* gel solution, which exhibited a lower TEER reduction effect. The decrease in TEER caused by the *A. vera* gel on the Caco-2 cell monolayers was inversely proportional to the concentration applied. This could probably be explained by the increase in the viscosity of the *A. vera* gel solutions, with each concentration increase, which may have decreased the diffusion of ions across the Caco-2 cell monolayers.

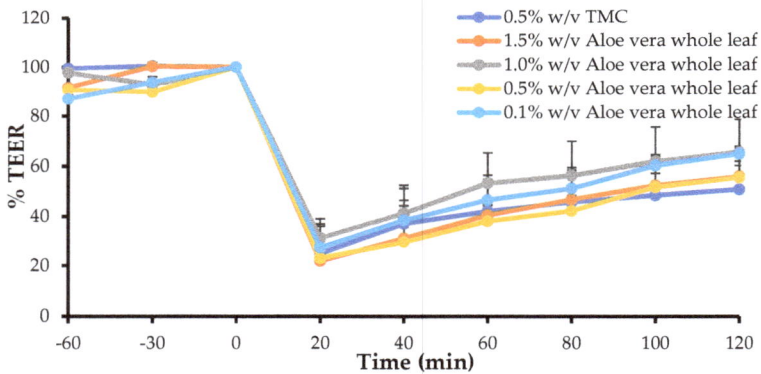

Figure 3. Percentage TEER of the Caco-2 cell monolayers after the application of the *A. vera* whole leaf, at different concentrations, and TMC (0.5% *w/v*, positive control) plotted as a function of time (*n* = 3) (Error bars represent SD).

From Figure 3, it is evident that the *A. vera* whole-leaf extract solutions caused a rapid and relatively large decrease in the TEER of the Caco-2 cell monolayers, which started to recover towards the initial value, over the period of 120 min. Furthermore, the decrease in TEER caused by some of the *A. vera* whole-leaf extract solutions, was larger than that of the positive control (0.5% *w/v* TMC). However, the reduction in TEER did not correlate, directly or inversely, with the concentration of the *A. vera* whole-leaf extract solutions.

Nonetheless, the TEER reduction results are in line with previous studies on the application of the *A. vera* gel and whole leaf extract on epithelial surfaces [32,33,35]. The TEER results indicated that the *A. vera* gel and whole-leaf extract were capable of opening tight junctions between the Caco-2 cells.

3.5. In Vitro Permeation Studies

The *A. vera* gel and whole-leaf extract showed the ability to enhance the transport of the FITC-dextran with a molecular weight of 4 kDa, across the Caco-2 cell monolayers, however, no transport could be detected for the FITC-dextran molecules, with molecular weights of 10 kDa (FD-10), 20 kDa (FD-20), and 40 kDa (FD-40), in the absence or presence of the *A. vera* gel and whole-leaf extract solutions, across the Caco-2 cell monolayers.

The transport curves and apparent permeability coefficient (P_{app}) values of the FD-4, across the Caco-2 cell monolayers, in the absence and presence of four different concentrations of the *A. vera* gel and whole-leaf extract, respectively, are shown in Figures 4–7.

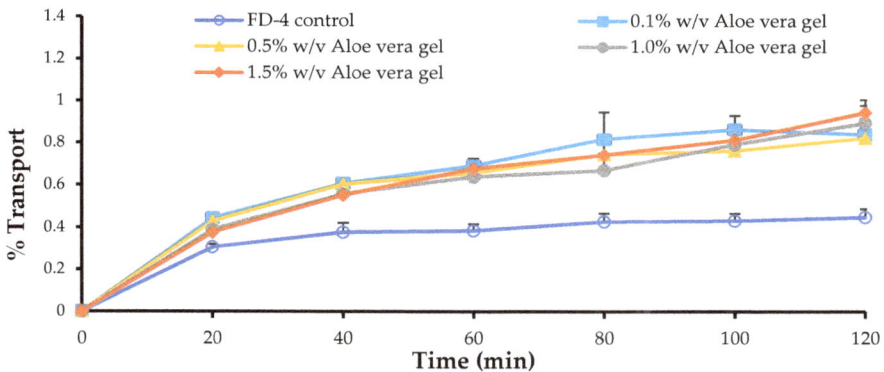

Figure 4. Percentage transport of the Fluorescein isothiocyanate (FITC)-dextran (FD) (FD-4 with MW of 4 kDa) plotted as a function of time, across the Caco-2 cell monolayers, in the absence (FD-4 control) and presence of the *Aloe vera* gel solutions, with different concentrations ($n = 3$; error bars represent SD).

From Figure 4, a clear increase in the percentage transport of FD-4, in relation to the negative control (FD-4 alone), can be seen for all concentrations of the *A. vera* gel solutions that were applied to the Caco-2 cell monolayers, with the FD-4. The transport of the FD-4, alone, showed an initial increase until 20 min, whereafter it reached a plateau, over the rest of the 120 min transport period. While in the presence of the *A. vera* gel it continued to be transported, albeit at a slower rate than the first 20 min.

A slightly higher than the two-fold increase in the transport of the FD-4 (R or permeation-enhancement ratio values indicated on Figure 5) in relation to the control group (FD-4 alone) was shown for all the concentrations of the *A. vera* gel solutions tested. The transport of the FD-4 was, statistically, significantly higher ($p < 0.05$) in the presence of all the *A. vera* gel solutions, compared to the transport of the control group (FD-4 alone). *A. vera* gel, therefore, showed the ability to significantly enhance the transport of a macromolecule (FD-4), across intestinal epithelial cell monolayers (Caco-2), which is in line with previous findings [32–34].

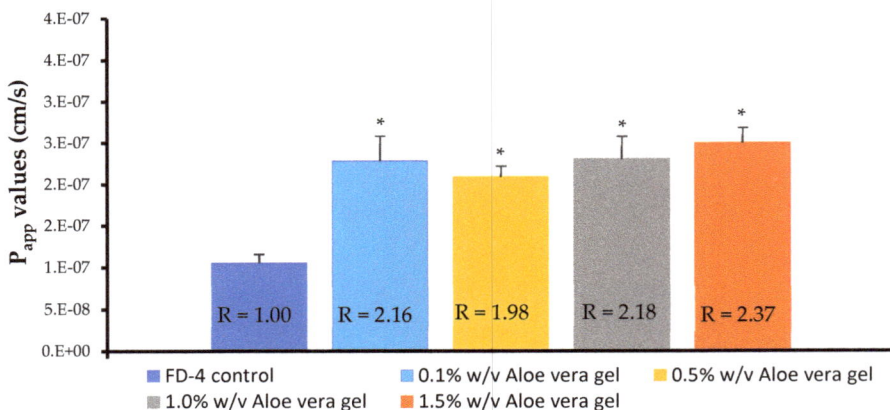

Figure 5. Apparent permeability coefficient (P_{app}) values of the FITC-dextran (FD-4 with MW of 4 kDa), across the Caco-2 cell monolayers, when co-applied with the *Aloe vera* gel solutions. Bars marked with an asterisk (*) indicate statistical significant differences from the control ($p < 0.05$) ($n = 3$; error bars represent SD) (R = permeation-enhancement ratio).

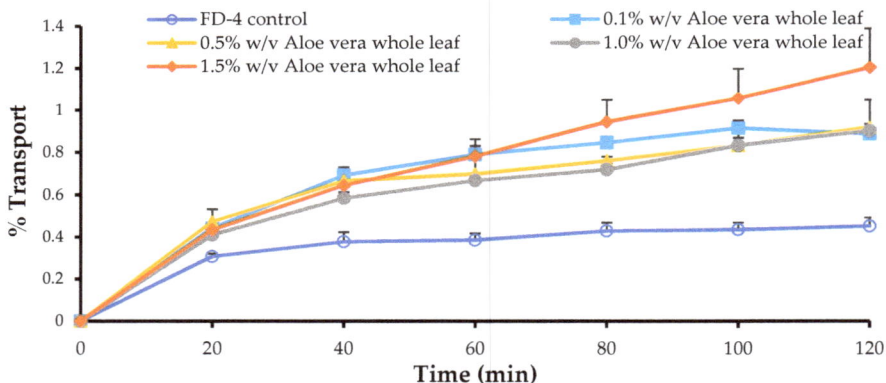

Figure 6. Percentage transport of the FITC-dextran (FD-4 with MW of 4 kDa) plotted as a function of time, across the Caco-2 cell monolayers, in the absence (FD-4 control) and presence of the *Aloe vera* whole-leaf extract solutions, with different concentrations ($n = 3$; error bars represent SD).

From Figure 6, a distinct increase in the FD-4 transport across the Caco-2 cell monolayers can be seen for all the concentrations of the *A. vera* whole-leaf extract solutions, when compared to the negative control group (FD-4 alone). The transport of the FD-4 alone (negative control) reached a plateau after 20 min, and only slightly increased, further, over the remainder of the transport period (120 min); while in the presence of the *A. vera* whole-leaf extract, it continued to be transported.

The transport of the FD-4 in the presence of all concentrations of the *A. vera* whole-leaf extract solutions, were significantly higher (Figure 7) than that of the control group (FD-4 alone) ($p < 0.05$). *A. vera* whole-leaf extract has, therefore, shown the ability to significantly enhance the transport of a macromolecular model compound (FD-4), across the intestinal epithelial cell monolayers (Caco-2), which is in line with previous findings [32–34]. The absorption-enhancing effect of the *A. vera* whole-leaf extract was in agreement with the TEER reduction results and can, therefore, most probably be attributed to its tight junction-modulating activities.

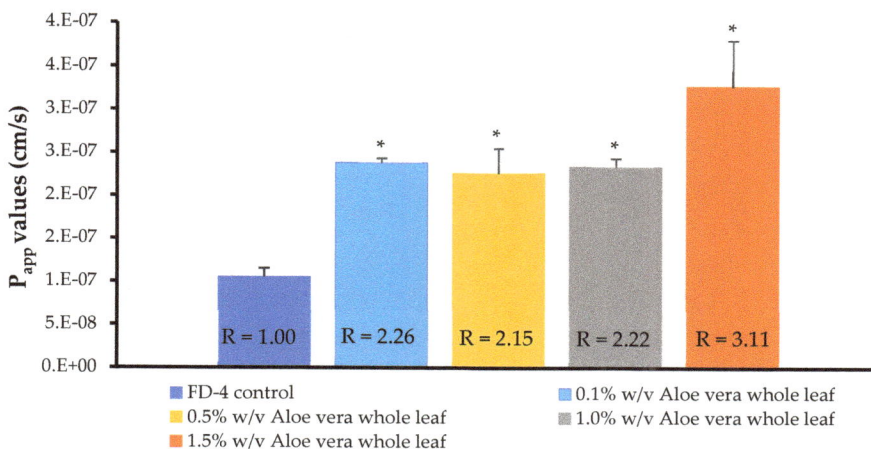

Figure 7. Apparent permeability coefficient (P_{app}) values of the FITC-dextran (FD-4 with MW of 4 kDa) across the Caco-2 cell monolayers, when co-applied with the *Aloe vera* whole-leaf extract solutions. Bars marked with an asterisk (*) indicate statistically significant differences from the negative control group ($p < 0.05$) ($n = 3$; error bars represent SD) (R = permeation-enhancement ratio).

3.6. Confocal Laser Scanning Microscopy (CLSM)

3.6.1. Visualization of the Transport Pathway

Figure 8 shows the top-view confocal micrograph images of the Caco-2 cell monolayers to which the FD-4 was applied, in the absence (negative control) and presence of the *A. vera* gel and whole-leaf extract, as well as TMC (positive control).

From the confocal micrograph images in Figure 8, the intercellular accumulation of FD-4 (green) between the Caco-2 cells can be observed, when it was applied with the absorption enhancers (Figure 8b–d), compared to no accumulation in the negative control (Figure 8a). This accumulation in the intercellular spaces between the cells indicated a movement of the FD-4 molecules, via the paracellular pathway. The CLSM image of the positive control (0.5% *w/v* TMC, a known tight junction modulator and paracellular absorption enhancer) is in accordance to previously published papers [58,59]. The lack of green fluorescence inside the cells, confirmed that the incubation with TMC, the *A. vera* gel, and *A. vera* whole-leaf extract, did not damage the cell membranes. The paracellular accumulation of the FD-4, in the presence of the *A. vera* gel and the whole-leaf extract, corresponded with the TEER reduction results and is most probably the result of their ability to modulate tight junctions.

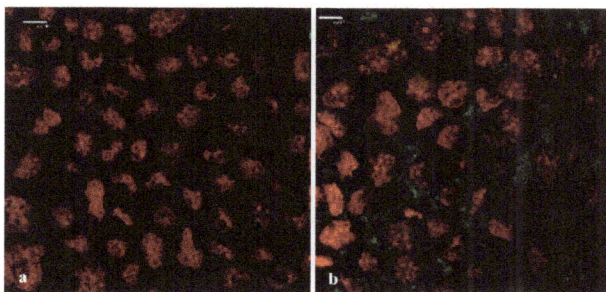

Figure 8. *Cont.*

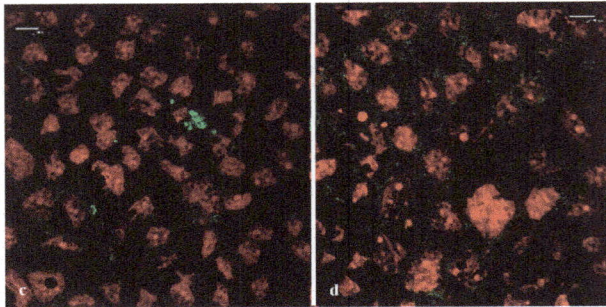

Figure 8. Top-view confocal micrograph images of the Caco-2 cell monolayers on which the FITC-dextran with MW of 4 kDa (FD-4) was applied (**green**: FD-4 and **red**: cell nuclei stained with propidium iodide). (**a**) Negative control (FD-4 alone), (**b**) positive control (0.5% w/v TMC), (**c**) *A. vera* gel (1.0% w/v), and (**d**) *A. vera* whole-leaf extract (1.0% w/v) (Scale bars represents 10 μm).

3.6.2. Visualization of the F-Actin Filaments in the Cytoskeleton

According to Ward et al. [11], disruption of the actin cytoskeleton through modulation of the F-actin structure can cause opening of the tight junctions and an increase in paracellular permeability. The re-arrangement of filamentous actin (F-actin) in the cytoskeleton of the Caco-2 cells was visualized, in order to determine the possible mechanism of action by which the *A. vera* gel and the whole-leaf extract increase the paracellular absorption. The CLSM images in Figure 9 show the F-actin expression in a Caco-2 cell monolayer, after incubation with the TMC (positive control), *A. vera* gel, and whole-leaf extract, and without an absorption enhancer (negative control).

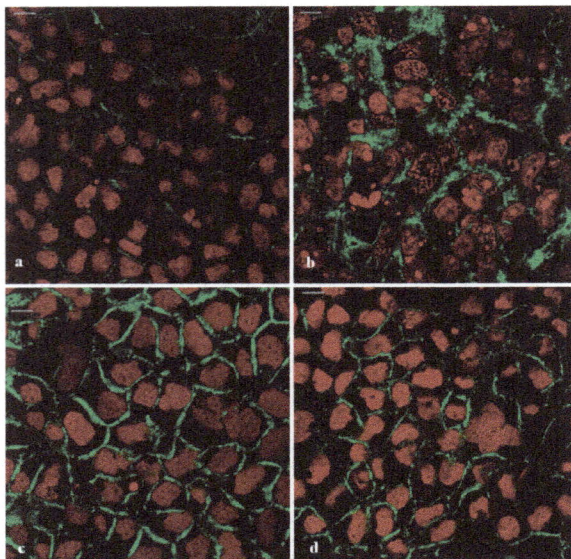

Figure 9. Confocal micrograph images of the filamentous actin (F-actin) distribution in the Caco-2 cell monolayers (**green**: F-actin stained with CytoPainter® Phalloidin iFluor 488 and **red**: cell nuclei stained with propidium iodide). (**a**) Negative control (untreated Caco-2 cell monolayer), (**b**) positive control (0.5% w/v TMC), (**c**) 1.0% w/v *A. vera* gel, and (**d**) 1.0% w/v *A. vera* whole-leaf extract (Scale bars represent 10 μm).

In the confocal micrograph images shown in Figure 9, the differences can be seen in the appearance of the F-actin when the Caco-2 cells were treated with *A. vera* gel, *A. vera* whole-leaf extract, and TMC (positive control), as compared to the negative control (untreated cells). The untreated Caco-2 cell monolayer (negative control) showed very little and irregular fluorescence (green) distribution of the F-actin, along the cell borders. In contrast to this, the F-actin fluorescence localization (green) in all the other images was visibly different (Figure 9b–d), which indicates that the F-actin distribution was re-arranged. The rearranged F-actin fluorescence pattern, seen in Figure 9b, is in congruence with previously published research on the effect of TMC (a known tight junction modulator) on the actin cytoskeleton of the Caco-2 cells [56]. The changed fluorescence patterns of the F-actin seen in the Caco-2 cells that were treated with *A. vera* gel (Figure 9c) and the *A. vera* whole-leaf extract (Figure 9d), were similar to that of the TMC. The changed F-actin distribution, therefore, indicates that tight junction modulation occurred in the presence of *A. vera* gel and *A. vera* whole-leaf extract.

4. Conclusions

Tight junction modulation by the *A. vera* gel and *A. vera* whole-leaf extract has previously been suggested, by Chen et al. [32], as a possible mechanism of its action for drug-absorption enhancement. The results obtained from this study confirmed tight junction modulation by the *A. vera* gel and *A. vera* whole-leaf extract, by means of different tests, including TEER reduction, transport enhancement of the FD-4, accumulation of FD-4 between the epithelial cells (i.e., in the intercellular spaces), and F-actin disruption, as determined with confocal laser scanning microscopy.

Author Contributions: Conceptualization, J.H. and L.d.P.; Methodology, A.H., C.W., J.H., and M.G.; Validation, A.H. and C.W.; Investigation, A.H., C.W., and M.G.; Supervision, J.H. and L.d.P.; Writing-Original Draft Preparation, A.H.; Writing-Review & Editing, C.W., M.G., L.d.P., and J.H.; Visualization, A.H. and M.G.; Funding Acquisition, J.H.

Funding: This research was funded by the National Research Foundation (NRF; grant nr 98939). Disclaimer: Any opinions, findings and conclusions, or recommendations expressed in this material are those of the authors and, therefore, the NRF does not accept any liability in regards, thereof.

Acknowledgments: Thank you to Improve USA Inc. (De Soto, TX, USA) for the kind donation of the *Aloe vera* gel and the whole-leaf extract (Daltonmax700®). Financial support by the North West University (NWU) is, hereby, acknowledged. We want to acknowledge Suria Ellis at the Statistical Service Department of NWU, for the statistical analysis of the permeation data.

Conflicts of Interest: The authors declare no conflict of interest.

References

1. Park, K.; Kwon, I.C.; Park, K. Oral protein delivery: Current status and future prospect. *React. Funct. Polym.* **2011**, *71*, 280–287. [CrossRef]
2. Griffin, B.T.; Guo, J.; Presas, E.; Donovan, M.D.; Alonso, M.J.; O'Driscoll, C.M. Pharmacokinetic, pharmacodynamic and biodistribution following oral administration of nanocarriers containing peptide and protein drugs. *Adv. Drug Deliv. Rev.* **2016**, *106*, 367–380. [CrossRef] [PubMed]
3. Muheem, A.; Shakeel, F.; Jahangir, M.A.; Anwar, M.; Mallick, N.; Jain, G.K.; Warsi, M.H.; Ahmad, F.J. A review on the strategies for the oral delivery of proteins and peptides and their clinical perspectives. *Saudi Pharm. J.* **2016**, *24*, 413–428. [CrossRef] [PubMed]
4. Sánchez-Navarro, M.; Garcia, J.; Giralt, E.; Teixidó, M. Using peptides to increase transport across the intestinal barrier. *Adv. Drug Deliv. Rev.* **2016**, *106*, 355–366. [CrossRef] [PubMed]
5. Zhu, H.; Li, B.V.; Uppoor, R.S.; Mehta, M.; Yu, L.X. Bioavailability and bioequivalence. In *Developing Solid Oral Dosage Forms: Pharmaceutical Theory & Practice*, 2nd ed.; Qiu, Y., Chen, Y., Zhang, G.G.Z., Yu, L., Mantri, R.V., Eds.; Elsevier: Amsterdam, The Netherlands, 2017; pp. 381–397, ISBN 978-01-2802-447-8.
6. Cabrera-Pérez, M.A.; Sanz, M.B.; Sanjuan, V.M.; González-Álvarez, M.; González-Álvarez, I. Importance and applications of cell- and tissue-based in vitro models for drug permeability screening in early stages of drug development. In *Concepts and Models for Drug Permeability Studies*, 1st ed.; Sarmento, B., Ed.; Woodhead Publishing: Cambridge, UK, 2016; pp. 3–29, ISBN 978-00-8100-094-6.

7. Rosenthal, R.; Günzel, D.; Finger, C.; Krug, S.M.; Richter, J.F.; Schulzke, J.; Fromm, M.; Amasheh, S. The effect of chitosan on transcellular and paracellular mechanisms in the intestinal epithelial barrier. *Biomaterials* **2012**, *33*, 2791–2800. [CrossRef] [PubMed]

8. Artursson, P.; Palm, K.; Luthman, K. Caco-2 monolayers in experimental and theoretical predictions of drug transport. *Adv. Drug Deliv. Rev.* **2001**, *46*, 27–43. [CrossRef]

9. Lin, Y.; Chen, C.; Liang, H.; Kulkarni, A.R.; Lee, P.; Chen, C.; Sung, H. Novel nanoparticles for oral insulin delivery via the paracellular pathway. *Nanotechnology* **2007**, *18*, 1–11. [CrossRef]

10. Tscheik, C.; Blasig, I.E.; Winkler, L. Trends in drug delivery through tissue barriers containing tight junctions. *Tissue Barriers* **2013**, *1*, e24565. [CrossRef]

11. Ward, P.D.; Tippin, T.K.; Thakker, D.R. Enhancing paracellular permeability by modulating epithelial tight junctions. *Pharm. Sci. Technol. Today* **2000**, *3*, 346–358. [CrossRef]

12. Lemmer, H.J.R.; Hamman, J.H. Paracellular drug absorption enhancement through tight junction modulation. *Expert Opin. Drug Deliv.* **2013**, *10*, 103–114. [CrossRef]

13. Matter, K.; Balda, M.S. Functional analysis of tight junctions. *Methods* **2003**, *30*, 228–234. [CrossRef]

14. Sun, H.; Chow, E.C.Y.; Liu, S.; Du, Y.; Pang, K.S. The Caco-2 cell monolayer: Usefulness and limitations. *Expert Opin. Drug Metab. Toxicol.* **2008**, *4*, 395–411. [CrossRef] [PubMed]

15. Maher, S.; Mrsny, R.J.; Brayden, D.J. Intestinal permeation enhancers for oral peptide delivery. *Adv. Drug Deliv. Rev.* **2016**, *106*, 277–319. [CrossRef] [PubMed]

16. Lakkireddy, H.R.; Urmannb, M.; Besenius, M.; Werner, U.; Haack, T.; Brun, P.; Alié, J.; Illel, B.; Hortala, L.; Vogel, R.; et al. Oral delivery of diabetes peptides—Comparing standard formulations incorporating functional excipients and nanotechnologies in the translational context. *Adv. Drug Deliv. Rev.* **2016**, *106*, 196–222. [CrossRef] [PubMed]

17. Renukuntla, J.; Vadlapudi, A.D.; Patel, A.; Boddu, S.H.S.; Mitra, A.K. Approaches for enhancing oral bioavailability of peptides and proteins. *Int. J. Pharm.* **2013**, *447*, 75–93. [CrossRef] [PubMed]

18. Mahato, R.I.; Narang, A.S.; Thoma, L.; Miller, D.D. Emerging trends in oral delivery of peptide and protein drugs. *Crit. Rev. Ther. Drug Carrier Syst.* **2003**, *20*, 153–214. [CrossRef]

19. Isoda, H.; Han, J.; Tominaga, M.; Maekawa, T. Effects of capsaicin on human intestinal cell line Caco-2. *Cytotechnology* **2001**, *36*, 155–161. [CrossRef]

20. Kesarwani, K.; Gupta, R. Bioavailability enhancers of herbal origin: An overview. *Asian Pac. J. Trop. Biomed.* **2013**, *3*, 253–266. [CrossRef]

21. Salama, N.N.; Eddington, N.D.; Fasano, A. Tight junction modulation and its relationship to drug delivery. *Adv. Drug Deliv. Rev.* **2006**, *58*, 15–28. [CrossRef]

22. Tatiraju, D.V.; Bagade, V.B.; Karambelkar, P.J.; Jadhav, V.M.; Kadam, V. Natural bioenhancers: An overview. *J. Pharmacogn. Phytochem.* **2013**, *2*, 55–60.

23. Werle, M.; Bernkop-Schnürch, A. Thiolated chitosans: Useful excipients for oral drug delivery. *J. Pharm. Pharmacol.* **2008**, *60*, 273–281. [CrossRef] [PubMed]

24. Vllasaliu, D.; Casettari, L.; Fowler, R.; Exposito-Harris, R.; Garnett, M.; Illum, L.; Stolnik, S. Absorption-promoting effects of chitosan in airway and intestinal cell lines: A comparative study. *Int. J. Pharm.* **2012**, *430*, 151–160. [CrossRef] [PubMed]

25. Boudreau, M.D.; Beland, F.A. An evaluation of the biological and toxicological properties of *Aloe barbadensis* (Miller), *Aloe vera*. *J. Environ. Sci. Health C* **2006**, *24*, 103–154. [CrossRef] [PubMed]

26. Sahu, P.K.; Giri, D.D.; Singh, R.; Pandey, P.; Gupta, S.; Shrivastava, A.K.; Kumar, A.; Pandey, K.D. Therapeutic and medicinal uses of *Aloe vera*: A review. *Pharmacol. Pharm.* **2013**, *4*, 599–610. [CrossRef]

27. Eshun, K.; He, Q. *Aloe vera*: A valuable ingredient for the food, pharmaceutical and cosmetic industries—A review. *Crit. Rev. Food Sci. Nutr.* **2004**, *44*, 91–96. [CrossRef]

28. Hamman, J.H. Composition and applications of *Aloe vera* leaf gel. *Molecules* **2008**, *13*, 1599–1616. [CrossRef]

29. Sánchez-Machado, D.I.; López-Cervantes, J.; Sendón, R.; Sanches-Silva, A. *Aloe vera*: Ancient knowledge with new frontiers. *Trends Food Sci. Technol.* **2017**, *61*, 94–102. [CrossRef]

30. Mascolo, N.; Izzo, A.A.; Borrelli, F.; Capasso, R.; Di Carlo, G.; Sautebin, L.; Capasso, F. Healing powers of aloes. In *Aloes: The genus Aloe*, 1st ed.; Reynolds, T., Ed.; CRC Press: Washington, DC, USA, 2004; pp. 209–238, ISBN 978-04-1530-672-0.

31. Vinson, J.A.; Al Kharrat, H.; Andreoli, L. Effect of *Aloe vera* preparations on the human bioavailability of vitamins C and E. *Phytomedicine* **2005**, *12*, 760–765. [CrossRef]

32. Chen, W.; Lu, Z.; Viljoen, A.; Hamman, J. Intestinal drug transport enhancement by *Aloe vera*. *Planta Med.* **2009**, *75*, 587–595. [CrossRef]

33. Beneke, C.; Viljoen, A.; Hamman, J.H. In vitro drug absorption enhancement effects of *Aloe vera* and *Aloe ferox*. *Sci. Pharm.* **2012**, *80*, 475–486. [CrossRef]

34. Beneke, C.; Viljoen, A.; Hamman, J.H. Modulation of drug efflux by aloe materials: An in vitro investigation across rat intestinal tissue. *Pharmacogn. Mag.* **2013**, *9*, 44–48. [CrossRef]

35. Lebitsa, T.; Viljoen, A.; Lu, Z.; Hamman, J. In vitro drug permeation enhancement potential of Aloe gel materials. *Curr. Drug Deliv.* **2012**, *9*, 297–304. [CrossRef] [PubMed]

36. Cole, L.; Heard, C. Skin permeation enhancement potential of *Aloe vera* and a proposed mechanism of action based upon size exclusion and pull effect. *Int. J. Pharm.* **2007**, *333*, 10–16. [CrossRef] [PubMed]

37. Fox, L.; Gerber, M.; Du Preez, J.L.; Du Plessis, J.; Hamman, J.H. Skin permeation enhancement effects of the gel and whole leaf materials of *Aloe vera*, *Aloe marlothii* and *Aloe ferox*. *J. Pharm. Pharmacol.* **2014**, *67*, 96–106. [CrossRef] [PubMed]

38. Ojewole, E.; Mackraj, I.; Akhundov, K.; Hamman, J.; Viljoen, A.; Olivier, E.; Wesley-Smith, J.; Govender, T. Investigating the effect of *Aloe vera* gel on the buccal permeability of didanosine. *Planta Med.* **2012**, *78*, 354–361. [CrossRef]

39. Djuv, A.; Nilsen, O.G. Caco-2 cell methodology and inhibition of the P-glycoprotein transport of digoxin by *Aloe vera* juice. *Phytother. Res.* **2008**, *22*, 1623–1628. [CrossRef]

40. Jiao, P.; Jia, Q.; Randel, G.; Diehl, B.; Weaver, S.; Milligan, G. Quantitative ^{1}H-NMR Spectrometry Method for Quality Control of *Aloe vera* Products. *J. AOAC Int.* **2010**, *93*, 842–848.

41. Sieval, A.B.; Thanou, M.; Kotzé, A.F.; Verhoef, J.C.; Brussee, J.; Junginger, H.E. Preparation and NMR characterization of highly substituted *N*-trimethyl chitosan chloride. *Carbohydr. Polym.* **1998**, *36*, 157–165. [CrossRef]

42. Hamman, J.H.; Stander, M.; Kotzé, A.F. Effect of the degree of quaternisation of *N*-trimethyl chitosan chloride of absorption enhancement: In vivo evaluation in rat nasal epithelia. *Int. J. Pharm.* **2002**, *232*, 235–242. [CrossRef]

43. Calatayud, M.; Devesa, V.; Montoro, R.; Vélez, D. In vitro study of intestinal transport of arsenite, monomethylarsonous acid, and dimethylarsinous acid by Caco-2 cell line. *Toxicol. Lett.* **2011**, *204*, 127–133. [CrossRef]

44. Bhushani, J.A.; Karthik, P.; Anandharamakrishnan, C. Nanoemulsion based delivery system for improved bioaccessibility and Caco-2 cell monolayer permeability of green tea extract. *Food Hydrocoll.* **2016**, *56*, 372–382. [CrossRef]

45. Alqahtani, S.; Mohamed, L.A.; Kaddoumi, A. Experimental models for predicting drug absorption and metabolism. *Expert Opin. Drug Metab. Toxicol.* **2013**, *9*, 1–14. [CrossRef] [PubMed]

46. Du Toit, T.; Malan, M.M.; Lemmer, H.J.R.; Gouws, C.; Aucamp, M.E.; Breytenbach, W.J.; Hamman, J.H. Combining chemical permeation enhancers for synergistic effects. *Eur. J. Drug Metab. Pharmacokinet.* **2016**, *41*, 575–586. [CrossRef] [PubMed]

47. Pick, D.; Degen, C.; Leiterer, M.; Jahreis, G.; Einax, J.W. Transport of selenium species in Caco-2 cells: Analytical approach employing the Ussing chamber technique and HPLC-ICP-MS. *Microchem. J.* **2013**, *110*, 8–14. [CrossRef]

48. Wahlang, B.; Pawar, Y.B.; Bansal, A.K. Identification of permeability-related hurdles in oral delivery of curcumin using the Caco-2 cell model. *Eur. J. Pharm. Biopharm.* **2011**, *77*, 275–282. [CrossRef] [PubMed]

49. Palumbo, P.; Picchini, U.; Beck, B.; van Gelder, J.; Delbar, N.; DaGaetano, A. A general approach to the apparent permeability index. *J. Pharmacokinet. Pharmacodyn.* **2008**, *35*, 235–248. [CrossRef] [PubMed]

50. Johnson, P.H.; Frank, D.; Costantino, H.R. Discovery of tight junction modulators: Significance for drug development and delivery. *Drug Discov. Today* **2008**, *13*, 261–267. [CrossRef] [PubMed]

51. Kotzé, A.F.; Leußen, H.L.; De Leeuw, B.J.; De Boer, B.G.; Verhoef, J.C.; Junginger, H.E. Comparison of the effect of different chitosan salts and *N*-trimethyl chitosan chloride on the permeability of intestinal epithelial cells (Caco-2). *J. Control Release* **1998**, *51*, 35–46. [CrossRef]

52. Abcam. Immunocytochemistry and Immunofluorescence Protocol: Procedure for Staining of Cell Cultures Using Immunofluorescence. Available online: http://www.abcam.com/protocols/immunocytochemistry-immunofluorescence-protocol (accessed on 9 November 2017).

53. Wu, S.; Don, T.; Lin, C.; Mi, F. Delivery of berberine using chitosan/fucoidan-taurine conjugate nanoparticles for treatment of defective intestinal epithelial tight junction barrier. *Mar. Drugs* **2014**, *12*, 5677–5697. [CrossRef]

54. Abcam. Protocol Booklet: CytoPainter Phalloidin-iFlour 488 Reagent: Instructions for Use for Staining F-Actin in Adherent or Suspension Cells. Available online: http://www.abcam.com/ps/products/176/ab176753/documents/ab176753%20CytoPainter%20Phalloidin-iFluor%20488%20Reagent%20protocol%20v3%20(website).pdf (accessed on 9 November 2017).

55. Dorkoosh, F.A.; Broekhuizen, C.A.N.; Borchard, G.; Rafiee-Tehrani, M.; Verhoef, J.C.; Junginger, H.E. Transport of octreotide and evaluation of mechanism of action of opening the paracellular tight junction using superporous hydrogel polymers in Caco-2 cell monolayers. *J. Pharm. Sci.* **2004**, *93*, 743–752. [CrossRef]

56. Hsu, L.; Ho, Y.; Chuang, E.; Chen, C.; Juang, J.; Su, F.; Hwang, S.; Sung, H. Effects of pH on molecular mechanisms of chitosan-integrin interactions and resulting tight-junction disruptions. *Biomaterials* **2013**, *34*, 784–793. [CrossRef] [PubMed]

57. Abcam. Product Datasheet: Fluoroshield Mounting Medium with Propidium Iodide ab104129. Available online: http://www.abcam.com/fluoroshield-mounting-medium-with-propidium-iodide-20ml-ab104129.html (accessed on 9 November 2017).

58. Kotzé, A.F.; Leußen, H.L.; De Leeuw, B.J.; De Boer, B.G.; Verhoef, J.C.; Junginger, H.E. *N*-trimethyl chitosan chloride as a potential absorption enhancer across mucosal surfaces: In vitro evaluation in intestinal epithelial cells (Caco-2). *Pharm. Res.* **1997**, *14*, 1197–1202. [CrossRef] [PubMed]

59. Thanou, M.; Verhoef, J.C.; Junginger, H.E. Oral drug absorption enhancement by chitosan and its derivatives. *Adv. Drug Deliv. Rev.* **2001**, *52*, 117–126. [CrossRef]

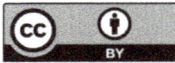

pharmaceutics

MDPI

Review

Drug Bioavailability Enhancing Agents of Natural Origin (Bioenhancers) that Modulate Drug Membrane Permeation and Pre-Systemic Metabolism

Bianca Peterson, Morné Weyers, Jan H. Steenekamp, Johan D. Steyn, Chrisna Gouws and Josias H. Hamman *

Centre of Excellence for Pharmaceutical Sciences (Pharmacen™), North-West University, Potchefstroom 2520, South Africa; bianca.peterson@nwu.ac.za (B.P.); weyers.morne@gmail.com (M.W.); jan.steenekamp@nwu.ac.za (J.H.S.); dewald.steyn@nwu.ac.za (J.D.S.); chrisna.gouws@nwu.ac.za (C.G.)
* Correspondence: sias.hamman@nwu.ac.za; Tel.: +27-18-299-4035

Received: 11 December 2018; Accepted: 24 December 2018; Published: 16 January 2019

Abstract: Many new chemical entities are discovered with high therapeutic potential, however, many of these compounds exhibit unfavorable pharmacokinetic properties due to poor solubility and/or poor membrane permeation characteristics. The latter is mainly due to the lipid-like barrier imposed by epithelial mucosal layers, which have to be crossed by drug molecules in order to exert a therapeutic effect. Another barrier is the pre-systemic metabolic degradation of drug molecules, mainly by cytochrome P450 enzymes located in the intestinal enterocytes and liver hepatocytes. Although the nasal, buccal and pulmonary routes of administration avoid the first-pass effect, they are still dependent on absorption of drug molecules across the mucosal surfaces to achieve systemic drug delivery. Bioenhancers (drug absorption enhancers of natural origin) have been identified that can increase the quantity of unchanged drug that appears in the systemic blood circulation by means of modulating membrane permeation and/or pre-systemic metabolism. The aim of this paper is to provide an overview of natural bioenhancers and their main mechanisms of action for the nasal, buccal, pulmonary and oral routes of drug administration. Poorly bioavailable drugs such as large, hydrophilic therapeutics are often administered by injections. Bioenhancers may potentially be used to benefit patients by making systemic delivery of these poorly bioavailable drugs possible via alternative routes of administration (i.e., oral, nasal, buccal or pulmonary routes of administration) and may also reduce dosages of small molecular drugs and thereby reduce treatment costs.

Keywords: bioenhancer; cytochrome P450; drug absorption enhancer; efflux; metabolism; P-glycoprotein; pharmacokinetic interaction; tight junction

---

1. Introduction

Drug absorption is the process whereby drug molecules are transferred from the site of administration across biological membranes into the systemic blood circulation to produce a systemic pharmacological effect. Biological cell membranes have a lipophilic nature due to their phospholipid bilayer structures. Molecules should therefore have sufficient hydrophilic properties to dissolve in the aqueous environments surrounding the biological membranes, but should also have sufficient lipophilic properties to partition into the membranes in order to achieve passive absorption via the transcellular pathway [1]. Adjacent epithelial/endothelial cells are connected by tight junctions, which are traversed by aqueous channels/fenestrae through which only small water-soluble molecules (<600 Da) can pass to get absorbed via the paracellular pathway [2].

A number of active transporter molecules (including both uptake transporters and efflux transporters) are present in various cell types in different organs. Drug efflux transporters found in the plasma membranes of intestinal epithelial cells can pump structurally diverse compounds from within the intestinal epithelial cells back to the gastro-intestinal lumen and thereby reduce drug bioavailability [3]. Efflux of compounds occurs by active transporters that need energy and this process is adenosine triphosphate (ATP)-dependent [4]. The ATP-binding cassette (ABC) transporter superfamily is among the largest and most broadly expressed efflux transporters discovered so far, consisting of P-glycoprotein (P-gp), the multidrug resistant protein (MRP) and the breast cancer resistance protein (BCRP) [5–7]. Another major determinant of oral drug bioavailability besides drug permeation across the epithelial cells is pre-systemic metabolism or first-pass metabolism, which is the metabolism that takes place during uptake before the drug molecules reach the systemic circulation, as observed for olanzapine treatment [8]. Pre-systemic metabolism occurs mainly in the enterocytes of the gastrointestinal epithelium and the hepatocytes of the liver. The cytochrome P450 (CYP) family of enzymes account for the majority of oxidative metabolic reactions of xenobiotics during pre-systemic and systemic metabolism. More than 30 different human CYP enzymes have been identified, of which CYP3A4 appears to be one of the most important drug-metabolizing enzymes in humans [9].

For the purpose of this paper, the term bioenhancer is reserved for molecules of natural origin that are capable of increasing the rate and/or extent at which co-administered drug molecules reach the systemic circulation unchanged (i.e., increased bioavailability). The main mechanisms that have been identified through which bioenhancers can improve the bioavailability of drug molecules include alteration of the plasma membrane fluidity to increase passive transcellular drug permeation; modulation of tight junctions to allow for increased paracellular diffusion; and active efflux transporter modulation, such as P-gp-related efflux inhibition. Inhibition of CYP enzymes in the intestinal epithelium and liver can significantly impact upon the bioavailability of drugs that are substrates of these enzymes by means of reducing pre-systemic metabolism [10–12].

The most popular route of drug administration remains the oral route [2]. As mentioned before, the oral bioavailability of a drug molecule is determined by its ability to penetrate the gastrointestinal epithelial membrane, which is mainly determined by its physico-chemical properties (e.g., pKa, lipophilicity, molecular size, charge, dissolution and solubility) [13], together with the extent of enzymatic metabolism during its movement to the systemic circulation (known as pre-systemic metabolism or the first-pass effect). Some other factors that may affect the oral bioavailability of a drug include the gastric emptying rate, pH of the gastrointestinal fluid, interactions with other compounds (e.g., other drugs, food or herbs) and its affinity for active transporters [2,14].

Drug administration via the nasal route can easily be accomplished by patients for both local and systemic drug delivery, which is non-invasive and painless. A relatively large epithelial surface is available that is highly permeable and offers a rapid onset of therapeutic effect. For drugs that target the central nervous system, direct nose-to-brain drug delivery is possible [13,15,16]. Additionally, intranasal drug administration bypasses hepatic first-pass metabolism [13,17,18]. However, the protective mucous layer and ciliary clearance may potentially have a negative impact on intranasal absorption [13,15].

The buccal route of administration is a good alternative for drugs that are unstable in gastric fluids and those that are severely affected by first-pass metabolism. However, absorption across the buccal mucosa is relatively slow due to the limited surface area, poor permeability of buccal epithelial tissue, removal of drug by saliva and the presence of peptidases within the buccal mucosa [15]. Hence this route of drug administration is mostly suited for highly potent, low dose drugs [15].

The pulmonary route of drug administration (i.e., administration via the lungs) is associated with rapid drug delivery due to the large surface area and abundant blood supply [2,15]. Pulmonary drug delivery can occur through different dosage forms, such as aerosol or nebulizer, for both local treatment (e.g., bronchodilators) or systemic drug delivery [2]. In the case of volatile anesthetics or for voluptuary drugs, the inhalation route is the preferred way of administration [2,19].

In this paper, discussions regarding drug absorption enhancing agents are restricted to bioenhancers of natural origin (therefore purely synthetic chemical permeation enhancers are excluded).

The selected bioenhancers are discussed in terms of their main effects on drug bioavailability as well as their mechanisms of action as elucidated by in vitro and in vivo studies. Furthermore, a comprehensive list of bioenhancers is included in Table 1 for each of the four selected routes of administration including the buccal, nasal, pulmonary and oral routes of drug administration.

2. Buccal Route of Administration

Figure 1 illustrates the main mechanisms of action of selected bioenhancers for improved drug delivery via the buccal route of administration.

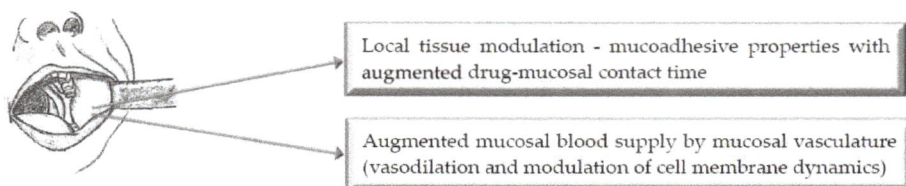

Local tissue modulation - mucoadhesive properties with augmented drug-mucosal contact time

Augmented mucosal blood supply by mucosal vasculature (vasodilation and modulation of cell membrane dynamics)

Figure 1. Illustration of the main mechanisms of action of bioenhancers for enhanced buccal drug delivery.

2.1. Aloe Vera

The effect of *Aloe vera* gel on the permeability of didanosine (ddI) across porcine buccal mucosae was investigated using Franz diffusion cells. The control solution contained ddI in phosphate buffer saline (PBS) at pH 7.4 alone (5, 10, 15, 20 mg/mL), and the test solutions contained ddI (20 mg/mL) in the presence of *A. vera* gel (0.25, 0.5, 1, 2, 4, and 6% *w/v*) [20].

At concentrations of 0.25 to 2% *w/v*, *A. vera* gel significantly enhanced the buccal permeability of ddI with enhancement ratios ranging from 5.09 (0.25% *w/v*) to 11.78 (2% *w/v*). However, at higher concentrations (4 and 6% *w/v*) of *A. vera* gel, decreased ddI permeability across the buccal tissue was observed. This may be attributed to the high viscosity of the *A. vera* gel at these high concentrations, which caused resistance to drug diffusion. *A. vera* gel may be used as a potential buccal permeation enhancer for ddI in the treatment of HIV and AIDS [20].

Table 1. Summary of selected natural bioenhancers and their main mechanisms of action on various drugs for enhanced nasal, oral, buccal and pulmonary drug delivery.

Route of Administration	Bioenhancer (Class)	Biological Source	Mechanism(s) of Action	Study Design Model	Research Compound	Reference(s)
Buccal	Aloe vera (gel, whole leaf)	Plant (*Aloe vera*)	Intercellular modulation	In vitro (Franz diffusion cells)	Didanosine: Antiviral reverse transcriptase inhibitor	[20]
Buccal	Chitosan (Biopolymer)	Deacetylated chitin from crustaceans and fungi	Mucoadhesion; changes in lipid organization and loosening of intercellular filaments	In vitro (T146 cells [1])	FITC–dextran: Hydrophilic polysaccharide	[21]
Buccal	Chitosan (Biopolymer)	Deacetylated chitin from crustaceans and fungi	Mucoadhesion; mucosal membrane modulation	Ex vivo (porcine buccal mucosa)	Hydrocortisone: Corticosteroid TGF-beta: Cytokine polypeptide	[22]
Buccal	Chitosan–TBA (Thiolated polymer)	Deacetylated chitin from crustaceans and fungi	Mucoadhesion; mucosal membrane modulation	Ex vivo (porcine buccal mucosa); in vivo (pig)	PACAP: Pituitary Adenylate Cyclase-activating Peptide	[23,24]
Buccal	Cod-liver oil extract (Fatty acid)	Animal (Cod fish)	No mechanism specified	Ex vivo (hamster cheek pouch)	Ergotamine tartrate: Ergopeptine alkaloid	[25]
Buccal	Menthol (Alcohol)	Plant (Corn mint, peppermint, or other mint oils)	No mechanism specified	Ex vivo (porcine buccal mucosa)	Dideoxycytidine: Nucleoside analog reverse transcriptase inhibitor (NRTI)	[26]
Buccal	Oleic acid, eicosapentaenoic acid, docosahexaenoic acid (Fatty acids)	Animal (Cod fish)	No mechanism specified	In vitro (membraneless dissolution test), in vivo (rat)	Insulin: Peptide hormone	[27]
Buccal	Sodium glycodeoxycholate (Bile salt)	Intestinal bacterial by-product	No mechanism specified	Ex vivo (porcine buccal mucosa)	Dideoxycytidine: Nucleoside analog reverse transcriptase inhibitor (NRTI)	[28]
Buccal	TMC (Cationic polymers)	Chemically modified chitosan (crustaceans, fungi)	Mucoadhesion; mucosal membrane modulation	Ex vivo (porcine buccal mucosa)	FD4: Hydrophilic polysaccharide	[29]
Nasal	Chitosan (Biopolymer)	Chemically modified chitosan (crustaceans, fungi)	Tight junction modulation	In vivo (sheep)	sCT: Endogenous polypeptide hormone	[30]
Nasal	Chitosan (Biopolymer)	Deacetylated chitin from crustaceans and fungi	Increased mucoadhesion; tight junction modulation	In vivo (sheep, human)	Morphine: Opium alkaloid	[31]
Nasal	Chitosan–TBA (Thiolated polymer)	Deacetylated chitin from crustaceans and fungi	Increased mucoadhesion; tight junction modulation	In vivo (rat)	Insulin: Peptide hormone	[32]

Table 1. *Cont.*

Route of Administration	Bioenhancer (Class)	Biological Source	Mechanism(s) of Action	Study Design Model	Research Compound	Reference(s)
Nasal	TMC (Cationic polymers)	Chemically modified chitosan (crustaceans and fungi)	Increased mucoadhesion; tight junction modulation	In vivo (rat)	Mannitol: Sugar alcohol	[33]
Oral	(-)-Epicatechin (Flavonoid)	Plant (woody plants)	Metabolism (glucuronidation) inhibition	Ex vivo (rat small intestine)	Alpha-naphtol: Organic fluorescent compound	[34]
Oral	*Aloe vera* (gel and whole leaf)	Plant (*Aloe vera*)	Tight junction modulation	Ex vivo (rat intestinal tissue)	Atenolol: Beta-receptor activity compound	[35]
Oral	Aloe vera (gel and whole leaf)	Plant (*Aloe vera*)	Tight junction modulation	In vitro (Caco-2 cells [2])	Insulin: Peptide hormone	[36]
Oral	Aloe vera (juice)	Plant (*Aloe vera*)	Local mucosal tissue modulation	In vivo (human)	Vitamin C and E: Ascorbic acid, tocopherols, tocotrienols.	[37]
Oral	Aloe vera (gel polysaccharides)	Plant (*Aloe vera*)	Metabolism inhibition; tight junction modulation	In vitro (Caco-2, LS180 cells [3], In vivo (rat)	Indinavir: Antiviral protease inhibitor	[38]
Oral	BHCl (Flavonoid)	Acidification of betaine Plant (beetroot: *Beta vulgaris*)	Metabolism enhancement (transient re-acidification of gastric pH)	In vivo (human)	Dasatinib: Protein kinase inhibitor	[39]
Oral	Caraway (Flavonoid)	Plant (meridian fennel/Persian cumin: *Carum carvi*)	Local mucosal tissue modulation	In vivo (human)	Rifampicin: Semisynthetic rifamycin derivative, Isoniazid: Isonicotinic acid derivative, pyrazinamide: nicotinamide pyrazine analogue	[40]
Oral	Chitosan (Biopolymer)	Deacetylated chitin from crustaceans and fungi	Tight junction modulation	In vitro (HT-29 clone B6 cells [4])	Heparin: Anticoagulant	[41]
Oral	Chitosan (Biopolymer)	Deacetylated chitin from crustaceans and fungi	Tight junction modulation	In vitro (Caco-2 cells [2])	Chitosan–(Lissamine–rhodamine labelled)	[42]
Oral	Chitosan–TBA (Thiolated polymer)	Deacetylated chitin from crustaceans and fungi	Mucoadhesion; tight junction modulation	Ex vivo (guinea pig small intestinal mucosa)	Cefadroxil: Cephalosporin	[43]
Oral	Chitosan–TBA (Thiolated polymer)	Deacetylated chitin from crustaceans and fungi	Mucoadhesion; tight junction modulation	In vivo (rat)	Insulin: Peptide hormone	[44]
Oral	Curcumin (Flavonoid)	Plant (turmeric: *Curcuma longa*)	Metabolism (UDP-glucuronyl transferase) inhibition	In vitro (rat microsomes)	Mycophenolic acid: Immunosuppressant	[45]
Oral	Curcumin (Flavonoid)	Plant (turmeric: *Curcuma longa*)	Efflux transporter inhibition; metabolism inhibition	In vivo (rabbit)	Norfloxacin: Fluoroquinolone	[46]
Oral	Curcumin (Flavonoid)	Plant (turmeric: *Curcuma longa*)	Metabolism (CYP3A4) inhibition	In vitro (human liver microsomes)	Midazolam: Benzodiazepine	[47]

173

Table 1. *Cont.*

Route of Administration	Bioenhancer (Class)	Biological Source	Mechanism(s) of Action	Study Design Model	Research Compound	Reference(s)
Oral	Curcumin (Flavonoid)	Plant (turmeric: *Curcuma longa*)	Efflux transporter (P-gp) inhibition; metabolism (CYP3A4) inhibition	In vivo (rat)	Midazolam: Benzodiazepine	[48]
Oral	Cyclosporine A (Immunosuppressant)	Fungi (*Tolypocladium inflatum* Gams)	Efflux transporter (P-gp) inhibition	In vivo (rat, dog)	Clopidogrel: Platelet aggregation inhibitor	[49]
Oral	Diosmin (Flavonoid)	Plant (citrus fruits)	Efflux transporter (P-gp) inhibition	In vitro (Caco-2 cells ^{2})	Digoxin: Digitalis glycoside	[50]
Oral	Emodin (Anthraquinone derivative)	Plant (senna: *Cassia angustifolia*, *Aloe vera* (syn *Aloe barbadensis*), rhubarb: *Rheum officinale*)	Efflux transporter (P-gp) inhibition	In vitro (MDR1-MDCKII cells ^{6}, Caco-2 cells ^{2})	Digoxin: Digitalis glycoside	[51]
Oral	Fulvic acid (Organic acid)	Plant (decomposed material)	Metabolism enhancement (enhanced drug water solubility)	In vivo (rat)	Glibenclamide: Sulfonylurea antidiabetic; Insulin: Peptide hormone; Pentazocin: Opioid analgesic	[52]
Oral	Gallic acid ester (Organic acid)	Plant (gallnuts, sumac, witch hazel, tea leaves, oak bark)	Metabolism (CYP3A) inhibition	In vitro (human liver microsomes)	Nifedipine: Calcium channel blocker	[53]
Oral	Genistein (Flavonoid)	Plant (soyabean: *Glycine max*, kudzu: *Pueraria lobata*)	Efflux transporter (MRP) inhibition	In vitro (HT-29 cells ^{4}), In vivo (rat)	Epigalllocatechin-3-gallate (EGCG); Phenolic antioxidant	[54]
Oral	Genistein (Flavonoid)	Plant (soyabean: *Glycine max*, kudzu: *Pueraria lobata*)	Efflux transporter (P-gp, BCRP, MRP2) inhibition; metabolism (CYP3A4) inhibition	In vivo (rat)	Paclitaxel: Tetracyclic diterpenoid	[55]
Oral	Gokhru extract (Herbal)	Plant (*Tribulus terrestris*)	Local mucosal tissue modulation	In vitro (goat everted sac)	Metformin: Biguanide	[56]
Oral	Gokhru extract (Herbal)	Plant (*Tribulus terrestris*)	Local mucosal tissue modulation	In vivo (chicken everted intestine)	Metformin: Biguanide	[57]
Oral	Grapefruit juice (Citrus fruit)	Plant (grapefruit: *Citrus paradisi*)	Efflux transporter (P-gp, MRP2); metabolism (CYP3A4) inhibition; renal uptake transporter (OATP) inhibition	Various	Various	[58]
Oral	LSC (Chitosan derivative)	Modified chitosan (crustaceans and fungi)	Increased mucoadhesion; tight junction modulation	In vitro (Caco-2 cells ^{2}), In vivo (rat), Ex vivo (rat intestine)	Insulin: Peptide hormone	[59]
Oral	Lycopene (Carotenoid)	Plant (red fruits and vegetables)	Dual carotenoid/LDL receptor mechanism for targeted hepatic delivery	In vivo (human)	Simvastatin: HMG–CoA reductase inhibitor	[60]

Table 1. *Cont.*

Route of Administration	Bioenhancer (Class)	Biological Source	Mechanism(s) of Action	Study Design Model	Research Compound	Reference(s)
Oral	Lysergol (Alkaloid)	Plant (morning glory plant: *Ipomoea* spp.)	Metabolism inhibition	In vivo (rat)	Berberine: Benzylisoquinoline alkaloid	[61]
Oral	Lysergol (Alkaloid)	Plant (morning glory plant: *Ipomoea* spp.)	Efflux transporter (BCRP) inhibition; metabolism inhibition	In vitro (rat liver microsomes)	Curcumin: Zingiberaceae Sulfasalazine: Aminosalicylic agent	[62]
Oral	Moringa oleifera pods (Traditional herbal medicine)	Plant (*Moringa oleifera*)	Metabolism (CYP450) inhibition	In vivo (mice)	Rifampicin: Semisynthetic rifamycin derivative	[63]
Oral	Naringin (Flavonoid glycoside)	Plant (grapefruit, apple, onion, tea)	Efflux transporter (P-gp) inhibition; metabolism inhibition	In vivo (rat)	Diltiazem: Benzothiazepine derivates	[64]
Oral	Naringin (Flavonoid glycoside)	Plant (grapefruit, apple, onion, tea)	Metabolism (CYP3A4) inhibition	In vivo (rat)	Tamoxifen: selective estrogen receptor modulator (SERM)	[65]
Oral	Naringin (Flavonoid glycoside)	Plant (grapefruit, apple, onion, tea)	Efflux transporter (P-gp) inhibition; metabolism (CYP3A4) inhibition	In vivo (rat)	Paclitaxel: Tetracyclic diterpenoid	[66]
Oral	Naringin (Flavonoid glycoside)	Plant (grapefruit, apple, onion, tea)	Efflux transporter (P-gp) inhibition; metabolism (CYP3A4) inhibition	Ex vivo (rat everted gut sac)	Clopidogrel: Platelet aggregation inhibitor	[67]
Oral	Naringin (Flavonoid glycoside)	Plant (grapefruit, apple, onion, tea)	Metabolism (CYP3A4) inhibition	In vivo (rabbit)	Verapamil: Calcium channel blocker	[68]
Oral	Palmitoyl carnitine chloride (Chelating agents)	Esterification of carnitinePlant/animal (various)	Tight junction modulation	In vitro (Caco-2 cells [2])	Clodronate: Bisphosphonate	[69]
Oral	Peppermint oil (Herbal)	Plant (peppermint: *Mentha piperita*)	Metabolism (CYP3A) inhibition	Ex vivo (rat intestinal tissue)	Cyclosporine: Immunosuppressant	[70]
Oral	Piperine (Alkaloid)	Plant (*Piper longum* and *Piper nigrum*)	Local mucosal tissue modulation; thermogenic activity	In vivo (human)	B-carotene: Terpenoid	[71]
Oral	Piperine (Alkaloid)	Plant (*Piper longum* and *Piper nigrum*)	Local mucosal tissue modulation; thermogenic activity	In vivo (human)	Coenzyme Q10: benzoquinone	[72]
Oral	Piperine (Alkaloid)	Plant (*Piper longum* and *Piper nigrum*)	Decreased elimination (gastrointestinal transit inhibition; gastric emptying inhibition)	In vivo (rat, mice)	Phenol red: Spheroid	[73]
Oral	Piperine (Alkaloid)	Plant (*Piper longum* and *Piper nigrum*)	Metabolism inhibition	In vivo (human)	Propanol: Beta-receptor activity compound, theophylline: methylxanthine	[74]

Table 1. *Cont.*

Route of Administration	Bioenhancer (Class)	Biological Source	Mechanism(s) of Action	Study Design Model	Research Compound	Reference(s)
Oral	Piperine (Alkaloid)	Plant (*Piper longum* and *Piper nigrum*)	Metabolism (CYP450) inhibition	In vivo (rat)	Nimesulide: Non-steroidal anti-inflammatory	[75]
Oral	Piperine (Alkaloid)	Plant (*Piper longum* and *Piper nigrum*)	Efflux transporter (P-gp) inhibition	In vivo (rat)	Fexofenadine: Terfenadine metabolite	[76]
Oral	Piperine (Alkaloid)	Plant (*Piper longum* and *Piper nigrum*)	Metabolism inhibition	In vivo (mice)	Resveratrol: Phytoalexin	[77]
Oral	Piperine (Alkaloid)	Plant (*Piper longum* and *Piper nigrum*)	Metabolism inhibition	In vivo (human)	Nevirapine: Non-nucleoside reverse transcriptase inhibitor	[78]
Oral	Piperine (Alkaloid)	Plant (*Piper longum* and *Piper nigrum*)	Metabolism inhibition	In vivo (mice)	Epigallocatechin-3-gallate (EGCG): Phenolic antioxidant	[79]
Oral	Piperine (Alkaloid)	Plant (*Piper longum* and *Piper nigrum*)	Metabolism inhibition	In vivo (rat)	Pentobarbitone: Barbiturate.	[80]
Oral	Piperine (Alkaloid)	Plant (*Piper longum* and *Piper nigrum*)	Metabolism (CYP3A4) inhibition	In vivo (human)	Carbamazepine: Carboxamide derivative	[81]
Oral	Piperine (Alkaloid)	Plant (*Piper longum* and *Piper nigrum*)	Metabolism (CYP450) inhibition	In vivo (rat)	Nateglinide: Meglitinide	[82]
Oral	Piperine (Alkaloid)	Plant (*Piper longum* and *Piper nigrum*)	Metabolism (hepatic and intestinal glucuronidation) inhibition	In vivo (rat, human)	Curcumin: Zingiberaceae agent	[83]
Oral	Piperine (Alkaloid)	Plant (*Piper longum* and *Piper nigrum*)	Metabolism inhibition	In vivo (hen)	Oxytetracycline: Bacterial protein synthesis inhibitor	[84]
Oral	Quercetin (Flavonoid)	Plant (citrus fruits, vegetables, leaves, grains)	Efflux transporter (P-gp) inhibition	In vivo (rat), Ex vivo (rat and chick everted intestinal sac)	Ranolazine: Piperazine derivative	[85]
Oral	Quercetin (Flavonoid)	Plant (citrus fruits, vegetables, leaves, grains)	Efflux transporter (P-gp) inhibition	In vivo (rat), In vitro (Caco-2 cells [2])	Irinotecan: Cytotoxic alkaloid	[86]
Oral	Quercetin (Flavonoid)	Plant (citrus fruits, vegetables, leaves, grains)	Efflux transporter (P-gp) inhibition	In vivo (rats), Ex vivo (rat intestinal everted sac)	Valsartan: Angiotensin II receptor antagonist	[87]
Oral	Quercetin (Flavonoid)	Plant (citrus fruits, vegetables, leaves, grains)	Metabolism (CYP3A) inhibition	In vivo (rabbit)	Verapamil: Calcium channel blocker	[88]
Oral	Quercetin (Flavonoid)	Plant (citrus fruits, vegetables, leaves, grains)	Efflux transporter (P-gp) inhibition; metabolism (CYP3A) inhibition	In vivo (rabbit)	Dilitiazem: Nondihydropyridine calcium channel blocker	[89]
Oral	Quercetin (Flavonoid)	Plant (citrus fruits, vegetables, leaves, grains)	Efflux transporter (P-gp) inhibition; metabolism (CYP3A) inhibition	In vivo (rat)	Doxorubicin: Daunorubicin precursor	[90]

Table 1. *Cont.*

Route of Administration	Bioenhancer (Class)	Biological Source	Mechanism(s) of Action	Study Design Model	Research Compound	Reference(s)
Oral	Quercetin (Flavonoid)	Plant (citrus fruits, vegetables, leaves, grains)	Efflux transporter (P-gp) inhibition	In vivo (human)	Fexofenadine: Terfenadine metabolite	[91]
Oral	Quercetin (Flavonoid)	Plant (citrus fruits, vegetables, leaves, grains)	Efflux transporter (P-gp) inhibition	In vivo (rat, dog)	Clopidogrel: Platelet aggregation inhibitor	[49]
Oral	Quercetin (Flavonoid)	Plant (citrus fruits, vegetables, leaves, grains)	Efflux transporter (P-gp) inhibition; metabolism (CYP3A) inhibition	In vivo (rat)	Etoposide: Podophyllotoxin derivative	[92]
Oral	Quercetin (Flavonoid)	Plant (citrus fruits, vegetables, leaves, grains)	Efflux transporter (P-gp) inhibition; metabolism (CYP3A) inhibition	Various	Epigalllocatechin-3-gallate (EGCG): Phenolic antioxidant	[93]
Oral	Quercetin (Flavonoid)	Plant (citrus fruits, vegetables, leaves, grains)	Efflux transporter (P-gp) inhibition	In vitro (human MCF-7 ADRr cells [7])	Doxorubicin: Daunorubicin precursor	[94]
Oral	Quercetin (Flavonoid)	Plant (citrus fruits, vegetables, leaves, grains)	Efflux transporter (MRP) inhibition; metabolism (CYP3A) inhibition	In vivo (rat)	Tamoxifen: selective estrogen receptor modulator (SERM)	[95]
Oral	Quercetin (Flavonoid)	Plant (citrus fruits, vegetables, leaves, grains)	Metabolism (CYP3A) inhibition	In vivo (rat)	Pioglitazone: Thiazolidinedione	[96]
Oral	Quinidine (Class I antiarrhythmic agent)	Chemically modified: stereoisomer of quinine Plant (cinchona tree: *Cinchona* sp.)	Efflux transporter (P-gp) inhibition	Ex vivo (everted rat gut sac)	Paeoniflorin: *Paeonia lactiflora* derivative	[97]
Oral	Resveratrol (Polyphenolic phytoalexin)	Plant (berries, grape skins, red wine)	Metabolism (CYP2C9, CYP2E1) inhibition	In vivo (human)	Diclofenac: NSAID	[98]
Oral	Resveratrol (Polyphenolic phytoalexin)	Plant (berries, grape skins, red wine)	Efflux transporter (P-gp, MRP-2) inhibition; reduced elimination; renal uptake transporter (OAT1, OAT3) inhibition	In vitro (Caco-2 cells [2], mock-MDCK, MDR1-MDCK [6], MRP2-MDCK [6], mock-HEK293, hOAT1-HEK293 [8] cells), Ex vivo (rat everted intestine, rat kidney slices), In vivo (rat)	Methotrexate: Immunosuppressant	[99]
Oral	Sinomenine (Alkaloid)	Plant (*Sinomenium acutum*)	Efflux transporter (P-gp) inhibition	Ex vivo (everted rat gut sac)	Paeoniflorin: *Paeonia lactiflora* derivative	[97]
Oral	Sinomenine (Alkaloid)	Plant (*Sinomenium acutum*)	Efflux transporter (P-gp) inhibition	In vivo (rat)	Paeoniflorin: *Paeonia lactiflora* derivative	[100]

Pharmaceutics **2019**, *11*, 33

Table 1. *Cont.*

Route of Administration	Bioenhancer (Class)	Biological Source	Mechanism(s) of Action	Study Design Model	Research Compound	Reference(s)
Oral	Sodium caprate (Fatty acid)	Chemically modified: salification of caproic acid Animal (fats and oils)	Tight junction modulation	In situ (recirculating intestinal perfusion), ex vivo (everted rat gut sacs), in vivo (rat)	Berberine: Antidiabetic plant alkaloid	[101]
Oral	Sodium cholate/phospholipid-mixed micelles (Bile salts)	Intestinal bacterial by-product	Mucosal membrane modulation	In vivo (dog)	Silybin, the major active component of silymarin (antihepatotoxic polyphenolic substance isolated from milk thistle plant, Silybum marianum)	[102]
Oral	Soybean phosphotidylcholine/ sodium deoxycholate (SPC/SDC) (Bile salts)	SPC: plant (soya bean: *Glycine max*) SDC: chemically modified: salification of deoxycholic acid (metabolic byproduct of intestinal bacteria)	Mucosal membrane modulation	In vivo (dog)	Fenofibrate	[103]
Oral	Tamarixetin (metabolite of quercetin) (Flavonoid)	Plant (hogweed/cow parsnip: *Heracleum stenopterum*)	Metabolism (CYP2C isozyme) inhibition	In vitro (rat liver microsomes), In vivo (rat)	Fluvastatin: HMG CoA reductase inhibitor	[104]
Oral	TMC (Cationic polymers)	Modified chitosan (crustaceans, fungi)	Mucoadhesion; tight junction modulation	In vitro (Caco-2 cells [2])	Mannitol: Sugar alcohol PEG 4000: Polyethylene glycol	[105]
Oral	TMC (Cationic polymers)	Modified chitosan (crustaceans, fungi)	Tight junction modulation	In vitro (Caco-2 cells [2])	Mannitol: Sugar alcohol FITC–dextran: Hydrophilic polysaccharide Buserelin: Gonadotropin-releasing hormone agonist	[106]
Oral	TMC (Cationic polymers)	Modified chitosan (crustaceans, fungi)	Tight junction modulation	In vitro (Caco-2 cells [2])	Clodronate: Bisphosphonate	[69]
Oral	ZOT (Toxins and venom extracts)	Bacteria (*Vibrio cholerae*)	Tight junction modulation	In vitro (Caco-2 cells [2])	PEG 4000: Polyethylene glycol FITC–dextran: Hydrophilic polysaccharide Inulin: Naturally occurring polysaccharide Paclitaxel: Tetracyclic diterpenoid Acyclovir: HSV-specified DNA polymerases inhibitor Cyclosporine: Immunosuppressant Doxorubicin: Daunorubicin precursor	[107]

Table 1. *Cont.*

Route of Administration	Bioenhancer (Class)	Biological Source	Mechanism(s) of Action	Study Design Model	Research Compound	Reference(s)
Pulmonary	Aprotinin, bestatin (Protease inhibitors)	Animal (bovine lung tissue), bacteria (*Streptomyces olivoreticuli*)	Metabolism inhibition	In vivo (rat)	rhG-CSF: Granulocyte-colony stimulating factor	[108]
Pulmonary	Chitosan (Biopolymer)	Chemically modified: deacetylation of chitin Animal (crustaceans), fungi	Tight junction modulation	In vitro (Calu-3 cells [5]); in vivo (rat)	Octreotide: Somatostatin analog	[109]
Pulmonary	Citric acid (Chelating agents)	Plant (citrus fruits and vegetables), fungi (*Aspergillus niger*)	Local mucosal tissue modulation; metabolism inhibition	In vivo (rat)	Insulin: Peptide hormone	[110]
Pulmonary	HPBCD, Crysmeb (Cyclodextrin derivatives)	Plant (starch)	Tight junction modulation	In vitro (Calu-3 cells [5])	Mannitol: Sugar alcohol	[111]
Pulmonary	Lanthanum, cerium, gadolinium (Lanthanides)	Natural elements	Drug targeting	In vivo (rat)	Insulin: Peptide hormone	[112]
Pulmonary	Sodium glycocholate (Bile salt)	Intestinal bacterial by-product	Tight junction modulation	Ex vivo (rabbit trachea and jejunum)	Thyrotropin-releasing hormone (TRH): Tripeptidal hypothalamus hormone Insulin: Peptide hormone	[113]
Pulmonary	Sodium taurocholate (Bile salt)	Intestinal bacterial by-product	Metabolism enhancement (dissociation of insulin hexamers); tight junction modulation; metabolism (enzymatic degradation) inhibition	In vitro (Caco-2 cells [2]), In vivo (dog)	Insulin: Peptide hormone	[114]
Pulmonary	Dideoxycytidine: Nucleoside analog reverse transcriptase inhibitor (NRTI)	Plant (Starch)	Tight junction modulation	In vitro (Calu-3 cells [5]), in vivo (rat)	Enoxaparin: Anticoagulant	[115]
Pulmonary	TMC (Cationic polymers)	Chemically modified: deacetylation of chitin Animal (crustaceans), fungi	Tight junction modulation	In vitro (Calu-3 cells [5]); in vivo (rat)	Octreotide: Octapeptide	[109]

[1] T146 cells: buccal epithelium cells. [2] Caco-2 cells: human epithelial colorectal adenocarcinoma cells. [3] LS180 cells: intestinal human colon adenocarcinoma cells. [4] HT-29 clone B6: human colon carcinoma cells. [5] Calu-3 cells: mammalian airway epithelium cells. [6] MDR1-MDCKII/MRP2-MDCK cells: Madin–Darby Canine Kidney cells with multidrug resistance 1 (MDR1) or multidrug resistance-associated protein 2 (MRP2) gene. [7] MCF-7 ADRr (re-designated NCI-ADR-RES) cells: ovarian tumor cells. [8] hOATP1/3-HEK293 cells: human embryonic kidney cells transfected with human organic anion-transporting polypeptide 1 or 3.

2.2. Bile Salts

The in vitro permeation of 2′,3′-dideoxycytidine (ddC) across porcine buccal mucosae was studied in the absence and presence of sodium glycocholate using in-line flow-through diffusion cells [28]. Fresh isotonic McIlvaine buffer solution (IMB, pH 7.4), which simulated gingival fluid without enzyme, with 10 mg/mL ddC, 0.01% (*w/v*) gentamicin and sodium glycocholate in concentrations varying from 0.6 to 50 mM, were added to the donor chambers. A flow rate of 0.8 mL/h was maintained, and samples were collected every 90 min for 22.5 h. Results demonstrated a concentration-dependent increase in ddC permeation across buccal mucosa as donor concentrations of ddC was increased from 1 to 20 mg/mL. This is indicative of passive diffusion [28]. In the presence of sodium glycocholate (4 mM), the permeability of ddC was significantly increased (~32-fold) to an apparent permeability coefficient (P_{app}) value of $5.11 \pm 1.46 \times 10^{-6}$ cm/s. At lower sodium glycocholate concentrations (<4 mM), a limited enhancement effect was observed, while the P_{app} value was only increased to $5.61 \pm 1.06 \times 10^{-6}$ cm/s at higher concentrations of sodium glycocholate (10 and 50 mM). Earlier studies indicated that 4 mM sodium glycocholate was close to the critical micelle concentration (CMC) of sodium glycocholate [116,117]. Since sodium glycocholate can solubilize the membrane lipids by incorporating them into sodium glycocholate micelles, a low enhancement effect was expected at sodium glycocholate concentrations below the CMC of 4 mM. On the other hand, interfacial saturation between sodium glycocholate micelles and lipid could explain the restricted enhancement effect observed with sodium glycocholate at concentrations beyond the CMC [28].

2.3. Chitosan and Derivatives

It was shown that chitosan could enhance the absorption of the transforming growth factor-β (TGF-β), a large bioactive peptide, across buccal mucosal tissue. A gel was prepared that consisted of 2% chitosan-H (MW: 1 400,000; degree of deacetylation: 80%) in dilute lactic acid solution. I125-labelled TGF-b (MW: ~25 Kda) was incorporated into the chitosan gel, as well as in a control solution of PBS. Continuous-flow perfusion chambers were used to study the permeability of TGF-β across porcine buccal mucosa dermatomed to a thickness of approximately 700 μm. Additionally, horizontal sectioning and counting was performed to determine the localization of TGF-β within the buccal mucosa [22]. Results demonstrated that chitosan enhanced the permeability of the TGF-β bioactive peptide in buccal mucosa six- to seven-fold, even though oral mucosa is relatively impermeable to TGF-β due to its large size [22].

Furthermore, compared to the control PBS solution, an increased amount of TGF-β was found in the superficial layers of the epithelium [22]. Enhanced penetration of TGF-β into buccal mucosa may be the result of increased retention of the drug at the application site due to the mucoadhesive nature of chitosan [22]. Another potential mechanism whereby chitosan improved drug transport across the buccal epithelium, is interference with the lipid organization in the intercellular regions of the epithelium [22].

Another in vitro study demonstrated decreased trans-epithelial electrical resistance (TEER) of the buccal epithelial TR146 cell culture model when chitosan was used as a bioenhancer for peptide and protein absorption. In this study, chitosan glutamate concentrations of 20 μg/mL and higher showed enhanced transport of large hydrophilic compounds, ^{3}H-mannitol and fluorescein isothiocyanate labeled dextrans (FITC–dextrans), at pH 6. ^{3}H-mannitol demonstrated the highest cellular permeability, and decreasing permeability was observed for FITC–dextran with molecular weight (MW) of 4000 Da (FD4), FD10 (MW of 10,000 Da), and FD20 (MW of 20,000 Da) as their molecular weights increased [21]. Enhanced permeability caused by chitosan of all the test substances, except FD20, was statistically significant. Compared to untreated cells, the TEER of the TR146 cell culture model was drastically reduced to ~30% in the presence of chitosan glutamate at concentrations of 20 μg/mL and higher [21]. Contrary to nasal and intestinal mucosal membranes, the buccal mucosal intercellular barrier is not based on tight junctions [22], therefore tight junction modulation cannot be the mechanism by which permeability enhancement proceeded. It was thus suggested that interference with the lipid organization in the buccal mucosa was responsible for improved drug transport in the presence of chitosan glutamate or also potential loosening of intercellular filaments [21].

Thiolated chitosans have shown the ability to significantly improve mucoadhesion and drug permeation [118]. A mucoadhesive buccal peptide drug delivery system with thiolated chitosan was designed and evaluated in vitro and in vivo as an approach for the buccal delivery of pituitary adenylate cyclase-activating polypeptide (PACAP) [23,24]. Chitosan-4-thiobutylamidine (chitosan–TBA) was synthesized and homogenized with enzyme inhibitor and permeation mediator glutathione (GSH), lyophilized and compressed into flat-faced discs. Two experimental formulations were prepared for in vivo evaluation, namely, formulation A that comprised chitosan–TBA (69.5 mg), GSH (3.75 mg), Brij 35 (0.75 mg), and PACAP (1 mg); whereas formulation B contained an innermost layer of chitosan–TBA (50 mg), GSH (2.5 mg), Brij 35 (2.5 mg), PACAP (1 mg) and an outermost layer of chitosan–TBA (50 mg). Additionally, formulation B contained a palm wax coating on one side to ensure unidirectional release of the drug toward buccal mucosa, whilst avoiding losses in the oral cavity [23]. Control formulations contained unmodified chitosan and PACAP (formulation C) or unmodified chitosan, Brij 35, and PACAP (formulation D). These test formulations were given to pigs via buccal administration for 6 h. An absolute bioavailability of 1% was obtained with formulations A and B, whereas the controls (formulations C and D) did not allow PACAP to even reach the systemic circulation [23].

In another study, trimethyl chitosan (TMC) with different quaternization degrees (QDs of 4%, 35% and 90%) showed increased mucoadhesive properties and enhanced permeation of FD4 (FITC–dextran with a molecular weight (MW) of 4000 Da) across porcine cheek mucosa [29]. The epithelium of the porcine cheek mucosa was peeled from the underlying tissues and mounted in Franz diffusion cells. TMC polymer solutions were prepared at 4% (*w/w*) concentration by gentle stirring at room temperature, followed by addition of FD4 at 0.2% (*w/w*) concentration [29]. A tensile stress tester was used to evaluate the mucoadhesive properties of the polymer solutions on cheek buccal mucosa and submaxillary bovine mucin. Results from the in vitro permeation studies demonstrated that permeation of FD4 across the excised cheek mucosal tissue was poor and difficult in the absence of a penetration enhancer. Mucoadhesive performance increased with increasing QD, regardless of media or biological substrate used. However, increased permeation of FD4 was only observed with pH 6.4 buffer, which can be attributed to increased polymer solubility. The best permeation enhancement results were obtained with low molecular weight TMCs with high QD [29].

2.4. Fatty Acids

A study investigated the effect of unsaturated fatty acids (including oleic acid, eicosapentaenoic acid (EPA), and docosahexaenoic acid (DHA)) when concomitantly administered with insulin in a Pluronic F-127 (PF-127) gel formulation [27]. PF-127 (MW: 12,500 Da) was used to prepare insulin gel formulations with or without unsaturated fatty acids. The final concentrations of PF-127 and unsaturated fatty acids were 20 and 5%, respectively. The control formulation consisted of a 20% PF-127 gel containing only insulin [27]. In vitro release studies were performed using membrane-less dissolution tests. In vivo studies were performed by buccally administering a volume of 0.2 mL of a formulation (insulin dose, 25 IU/kg) to anesthetized rats. Blood samples were taken before and after buccal dosing to determine the serum glucose levels [27].

A decreased rate of insulin release together with a remarkable and continuous hypoglycemic effect was observed with PF-127 gels (insulin dose, 25 IU/kg) containing unsaturated fatty acids. The reduced release rate may be partly due to reductions in the numbers and dimensions of the aqueous channels through which the hydrophilic solutes diffuse, or it may be due to the viscosity of the formulations [27]. The serum glucose levels were significantly reduced with all formulations containing unsaturated fatty acids. Results demonstrated that PF-127 gels containing oleic acid yielded the highest bioavailability (15.9 ± 7.9%) of insulin relative to subcutaneous administration. In comparison, EPA and DHA yielded bioavailabilities of 3.4 ± 1.2% and 4.1 ± 3.4%, respectively. However, increased bioavailability observed in the presence of DHA was not statistically significant [27].

Similarly, a study investigated the effect of cod-liver oil extract (CLOE) and hydrogenated castor oil (HCO) on the buccal permeation of ergotamine tartrate (ET) [25]. Hamster cheek pouch was used as a model membrane for the in vitro permeation study using a two-chamber diffusion cell (37 °C). The buccal membrane was pre-treated for 1 or 3 h with a solution of phosphate buffer (PB, pH 7.4) and propylene glycol (PG) (PB:PG, 1:1) containing 5% of each of the permeation enhancers which was each added to the donor cell. After pre-treatment, the solutions in both cells were removed and the cells were rinsed multiple times using a fresh PG/PB mixture. This was immediately followed by the permeation experiment where the donor cell was filled with a suspension of ET in PG/PB, and the receiver cell was filled with the PG/PB mixture only [25]. Results from the permeation study demonstrated that the permeation rate of ET was markedly increased in the presence of each of the permeation enhancers (5%). In the presence of HCO, the solubility of ET was noticeably increased, which resulted in a relatively low flux of ET due to a decrease in the partitioning of ET to the mucosa [25]. On the other hand, the solubility of ET increased ~2-fold in the presence of CLOE, which produced a ~8-fold increase in the flux of ET. These results suggest that CLOE has a direct action on the mucosa in addition to the solubilizing effect it has on ET [25]. Increasing concentrations of CLOE did not enhance the permeation of ET greatly, and 3% concentration of CLOE was considered to be sufficient to exhibit the enhancing action. Furthermore, the flux of ET was almost constant with or without pre-treatment, and an extended period of pre-treatment had no effect on the flux of ET. These findings suggest that CLOE exhibits a transient enhancing effect [25].

The permeation study was repeated on four of the major fatty acids in CLOE, namely palmitic acid, oleic acid, eicosapentaenoic acid (EPA), and docosahexaenoic acid (DHA). However, the concentration of each fatty acid in the donor solution was calculated according to its composition ratios in CLOE. Results from this permeation study revealed that the individual fatty acids had a significantly lower effect on the flux of ET than that of 5% CLOE, of which oleic acid showed the greatest enhancing action. This suggests that the synergistic action of the individual fatty acids in CLOE likely contributes to the greater enhancing action of CLOE [25].

2.5. Menthol

A study of the trans-buccal permeation of dideoxycytidine (ddC) using menthol as an enhancer demonstrated a significant increase in ddC permeability. Porcine buccal tissue was used for the permeation experiments using side-bi-side flow-through diffusion cells at 37 °C. The P_{app} of ddC across the buccal mucosa increased 2.02 times at a menthol concentration of 0.3 mg/mL. However, no significant difference was observed between the permeation enhancement of ddC in the presence of lower concentrations (0.1 and 0.2 mg/mL) of l-menthol. This may be due to the limited effect of menthol on the intercellular lipid extraction over the range of concentrations studied [26]. It was suggested that the observed enhancement in ddC permeation may be partly due to the partition coefficient enhancing effects of l-menthol [26].

3. Nasal Route of Administration

Figure 2 illustrates the main mechanisms of action of selected bioenhancers for improved drug delivery via the nasal route of administration.

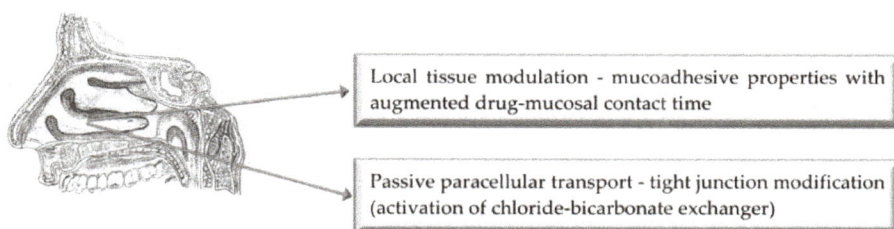

Figure 2. Illustration of the main mechanisms of action of bioenhancers for enhanced nasal drug delivery.

3.1. Bile Salts

The bioavailability of insulin from a nasal formulation with 5% glycofurol (GF) was studied in rabbits [119]. Zinc-free human insulin, Novolin® Nasal (Novo Nordisc) and glycofurol 75 (Hoffman La-Roche) were used in this study. Preparation of intranasal formulations consisted of 6.6 mg insulin dissolved in 1 mL phosphate buffer (12.5 mM, pH 7.4) containing 5% glycofurol. The dosage administered was 50 μL of the nasal solution within each nostril equivalent to 0.66 mg insulin (15.8 IU). Blood glucose was determined in blood collected at pre-determined time intervals. The frog palate model described by Gizurarson, et al. [120] was used to test local toxicity on mucocilliary clearance with phosphate buffer (12.5 mM) at pH 7.4 and 5% glycofurol. The results demonstrated greater decreased plasma glucose levels when glycofurol was included in the nasal formulation, which were comparable with previously published results [121]. Although the absorption enhancing mechanism of glycofurol is not known, the results demonstrated rapid insulin absorption with 90% reduction in the initial glucose blood concentration after 15 min. Furthermore, the plasma glucose was still suppressed with 85% of the initial value at a time interval of 120 min. The results are indicative of glycofurol having the ability to enhance insulin absorption in rats with enduring suppression of blood glucose levels.

Bagger, et al. [122] investigated the absolute nasal bioavailability of peptide T in rabbits when administered with sodium glycocholate and glycofurol. Previous nasal absorption studies with the bile salt sodium glycocholate as a drug absorption enhancer of peptide and peptide-like compounds has shown apparent bioenhancing effects [123–127]. In this study, the absorption enhancing action of sodium glycocholate and glycofurol was investigated by using T_{max}, C_{max} and time-dependent concentration profiles of peptide T. The bioavailability of peptide T administered with the selected bioenhancers was compared to a control formulation consisting of peptide T in water, which gave a bioavailability of 5.9%. Sodium glycocholate showed the highest increase in the bioavailability of peptide T (59%), while glycofurol also increased its bioavailability (22%). On the other hand, when the two bioenhancers were combined (i.e., glyceforol and sodium glycocholate), a bioavailability of 29% was obtained for peptide T. Furthermore, when peptide T was co-administered with sodium glycocholate, the bioenhancing effect was characterized by rapid absorption but relatively short duration of action. The glycofurol showed a lower absorption enhancement effect, but with a longer duration of action [122].

3.2. Chitosan and Derivatives

Chitosan is a polysaccharide obtained from deacetylation of chitin, the second most abundant natural polymer that is contained in the exoskeletons of insects and crustaceans. Illum and co-workers were the first to demonstrate the nasal drug absorption enhancement effects of chitosan. Chitosan showed, for example, the ability to increase the C_{max} of insulin in sheep from 34 mIU/L to 191 mIU/L, while the AUC was elevated 7-fold [128]. The use of chitosan as a novel absorption enhancer for peptide drugs has been described previously [129], while its use in nasal delivery systems for a range of therapeutics has recently been comprehensively reviewed [130]. Selected studies will briefly be discussed below as illustration of the nasal drug delivery enhancement potential of the natural polymer, chitosan.

Illum, Watts, Fisher, Hinchcliffe, Norbury, Jabbal–Gill, Nankervis and Davis [31] showed that the co-administration of either chitosan in solution or chitosan formulated in microspheres can improve the bioavailability of morphine hydrochloride after nasal administration in sheep. Chitosan caused an increase in the C_{max} of morphine from 151 nM in the control group (morphine alone) to 657 nM, and improved the bioavailability of morphine from 10.0% (control group) to 26.6%. Furthermore, the rate of absorption was increased as indicated by the T_{max} of 14 min as opposed to 20 min in the control group. Chitosan formulated into microspheres even further improved the bioavailability parameters of morphine with a C_{max} of 1,010 nM and bioavailability of 54.65%. The rate of absorption was also improved with a T_{max} of 8 min, which was statistically significantly different from that of the control [128].

Hinchcliffe, Jabbal–Gill and Smith [30] investigated the pharmacokinetic effects of a chitosan-based intranasal delivery system on salmon calcitonin within a sheep model. A control nasal solution containing salmon calcitonin (2200 IU/mL) only was compared to a salmon calcitonin solution containing chitosan glutamate (5 mg/mL) as well as to Miacalcin®, a commercially available salmon calcitonin containing nasal spray. A C_{max} value of 99 pg/mL (range 50–107 pg/mL) was obtained for the salmon calcitonin solution containing chitosan compared to 33 pg/mL (range 13–49 pg/mL) for the salmon calcitonin control solution and 42 pg/mL (range 15–79 pg/mL) for the Miacalcin® nasal spray. Furthermore, the average AUC value of the chitosan-containing solution of 3220 pg/mL/min (range 1606–4972 pg/mL/min) demonstrated a 3.5-fold increase compared to that of the control salmon calcitonin solution (943 pg/mL/min, range 198–2519 pg/mL/min) and 2-fold increase towards that of the Miacalcin® nasal spray (1636 pg/mL/min, range 87–3792 pg/mL/min) [30].

Since chitosan is only soluble at acidic pH values below its pKa value, chemically modified derivatives, such as N-trimethyl chitosan chloride (TMC), have been synthesized to improve solubility at more neutral pH values [131]. In a study where TMC polymers with different quaternisation degrees (QD) was nasally administered with ^{14}C-mannitol to rats, it was shown that the QD of TMC played an important role at a neutral environment (pH 7.4) in terms of its nasal absorption enhancement effects. The nasal delivery of ^{14}C-mannitol increased with an increase in QD until a threshold value was reached at 45% [33].

3.3. Starch Microspheres

In vivo studies in sheep found augmented nasal drug absorption for bioadhesive starch microsphere delivery systems, which could be improved synergistically by combination with other absorption enhancing agents. The comparison of control solutions with starch microspheres containing insulin and gentamicin showed 5-fold and 10-fold increases in absorption efficiency, respectively [132–134]. Similar starch microsphere formulations and drug compounds demonstrated approximately 30-fold increases in the bioavailability of the drugs when administered nasally to rats [135].

4. Oral Route of Administration

Figure 3 illustrates the main mechanisms of action of selected bioenhancers for improved drug delivery via the oral route of administration.

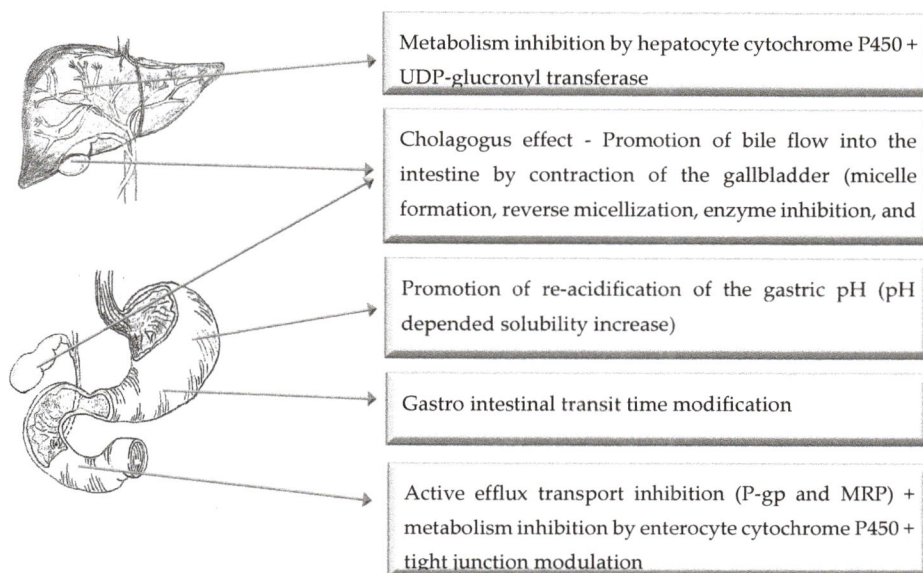

	Metabolism inhibition by hepatocyte cytochrome P450 + UDP-glucronyl transferase
	Cholagogus effect - Promotion of bile flow into the intestine by contraction of the gallbladder (micelle formation, reverse micellization, enzyme inhibition, and
	Promotion of re-acidification of the gastric pH (pH depended solubility increase)
	Gastro intestinal transit time modification
	Active efflux transport inhibition (P-gp and MRP) + metabolism inhibition by enterocyte cytochrome P450 + tight junction modulation

Figure 3. Illustration of the main mechanisms of action of bioenhancers for enhanced oral drug delivery.

4.1. Aloe Vera

Aloe vera leaf materials and extracts have been found to modify in vitro drug transport and in vivo drug bioavailability. In a double-blind, cross-over clinical study investigating the effect of *A. vera* liquid products on the absorption of vitamins C and E in human subjects, both *A. vera* gel product (AVG) and *A. vera* whole leaf product (AVWL) were investigated. AVG caused a 3.7-fold and AVWL a 2-fold increase in the bioavailability of vitamin C in comparison to the control (i.e., vitamin C administered with water). With respect to the influence on the bioavailability of vitamin E, both *Aloe* products caused a statistically significant increase in the baseline levels of vitamin E at 6 and 8 h post administration. However, due to large inter-individual variation, the AUC values between the different treatments were not statistically significant. The authors attributed the improvement in the bioavailability of vitamins C and E by the *A. vera* products to a protective action against degradation in the gastrointestinal tract, however, this was not proven in the study [37].

Both *A. vera* gel and whole leaf materials increased insulin transport extensively across Caco-2 cell monolayers over a concentration range of 0.1 to 5% *w/v* at two different pH values of 5.8 and 7.4. The *Aloe* materials decreased the TEER of the Caco-2 cell monolayers markedly at concentrations higher than 0.5% *w/v*, which was reversible [36]. A study was conducted using *A. ferox* and *A. vera* gel material, whole leaf material as well as precipitated polysaccharides (from these materials) in a concentration of 2% *w/v* in combination with atenolol as model drug across excised rat intestinal tissues in diffusion chambers. All the *Aloe* materials lowered the TEER of the excised rat intestinal tissues statistically significantly ($p < 0.05$) in comparison to the control (atenolol alone) and to a larger extent than the positive control (0.2% *w/v* sodium lauryl sulfate). In this study, it was also shown that some precipitated polysaccharides resulted in a higher decrease in TEER than their corresponding gel and whole leaf material counterparts. This reduction in TEER was indicative of the ability of the *Aloe* leaf materials to open tight junctions and consequently enhance paracellular transport of hydrophilic drug molecules such as atenolol. Only the precipitated polysaccharide fraction from dehydrated *A. vera* gel (Daltonmax 700®) material could enhance the transport of atenolol across intestinal rat tissue statistically significantly in comparison to the control. Although not statistically significant in comparison to the control, the polysaccharide fraction obtained from the *A. vera* whole leaf extract (Daltonmax 700®) caused a substantial increase in atenolol transport. The *A. ferox* materials were, however, not able to enhance the transport of atenolol across the excised rat intestinal tissues [35].

In a study by Wallis, Malan, Gouws, Steyn, Ellis, Abay, Wiesner, P Otto and Hamman [38], the effect of *A. vera* gel and polysaccharides (i.e., crude polysaccharides as well as fractionated polysaccharides based on molecular weight) on the bioavailability of indinavir was investigated in Sprague–Dawley rats. As part of this study, the effect of the selected *Aloe* materials was also investigated on the TEER of Caco-2 cell monolayers as well as their influence on the metabolism of indinavir in LS 180 cells. The results of this study indicated that all of the *Aloe* materials decreased the TEER of the Caco-2 cell monolayers indicating opening of tight junctions. The precipitated polysaccharides decreased the TEER to a larger extent than the gel material. However, no clear correlation between the different molecular weight fractions of the polysaccharides and TEER reduction could be made. All of the *Aloe* materials exhibited enzyme inhibitory effects, although not statistically significant, in comparison to the control (indinavir alone). With respect to the influence on the bioavailability of indinavir as indicated by AUC, all the investigated *Aloe* materials rendered an increase in bioavailability although not statistically significant. The increase in indinavir bioavailability caused by the crude precipitated polysaccharide and polysaccharide fractions were higher than that seen for the *A. vera* gel. The increase in bioavailability of indinavir in this study was attributed to a combination of mechanisms including the opening of the tight junctions (as indicated by a reduction in TEER) and an inhibition in the metabolism of indinavir (as indicated by the metabolite plasma concentration). Furthermore, from the results of this study, it is evident that the biologically active components responsible for the modulation of drug pharmacokinetics and absorption are most probably concentrated in the polysaccharide component of the *A. vera* gel material although it cannot be directly correlated with the molecular size of the polysaccharide component [38].

4.2. Bile Salts

The ability of bile salts to enhance the oral bioavailability of compounds, especially poorly water-soluble drugs, has been discovered many years ago [136–138].

The study by Yu, Zhu, Wang, Peng, Tong, Cao, Qiu and Xu [102] investigated the bioavailability of silybin when mixed with bile salt micelles compared with silybin-N-methylglucamine alone after oral administration in dogs. The prepared mixed bile salt micelles showed a mean particle size of 75.9 ± 4.2 nm. Silybin-sodium cholate/phospholipid-mixed micelles revealed a very slow release of the silybin, only 17.5% (*w/w*) over 72 h in phosphate buffer (pH 7.4) and 15.6% (*w/w*) in HCl solution (pH 1.2). In spite of this slow release, the relative bioavailability of silybin in the mixed micelles versus silybin-N-methylglucamine in dogs was 252% [102].

An in vivo study in diabetic rats was used to investigate the regional-specific intestinal delivery of insulin by co-administration of sodium glycocholate [139]. Insulin (10 UI/kg) was administered intestinally (duodenum, jejunum and ileum) to rats by surgical technique without (control) and with 5% sodium glycocholate. Insulin absorbed from the gastrointestinal tract was investigated by measuring the hypoglycemic effect in the rats at 45 and 60 min post administration. The hypoglycemic effect (100%) of the positive control was specified at 77.9 mg/100 mL glucose at 45 min and 70.5 mg/100 mL glucose at 60 min. For the duodenum region, the insulin control showed a hypoglycemic effect of 71% at 45 min and 84% at 60 min, while the insulin with sodium glycocholate showed hypoglycemic effects of 90% and 95% at 45 and 60 min post administration, respectively. For the jejunum region, the insulin control showed 34% and 54% hypoglycemic effects, while the insulin with sodium glycocholate showed 39% and 60% hypoglycemic effects at 45 and 60 min post administration, respectively. However, administration within the ileum of rats did not demonstrate a significant decrease in blood glucose concentration profiles compared to control. For the ileum, the insulin control showed 9% and 5%, while insulin with sodium glycocholate showed 5% and 8% at 45 and 60 min post administration, respectively [139].

These effects could be contributed to the increased insulin absorption in the presence of the bile salt, potentially by mechanisms of mucus layer modification as well as tight junction modulation [140,141]. Finally, the effects of sodium glycocholate on the intestinal absorption enhancement of insulin demonstrated site-dependent effects with duodenum being the optimal site for insulin oral delivery [139].

4.3. Black Cumin

Nigella sativa, commonly known as black cumin/caraway, was previously evaluated as a bioenhancer for amoxicillin [142]. *N. sativa* extracts were prepared by cleaning, milling and sieving seeds, followed by extractions with methanol and hexane for 6 h [142]. Everted rat intestinal sacs were used to study the transfer of amoxicillin (6 mg/mL) in PBS (pH 7.4) with or without methanol (3 mg) and hexane (6 mg) extract of *N. sativa* seeds. The amount of amoxicillin transported across the gut was quantified spectrophotometrically at 273 nm [142]. For in vivo studies, amoxicillin (25 mg/kg) was orally co-administered with *N. sativa* hexane extract (25 mg/kg) to rats. Blood samples were collected at 0, 0.25, 0.5, 0.75, 1, 1.5, 2, 4, 6 and 8 h post-dosing, after which UPLC-MS/MS was used to quantify the amount of amoxicillin in rat plasma [142].

Results from the in vitro study demonstrated that both the methanol and hexane extracts of *N. sativa* significantly increased the permeation of amoxicillin, with the latter showing the greatest increase [142]. Hence, hexane extract was selected for in vivo evaluation. Results from the in vivo study also demonstrated a significant increase in amoxicillin plasma concentration in rats. *N. sativa* extract increased the rate and extent of amoxicillin absorption, increasing the C_{max} from 4138.251 ± 156.93 to 5995.045 ± 196.28 ng/mL, while $AUC_{0 \to t}$ increased from 8890.40 ± 143.33 to 13483.46 ± 152.45 ng/mL·h. It was suggested that this permeation enhancing effect of *N. sativa* might be attributed to the presence of fatty acids [142]. It has previously been demonstrated that fatty acids are able to enhance permeation of low permeable drugs by increasing the fluidity of the apical and basolateral membranes [143]. A similar in vivo study performed on rabbits yielded opposite results. In that study, the C_{max} and $AUC_{0-\infty}$ of cyclosporine (30 mg/kg) significantly decreased by 35.5% and 55.9%, respectively, after pretreatment with *Nigella* (200 mg/kg). However, a significant increase in cyclosporine clearance (~2-fold) was observed, thus suggesting that intestinal P-gp and/or CYP3A4 are activated in the presence of *N. sativa* [144].

4.4. Capsaicin

In vitro, in situ and in vivo evaluations of the effect of capsaicin pre-treatment on fexofenadine showed significantly enhanced intestinal absorption of fexofenadine [145]. Non-everted intestinal sacs of rats were employed in the in vitro study, while an in situ single-pass intestinal perfusion study was conducted on rats where the ileal segment (~8–12 cm) was isolated and cannulated. For the in vivo study, the same pre-treatment was applied for 7 days in rats. Results from the non-everted sac study indicated a significant increase in the intestinal transport and P_{app} of fexofenadine in the presence of capsaicin. It was suggested that P-gp efflux inhibition in intestine of rats was the action mechanism, since the results obtained with capsaicin pre-treatment and verapamil, a standard P-gp inhibitor, were comparable [145]. In situ single-pass intestinal perfusion results demonstrated a significant increase in the absorption rate constant, fraction absorbed, and effective permeability of fexofenadine in rats pre-treated with capsaicin and verapamil in comparison with control group [145]. In vivo results showed a significant increase in the AUC and C_{max} of fexofenadine orally administered to rats pretreated with capsaicin. Additionally, the apparent oral clearance of fexofenadine was significantly decreased, while t_{max} and $t_{1/2}$ were unchanged. Findings from this study thus provide in vivo evidence that capsaicin might increase the bioavailability of fexofenadine via the inhibition of P-gp-mediated drug efflux [145].

4.5. Caraway

Caraway is obtained from the dried ripe fruit of the plant *Carum carvi*. In an open-label, cross-over in vivo study, the bioenhancing effect of *C. carvi* (Caraway) extract (100 mg) on the pharmacokinetics of rifampicin, isoniazid and pyrazinamide administered as a fixed-dose combination (FDC) was investigated. The Caraway extract increased both C_{max} and AUC as indicators of bioavailability for all three drugs, statistically significantly. The increase in C_{max} was 32.22%, 36.01% and 33.22% for rifampicin, isoniazid and pyrazinamide, respectively, while the increase in $AUC_{0-24\,h}$ was 32.16%, 29.06% and 27.92% for rifampicin, isoniazid and pyrazinamide, respectively. According to the authors, the improvement in bioavailability caused by Caraway extract may be attributed to an enhancement of mucosal to serosal permeation as well as its influence on P-gp efflux [40]. Caraway was shown to act as an inhibitor of P-gp efflux and the main active components were found to be carvone and limonene [146].

4.6. Cylcosporine A

Cyclosporine A is a polypeptide consisting of 11 amino acids and was initially derived from a fungus, *Tolypocladium inflatum Gams* [147]. Cyclosporine A is used amongst other indications as an immunosuppresive agent during organ transplantation, to treat autoimmune diseases and in the treatment of certain viral diseases such as Hepatitis C, to name but a few uses. Cyclosporine A has been shown to act as an inhibitor of the efflux transporter, P-gp and as a result may increase the bioavailability of drugs that are substrates for this active efflux transporter [51]. Cyclosporine A has been shown to improve the bioavailability of clopidogrel, an antiplatelet drug, in rats. Co-administration of a dose of 10 mg/kg of cyclosporine A and 30 mg/kg of clopidogrel resulted in a 3.48-fold and 2.83-fold increase in the AUC and C_{max} of clopidogrel, respectively. The authors attributed this increase in bioavailability to the inhibition of P-gp-mediated efflux [49].

4.7. Chitosan and Derivatives

The oral drug absorption enhancing effects of chitosan and its derivatives have previously been reviewed extensively [148,149]. In brief, several studies have shown that chitosan (including chitosan salts such as chitosan hydrochloride and chitosan glutamate) is an effective oral drug absorption enhancer across in vitro cell models as well as in vivo animal models [42,150–152]. The major mechanism of drug absorption enhancement has been shown to involve tight junction modulation to allow for enhanced paracellular uptake of hydrophilic and macromolecular drug compounds. Although a number of studies indicated interactions of chitosan with epithelial cells to open tight junctions [153] through redistribution of F-actin and ZO-1 [148,154], it was shown on HT-29/B6 cells with two-path impedance spectroscopy that the tight junction opening effect of chitosan was due to changes in intracellular pH caused by the activation of a chloride-bicarbonate exchanger [155].

To improve some of the characteristics of chitosan, several derivatives and chemically modified chitosans have been investigated for their drug delivery potential including trimethyl-chitosans, thiolated chitosans, carboxymethyl chitosan and derivatives, hydrophobic chitosans, chitosan succinate and phthalate, PEGylated chitosans and chitosan-enzyme inhibitor conjugates, which have been published in a review previously [156].

4.8. Curcumin

Curcumin (diferuloylmethane) is the major curcuminoid contained in the rhizome of *Curcuma longa* L. (turmeric) that has been shown to have several biological and pharmacological activities [157]. A previously published review on pharmacokinetic interactions of curcuminoids with conventional drugs revealed potential interactions via modulation of CYP450 and phase II enzymes as well as P-gp efflux inhibition and potential effects on organic anion transporting polypeptides (OATP).

Unfortunately, contrasting results were obtained by different studies ranging from drug absorption enhancement to drug absorption reduction by curcumin [158].

An example of a study where curcumin was found to significantly increase drug bioavailability is an in vivo study in Sprague–Dawley rats that received curcumin (60 mg/kg) for four days prior to drug administration (pre-treatment group), while another group received curcumin (60 mg/kg) once only concomitantly with the drug and the control group received no curcumin. The bioavailability of celiprolol increased statistically significantly in the curcumin pre-treated rats, but not in rats where it was co-administered once only with curcumin. Although the bioavailability of midazolam increased in both the pre-treatment group as well as the co-administered group, it was only statistically significant in the pre-treatment group. Western blot analyses revealed that intestinal P-gp protein expression reduced by 49%, while CYP3A protein content reduced by 42% after 4 days of pre-treatment with curcumin. On the other hand, the hepatic P-gp protein expression increased by 144% and the CYP3A protein content was increased by 91%. Renal P-gp protein levels remained unchanged, but renal CYP3A was enhanced by 41%. Since celiprolol is a P-gp substrate and midazolam is extensively metabolized by CYP3A enzymes, it was deduced from this study that the pharmacokinetics of these two drugs have been changed by curcumin due to down regulation of P-gp and CYP3A in the small intestine [48]. Furthermore, when curcumin was administered at a dose of 10 mg/kg with tamoxifen to rats, the AUC and C_{max} values of tamoxifen were significantly increased (i.e., by 64% and 71%, respectively) [159]. Pre-treatment of broiler chickens with 100 mg/kg curcumin for ten days enhanced the absolute and relative bioavailabilities of marbofloxacin in these animals [160]. The P-gp inhibiting effects of curcumin was confirmed in an in vitro study on a human P-gp overexpressing cell line (LLC-GA5-COL300) where the uptake of calcein-AM was increased [161].

4.9. Diosmin

Certain flavones (e.g., tangeretin, nobiletin and bergamottin) from citrus fruits have shown P-gp inhibitory effects, which caused pharmacokinetic interactions with drugs that are substrates for this efflux transporter. Diosmin, a flavonoid contained in citrus fruit, was investigated in the Caco-2 cell model for P-gp inhibitory effects using rhodamine 123 and digoxin as model compounds. Rhodomine 123 accumulation in the Caco-2 cells was investigated in the absence and presence of diosmin. At a concentration of 50 μM, diosmin caused a 494 ± 8.4% increase in the cellular accumulation of rhodamine 123 in reference to the control. To further investigate the initial observation of P-gp-mediated efflux inhibition by diosmin, bi-directional transport (i.e., in the apical-to-basolateral [A-B] and basolateral-to-apical [B-A] direction) of digoxin across Caco-2 cell monolayers was conducted in the absence and presence of diosmin. At a concentration of 50 μM diosmin, the $P_{app\,(A-B)}$ was significantly increased from $2.8 \pm 0.07 \times 10^{-6}$ cm/s to $9.5 \pm 0.06 \times 10^{-6}$ cm/s, while the $P_{app\,(B-A)}$ was significantly decreased from $41.1 \pm 1.20 \times 10^{-6}$ cm/s to $17.1 \pm 0.10 \times 10^{-6}$ cm/s. These P_{app} values corresponded to transport ratio values of 15.2 in the absence and 2.3 in the presence of diosmin. Based on the results of this study, it is clear that diosmin act as a P-gp efflux transport inhibitor and as such has the potential to improve the bioavailability of drugs that are substrates for P-gp [50].

In a more recent study, the effect of diosmin on the in vivo pharmacokinetics of fexofenadine in rats was investigated. In this study, rats were pre-treated for 7 days with diosmin (50 mg/kg) where after fexofenadine (10 mg/kg) was administered on day 8. Pre-treatment with diosmin resulted in a 2.5- and 2.2-fold increase in C_{max} and $AUC_{0-\infty}$, respectively. The enhanced bioavailability of fexofenadine in this study was attributed to the fact that diosmin is a potent P-gp inhibitor [162].

4.10. Emodin

Anthraquinones such as emodin (1,3,8-trihydroxy-6-methyl-anthraquinone) occur naturally in a wide variety of plants and herbs such as *Rheum palmatum* [163], *Polygonum multiflorum* [164], *Polygonum cuspidatum* [165], *Cassia obtusifolia* [166] and *Aloe vera* [167]. Administration of emodin may lead to synergistic and/or inhibitory effects on P-gp-related efflux and/or modulation of multidrug-resistance associated protein 1, 2 and 3 (MRP1, MRP2 and MRP3) and these effects may have a profound effect on the bioavailability of co-administered substrate molecules [163,168–171].

In an extensive study conducted by Min, et al. [172], potential interactions between emodin and rhodamine 123 were investigated in various in vitro models. In this study, human myelogenous myeloid leukemia cells (K562), the P-gp over-expressing adriamycin resistant K562 cells (K562/ADM) and Caco-2 cells were used as in vitro models to investigate if the co-administration of emodin at various concentrations had any significant effect on the intracellular accumulation of rhodamine 123 (1 µM). The results showed that addition of emodin increased the intracellular accumulation of rhodamine 123 in a concentration-dependent manner in both the Caco-2 and K562/ADM cell models. The extent of the accumulation of rhodamine 123 in Caco-2 cells by emodin (20 µM) was comparable to that of a much higher verapamil concentration (200 µM). Binding site competition between emodin and rhodamine 123 on P-gp was also investigated. The results showed that the calculated K_i values increased consistently in conjunction with increasing rhodamine 123 concentrations (0 to 20 µM), which indicated that a competitive interaction occurred between emodin and rhodamine 123. It was concluded that emodin and rhodamine 123 shared the same R-binding site on P-gp [172].

An MTT method was also used in conjunction with the K562/ADM cell line to investigate if the addition of emodin could potentially reverse P-gp-mediated MDR. The results showed that the addition of emodin (20 µM), alone or in combination with 10 µM adriamycin, exerted down regulation of P-gp expression in comparison to the control group. The authors concluded that emodin could potentially reverse P-gp-mediated MDR due to inhibition of P-gp expression in K562/ADM cells and also by competitive interactions between emodin and rhodamine 123 at the R-binding site of P-gp. The results confirmed that emodin is an effective inhibitor of P-gp and its effects are mediated either by direct binding to P-gp and subsequent weakening of the P-gp-mediated efflux function or by indirect mechanisms related to a reduction in P-gp expression [172].

In another study, it was also shown that the addition of emodin to the Caco-2 cell model had the ability to decrease P-gp-mediated efflux, but additionally it was also reported that P-gp expression was mediated via the MAPK/AP-1 pathway by means of COX-2 inhibition [173]. An in vitro transport study across rat intestinal tissues using an Ussing-chamber technique showed that the transport of digoxin was decreased in the presence of emodin while the transport of teniposide was increased in the presence of emodin. The authors concluded that emodin was an inducer of P-gp-related efflux and also an inhibitor of MRP3 [174].

4.11. Gallic Acid Ester

Gallic acid is a water soluble phenolic acid which is found in grapes and in the leaves of various plants and forms part of a larger group of plant polyphenols known as gallotannins [175]. Gallotannins are transformed in the gastrointestinal tract by hydrolysis to form free gallic acid [176]. Various health benefits are associated with the intake of gallic acid and it is reported in the literature to exert anti-cancer, anti-inflammatory, cardio-protective and anti-diabetic properties [175]. Gallic acid has been reported to exhibit inhibitory effects on P-gp-mediated drug efflux and also on CYP450-related isozymes such as CYP3A4 [177–179].

In vitro and in situ transport studies were conducted to investigate the effects of gallic acid on the transport of diltiazem. The in vitro studies entailed the use of non-everted gut sacs from Wistar rat intestinal tissue. The results from the in vitro study showed that the apparent permeability of diltiazem had increased in the presence of gallic acid by 4.4-, 5.1- and 4.9-fold in the respective segments of the duodenum, jejunum and ileum of non-everted intestinal gut sacs when compared with the control group [180].

For the in situ single-pass intestinal perfusion study, rats were randomly divided into four groups ($n = 5$) (control, standard inhibitor, and pre-treated with either gallic acid or ellagic acid). Perfusion of the cannulated intestinal segment was performed using phosphate buffered saline (pH = 7.2) containing diltiazem (100 µg/mL) and phenol red (50 mg/mL). A constant flow rate of 0.2 mL/min was maintained for a period of 90 min and samples were collected at 10 min intervals. The results from the in situ study showed that pre-treatment with gallic acid (50 mg/kg) for 7 days resulted in a significant ($p < 0.05$) increase in diltiazem transport in rats when compared to the control group (diltiazem alone) following pre-treatments with gallic acid for 7 days. The C_{max}, AUC_{0-t}, and $AUC_{0-\infty}$ of diltiazem were increased by 1.90-, 2.06- and 2.08-fold, respectively (Athukuri and Neerati., 2018). Based on these results, it was suggested that gallic acid was most likely a dual inhibitor of both P-gp and CYP3A4 and that this dualistic effect may have resulted in the significant enhancement in the bioavailability of diltiazem [180].

The transport of metoprolol was assessed in a similar in situ single-pass intestinal perfusion study to evaluate the pharmacokinetic parameters of orally administered metoprolol in Wistar rats. The rats were pre-treated with gallic acid (50 mg/kg) for 7 days before the start of the study. A significant increase in the C_{max} and AUC values of metoprolol were evident. It was concluded that gallic acid had enhanced the oral bioavailability by inhibiting CYP2D6 activity in the liver, which caused reduced metabolism of metoprolol [181].

4.12. Genistein

The flavonoid genistein (5,7-Dihydroxy-3-(4-hydroxyphenyl)chromen-4-one) is a plant-derived (*Glycine max* and *Pueraria lobata*) isoflavone and a phytoestrogen, frequently ingested by humans [54,55,182]. Genistein has very poor bioavailability in itself and although some studies have suggested that genistein may have anticancer effects, these effects could not be obtained in clinical studies because of its low bioavailability [183]. Genistein is purported to be an enhancer of bioavailability of drugs, since it has been shown to inhibit efflux of P-gp, BCRP and MRP2 transporters. These properties were investigated in a Caco-2 antiparasitic agent transport study, where taxol (a P-gp substrate) was applied in combination with 33 or 100 μM genistein [184]. Although no inhibition of transport could be measured for 33 μM genistein, 100 μM genistein resulted in 20% inhibition. It was subsequently determined that although genistein inhibited P-gp, it did not appear to be a substrate of P-gp. Another study showed 10–30 μM genistein increased sensitivity of a P-gp hyper-expressing drug resistant human cervical carcinoma cell line (KB-V1) to vinblastine and paclitaxel, while reducing efflux of Rhodamine 123 and vinblastine in a dose-dependent manner (10–200 μM) [185]. However, no correlating change in P-gp expression was observed following exposure to genistein, indicating only P-gp activity was modulated. Li and Choi [55] later demonstrated that a single oral dose of 30 mg/kg paclitaxel 30 min after ingesting 3.3 mg/kg or 10 mg/kg genistein, significantly increased the AUC by 54.7% in male Sprague–Dawley rats. This was as a result of decreased plasma clearance (35.2%), thereby increasing systemic exposure. The same effect was seen when the paclitaxel was administered intravenously (3.3 mg/kg). It was proposed that the genistein inhibited the efflux transporters and metabolic enzymes for which paclitaxel is known to be a substrate, probably being P-gp and CYP3A [55,182].

Genistein also inhibited efflux of 2′,7′-bis-(carboxypropyl)-5(6)-carboxyfluorescein (BCPCF), an MRP1 substrate, from human erythrocytes. Genistein displayed an IC_{50} concentration of 50–70 μM for BCPCF efflux. It was reported that genistein inhibited MRP1 efflux transporters, but that this modulation was substrate sensitive [186].

Genistein has been shown to inhibit the biotransformation and intestinal efflux of (-)-epigallocatechin-3-gallate (EGCG) in more recent studies. EGCG is a flavonoid in various foods and beverages, but especially in *Camellia sinensis* (green tea), and has been shown to have several therapeutic effects such as anti-cancer, anti-viral and anti-inflammatory effects, but it has very poor oral systemic absorption [187]. Lambert, Kwon, Ju, Bose, Lee, Hong, Hao and Yang [54] demonstrated an increase in cytosolic EGCG of 2- to 5-fold in the presence of genistein (20 μM), in HT-29 human colon cancer cells. They also treated CF-1 mice with 200 mg/kg genistein and 75 mg/kg EGCG, resulting in increased plasma half-life and maximal concentration of the EGCG. However, in a male adenomatous polyposis coli (APC) min/+ mouse model, this combination also enhanced tumor genesis.

An in vitro and in vivo study treated Mardin-Darby canine kidney (MDCK-II) cells and Assaf sheep with the antibacterial fluoroquinolone, danofloxacin, concomitantly with genistein [188]. Danofloxasin is exclusive for animal use and is actively secreted into milk. The in vitro transport study showed that genistein inhibited BCRP transport of danofloxasin efficiently, while the in vivo study indicated no change in danofloxasin plasma levels following isoflavone supplementation. A prolonged diet of soy, however, did reduce antimicrobial concentrations in the milk.

Important to note are the findings of Chen, et al. [189], which indicated that genistein can induce the phase II drug-metabolizing enzyme, sulfotransferase. Enzymatic activity, protein levels and mRNA expression were evaluated in a transformed human liver cell line (HepG2) and a colon carcinoma cell line (Caco-2). It was concluded that gene expression (SULT1A1 and SULT2A1) was induced by genistein in a time and dose-dependent (0–25 μM) manner. Contrary, approximately 0.1 μM genistein inhibited human liver phenol sulfotransferase by 50% in a competitive manner [190].

4.13. Gokhru Extract

Gokhru extract, a popular plant extract used in Ayurvedic medicines, is derived from *Tribulus terrestris* Linn (Zygophyllaceae) [56,191]. Some of the phytochemicals previously identified in *T. terrestris* include saponins, steroids, flavonoids and carboline alkaloids. Gokhru extract is traditionally used as a diuretic, anti-inflammatory, anabolic, spasmolytic, muscle relaxant, hypotensive, and hypoglycemic agent, but it has been reported to influence bioavailability of co-administered drugs.

One study investigated the effect of Gokhru extract on the absorption of metformin hydrochloride (HCl) in an everted sac model [56]. Metformin is an anti-diabetic drug that is known to be highly soluble, but poorly membrane permeable (BCS class III). In this study, the extract was prepared from dried plant material (fresh fruits, leaves and stems) with hot ethanol. The results showed increased absorption of metformin in the presence of the Gokhru extract, and the authors suggested the major saponin component in the extract may have contributed largely to this increase in drug transport. Saponins consist of one or more sugar chains, connected to a steroid or triterpenoid aglycon. It can solubilize cholesterol, while maintaining most of the structure of the cell membranes, thereby permeabilizing it to increase membrane permeability [57].

A similar study formulated metformin HCl tablets (175–500 mg) with varying concentrations Gokhru extract (0–100 mg), which were then investigated using a chicken intestine everted sac model. In this study, the drug absorption enhancement properties of Gokhru extract was confirmed with increased metformin permeation across the chicken intestinal membranes from 29% to 54% [57].

A methanol extract was prepared from dried *T. terrestris* leaves and applied together with salicylic acid (aspirin) to the mucosal side of the goat intestinal tissues used in an everted sac technique. The Gokhru extract increased aspirin transport and it was proposed that the permeability enhancing action was a result of the saponins effects on the membranes [191].

4.14. Grapefruit Juice

The pharmacokinetic interaction between grapefruit (*Citrus paradisi*) juice and the calcium channel antagonist, felodipine, was discovered serendipitously during an in vivo clinical study in 1989 that was designed to evaluate the potential interaction between ethanol and felodipine. Grapefruit juice was used to mask the taste of ethanol in this study. Concomitant intake of felodipine with grapefruit juice caused higher anti-hypertensive effects as well as higher felodipine plasma concentrations. This observation led to a follow-up pilot study in a single volunteer where felodipine plasma concentrations were found to be more than 5-fold higher when it was taken with grapefruit juice than with water [192]. Since this initial discovery, more than 85 drugs have shown to interact with grapefruit juice in terms of pharmacokinetics of which most experienced increased plasma concentrations [193].

In a study on borderline hypertensive patients where the effect of different fruit juices was evaluated on felodipine pharmacokinetics, it was shown that grapefruit juice, but not orange juice, could markedly increase felodipine's bioavailability parameters (both C_{max} and AUC were increased).

In addition, grapefruit juice reduced the ratio of dehydrofelodipin (the primary metabolite of felodipine produced by CYP3A4) to felodipine. This effect was not observed for intravenous administration of felodipine with grapefruit juice, which indicated selective inhibition of pre-systemic metabolism involving CYP3A4 [194].

Several studies showed that three groups could be distinguished with respect to the effect of grapefruit juice on the pharmacokinetic parameters of drugs, namely "increase", "decrease" and "no change" [195]. The uptake and bioavailability enhancement effect of grapefruit juice was shown in a study where both in vitro and in vivo models were used. Lyophilized freshly-prepared grapefruit juice significantly increased the uptake of doxorubicin into human uterine sarcoma (MES-SA/DX5) cells and significantly increased the bioavailability of timolol maleate in rabbits [196]. However, it was shown that both regular strength and double strength grapefruit juice did not have a significant effect on the pharmacokinetic parameters of simvastatin when administered concomitantly to Sprague–Dawley rats in a dose of 20 mg/kg over 28 days. On the other hand, simvastatin plasma concentrations were elevated by double strength grapefruit juice when the drug was administered at a dose of 80 mg/kg [197], indicating a dose-dependent pharmacokinetic interaction. In another in vivo study, grapefruit juice decreased the oral bioavailability of fexofenadine [58].

Results from different studies revealed, over time, that the pharmacokinetic effect of several forms of grapefruit (i.e., whole fruit, fresh fruit juice or frozen concentrate) is drug-specific and it may in some cases be concentration-dependent. It was also shown that the lower the inherent bioavailability of the drug due to pre-systemic metabolism, the higher the chance is that the interaction with grapefruit can be dangerous [193].

One of the main mechanisms of action of grapefruit juice by which the bioavailability of drugs (e.g., felodipine) is increased, is by mechanism-based inhibition of CYP3A4 in the enterocytes of the small intestine and hepatocytes of the liver [58,198]. It was also shown that grapefruit juice could inhibit the P-gp efflux transporter and thereby increase the bioavailability of drugs that are substrates for this efflux transporter (e.g., talinolol) [199,200]. Furthermore, a study on 10 volunteers that received grapefruit juice three times a day for 6 days revealed that their small intestinal CYP3A4 protein expression reduced by 62%, but not their liver CYP3A4 protein expression. This selective down regulation of CYP3A4 correlated well with the C_{max} increase of felodipine after grapefruit juice consumption relative to that taken with water [201]. On the other hand, it was found that grapefruit juice has the ability to inhibit uptake transporters such as OATP, specifically OATP1A2 and OATP2B1, and thereby it can decrease the absorption of certain drugs (e.g., fexofenadine) [202,203].

4.15. Lycopene

The effect of a lycopene-containing nano-formulation containing simvastatin on low density lipoprotein (LDL) was investigated in mildly hypercholesterolemic patients [60]. The aim of this study was to evaluate lycopene as a vector of intrahepatic transport to specifically enhance the hepatic bioavailability of simvastatin. This is important, since hepatic cholesterologenesis is the main site of statin action. Furthermore, the plasma lipid profile is not affected by extrahepatic inhibition of HMG-CoA reductase, and extrahepatic toxicity is observed with increasing statin concentrations [60]. A total of 10 patients with moderately increased plasma LDL levels (150 to 200 mg/dL) received 20 mg of either unmodified simvastatin or lycosome-formulated statin (Lyco–Simvastatin) daily. Plasma samples were obtained after 30-day treatment and analyzed for lipids. The results demonstrated that the solubilized lycosome nanoparticles increased the intestinal absorption rate in comparison with unmodified simvastatin and were able to bind hepatocyte membranes. The lycopene-containing simvastatin formulation significantly ($p = 0.0049$) reduced LDL levels in the hypercholesterolemic patients as compared to unmodified simvastatin [60].

The mechanism of action of lycopene is enhanced hepatic uptake via a dual carotenoid/LDL receptor-mediated mechanism [60]. It was shown that lycopene crystals and/or lycopene-containing nanoparticles (lycosomes) became incorporated into chylomicrons upon absorption. The chylomicrons are then distributed by lymph and likely undergo a dual receptor-mediated uptake associated with the lycopene core. The latter is a powerful ligand for carotenoid receptors that are expressed by hepatocytes and therefore promoted intrahepatic delivery of lycosome-formulated statins [60]. Enhanced hepatic uptake of lycostatin is also possible due to a second pathway of intrahepatic uptake involving an LDL-receptor mechanism. Chylomicrons and their enzymatically degraded products, LDL and very low density lipoprotein (VLDL), contain ApoB that mediates their transport inside hepatocytes using the LDL receptor [60]. Although further research related to the pharmacology of Lyco-Simvastatin is needed, lycopene seems to a promising bioenhancer for targeted hepatic delivery of simvastatin [60].

4.16. Lysergol

Lysergol (9,10-Didehydro-6-methylergoline-8-O-methanol) is a compound present in several higher plants (e.g., *Ipomoea violacea*, *I. muricata* and *Rivea corymbosa*) and lower fungi (e.g., *Claviceps*, *Penicillium* and *Rhizopus*) [182,204]. Lysergol is traditionally used as a psychotropic, analgesic, analeptic, hypotensive and immuno-stimulant. It usually maintains normal blood flow through its vaso-activity and can promote drug absorption from the gastrointestinal tract [205]. An in vivo study by Shukla, Malik, Jaiswal, Sharma, Tanpula, Goyani and Lal [62] indicated that lysergol increased the bioavailability and decreased the clearance of curcumin significantly. This was followed by in vitro mechanistic studies using rat liver microsomes and probe substrates for P-gp and BCRP transporter proteins. The results suggested that BCRP, rather than P-gp, was inhibited by lysergol. In situ single-pass intestinal perfusion studies of the P-gp substrate, digoxin, and the BCRP substrate, sulfasalazine, were then performed in Sprague–Dawley rats following pre-treatment with 20 mg/kg lysergol. These studies supported the conclusion that P-gp was not involved in the permeation-enhancing effect of lysergol, but that BCRP was inhibited [62].

Lysergol (2–10 µg/mL) isolated from *I. muricata* seeds with methyl alcohol has been shown to act as a bioenhancer of antibiotics. The authors showed that rifampicin and tetracycline intestinal transport could be enhanced (2.96–8.53 fold) by lysergol in vitro [204]. Lysergol also increased the oral bioavailability of the quaternary protoberberine alkaloid, berberine, in male Sprague–Dawley rats. Berberine is used for numerous ailments, including bacterial infection, intestinal parasitic infection and diarrhea, but it is very poorly absorbed in the intestines and extensively metabolized. The study indicated that 20 mg/kg lysergol could increase the bioavailability of the berberine [61].

4.17. Naringin and Bergamottin

Certain phytochemicals such as naringin (a flavonoid) and bergamottin (a furanocoumarin) contained in grapefruit have been associated with the pharmacokinetic interactions observed for grapefruit juice co-administered with certain drugs [195]. When paclitaxel has been orally co-administered with naringin to Sprague–Dawley rats, the paclitaxel plasma concentrations increased statistically significantly. Since naringin affected the bioavailability of paclitaxel similar to that of quercetin, a known inhibitor of CYP3A and P-gp, it was deduced that naringin enhanced the bioavailability of paclitaxel by means of inhibition of CYP3A metabolism and P-gp efflux transporters [66]. Similarly, the pharmacokinetic parameters of diltiazem (AUC and C_{max}) were increased by 2-fold when the rats were pre-treated with naringin (administered 30 min prior to diltiazem) compared to the control group. In addition, the AUC metabolite-to-parent ratio decreased by 30% in the presence of naringin compared to the control. This confirmed the ability of naringin to inhibit metabolism of diltiazem [64].

The CYP3A4 inhibition activities of bergamottin and 6′,7′-dihydroxybergamottin were investigated in a human intestinal microsome study on two model compounds namely testosterone and midazolam. Bergamottin was identified as a substrate-dependent reversible inhibitor, but a substrate-independent mechanism-based inhibitor of CYP3A4. On the other hand, 6′,7′-dihydroxybergamottin was found to be a substrate-independent reversible and mechanism-based CYP3A4 inhibitor [206].

4.18. Palmitoyl Carnitine Chloride

Initial drug absorption enhancement studies on palmitoyl carnitine, a fatty acid ester of carnitine, showed that it is capable of intestinal drug absorption enhancement by means of tight junction opening (paracellular transport) and disruption of brush-border membrane lipids (transcellular transport) [207,208]. An in depth study on Caco-2 cell monolayers indicated that lytic effects and reduction in cell viability accompanied transport enhancement of hydrophilic macromolecules at all concentrations of palmitoyl carnitine that were investigated. It was concluded that the alteration of the tight junctional network, which was shown by TEER reduction and confocal laser scanning microscopic localization of ZO-1, occurred secondary to the interaction of palmitoyl carnitine with the membrane. Since complete recovery of TEER could not be obtained, the use of palmitoyl carnitine for drug absorption enhancement should be considered with caution [209].

4.19. Piperine

Piperine is an alkaloid contained in black pepper (*Piper nigrum*) and long pepper (*Piper longum*) [11]. Piperine can probably be considered as one of the world's first bioenhancers since its use dates as far back as the 7th century BC [205,210]. Piperine is traditionally used for its anti-inflammatory, anti-pyretic, anti-fungal, anti-diarrheal and anti-cancer effects [211]. Possible mechanisms by which piperine caused bioenhancing effects include alteration of membrane dynamics, inhibition of P-gp efflux, and inhibition of gastrointestinal and hepatic metabolism [11,83,210].

A study that investigated the effects of piperine on the serum levels of resveratrol (3,5,4'-trihydroxystilbene) when orally co-administered to C57BL mice, showed that AUC and C_{max} were increased by 229% and 1,544%, respectively [77]. Jin and Han [76] investigated the bioavailability changing effects of orally administered piperine in rats when co-administering fexofenadine either orally (10 mg/kg) or intravenously (5 mg/kg). The results suggested that there were no significant variations in the C_{max} of fexofenadine or its half-life, but the oral exposure (AUC) of fexofenadine was almost doubled. It was deduced from this study that the effects of piperine are more prominent after oral administration (likely due to the P-gp-mediated efflux inhibition and metabolism inhibition in the gastrointestinal epithelium) than after intravenous administration (due to hepatic metabolism inhibition) [76].

4.20. Quercetin

Quercetin, which is a CYP3A4 and P-gp inhibitor, has shown the ability to significantly enhance the bioavailability of orally administered tamoxifen and 4-hydroxytamoxifen in rats [95]. In that study, tamoxifen (10 mg/kg) was orally administered with or without quercetin (2.5, 7.5 and 15 mg/kg) in rats. Tamoxifen (10 mg/kg) was added to 1.5 mL distilled water for the control solution, whereas the required quercetin dose was dissolved in 1 mL distilled water to prepare quercetin suspensions for oral administration. Plasma concentrations of tamoxifen were measured in blood samples (0.5 mL) collected at 0, 0.5, 1, 2, 3, 4, 5, 6, 8, 12, 24 and 36 h after tamoxifen administration using HPLC [95].

The relative bioavailability of tamoxifen was 1.35- and 1.61-fold higher, with an absolute bioavailability of 20.2% and 24.1% with 2.5 and 7.5 mg/kg quercetin, respectively. These changes in bioavailability were significant ($p < 0.05$). Interestingly, higher concentrations of quercetin (15 mg/kg) did not induce any significant changes. No significant changes in the terminal half-life ($t_{1/2}$) and the time to reach the peak concentration (T_{max}) of tamoxifen was observed when co–administered with quercetin. When 4-hydroxytamoxifen, one of tamoxifen's metabolites, were co-administered with quercetin (7.5 mg/kg), a significant increase in the AUC of 4-hydroxytamoxifen was observed. These results suggested that MDR efflux and first-pass metabolism of tamoxifen was inhibited by quercetin [95].

Another in vivo study demonstrated an inhibitory effect on P-gp efflux of fexofenadine when it was co-administered with quercetin [91]. Twelve healthy subjects received an oral dose of quercetin

(500 mg) or placebo 3 times daily for 7 days. On the 7th day, a single dose of 60 mg fexofenadine was administered orally with 240 mL water under fasting conditions of more than 10 h. The healthy volunteers received the oral administration of fexofenadine while in the sitting position, and remained seated for 4 h [91]. Four and 10 h after dosing, subjects received standardized meals with only minor amounts of flavonoids, so as not to influence the absorption of fexofenadine or quercetin. Subsequently, blood samples were drawn immediately before, as well as 0.25, 0.5, 1, 1.5, 2, 2.5, 3, 4, 6, 8, 12, and 24 h after fexofenadine administration. Urine samples were collected during time intervals of 0–2, 2–4, 4–8, 8–12, and 12–24 h after dosing. Plasma and urinary fexofenadine concentrations were quantified using HPLC [91].

Results indicated that quercetin significantly enhanced the mean plasma concentrations of fexofenadine. The AUC of plasma fexofenadine increased by 55% from 2,005.3 to 3,098.6 ng.h/nL ($p < 0.001$) in the presence of quercetin. The C_{max} was similarly increased by 68% from 295.3 to 480.3 ng/mL ($p = 0.006$) when co-administered with quercetin. After quercetin treatment, the oral clearance of fexofenadine was significantly decreased by 37% from 61.4 to 38.7 L/h ($p < 0.001$). However, no differences in the renal clearance and half-life were observed between the groups receiving placebo versus quercetin [91].

In summary, quercetin can be used as a bioenhancer for enhanced intestinal absorption, and hence bioavailability, of tamoxifen [95] and fexofenadine [91]. The action mechanisms employed by quercetin are MDR transporter efflux inhibition, as well as first-pass metabolism inhibition [95]. If the results obtained with tamoxifen from the rats' model is confirmed in the clinical trials, the dose of tamoxifen should be adjusted for potential drug interactions when quercetin or the quercetin-containing dietary supplements are simultaneously consumed with this drug [95]. Although the inhibitory effect of quercetin on P-gp-mediated efflux of fexofenadine was demonstrated in the short-term (7 days), it is uncertain whether long-term use of quercetin will yield the same results [91].

4.21. Quinidine

A research study using everted gut sacs demonstrated that quinidine could significantly enhance the absorption of paeoniflorin (20 μM) [97]. Increased absorption of paeoniflorin was observed with an increase of incubation time, indicating that the absorption of this compound was time-dependent. In addition, the absorptive profiles with different concentrations of paeoniflorin indicated that absorption increased with increasing concentrations, but saturation of the in vitro gut sac system was observed at a concentration of ~80 μM. This saturation indicates that transport of paeoniflorin might be facilitated by an active transporter or carrier [97]. Co-administration of quinidine (1.3 mM) and paeoniflorin (20 μM) yielded a 1.5-fold increase in the absorption of paeoniflorin after 45 min of incubation. Absorption of paeoniflorin in the intestine could thus be significantly enhanced by co-administration of quinidine [97].

4.22. Resveratrol

A recent study demonstrated that resveratrol could significantly increase rat intestinal absorption of methotrexate in vivo and in vitro [99]. Furthermore, resveratrol was also able to inhibit efflux transport and decrease renal clearance of methotrexate. The bidirectional transport of methotrexate across mock-MDCK, MDR1-MDCK, and MRP2-MDCK cell monolayers were evaluated using an experimental buffer solution containing methotrexate (10 μM) and/or resveratrol (10 μM). This experimental buffer solution was added to the donor chamber, either 400 μL apical or 600 μL basolateral chamber, respectively. At time intervals of 0.5, 1, 2, and 3 h, 50 μL samples were removed from the opposite (receiver) chamber and replenished with 50 μL fresh Hanks' balanced salt solution (HBSS, pH 7.4) [99].

Additionally, the in vitro uptake of methotrexate in the absence and presence of resveratrol in kidney slices and Caco-2 cells were determined by liquid chromatography-tandem mass spectrometry (LC-MS/MS). To clarify the action mechanism of resveratrol, transporter uptake assays were similarly performed using mock-human embryonic kidney (HEK) 293 cells, human organic anion transport 1 (hOAT1)-HEK293 cells and hOAT3-HEK293 cells. The transport buffer contained 10 µM methotrexate, *p*-amino hippuric acid (PAH), Penicillin G (PCG) or resveratrol. PAH and PCG are specific substrates of OAT1 and OAT3, respectively [99].

The in vivo absorption experiment in rats entailed an oral administration of 5 mg/kg methotrexate dissolved in 2% sodium bicarbonate with or without resveratrol (100 mg/kg, dissolved in 0.5% sodium carboxymethyl cellulose) and brought up to volume with normal saline. Blood samples were collected at 5, 10, 20, 30, 60, 120, 240, 360, 480, and 600 min to determine plasma concentrations of methotrexate. In order to establish the renal excretion of methotrexate, a solution of methotrexate (5 mg/kg) and/or resveratrol (10 mg/kg) dissolved in normal saline solution of hydroxypropyl-β-cyclodextrin was intravenously administered to rats. Again, blood samples were collected at the specified times to determine the plasma concentration of methotrexate. Furthermore, urine was collected at 2, 4, 6, 8, 10, 12, 16, and 24 h after dosing to determine the concentration of methotrexate excreted through urine [99].

In vivo results indicated that a significant increase in the plasma exposure of methotrexate was observed when methotrexate was orally or intravenously co-administered. In vitro results using the rat everted gut sac model demonstrated that serosal concentrations of methotrexate increased significantly in the presence of resveratrol, as well as verapamil and/ or CDF, inhibitors of P-gp and MRP2, respectively. These results thus suggest that resveratrol can enhance methotrexate intestinal absorption by inhibiting P-gp or MRP2. Furthermore, co-administration of methotrexate and resveratrol resulted in a 37.3% decreased cumulative urinary excretion of methotrexate, indicating that resveratrol could inhibit renal excretion of methotrexate. To clarify the action mechanism of the latter, methotrexate uptake experiments were conducted using rat kidney slices. Results from this experiment showed significantly decreased uptake of methotrexate in the presence of resveratrol and probenecid, a well-known inhibitor of OATs. Furthermore, PAH and PCG (substrates of OAT1 and OAT3, respectively), as well as methotrexate uptake was significantly inhibited by resveratrol in hOAT1-HEK293 or hOAT3-HEK293 cells. These results indicated that resveratrol was able to inhibit OAT1/3, which were target transporters involved in drug-drug interactions between methotrexate and resveratrol in the kidney. The rate of basal-to-apical transepithelial methotrexate transport in MDR1-MDCK and MRP2-MDCK cells increased 32.5- and 20.8-fold, respectively, in the presence of resveratrol. These results thus indicated that P-gp and MRP2 are also target transporters of methotrexate, which is inhibited by resveratrol [99].

In vivo and in vitro results indicated that resveratrol could significantly increase the absorption of methotrexate in the intestine, and also decreased methotrexate renal clearance. Uptake, transport and renal clearance studies confirmed that the mechanisms of action of resveratrol entailed inhibition of P-gp, MRP2, OAT1 and OAT3. This corresponds with previous studies demonstrating that methotrexate is mainly eliminated rapidly by OAT1 and OAT3 in the unchanged form into urine [212,213].

A recent study demonstrated contradictory results where resveratrol stimulated P-gp efflux of saquinavir in MDR1-expressing Madin–Darby canine kidney (MDCKII-MDR1) cells [214]. In this study, MDCKII-MDR1 cells were incubated with 50 µM saquinavir and/or resveratrol (1, 10, 33, and 100 µM) or verapamil (50 µM) at 37 °C for 4 h. Verapamil, a P-gp inhibitor, served as the positive control. Additionally, an in vitro metabolism experiment in microsomes assessed the effect of resveratrol on the intestinal CYP3A-mediated metabolism of saquinavir. In order to assess the effects of resveratrol on the pharmacokinetic profiles of saquinavir, 30 mg/kg saquinavir was orally administered, with or without resveratrol (20 mg/kg), to rats. Saquinavir was suspended in solvent (20% ethanol, 30% propylene glycol, and 50% saline) at a concentration of 6 mg/mL, whereas resveratrol was suspended in saline with 30% polyethylene glycol 400 at 20 mg/mL concentration. Subsequently, blood samples were collected at 0, 0.25, 0.5, 1, 2, 4, 8, 12, and 24 h after drug administration, and analyzed with LC-MS/MS [214].

Results demonstrated significantly decreased saquinavir intracellular concentrations in the presence of resveratrol in a concentration-dependent manner, which indicated that resveratrol stimulated P-gp-mediated efflux of saquinavir. Results from the metabolism experiment demonstrated a significant increase in residual saquinavir in the presence of resveratrol in a dose-dependent manner. This suggests that resveratrol has a concentration-dependent inhibitory effect on the intestinal CYP3A-mediated metabolism of saquinavir. Oral co-administration of resveratrol (20 mg/kg) decreased the mean $AUC_{0-\infty}$ of saquinavir by ~31%, while the mean apparent systemic clearance (CL/F) was increased by ~51%. However, both these changes were not statistically significant ($p > 0.05$) [214].

4.23. Sinomenine

Previous research using everted gut sacs demonstrated that sinomenine at 16 and 136 µM concentrations could significantly enhance the absorption of paeoniflorin (20 µM) by 1.5- and 2.5-fold, respectively [97]. Similarly, the absorption of digoxin (13 µM) could significantly be enhanced by 2.5-fold in the presence of sinomenine (136 µM). Increased absorption of paeoniflorin was observed with increase of incubation time, indicating that the absorption of this compound was time-dependent. In contrast, absorptive profiles with different concentrations of paeoniflorin indicated that absorption increased with increasing concentrations, but saturation of the in vitro gut sac system was observed at a concentration of ~80 µM [97]. This saturation indicated that transport of paeoniflorin might be facilitated by an energy-dependent carrier. Enhanced bioavailability of paeoniflorin (150 mg/kg) in the presence of sinomenine (90 mg/kg) has also previously been demonstrated in vivo in rats, yielding a 12-fold increase [100].

In order to investigate the potential mechanism underlying the observed enhanced absorption of paeoniflorin, two Pg-inhibitors (verapamil or quinidine) and a P-gp substrate (digoxin) was employed. Co-administration of verapamil (20 µM) and paeoniflorin (20 µM) yielded a 2.1-fold increase in the absorption of paeniflorin after 45 min of incubation. Similarly, when quinidine (1.3 mM) was co-administered, a 1.5-fold increase in the absorption of paeoniflorin was observed. Transportation and absorption of paeoniflorin in the intestine could thus be significantly enhanced by inhibition of P-gp by verapamil and quinidine [97]. Sinomenine (136 µM) was also able to significantly enhance the absorption of 13 µM digoxin, which is a well-known P-gp substrate-like drug, by 2.5-fold after 45 min of incubation.

4.24. Sodium Caprate (Fatty Acid)

Enhancement of sodium caprate on the intestinal absorption of berberine has been studied by in situ, in vitro and in vivo experiments [101]. Results from the recirculating perfusion model demonstrated an increased absorption rate of berberine (50 µmol/L) at 4 h from 9.3% to 18.5% in the presence of sodium caprate. In comparison, 100 µmol/L and 200 µmol/L berberine with sodium caprate (0.2% *w/v*) showed increased absorption rates of 13.1% and 20.1%, respectively. The in vitro everted rat gut sac experimental results showed that small amounts of berberine is absorbed in the intestine, with the highest and lowest amounts being absorbed in the jejunum and ileum, respectively. In the presence of sodium caprate, absorption of berberine was rapidly and significantly increased after 90 min incubation. Sodium caprate also resulted in an enhanced P_{app}. The greatest absorption of berberine in the presence of sodium caprate, was in the ileum (ER = 3.49), which showed the weakest absorption in the absence of sodium caprate. The duodenum and jejunum showed enhancement ratios (ERs) of 2.08 and 1.49, respectively. In vivo studies demonstrated that the bioavailability of berberine could be improved by co-administration of sodium caprate. A significant increase in the peak plasma concentration (from 721.39 ± 53.46 to 988.84 ± 135.56 ng/mL) of berberine in rats was observed, together with delayed peak time (from 30 to 60 min) and increased $AUC_{0-6\,h}$ (28%). Compared with the berberine treatment group, berberine with sodium caprate remarkably decreased the blood glucose levels and the areas under the glucose curves, thus enhancing the antidiabetic activity of insulin [101].

It is suggested that the low bioavailability of berberine is due to P-gp efflux. It has previously been demonstrated that sodium caprate can inhibit P-gp efflux [215].

4.25. Zonula Occludens Toxin (Zot)

Research demonstrated that the permeability of high molecular weight markers and poorly bioavailable compounds can be increased across Caco-2 cell monolayers by co-administration of the absorption enhancer Zonula occludens toxin (Zot, MW: 45 kDa), a toxin produced by the *Vibrio cholerae* bacteria [107]. During this study, the transport of hydrophilic high molecular weight markers (i.e., PEG4000, FITC–dextran 10,000, and inulin) and hydrophobic therapeutic agents (i.e., acyclovir, cyclopsorin, paclitaxel, and doxorubicin) were evaluated with Zot using Caco-2 cell monolayers. It has previously been established that Zot can reversibly open tight junctions between intestinal epithelial cells by binding to a specific receptor on the luminal surface of the intestine [216]. After cell monolayers were pre-incubated with Zot (0, 1, 2, and 4 µg/mL) for 30 min, markers or therapeutic agents were added to inserts at time 0 and samples were collected over 120 min from the basolateral chamber. Radio-graphic or HPLC methods were used for transport analysis, and TEER values were monitored over a 3 h period. Results indicated that 4 µg/mL Zot significantly enhanced the transport of markers with MW < 5 kDa by 6.2-fold. Similarly, Zot significantly increased transport of therapeutic agents at a concentration of 4 µg/mL, yielding enhancement ratios of 1.8 and 3.13 for acyclovir and paclitaxel, respectively. Significantly lower TEER values were observed between 0.5 and 2 h, although this effect of Zot on TEER across Caco-2 cell monolayers was reversible.

Caco-2 transport studies with the transcellular marker propranolol indicated that Zot does not significantly modulate the transcellular pathway [107]. Furthermore, a lactate dehydrogenase (LDH) assay demonstrated no significant difference in LDH activity in the presence of Zot, thus suggesting Zot is non-cytotoxic at the effective concentration level after a 3 h incubation period [107]. The permeation of FITC was not significantly enhanced, whereas a significant increase (6.3-fold) in permeability of inulin from 7×10^{-7} cm/s (control) to 4.37×10^{-6} cm/s (4 µg/mL) was observed. It was suggested that the compact cylindrical configuration of inulin results in higher permeability of inulin vs. PEG4000, even though inulin has a higher molecular weight [107]. The in vitro results with the therapeutic agents displayed a range of permeation increase by Zot from 20–300%. The rank order of permeability enhancement observed with the therapeutic agents in the presence of Zot was paclitaxel > doxorubicin > acyclovir > cyclosporine A. Paclitaxel and cyclosporine A demonstrated P_{app} enhancement ratios of 3.13 and 1.2, respectively [107].

5. Pulmonary Route of Administration

Figure 4 illustrates the main mechanisms of action of selected bioenhancers for improved drug delivery via the pulmonary route of administration.

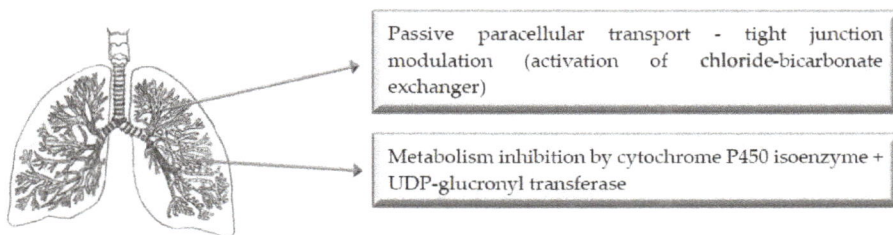

Figure 4. Illustration of the main mechanisms of action of bioenhancers for enhanced pulmonary drug delivery.

5.1. Bile Salts

A research study demonstrated that the tracheal permeability of thyrotropin-releasing hormone (TRH, MW: 362 Da) and insulin (MW: 5814 Da) was significantly increased by sodium glycocholate [113]. Non-everted sac segments of excised rabbit trachea were used. In addition to the transport study, the peptidase activities in the trachea and jejunum were measured and compared to examine the enzymatic barrier for TRH and insulin permeation across rabbit tracheal epithelium [113]. Results demonstrated that the permeability of both TRH (5 mM) and insulin (10 IU/mL) significantly increased in the presence of 10 mM glycocholate. The P_{app} values for TRH (5 and 10 mM) were $2.51 \pm 0.31 \times 10^{-7}$ and $3.54 \pm 0.87 \times 10^{-7}$ cm/s, respectively. Sodium glycocholate (10 mM) increased the tracheal permeability of TRH ~3-fold [113]. The P_{app} value for insulin (10 IU/mL) was $6.66 \pm 0.11 \times 10^{-9}$ cm/s. However, the half-life of insulin was about 14 h, and only showed slight degradation by luminal secreted enzymes for the duration (150 min) of the experiment. The tracheal and jejunal peptidases showed the following decreasing order of activity: DPP IV > Leu-aminopeptidase > cathepsin-B > trypsin [113]. These four peptidases had significantly lower activities in the tracheal epithelial cells compared to jejunal epithelial cells. Since TRH had no metabolites during tracheal permeation, a potential action mechanism of tight junction modulation and therefore enhanced paracellular permeability is suggested for sodium glycocholate [113]. Glycocholate is known to be a Leu-aminopeptidase inhibitor. However, insulin was slightly degraded during tracheal permeation. It is therefore suggested that insulin (MW: 5814 Da) is mainly transported via paracellular diffusion with slight metabolism by proteolytic enzymes such as trypsin-like and aminopeptidase-like enzymes through isolated rabbit tracheal epithelium [113].

Similarly, previous in vitro and in vivo research indicated that absorption of inhaled insulin could be enhanced by the bile salt sodium taurocholate [114]. For the in vivo study, beagle dogs were starved for at least 16 h, after which they were intubated and exposed to insulin or insulin-sodium taurocholate aerosols for differing times. As an intravenous reference, insulin in 0.9% NaCl was infused for 5 min (0.2 U/kg, 0.5 U/mL, 0.08 mL/kg per min) in the right foreleg vein. The insulin–sodium taurocholate solutions were aerosolized by a PARI LC jet nebulizer. The flow from the nebulizer was 3.2 L/min (1 Bar) and the target inhaled dose of insulin was 1 U/kg. Blood samples were collected before dosing and at 5, 10, 15, 25, 35, 50, 65, 95, 125 and 245 min after start ($t = 0$) of inhalation [114]. The bioavailability of pure insulin was $2.6 \pm 3\%$, while the bioavailability of nebulized insulin solutions increased to $23.2 \pm 4.4\%$ with addition of 32 mM sodium taurocholate. In comparison, a $3.81 \pm 1.12\%$ bioavailability of insulin was obtained when aerosolized powder was administered to the lungs. In vitro results indicated increased insulin transport, accompanied by reduced TEER, at sodium taurocholate concentrations between 25 and 30 mM. Unfortunately, the viability of cell layers was approximately zero at sodium taurocholate concentrations exceeding 32 mM [114].

5.2. Chitosan and Derivatives

The enhancement of bronchial octreotide absorption by chitosan and N-trimethyl chitosan (TMC) was evaluated with an integral in vitro/in vivo correlation approach [109]. The TMC derivatives with 20% and 60% QD (TMC20 and TMC60) were synthesized by alkaline methylation of chitosan. Chitosan was dissolved at 1.5% (*w/v*) in HBSS, buffered with 30 mM HEPES at pH 5.5. TMC20 and TMC60 were dissolved at 1.5% (*w/v*) in HBSS/HEPES at pH 7.4. Two hours prior to the TEER studies, the culture medium was removed and Calu-3 cells were equilibrated in 1 ml HBSS/HEPES at pH 7.4 in the basolateral chamber and 200 µL HBSS/HEPES, at pH 5.5 or pH 7.4, in the apical compartment. At $t = 0$, the apical medium was replaced by 200 µL chitosan, TMC20 or TMC60 formulations or by 200 µL HBSS/HEPES at pH 5.5 or pH 7.4 that served as controls. The TEER was measured at $t = 120$ and 60 before administration and $t = 0, 30, 60, 90, 120, 150, 210$ and 240 min after administration.

Octreotide was dissolved to an end concentration of 0.97 mM in 0.9% saline containing 1.5% chitosan (pH 5.5), TMC20 (pH 7.4) or TMC60 (pH 7.4). Control solutions contained octreotide in 0.9% saline of pH 5.5 and 7.4. From these solutions, 200 µL were instilled into the trachea of rats.

Intratracheal instillation was employed to ensure dose deposition in bronchial region of rats. Blood samples of 200 µL were collected initially, and every 30 min thereafter for 4 h. A group of 6 rats received a 200 µL intravenous bolus containing 190 µM octreotide in 0.9% saline in order to determine the absolute bioavailability of octreotide [109].

A significant, but reversible, reduction in TEER was observed in the presence of chitosan, TMC20 and TMC60, accompanied by 21-, 16- and 30-fold enhanced octreotide permeation, respectively. The bioavailability was enhanced by 2.4-, 2.5- and 3.9-fold, respectively. TMC60 induced a strong decrease in TEER, which suggested that pH, solubility and cationic charge density are important factors for paracellular barrier modulation [109]. A linear in vitro/in vivo correlation was observed between calculated absorption rates (R^2 = 0.93), which suggested that an analogous mechanism causes permeation enhancement by the polymers, both in vitro and in vivo. The permeation studies showed zero order kinetic profiles, suggesting that the polymers altered the structural integrity of tight junctions to facilitate passive paracellular diffusion of octreotide [109].

5.3. Citric Acid (Chelating Agent)

The effect of additives on the pulmonary absorption of insulin from solutions and dry powders was examined in male Sprague–Dawley rats [110]. Results from this study demonstrated a slight hypoglycemic effect in the absence of citric acid [110]. In the presence of citric acid, a significant and extended dose-dependent hypoglycemic effect was observed after insulin administration. Bioavailabilities of 43% and 57% were obtained with the citrate buffer solutions (0.19 mg/dose of citric acid in 0.1 mL) at pH 5 and 3, respectively. However, a greater hypoglycemic effect was achieved with citrate in dry powder than in solution. For the 0.2% (0.036 mg/dose) citric acid formulation, the blood glucose level rapidly decreased after insulin dry powder administration and the effect continued for the duration of the experiment [110]. An absolute bioavailability greater than 50% was achieved. LDH activity, which is a sensitive indicator of acute toxicity to lung cells, was as low for 0.2% citric acid as it was for PBS administration. This suggested that citric acid is a safe absorption enhancing additive. Possible action mechanisms proposed for citric acid included altered epithelium membrane integrity of the lungs, decreased insulin degradation by suppressing enzyme activity and phagocytic activity of alveolar macrophages [110].

5.4. Cyclodextrins (CDs)

An in vitro permeability study of chemically modified cyclodextrins (CDs), namely hydroxypropyl-β-cyclodextrin (HPβCD), hydroxypropyl-γ-cyclodextrin (HPγCD), randomly methylated β-cyclodextrin (Rameb), and 2-0-methyl-β-cyclodextrin (Crysmeb), was conducted using Calu-3 cells [111]. Results from this study showed a concentration-dependent increase in ^{14}C-mannitol flux across Calu-3 layers in the presence of each of the βCD derivatives, while no change in permeability was caused by HPγCD. Rameb was the only CD that enhanced mannitol transport at the lowest concentration (10 mM), whilst increasing mannitol flux 10-fold at the highest concentration (50 mM). Crysmeb and HPβCD were able to increase mannitol permeability at 25 and 50 mM. A reduction in TEER was observed for all increases in mannitol transport across the Calu-3 cell layers. Confocal microscopy revealed that Crysmeb (25 mM) was able to reversibly disrupt the tight junctional complexes [111].

Similarly, a previous study demonstrated that tetradecyl-β-maltoside (TDM) and dimethyl-β-cyclodextrin (DMβCD) could enhance the pulmonary absorption of low molecular weight heparin (LMWH) both in vitro and in vivo, mainly by acting on the membrane rather than interacting with the drug [115]. Calu-3 cells were used to conduct transport studies with ^{3}H-enoxaparin and ^{14}C-mannitol with or without different concentrations (0.0625%, 0.125%, and 0.25% (*w/v*)) of TDM or DMβCD at pH 7.4. TEER was measured during the transport experiments. For the in vivo pulmonary absorption studies, TDM and DMβCD were dissolved in saline to prepare 1% stock solutions of each. Enoxaparin, dalteparin (MW: 5000 Da), and unfractionated heparin (MW: 15,000–20,000 Da) were respectively mixed with either saline or TDM and DMβCD (0.0625%, 0.125%, and 0.25% (w/v)) to yield a final concentration of 15 U of anti-factor Xa activity per 100 μL formulation. These formulations (50 U/kg) were intratracheally or subcutaneously administered to rats for the absorption and bioavailability studies, respectively. Subsequently, blood samples (300 μL) were collected at 0, 15, 30, 60, 120, 240, 360, and 480 min. Enoxaparin absorption was determined by measuring plasma anti-factor Xa levels using a colorimetric assay, followed by standard pharmacokinetic analysis [115].

Results demonstrated a dose-dependent increase in enoxaparin in the presence of TDM or DMCD (0.0625–0.25%) in the apical fluid. With an increase in TDM concentration from 0.0625% to 0.25%, a statistically significant 4-fold increase in the P_{app} of enoxaparin was observed. Similar results were obtained with the transport of mannitol. Increase in the overall permeability of mannitol in the presence of TDM or DMβCD suggest that the action mechanism is loosening of tight junctions and therefore enhanced paracellular transport. This was confirmed with TEER values that were decreased to 51.9% and 70.7% of the initial value in the presence of 0.25% TDM and 0.25% DMβCD, respectively, after 2 h. However, the effect on TEER reduction was reversible, indicating that these bioenhancers are not likely to cause extensive damage or cellular toxicity in respiratory epithelial cells. Increased concentrations of TDM and DMβCD resulted in increased C_{max} and decreased T_{max} for enoxaparin. Altogether, results from the pharmacokinetic analysis suggested that TDM enhanced pulmonary absorption of enoxaparin. Bioavailability data showed that TDM was more efficacious in enhancing pulmonary absorption of LMWH when compared to DMβCD. Interestingly, pharmacokinetic profiles of pulmonary administered enoxaparin showed a quicker onset of anti-factor Xa activity compared to subcutaneous enoxaparin. Dalteparin also increased the anti-factor Xa levels rapidly and substantially in the presence of 0.125% TDM or DMβCD, whereas unfractionated heparin only produced a modest increase in anti-factor Xa activity. Reduced absorption of unfractionated heparin was observed, which could be due to the fact that it is larger and bulkier than LMWHs (enoxaparin and dalteparin). Results from this study are in agreement with previous studies on the nasal delivery of LMWHs [217]. Furthermore, comparative analysis demonstrated that the relative bioavailability of enoxaparin was 4- to 6-fold higher with pulmonary administration compared to nasally administered enoxaparin, and the amounts of bioenhancers required to produce therapeutic anti-factor Xa activity from pulmonary administered LMWHs were 2-5 times less [115].

5.5. Lanthanides

The absorption of insulin pre-administered or co-administered with lanthanides (Ln^{3+}), namely lanthanum, cerium and gadolinium, from rat lung was investigated by means of an in situ pulmonary absorption experiment [112]. Lanthanide ion solutions were prepared by dissolving the oxide in 5 mol/L HCl solution, followed by heating to deplete excess acid. Residue was then diluted with saline water and Ln^{3+} concentrations were determined. For pre-administered intratracheal drug delivery, Ln^{3+} (0.2 mg/kg) in 25 μL saline water (pH 7) was first injected, followed by insulin (1 IU/kg in 40 μL saline water, pH 7) administration 30 min later. In the other experiments, insulin and Ln^{3+} were co-administered. Blood samples (0.5 mL) were collected at predetermined time intervals after insulin administration, and serum insulin levels were measured [112].

Results demonstrated that serum insulin levels increased significantly in the presence of $CeCl_3$ and $GdCl_3$, with relative bioavailabilities of 57.9% and 59.5%, respectively. Furthermore, the anionic form of gadolinium showed greater enhancement of pulmonary insulin absorption than its cationic form (Gd^{3+}). The relative bioavailabilities of co-administered and pre-administered $GdCl_3$ were 80.1% and 59.5%, respectively. In comparison, $LaCl_3$ showed weak enhancement in pulmonary absorption of insulin, with a relative bioavailability of 30.9%, while $LuCl_3$ had no enhancing effect [112]. Co-administration of Gd^{3+} (0.2 mg/kg) with insulin (Fr = 80.1%) showed the greatest insulin absorption enhancement from the lung. Interestingly, higher concentrations of Gd^{3+} (0.6 mg/kg) showed decreased insulin absorption, possibly due to partial hydrolysis of Gd^{3+} upon entrance of the lung. The action mechanism proposed for Ln^{3+} is local mucosal tissue modulation, whereby lanthanides bind to membrane lipids and proteins to induce conformational changes and micropore formation to enhance the permeability of intracellular and exogenous matter flux [218,219]. Another action mechanism is the favorable absorption of insulin from the lung when a conformational change of insulin is induced when Ln^{3+} binds to zinc(II) binding sites. Additionally, increased interaction of insulin with its receptor in the cell membrane might be increased with insulin-bound Ln^{3+} in the serum [112].

5.6. Protease Inhibitors

The effects of protease inhibitors were evaluated as absorption enhancers for the pulmonary absorption of recombinant human colony-stimulating factor (rhG-CSF) in rats [108]. Protease inhibitors included (*p*-amidinophenyl) methanesulfonyl fluoride-HCl (*p*-APMSF), aprotinin and bestatin. The respective protease inhibitors (10 mM *p*-APMSF, 500 IU/mL aprotinin, 1 mM bestatin) were added to rhG-CSF solution (pH 6.5), after which the final rhG-CSF concentration was adjusted to 250 µg/mL. After intravenous, subcutaneous and intratracheal administration of the test solutions (containing protease inhibitors) and the control solution (rhG-CSF only), blood samples were collected periodically for 8h to determine the rhG-CSF plasma concentration by enzyme immunoassay.

The plasma rhG-CSF concentration was greatly enhanced in the presence of protease inhibitors, with *p*-APMSF showing the greatest enhancement with a ~3-fold increase in plasma rhG-CSF concentration from 3.9 to 11.7 ng/mL 30 min after intratracheal administration [108]. In order to determine the mechanism of enhanced absorption, a surfactant, polyoxyethylene 9-lauryl ether (Laureth-9) and the protease inhibitor *p*-APMSF were administered with rhG-CSF. The rhG-CSF concentration increased ~123-fold from 3.9 ± 1.4 ng/mL to 481.5 ± 96.7 ng/mL with the simultaneous intratracheal administration of Laureth-9 and *p*-APMSF. As a result, the proposed mechanism of action entails enhanced membrane permeation and inhibition of enzymatic degradation of rhG-CSF [108].

Similarly, a previous study demonstrated that the tracheal permeability of insulin was significantly increased by bestatin (aminopeptidase B and leucine aminopeptidase inhibitor), and aprotinin (trypsin and chymotrypsin inhibitor) [113]. Non-everted sac (2 cm) segments of excised rabbit trachea were used. Briefly, test solutions, with or without protease inhibitors (0.1 and 1 mM bestatin; 1000 and 10,000 KIU/mL aprotinin), in HEPES-buffered solution (0.2 mL, pH 7.4) was infused into the sac mucosal side, which was then placed in serosal medium consisting of oxygenated (O_2/CO_2, 95%:5%) HEPES (7 mL, pH 7.4). Samples (0.2 mL) were removed from the serosal fluid at pre-determined times for 150 min, and replaced with 0.2 mL fresh fluid. In another experiment, 10 µL samples were removed from the mucosal fluid at pre-determined times to calculate the degradation rate of insulin in the mucosal fluid of the trachea using the RIA method. Additionally, the peptidase activities in the trachea and jejunum were measured and compared to examine the enzymatic barrier for TRH and insulin permeation across rabbit tracheal epithelium [113].

Results demonstrated that the permeability of insulin (10 IU/mL) significantly increased in the presence of 1 mM bestatin and 10,000 KIU/mL aprotinin. However, the half-life of insulin was about 14 h, and only showed slight degradation by luminal secreted enzymes for the duration (150 min) of the experiment [113]. The tracheal and jejunal peptidases showed the following decreasing order of activity: DPP IV > Leu-aminopeptidase > cathepsin-B > trypsin. These four peptidases had significantly lower activities in the tracheal epithelial cells compared to jejunal epithelial cells. However, insulin was slightly degraded during tracheal permeation. It is suggested that insulin (MW: 5814 Da) is mainly transported via paracellular diffusion with slight metabolism by proteolytic enzymes such as trypsin-like and aminopeptidase-like enzymes through isolated rabbit tracheal epithelium. In summary, pulmonary administration of some peptide drugs, such as insulin, by intratracheal insufflation and instillation may contribute to the systemic absorption of these drugs [113].

5.7. Surfactants

The effects of surfactants of natural origin were evaluated as absorption enhancers for the pulmonary absorption of recombinant human colony-stimulating factor (rhG-CSF) in rats [108].

Surfactants included polyoxyethylene 9-lauryl ether (Laureth-9) and sodium glycocholate (SGC). Surfactants (1% *w/v*) were respectively added to rhG-CSF solution (pH 6.5), after which the final rhG-CSF concentration was adjusted to 250 µg/mL. After intravenous and intratracheal administration of the test solutions (containing surfactants) and the control solution (rhG-CSF only), blood samples were collected periodically for 8 h to determine the rhG-CSF plasma concentration by enzyme immunoassay.

The plasma rhG-CSF concentration was greatly enhanced in the presence of the surfactants. Relative bioavailabilities of rhG-CSF achieved with intravenous and intratracheal administration of Laureth-9 and SGC were 37% (intravenous), 88% (intratracheal), 84% (intravenous), and 197% (intratracheal), respectively [108]. In order to determine the mechanism of enhanced absorption, both the surfactant Laureth-9 and a protease inhibitor (*p*-amidinophenyl) methanesulfonyl fluoride-HCl (*p*-APMSF) were administered with rhG-CSF. The rhG-CSF concentration increased ~123-fold from 3.9 ± 1.4 ng/mL to 481.5 ± 96.7 ng/mL with the simultaneous intratracheal administration of Laureth-9 and *p*-APMSF. As a result, the proposed mechanism of action entails enhanced membrane permeation and inhibition of enzymatic degradation of rhG-CSF [108].

6. Conclusions

A comprehensive list of bioenhancers of natural origin is given in Table 1 with their mechanisms of action for four specific routes of drug administration, namely nasal, buccal, pulmonary, and oral. From all the described bioenhancing studies it is evident that inhibition of pre-systemic metabolism as well as efflux transporters and tight junction modulation is the predominant mechanism of drug bioavailability enhancement for the oral route of drug administration. Tight junction modulation and membrane disruption are the pre-dominant mechanisms of drug absorption enhancement for the nasal, buccal and pulmonary routes of administration. Since various factors can influence dissolution and absorption of drugs across different mucosal surfaces, studies on bioenhancers should be conducted for each specific drug for which bioavailability enhancement is needed. Although many studies have shown the potential of absorption enhancing agents, very few have been included in commercially available drugs.

Author Contributions: Conceptualization, J.H.H.; writing-original draft preparation, B.P., M.W., C.G., J.D.S., J.H.S. and J.H.H.; writing-review and editing, B.P. and J.H.H.; supervision, J.H.S., J.D.S. and J.H.H.

Funding: This research received no external funding.

Acknowledgments: The authors would like to thank Marioné van der Merwe for drawing the anatomical figures.

Conflicts of Interest: The authors declare no conflict of interest.

References

1. Navia, M.A.; Chaturvedi, P.R. Design principles for orally bioavailable drugs. *Drug Discov. Today* **1996**, *1*, 179–189. [CrossRef]
2. Chillistone, S.; Hardman, J. Factors affecting drug absorption and distribution. *Anaesth. Intensive Care Med.* **2008**, *9*, 167–171. [CrossRef]
3. Klein, I.; Sarkadi, B.; Váradi, A. An inventory of the human abc proteins. *Biochim. Biophys. Acta* **1999**, *1461*, 237–262. [CrossRef]
4. Higgins, C.F.; Gottesman, M.M. Is the multidrug transporter a flippase? *Trends Biochem. Sci.* **1992**, *17*, 18–21. [CrossRef]
5. Sikic, B.I. Modulation of multidrug resistance: A paradigm for translational clinical research. *Oncology* **1999**, *13*, 183–187. [PubMed]
6. Juliano, R.L.; Ling, V. A surface glycoprotein modulating drug permeability in chinese hamster ovary cell mutants. *Biochim. Biophys. Acta* **1976**, *455*, 152–162. [CrossRef]

7. Maliepaard, M.; Scheffer, G.L.; Faneyte, I.F.; van Gastelen, M.A.; Pijnenborg, A.C.; Schinkel, A.H.; van de Vijver, M.J.; Scheper, R.J.; Schellens, J.H. Subcellular localization and distribution of the breast cancer resistance protein transporter in normal human tissues. *Cancer Res.* **2001**, *61*, 3458–3464.

8. Lazzari, P.; Serra, V.; Marcello, S.; Pira, M.; Mastinu, A. Metabolic side effects induced by olanzapine treatment are neutralized by cb1 receptor antagonist compounds co-administration in female rats. *Eur. Neuropsychopharmacol.* **2017**, *27*, 667–678. [CrossRef]

9. Dresser, G.K.; Spence, J.D.; Bailey, D.G. Pharmacokinetic-pharmacodynamic consequences and clinical relevance of cytochrome p450 3a4 inhibition. *Clin. Pharmacokinet.* **2000**, *38*, 41–57. [CrossRef]

10. Schinkel, A.H.; Jonker, J.W. Mammalian drug efflux transporters of the atp binding cassette (abc) family: An overview. *Adv. Drug Deliv. Rev.* **2012**, *64*, 138–153. [CrossRef]

11. Khajuria, A.; Thusu, N.; Zutshi, U. Piperine modulates permeability characteristics of intestine by inducing alterations in membrane dynamics: Influence on brush border membrane fluidity, ultrastructure and enzyme kinetics. *Phytomedicine* **2002**, *9*, 224–231. [CrossRef] [PubMed]

12. Kumar-Sarangi, M.; Chandra-Joshi, B.; Ritchie, B. Natural bioenhancers in drug delivery: An overview. *Puerto Rico Health Sci. J.* **2018**, *37*, 12–18.

13. Bitter, C.; Suter-Zimmermann, K.; Surber, C. Nasal drug delivery in humans. *Curr. Probl. Dermatol.* **2011**, *40*, 20–35. [PubMed]

14. Liu, Z.; Wang, S.; Hu, M. Oral absorption basics: Pathways, physico-chemical and biological factors affecting absorption. In *Developing Solid Oral Dosage Forms*; Elsevier: Amsterdam, The Netherlands, 2009; pp. 263–288.

15. Crowley, P.; Martini, L. Optimising drug delivery: The challenges and opportunities. *Ondrugdelivery* **2015**, *2015*, 4–11.

16. Mastinu, A.; Premoli, M.; Maccarinelli, G.; Grilli, M.; Memo, M.; Bonini, S.A. Melanocortin 4 receptor stimulation improves social deficits in mice through oxytocin pathway. *Neuropharmacology* **2018**, *133*, 366–374. [CrossRef] [PubMed]

17. Sarkar, M.A. Drug metabolism in the nasal mucosa. *Pharm. Res.* **1992**, *9*, 1–9. [CrossRef] [PubMed]

18. Johnson, P.H.; Quay, S.C. Advances in nasal drug delivery through tight junction technology. *Expert Opin. Drug Deliv.* **2005**, *2*, 281–298. [CrossRef]

19. Bonini, S.A.; Premoli, M.; Tambaro, S.; Kumar, A.; Maccarinelli, G.; Memo, M.; Mastinu, A. Cannabis sativa: A comprehensive ethnopharmacological review of a medicinal plant with a long history. *J. Ethnopharmacol.* **2018**, *227*, 300–315. [CrossRef]

20. Ojewole, E.; Mackraj, I.; Akhundov, K.; Hamman, J.; Viljoen, A.; Olivier, E.; Wesley-Smith, J.; Govender, T. Investigating the effect of aloe vera gel on the buccal permeability of didanosine. *Planta Med.* **2012**, *78*, 354–361. [CrossRef]

21. Portero, A.; Remuñán-López, C.; Nielsen, H.M. The potential of chitosan in enhancing peptide and protein absorption across the tr146 cell culture model—An in vitro model of the buccal epithelium. *Pharm. Res.* **2002**, *19*, 169–174. [CrossRef]

22. Şenel, S.; Kremer, M.; Kaş, S.; Wertz, P.; Hıncal, A.; Squier, C. Enhancing effect of chitosan on peptide drug delivery across buccal mucosa. *Biomaterials* **2000**, *21*, 2067–2071. [CrossRef]

23. Langoth, N.; Kahlbacher, H.; Schöffmann, G.; Schmerold, I.; Schuh, M.; Franz, S.; Kurka, P.; Bernkop-Schnürch, A. Thiolated chitosans: Design and in vivo evaluation of a mucoadhesive buccal peptide drug delivery system. *Pharm. Res.* **2006**, *23*, 573–579. [CrossRef] [PubMed]

24. Langoth, N.; Bernkop-Schnürch, A.; Kurka, P. In vitro evaluation of various buccal permeation enhancing systems for pacap (pituitary adenylate cyclase-activating polypeptide). *Pharm. Res.* **2005**, *22*, 2045. [CrossRef] [PubMed]

25. Tsutsumi, K.; Obata, Y.; Takayama, K.; Loftsson, T.; Nagai, T. Effect of cod-liver oil extract on the buccal permeation of ergotamine tartrate. *Drug Dev. Ind. Pharm.* **1998**, *24*, 757–762. [CrossRef] [PubMed]

26. Shojaei, A.H.; Khan, M.; Lim, G.; Khosravan, R. Transbuccal permeation of a nucleoside analog, dideoxycytidine: Effects of menthol as a permeation enhancer. *Int. J. Pharm.* **1999**, *192*, 139–146. [CrossRef]

27. Morishita, M.; Barichello, J.M.; Takayama, K.; Chiba, Y.; Tokiwa, S.; Nagai, T. Pluronic® f-127 gels incorporating highly purified unsaturated fatty acids for buccal delivery of insulin. *Int. J. Pharm.* **2001**, *212*, 289–293. [CrossRef]

28. Xiang, J.; Fang, X.; Li, X. Transbuccal delivery of 2′, 3′-dideoxycytidine: In vitro permeation study and histological investigation. *Int. J. Pharm.* **2002**, *231*, 57–66. [CrossRef]

29. Sandri, G.; Rossi, S.; Bonferoni, M.C.; Ferrari, F.; Zambito, Y.; Di Colo, G.; Caramella, C. Buccal penetration enhancement properties of n-trimethyl chitosan: Influence of quaternization degree on absorption of a high molecular weight molecule. *Int. J. Pharm.* **2005**, *297*, 146–155. [CrossRef] [PubMed]

30. Hinchcliffe, M.; Jabbal-Gill, I.; Smith, A. Effect of chitosan on the intranasal absorption of salmon calcitonin in sheep. *J. Pharm. Pharmacol.* **2005**, *57*, 681–687. [CrossRef]

31. Illum, L.; Watts, P.; Fisher, A.; Hinchcliffe, M.; Norbury, H.; Jabbal-Gill, I.; Nankervis, R.; Davis, S. Intranasal delivery of morphine. *J. Pharmacol. Exp. Ther.* **2002**, *301*, 391–400. [CrossRef] [PubMed]

32. Krauland, A.H.; Guggi, D.; Bernkop-Schnürch, A. Thiolated chitosan microparticles: A vehicle for nasal peptide drug delivery. *Int. J. Pharm.* **2006**, *307*, 270–277. [CrossRef] [PubMed]

33. Hamman, J.; Stander, M.; Kotze, A. Effect of the degree of quaternisation of *N*-trimethyl chitosan chloride on absorption enhancement: In vivo evaluation in rat nasal epithelia. *Int. J. Pharm.* **2002**, *232*, 235–242. [CrossRef]

34. Mizuma, T.; Awazu, S. Dietary polyphenols (−)-epicatechin and chrysin inhibit intestinal glucuronidation metabolism to increase drug absorption. *J. Pharm. Sci.* **2004**, *93*, 2407–2410. [CrossRef] [PubMed]

35. Beneke, C.; Viljoen, A.; Hamman, J.H. In vitro drug absorption enhancement effects of aloe vera and aloe ferox. *Sci Pharm.* **2012**, *80*, 475–486. [CrossRef] [PubMed]

36. Chen, W.; Lu, Z.; Viljoen, A.; Hamman, J. Intestinal drug transport enhancement by aloe vera. *Planta Med.* **2009**, *75*, 587–595. [CrossRef] [PubMed]

37. Vinson, J.A.; Al Kharrat, H.; Andreoli, L. Effect of aloe vera preparations on the human bioavailability of vitamins c and e. *Phytomedicine* **2005**, *12*, 760–765. [CrossRef] [PubMed]

38. Wallis, L.; Malan, M.; Gouws, C.; Steyn, D.; Ellis, S.; Abay, E.; Wiesner, L.; P Otto, D.; Hamman, J. Evaluation of isolated fractions of aloe vera gel materials on indinavir pharmacokinetics: In vitro and in vivo studies. *Curr. Drug Deliv.* **2016**, *13*, 471–480. [CrossRef]

39. Yago, M.R.; Frymoyer, A.; Benet, L.Z.; Smelick, G.S.; Frassetto, L.A.; Ding, X.; Dean, B.; Salphati, L.; Budha, N.; Jin, J.Y. The use of betaine hcl to enhance dasatinib absorption in healthy volunteers with rabeprazole-induced hypochlorhydria. *AAPS J.* **2014**, *16*, 1358–1365. [CrossRef]

40. Choudhary, N.; Khajuria, V.; Gillani, Z.H.; Tandon, V.R.; Arora, E. Effect of carum carvi, a herbal bioenhancer on pharmacokinetics of antitubercular drugs: A study in healthy human volunteers. *Perspect. Clin. Res.* **2014**, *5*, 80.

41. Rosenthal, R.; Günzel, D.; Finger, C.; Krug, S.M.; Richter, J.F.; Schulzke, J.-D.; Fromm, M.; Amasheh, S. The effect of chitosan on transcellular and paracellular mechanisms in the intestinal epithelial barrier. *Biomaterials* **2012**, *33*, 2791–2800. [CrossRef]

42. Schipper, N.G.; Olsson, S.; Hoogstraate, J.A.; Vårum, K.M.; Artursson, P. Chitosans as absorption enhancers for poorly absorbable drugs 2: Mechanism of absorption enhancement. *Pharm. Res.* **1997**, *14*, 923–929. [CrossRef] [PubMed]

43. Bernkop-Schnürch, A.; Guggi, D.; Pinter, Y. Thiolated chitosans: Development and in vitro evaluation of a mucoadhesive, permeation enhancing oral drug delivery system. *J. Control. Release* **2004**, *94*, 177–186. [CrossRef] [PubMed]

44. Krauland, A.H.; Guggi, D.; Bernkop-Schnürch, A. Oral insulin delivery: The potential of thiolated chitosan-insulin tablets on non-diabetic rats. *J. Control. Release* **2004**, *95*, 547–555. [CrossRef] [PubMed]

45. Basu, N.K.; Kole, L.; Kubota, S.; Owens, I.S. Human udp-glucuronosyltransferases show atypical metabolism of mycophenolic acid and inhibition by curcumin. *Drug Metab. Dispos.* **2004**, *32*, 768–773. [CrossRef] [PubMed]

46. Pavithra, B.; Prakash, N.; Jayakumar, K. Modification of pharmacokinetics of norfloxacin following oral administration of curcumin in rabbits. *J. Vet. Sci.* **2009**, *10*, 293–297. [CrossRef] [PubMed]

47. Zhang, W.; Lim, L.-Y. Effects of spice constituents on p-gp-mediated transport and cyp3a4-mediated metabolism in vitro. *Drug Metab. Dispos.* **2008**, *36*, 1283–1290. [CrossRef] [PubMed]

48. Zhang, W.; Tan, T.M.C.; Lim, L.-Y. Impact of curcumin-induced changes in p-glycoprotein and cyp3a expression on the pharmacokinetics of peroral celiprolol and midazolam in rats. *Drug Metab. Dispos.* **2007**, *35*, 110–115. [CrossRef]

49. Lee, J.H.; Shin, Y.-J.; Oh, J.-H.; Lee, Y.-J. Pharmacokinetic interactions of clopidogrel with quercetin, telmisartan, and cyclosporine a in rats and dogs. *Arch. Pharm. Res.* **2012**, *35*, 1831–1837. [CrossRef]

50. Yoo, H.H.; Lee, M.; Chung, H.J.; Lee, S.K.; Kim, D.-H. Effects of diosmin, a flavonoid glycoside in citrus fruits, on p-glycoprotein-mediated drug efflux in human intestinal caco-2 cells. *J. Agric. Food Chem.* **2007**, *55*, 7620–7625. [CrossRef]

51. Li, X.; Hu, J.; Wang, B.; Sheng, L.; Liu, Z.; Yang, S.; Li, Y. Inhibitory effects of herbal constituents on p-glycoprotein in vitro and in vivo: Herb–drug interactions mediated via p-gp. *Toxicol. Appl. Pharmacol.* **2014**, *275*, 163–175. [CrossRef]

52. Ghosal, S. Delivery System for Pharmaceutical, Nutritional and Cosmetic Ingredients. U.S. Patent 6,558,712, 6 May 2003.

53. Wacher, V.J.; Benet, L.Z. Use of Gallic Acid Esters to Increase Bioavailability of Orally Administered Pharmaceutical Compounds. U.S. Patent 5,962,522, 5 October 1999.

54. Lambert, J.D.; Kwon, S.-J.; Ju, J.; Bose, M.; Lee, M.-J.; Hong, J.; Hao, X.; Yang, C.S. Effect of genistein on the bioavailability and intestinal cancer chemopreventive activity of (−)-epigallocatechin-3-gallate. *Carcinogenesis* **2008**, *29*, 2019–2024. [CrossRef] [PubMed]

55. Li, X.; Choi, J.-S. Effect of genistein on the pharmacokinetics of paclitaxel administered orally or intravenously in rats. *Int. J. Pharm.* **2007**, *337*, 188–193. [CrossRef] [PubMed]

56. Ayyanna, C.; Mohan Rao, G.; Sasikala, M.; Somasekhar, P.; Arun Kumar, N.; Pradeep Kumar, M. Absorption enhancement studies of metformin hydrochloride by using tribulus terrestris plant extract. *Int. J. Pharm. Technol.* **2012**, *4*, 4119–4125.

57. Kumar, A.; Bansal, M. Formulation and evaluation of antidiabetic tablets: Effect of absorption enhancser. *World J. Pharm. Res.* **2014**, *3*, 1426–1445.

58. Dresser, G.; Bailey, D. The effects of fruit juices on drug disposition: A new model for drug interactions. *Eur. J. Clin. Investig.* **2003**, *33*, 10–16. [CrossRef]

59. Rekha, M.; Sharma, C.P. Synthesis and evaluation of lauryl succinyl chitosan particles towards oral insulin delivery and absorption. *J. Control. Release* **2009**, *135*, 144–151. [CrossRef]

60. Petyaev, I.M. Improvement of hepatic bioavailability as a new step for the future of statin. *Arch. Med Sci.* **2015**, *11*, 406. [CrossRef]

61. Patil, S.; Dash, R.P.; Anandjiwala, S.; Nivsarkar, M. Simultaneous quantification of berberine and lysergol by hplc-uv: Evidence that lysergol enhances the oral bioavailability of berberine in rats. *Biomed. Chromatogr.* **2012**, *26*, 1170–1175. [CrossRef]

62. Shukla, M.; Malik, M.; Jaiswal, S.; Sharma, A.; Tanpula, D.; Goyani, R.; Lal, J. A mechanistic investigation of the bioavailability enhancing potential of lysergol, a novel bioenhancer, using curcumin. *RSC Adv.* **2016**, *6*, 58933–58942. [CrossRef]

63. Pal, A.; Bawankule, D.U.; Darokar, M.P.; Gupta, S.C.; Arya, J.S.; Shanker, K.; Gupta, M.M.; Yadav, N.P.; Singh Khanuja, S.P. Influence of moringa oleifera on pharmacokinetic disposition of rifampicin using hplc-pda method: A pre-clinical study. *Biomed. Chromatogr.* **2011**, *25*, 641–645. [CrossRef]

64. Choi, J.-S.; Han, H.-K. Enhanced oral exposure of diltiazem by the concomitant use of naringin in rats. *Int. J. Pharm.* **2005**, *305*, 122–128. [CrossRef] [PubMed]

65. Choi, J.-S.; Kang, K.W. Enhanced tamoxifen bioavailability after oral administration of tamoxifen in rats pretreated with naringin. *Arch. Pharm. Res.* **2008**, *31*, 1631–1636. [CrossRef] [PubMed]

66. Choi, J.-S.; Shin, S.-C. Enhanced paclitaxel bioavailability after oral coadministration of paclitaxel prodrug with naringin to rats. *Int. J. Pharm.* **2005**, *292*, 149–156. [CrossRef] [PubMed]

67. Lassoued, M.A.; Sfar, S.; Bouraoui, A.; Khemiss, F. Absorption enhancement studies of clopidogrel hydrogen sulphate in rat everted gut sacs. *J. Pharm. Pharmacol.* **2012**, *64*, 541–552. [CrossRef] [PubMed]

68. Yeum, C.-H.; Choi, J.-S. Effect of naringin pretreatment on bioavailability of verapamil in rabbits. *Arch. Pharm. Res.* **2006**, *29*, 102. [CrossRef] [PubMed]

69. Raiman, J.; Törmälehto, S.; Yritys, K.; Junginger, H.E.; Mönkkönen, J. Effects of various absorption enhancers on transport of clodronate through caco-2 cells. *Int. J. Pharm.* **2003**, *261*, 129–136. [CrossRef]

70. Wacher, V.J.; Wong, S.; Wong, H.T. Peppermint oil enhances cyclosporine oral bioavailability in rats: Comparison with D-α-tocopheryl poly (ethylene glycol 1000) succinate (tpgs) and ketoconazole. *J. Pharm. Sci.* **2002**, *91*, 77–90. [CrossRef] [PubMed]

71. Badmaev, V.; Majeed, M.; Norkus, E.P. Piperine, an alkaloid derived from black pepper increases serum response of β-carotene during 14-days of oral β-carotene supplementation. *Nutr. Res.* **1999**, *19*, 381–388. [CrossRef]

72. Badmaev, V.; Majeed, M.; Prakash, L. Piperine derived from black pepper increases the plasma levels of coenzyme q10 following oral supplementation. *J. Nutr. Biochem.* **2000**, *11*, 109–113. [CrossRef]
73. Bajad, S.; Bedi, K.; Singla, A.; Johri, R. Piperine inhibits gastric emptying and gastrointestinal transit in rats and mice. *Planta Med.* **2001**, *67*, 176–179. [CrossRef]
74. Bano, G.; Raina, R.; Zutshi, U.; Bedi, K.; Johri, R.; Sharma, S. Effect of piperine on bioavailability and pharmacokinetics of propranolol and theophylline in healthy volunteers. *Eur. J. Clin. Pharmacol.* **1991**, *41*, 615–617. [CrossRef]
75. Gupta, S.; Bansal, P.; Bhardwaj, R.; Velpandian, T. Comparative anti-nociceptive, anti-inflammatory and toxicity profile of nimesulide vs nimesulide and piperine combination. *Pharmacol. Res.* **2000**, *41*, 657–662. [CrossRef]
76. Jin, M.J.; Han, H.K. Effect of piperine, a major component of black pepper, on the intestinal absorption of fexofenadine and its implication on food–drug interaction. *J. Food Sci.* **2010**, *75*, H93–H96. [CrossRef]
77. Johnson, J.J.; Nihal, M.; Siddiqui, I.A.; Scarlett, C.O.; Bailey, H.H.; Mukhtar, H.; Ahmad, N. Enhancing the bioavailability of resveratrol by combining it with piperine. *Mol. Nutr. Food Res.* **2011**, *55*, 1169–1176. [CrossRef]
78. Kasibhatta, R.; Naidu, M. Influence of piperine on the pharmacokinetics of nevirapine under fasting conditions. *Drugs R D* **2007**, *8*, 383–391. [CrossRef]
79. Lambert, J.D.; Hong, J.; Kim, D.H.; Mishin, V.M.; Yang, C.S. Piperine enhances the bioavailability of the tea polyphenol (−)-epigallocatechin-3-gallate in mice. *J. Nutr.* **2004**, *134*, 1948–1952. [CrossRef]
80. Mujumdar, A.; Dhuley, J.; Deshmukh, V.; Raman, P.; Thorat, S.; Naik, S. Effect of piperine on pentobarbitone induced hypnosis in rats. *Indian J. Exp. Boil.* **1990**, *28*, 486–487.
81. Pattanaik, S.; Hota, D.; Prabhakar, S.; Kharbanda, P.; Pandhi, P. Pharmacokinetic interaction of single dose of piperine with steady-state carbamazepine in epilepsy patients. *Phytother. Res. Int. J. Devoted Pharmacol. Toxicol. Eval. Nat. Prod. Deriv.* **2009**, *23*, 1281–1286. [CrossRef]
82. Sama, V.; Nadipelli, M.; Yenumula, P.; Bommineni, M.; Mullangi, R. Effect of piperine on antihyperglycemic activity and pharmacokinetic profile of nateglinide. *Arzneimittelforschung* **2012**, *62*, 384–388. [CrossRef]
83. Shoba, G.; Joy, D.; Joseph, T.; Majeed, M.; Rajendran, R.; Srinivas, P. Influence of piperine on the pharmacokinetics of curcumin in animals and human volunteers. *Planta Med.* **1998**, *64*, 353–356. [CrossRef]
84. Singh, M.; Varshneya, C.; Telang, R.; Srivastava, A. Alteration of pharmacokinetics of oxytetracycline following oral administration of piper longum in hens. *J. Vet. Sci.* **2005**, *6*, 197–200.
85. Babu, P.R.; Babu, K.N.; Peter, P.H.; Rajesh, K.; Babu, P.J. Influence of quercetin on the pharmacokinetics of ranolazine in rats and in vitro models. *Drug Dev. Ind. Pharm.* **2013**, *39*, 873–879. [CrossRef]
86. Bansal, T.; Awasthi, A.; Jaggi, M.; Khar, R.K.; Talegaonkar, S. Pre-clinical evidence for altered absorption and biliary excretion of irinotecan (cpt-11) in combination with quercetin: Possible contribution of p-glycoprotein. *Life Sci.* **2008**, *83*, 250–259. [CrossRef]
87. Challa, V.R.; Ravindra Babu, P.; Challa, S.R.; Johnson, B.; Maheswari, C. Pharmacokinetic interaction study between quercetin and valsartan in rats and in vitro models. *Drug Dev. Ind. Pharm.* **2013**, *39*, 865–872. [CrossRef]
88. Choi, J.S.; Han, H.K. The effect of quercetin on the pharmacokinetics of verapamil and its major metabolite, norverapamil, in rabbits. *J. Pharm. Pharmacol.* **2004**, *56*, 1537–1542. [CrossRef]
89. Choi, J.-S.; Li, X. Enhanced diltiazem bioavailability after oral administration of diltiazem with quercetin to rabbits. *Int. J. Pharm.* **2005**, *297*, 1–8. [CrossRef]
90. Choi, J.-S.; Piao, Y.-J.; Kang, K.W. Effects of quercetin on the bioavailability of doxorubicin in rats: Role of cyp3a4 and p-gp inhibition by quercetin. *Arch. Pharm. Res.* **2011**, *34*, 607–613. [CrossRef]
91. Kim, K.-A.; Park, P.-W.; Park, J.-Y. Short-term effect of quercetin on the pharmacokinetics of fexofenadine, a substrate of p-glycoprotein, in healthy volunteers. *Eur. J. Clin. Pharmacol.* **2009**, *65*, 609–614. [CrossRef]
92. Li, X.; Choi, J.-S. Effects of quercetin on the pharmacokinetics of etoposide after oral or intravenous administration of etoposide in rats. *Anticancer. Res.* **2009**, *29*, 1411–1415.
93. Nijveldt, R.J.; Van Nood, E.; Van Hoorn, D.E.; Boelens, P.G.; Van Norren, K.; Van Leeuwen, P.A. Flavonoids: A review of probable mechanisms of action and potential applications. *Am. J. Clin. Nutr.* **2001**, *74*, 418–425. [CrossRef]

94. Scambia, G.; Ranelletti, F.; Panici, P.B.; De Vincenzo, R.; Bonanno, G.; Ferrandina, G.; Piantelli, M.; Bussa, S.; Rumi, C.; Cianfriglia, M. Quercetin potentiates the effect of adriamycin in a multidrug-resistant mcf-7 human breast-cancer cell line: P-glycoprotein as a possible target. *Cancer Chemother. Pharmacol.* **1994**, *34*, 459–464. [CrossRef]

95. Shin, S.-C.; Choi, J.-S.; Li, X. Enhanced bioavailability of tamoxifen after oral administration of tamoxifen with quercetin in rats. *Int. J. Pharm.* **2006**, *313*, 144–149. [CrossRef]

96. Umathe, S.N.; Dixit, P.V.; Bansod, K.U.; Wanjari, M.M. Quercetin pretreatment increases the bioavailability of pioglitazone in rats: Involvement of cyp3a inhibition. *Biochem. Pharmacol.* **2008**, *75*, 1670–1676. [CrossRef]

97. Chan, K.; Liu, Z.Q.; Jiang, Z.H.; Zhou, H.; Wong, Y.F.; Xu, H.-X.; Liu, L. The effects of sinomenine on intestinal absorption of paeoniflorin by the everted rat gut sac model. *J. Ethnopharmacol.* **2006**, *103*, 425–432. [CrossRef]

98. Bedada, S.K.; Yellu, N.R.; Neerati, P. Effect of resveratrol treatment on the pharmacokinetics of diclofenac in healthy human volunteers. *Phytother. Res.* **2016**, *30*, 397–401. [CrossRef]

99. Jia, Y.; Liu, Z.; Wang, C.; Meng, Q.; Huo, X.; Liu, Q.; Sun, H.; Sun, P.; Yang, X.; Ma, X. P-gp, mrp2 and oat1/oat3 mediate the drug-drug interaction between resveratrol and methotrexate. *Toxicol. Appl. Pharmacol.* **2016**, *306*, 27–35. [CrossRef]

100. Liu, Z.Q.; Zhou, H.; Liu, L.; Jiang, Z.H.; Wong, Y.F.; Xie, Y.; Cai, X.; Xu, H.X.; Chan, K. Influence of co-administrated sinomenine on pharmacokinetic fate of paeoniflorin in unrestrained conscious rats. *J. Ethnopharmacol.* **2005**, *99*, 61–67. [CrossRef]

101. Lv, X.-Y.; Li, J.; Zhang, M.; Wang, C.-M.; Fan, Z.; Wang, C.-Y.; Chen, L. Enhancement of sodium caprate on intestine absorption and antidiabetic action of berberine. *AAPS Pharm.* **2010**, *11*, 372–382. [CrossRef]

102. Yu, J.-N.; Zhu, Y.; Wang, L.; Peng, M.; Tong, S.-S.; Cao, X.; Qiu, H.; Xu, X.-M. Enhancement of oral bioavailability of the poorly water-soluble drug silybin by sodium cholate/phospholipid-mixed micelles. *Acta Pharmacol. Sin.* **2010**, *31*, 759. [CrossRef]

103. Chen, Y.; Lu, Y.; Chen, J.; Lai, J.; Sun, J.; Hu, F.; Wu, W. Enhanced bioavailability of the poorly water-soluble drug fenofibrate by using liposomes containing a bile salt. *Int. J. Pharm.* **2009**, *376*, 153–160. [CrossRef]

104. Wang, H.-J.; Pao, L.-H.; Hsiong, C.-H.; Shih, T.-Y.; Lee, M.-S.; Hu, O.Y.-P. Dietary flavonoids modulate cyp2c to improve drug oral bioavailability and their qualitative/quantitative structure–activity relationship. *AAPS J.* **2014**, *16*, 258–268. [CrossRef]

105. Hamman, J.; Schultz, C.; Kotzé, A. N-trimethyl chitosan chloride: Optimum degree of quaternization for drug absorption enhancement across epithelial cells. *Drug Dev. Ind. Pharm.* **2003**, *29*, 161–172. [CrossRef]

106. Kotzé, A.R.; Lueßen, H.L.; de Leeuw, B.J.; Verhoef, J.C.; Junginger, H.E. N-trimethyl chitosan chloride as a potential absorption enhancer across mucosal surfaces: In vitro evaluation in intestinal epithelial cells (caco-2). *Pharm. Res.* **1997**, *14*, 1197–1202. [CrossRef]

107. Cox, D.S.; Raje, S.; Gao, H.; Salama, N.N.; Eddington, N.D. Enhanced permeability of molecular weight markers and poorly bioavailable compounds across caco-2 cell monolayers using the absorption enhancer, zonula occludens toxin. *Pharm. Res.* **2002**, *19*, 1680–1688. [CrossRef]

108. Machida, M.; Hayashi, M.; Awazu, S. The effects of absorption enhancers on the pulmonary absorption of recombinant human granulocyte colony-stimulating factor (rhg-csf) in rats. *Boil. Pharm. Bull.* **2000**, *23*, 84–86. [CrossRef]

109. Florea, B.I.; Thanou, M.; Junginger, H.E.; Borchard, G. Enhancement of bronchial octreotide absorption by chitosan and n-trimethyl chitosan shows linear in vitro/in vivo correlation. *J. Control. Release* **2006**, *110*, 353–361. [CrossRef]

110. Todo, H.; Okamoto, H.; Iida, K.; Danjo, K. Effect of additives on insulin absorption from intratracheally administered dry powders in rats. *Int. J. Pharm.* **2001**, *220*, 101–110. [CrossRef]

111. Salem, L.B.; Bosquillon, C.; Dailey, L.; Delattre, L.; Martin, G.; Evrard, B.; Forbes, B. Sparing methylation of β-cyclodextrin mitigates cytotoxicity and permeability induction in respiratory epithelial cell layers in vitro. *J. Control. Release* **2009**, *136*, 110–116. [CrossRef]

112. Shen, Z.-C.; Cheng, Y.; Zhang, Q.; Wei, S.-L.; Li, R.-C.; Wang, K. Lanthanides enhance pulmonary absorption of insulin. *Boil. Trace Element Res.* **2000**, *75*, 215–225. [CrossRef]

113. Morimoto, K.; Uehara, Y.; Iwanaga, K.; Kakemi, M. Effects of sodium glycocholate and protease inhibitors on permeability of trh and insulin across rabbit trachea. *Pharm. Acta Helv.* **2000**, *74*, 411–415. [CrossRef]

114. Johansson, F.; Hjertberg, E.; Eirefelt, S.; Tronde, A.; Bengtsson, U.H. Mechanisms for absorption enhancement of inhaled insulin by sodium taurocholate. *Eur. J. Pharm. Sci.* **2002**, *17*, 63–71. [CrossRef]

115. Yang, T.; Mustafa, F.; Bai, S.; Ahsan, F. Pulmonary delivery of low molecular weight heparins. *Pharm. Res.* **2004**, *21*, 2009–2016. [CrossRef]
116. Martin, G.P.; El-Hariri, L.M.; Marriott, C. Bile salt-and lysophosphatidylcholine-induced membrane damage in human erythrocytes. *J. Pharm. Pharmacol.* **1992**, *44*, 646–650. [CrossRef]
117. Gibaldi, M.; Feldman, S. Mechanisms of surfactant effects on drug absorption. *J. Pharm. Sci.* **1970**, *59*, 579–589. [CrossRef]
118. Bernkop-Schnürch, A.; Hornof, M.; Zoidl, T. Thiolated polymers—Thiomers: Synthesis and in vitro evaluation of chitosan–2-iminothiolane conjugates. *Int. J. Pharm.* **2003**, *260*, 229–237. [CrossRef]
119. Bechgaard, E.; Gizurarson, S.; Hjortkjær, R.K.; Sørensen, A.R. Intranasal administration of insulin to rabbits using glycofurol as an absorption promoter. *Int. J. Pharm.* **1996**, *128*, 287–289. [CrossRef]
120. Gizurarson, S.; Marriott, C.; Martin, G.P.; Bechgaard, E. The influence of insulin and some excipients used in nasal insulin preparations on mucociliary clearance. *Int. J. Pharm.* **1990**, *65*, 243–247. [CrossRef]
121. Sørensen, A.; Drejer, K.; Engesgaard, A.; Guldhammer, B.; Hansen, P.; Hjortekjaer, R.; Mygind, N. Rabbit model for studies of nasal administration of insulin and glucagon. *Diabet. Res. Clin. Pract. Suppl.* **1988**, *1*, S165.
122. Bagger, M.A.; Nielsen, H.W.; Bechgaard, E. Nasal bioavailability of peptide T in rabbits: Absorption enhancement by sodium glycocholate and glycofurol. *Eur. J. Pharm. Sci.* **2001**, *14*, 69–74. [CrossRef]
123. Shinichiro, H.; Takatsuka, Y.; Hiroyuki, M. Mechanisms for the enhancement of the nasal absorption of insulin by surfactants. *Int. J. Pharm.* **1981**, *9*, 173–184. [CrossRef]
124. Pontiroli, A.; Alberetto, M.; Pajetta, E.; Calderara, A.; Pozza, G. Human insulin plus sodium glycocholate in a nasal spray formulation: Improved bioavailability and effectiveness in normal subjects. *Diabete Metab.* **1987**, *13*, 441–443.
125. Pontiroli, A.; Alberetto, M.; Calderara, A.; Pajetta, E.; Pozza, G. Nasal administration of glucagon and human calcitonin to healthy subjects: A comparison of powders and spray solutions and of different enhancing agents. *Eur. J. Clin. Pharmacol.* **1989**, *37*, 427–430. [CrossRef] [PubMed]
126. Aungst, B.J.; Rogers, N.J.; Shefter, E. Comparison of nasal, rectal, buccal, sublingual and intramuscular insulin efficacy and the effects of a bile salt absorption promoter. *J. Pharmacol. Exp. Ther.* **1988**, *244*, 23–27. [PubMed]
127. Lee, V.H. Mucosal penetration enhancers for facilitation of peptide and protein drug absorption. *Crit. Rev. Ther. Drug Carr. Syst.* **1991**, *8*, 91–192.
128. Illum, L. Nasal drug delivery: New developments and strategies. *Drug Discov. Today* **2002**, *7*, 1184–1189. [CrossRef]
129. Illum, L.; Farraj, N.F.; Davis, S.S. Chitosan as a novel nasal delivery system for peptide drugs. *Pharm. Res.* **1994**, *11*, 1186–1189. [CrossRef] [PubMed]
130. Casettari, L.; Illum, L. Chitosan in nasal delivery systems for therapeutic drugs. *J. Control. Release* **2014**, *190*, 189–200. [CrossRef]
131. Kotze, A.; Luessen, H.; De Boer, A.; Verhoef, J.; Junginger, H. Chitosan for enhanced intestinal permeability: Prospects for derivatives soluble in neutral and basic environments. *Eur. J. Pharm. Sci.* **1999**, *7*, 145–151. [CrossRef]
132. Farraj, N.; Johansen, B.; Davis, S.; Illum, L. Nasal administration of insulin using bioadhesive microspheres as a delivery system. *J. Control. Release* **1990**, *13*, 253–261. [CrossRef]
133. Illum, L. Chitosan and its use as a pharmaceutical excipient. *Pharm. Res.* **1998**, *15*, 1326–1331. [CrossRef]
134. Illum, L.; Fisher, A.; Jabbal-Gill, I.; Davis, S. Bioadhesive starch microspheres and absorption enhancing agents act synergistically to enhance the nasal absorption of polypeptides. *Int. J. Pharm.* **2001**, *222*, 109–119. [CrossRef]
135. Björk, E.; Edman, P. Characterization of degradable starch microspheres as a nasal delivery system for drugs. *Int. J. Pharm.* **1990**, *62*, 187–192. [CrossRef]
136. Sallee, V.L.; Dietschy, J.M. Determinants of intestinal mucosal uptake of short-and medium-chain fatty acids and alcohols. *J. Lipid Res.* **1973**, *14*, 475–484.
137. Westergaard, H.; Dietschy, J.M. The mechanism whereby bile acid micelles increase the rate of fatty acid and cholesterol uptake into the intestinal mucosal cell. *J. Clin. Investig.* **1976**, *58*, 97–108. [CrossRef] [PubMed]
138. Wilson, F.A. Intestinal transport of bile acids. *Am. J. Physiol.-Gastrointest. Liver Physiol.* **1981**, *241*, G83–G92. [CrossRef] [PubMed]

139. Jalali, A.; Moghimipour, E.; Akhgari, A. Enhancing effect of bile salts on gastrointestinal absorption of insulin. *Trop. J. Pharm. Res.* **2014**, *13*, 1797–1802. [CrossRef]

140. Hersey, S.; Jackson, R. Effect of bile salts on nasal permeability in vitro. *J. Pharm. Sci.* **1987**, *76*, 876–879. [CrossRef]

141. Scott-Moncrieff, J.C.; Shao, Z.; Mitra, A.K. Enhancement of intestinal insulin absorption by bile salt–fatty acid mixed micelles in dogs. *J. Pharm. Sci.* **1994**, *83*, 1465–1469. [CrossRef] [PubMed]

142. Ali, B.; Amin, S.; Ahmad, J.; Ali, A.; Ali, M.; Mir, S.R. Bioavailability enhancement studies of amoxicillin with nigella. *Indian J. Med Res.* **2012**, *135*, 555. [PubMed]

143. Sinha, V.; Kaur, M.P. Permeation enhancers for transdermal drug delivery. *Drug Dev. Ind. Pharm.* **2000**, *26*, 1131–1140. [CrossRef]

144. Al-Jenoobi, F.; Al-Suwayeh, S.; Muzaffar, I.; Alam, M.A.; Al-Kharfy, K.M.; Korashy, H.M.; Al-Mohizea, A.M.; Ahad, A.; Raish, M. Effects of nigella sativa and lepidium sativum on cyclosporine pharmacokinetics. *BioMed Res. Int.* **2013**, *2013*. [CrossRef] [PubMed]

145. Bedada, S.K.; Appani, R.; Boga, P.K. Capsaicin pretreatment enhanced the bioavailability of fexofenadine in rats by p-glycoprotein modulation: In vitro, in situ and in vivo evaluation. *Drug Dev. Ind. Pharm.* **2017**, *43*, 932–938. [CrossRef] [PubMed]

146. Tatiraju, D.V.; Bagade, V.B.; Karambelkar, P.J.; Jadhav, V.M.; Kadam, V. Natural bioenhancers: An overview. *J. Pharm. Phytochem.* **2013**, *2*, 55–60.

147. Survase, S.A.; Kagliwal, L.D.; Annapure, U.S.; Singhal, R.S. Cyclosporin A—A review on fermentative production, downstream processing and pharmacological applications. *Biotechnol. Adv.* **2011**, *29*, 418–435. [CrossRef] [PubMed]

148. Thanou, M.; Verhoef, J.; Junginger, H. Oral drug absorption enhancement by chitosan and its derivatives. *Adv. Drug Deliv. Rev.* **2001**, *52*, 117–126. [CrossRef]

149. Prego, C.; Torres, D.; Alonso, M.J. The potential of chitosan for the oral administration of peptides. *Expert Opin. Drug Deliv.* **2005**, *2*, 843–854. [CrossRef] [PubMed]

150. Lueßen, H.L.; de Leeuw, B.J.; Langemeÿer, M.W.; de Boer, A.B.G.; Verhoef, J.C.; Junginger, H.E. Mucoadhesive polymers in peroral peptide drug delivery. Vi. Carbomer and chitosan improve the intestinal absorption of the peptide drug buserelin in vivo. *Pharm. Res.* **1996**, *13*, 1668–1672. [CrossRef]

151. Schipper, N.G.; Vårum, K.M.; Artursson, P. Chitosans as absorption enhancers for poorly absorbable drugs. 1: Influence of molecular weight and degree of acetylation on drug transport across human intestinal epithelial (caco-2) cells. *Pharm. Res.* **1996**, *13*, 1686–1692. [CrossRef]

152. Kotzé, A.F.; Lueßen, H.L.; de Leeuw, B.J.; Verhoef, J.C.; Junginger, H.E. Comparison of the effect of different chitosan salts and n-trimethyl chitosan chloride on the permeability of intestinal epithelial cells (caco-2). *J. Control. Release* **1998**, *51*, 35–46. [CrossRef]

153. Borchard, G.; Lueßen, H.L.; de Boer, A.G.; Verhoef, J.C.; Lehr, C.-M.; Junginger, H.E. The potential of mucoadhesive polymers in enhancing intestinal peptide drug absorption. Iii: Effects of chitosan-glutamate and carbomer on epithelial tight junctions in vitro. *J. Control. Release* **1996**, *39*, 131–138. [CrossRef]

154. Smith, J.; Wood, E.; Dornish, M. Effect of chitosan on epithelial cell tight junctions. *Pharm. Res.* **2004**, *21*, 43–49. [CrossRef] [PubMed]

155. Rosenthal, R.; Heydt, M.S.; Amasheh, M.; Stein, C.; Fromm, M.; Amasheh, S. Analysis of absorption enhancers in epithelial cell models. *Ann. N. Y. Acad. Sci.* **2012**, *1258*, 86–92. [CrossRef] [PubMed]

156. Werle, M.; Takeuchi, H.; Bernkop-Schnürch, A. Modified chitosans for oral drug delivery. *J. Pharm. Sci.* **2009**, *98*, 1643–1656. [CrossRef] [PubMed]

157. Cavaleri, F.; Jia, W. The true nature of curcumin's polypharmacology. *J. Prev. Med.* **2017**, *2*, 5. [CrossRef]

158. Bahramsoltani, R.; Rahimi, R.; Farzaei, M.H. Pharmacokinetic interactions of curcuminoids with conventional drugs: A review. *J. Ethnopharmacol.* **2017**, *209*, 1–12. [CrossRef] [PubMed]

159. Cho, Y.; Lee, W.; Choi, J. Effects of curcumin on the pharmacokinetics of tamoxifen and its active metabolite, 4-hydroxytamoxifen, in rats: Possible role of cyp3a4 and p-glycoprotein inhibition by curcumin. *Die Pharm. Int. J. Pharm. Sci.* **2012**, *67*, 124–130.

160. Abo-El-Sooud, K.; Samar, M.; Fahmy, M. Curcumin ameliorates the absolute and relative bioavailabilities of marbofloxacin after oral administrations in broiler chickens. *Wulfenia* **2017**, *24*, 284–297.

161. Ampasavate, C.; Sotanaphun, U.; Phattanawasin, P.; Piyapolrungroj, N. Effects of curcuma spp. On p-glycoprotein function. *Phytomedicine* **2010**, *17*, 506–512. [CrossRef]

162. Neerati, P.; Bedada, S.K. Effect of diosmin on the intestinal absorption and pharmacokinetics of fexofenadine in rats. *Pharmacol. Rep.* **2015**, *67*, 339–344. [CrossRef]

163. Wang, J.-B.; Zhao, H.-P.; Zhao, Y.-L.; Jin, C.; Liu, D.-J.; Kong, W.-J.; Fang, F.; Zhang, L.; Wang, H.-J.; Xiao, X.-H. Hepatotoxicity or hepatoprotection? Pattern recognition for the paradoxical effect of the chinese herb rheum palmatum l. In treating rat liver injury. *PLoS ONE* **2011**, *6*, e24498. [CrossRef]

164. Lee, M.-H.; Kao, L.; Lin, C.-C. Comparison of the antioxidant and transmembrane permeative activities of the different polygonum cuspidatum extracts in phospholipid-based microemulsions. *J. Agric. Food Chem.* **2011**, *59*, 9135–9141. [CrossRef] [PubMed]

165. Wang, M.; Zhao, R.; Wang, W.; Mao, X.; Yu, J. Lipid regulation effects of polygoni multiflori radix, its processed products and its major substances on steatosis human liver cell line l02. *J. Ethnopharmacol.* **2012**, *139*, 287–293. [CrossRef] [PubMed]

166. Yang, Y.-C.; Lim, M.-Y.; Lee, H.-S. Emodin isolated from cassia obtusifolia (leguminosae) seed shows larvicidal activity against three mosquito species. *J. Agric. Food Chem.* **2003**, *51*, 7629–7631. [CrossRef] [PubMed]

167. Naqvi, S.; Ullah, M.; Hadi, S. *DNA Degradation by Aqueous Extract of Aloe Vera in the Presence Of Copper Ions*; CSIR: New Delhi, India, 2010.

168. Yang, T.; Kong, B.; Kuang, Y.; Cheng, L.; Gu, J.; Zhang, J.; Shu, H.; Yu, S.; Yang, X.; Cheng, J. Emodin plays an interventional role in epileptic rats via multidrug resistance gene 1 (mdr1). *Int. J. Clin. Exp. Pathol.* **2015**, *8*, 3418. [PubMed]

169. Ko, J.-C.; Su, Y.-J.; Lin, S.-T.; Jhan, J.-Y.; Ciou, S.-C.; Cheng, C.-M.; Chiu, Y.-F.; Kuo, Y.-H.; Tsai, M.-S.; Lin, Y.-W. Emodin enhances cisplatin-induced cytotoxicity via down-regulation of ercc1 and inactivation of erk1/2. *Lung Cancer* **2010**, *69*, 155–164. [CrossRef] [PubMed]

170. Tan, W.; Lu, J.; Huang, M.; Li, Y.; Chen, M.; Wu, G.; Gong, J.; Zhong, Z.; Xu, Z.; Dang, Y. Anti-cancer natural products isolated from chinese medicinal herbs. *Chin. Med.* **2011**, *6*, 27. [CrossRef] [PubMed]

171. Guo, J.; Li, W.; Shi, H.; Xie, X.; Li, L.; Tang, H.; Wu, M.; Kong, Y.; Yang, L.; Gao, J. Synergistic effects of curcumin with emodin against the proliferation and invasion of breast cancer cells through upregulation of mir-34a. *Mol. Cell. Biochem.* **2013**, *382*, 103–111. [CrossRef]

172. Min, H.; Niu, M.; Zhang, W.; Yan, J.; Li, J.; Tan, X.; Li, B.; Su, M.; Di, B.; Yan, F. Emodin reverses leukemia multidrug resistance by competitive inhibition and downregulation of p-glycoprotein. *PLoS ONE* **2017**, *12*, e0187971. [CrossRef]

173. Choi, R.J.; Ngoc, T.M.; Bae, K.; Cho, H.-J.; Kim, D.-D.; Chun, J.; Khan, S.; Kim, Y.S. Anti-inflammatory properties of anthraquinones and their relationship with the regulation of p-glycoprotein function and expression. *Eur. J. Pharm. Sci.* **2013**, *48*, 272–281. [CrossRef]

174. Huang, J.; Guo, L.; Tan, R.; Wei, M.; Zhang, J.; Zhao, Y.; Gong, L.; Huang, Z.; Qiu, X. Interactions between emodin and efflux transporters on rat enterocyte by a validated ussing chamber technique. *Front. Pharmacol.* **2018**, *9*, 646. [CrossRef]

175. Mansouri, M.T.; Soltani, M.; Naghizadeh, B.; Farbood, Y.; Mashak, A.; Sarkaki, A. A possible mechanism for the anxiolytic-like effect of gallic acid in the rat elevated plus maze. *Pharmacol. Biochem. Behav.* **2014**, *117*, 40–46. [CrossRef] [PubMed]

176. Stupans, I.; Stretch, G.; Hayball, P. Olive oil phenols inhibit human hepatic microsomal activity. *J. Nutr.* **2000**, *130*, 2367–2370. [CrossRef] [PubMed]

177. Okuda, T.; Yoshida, T.; Hatano, T. Hydrolyzable tannins and related polyphenols. In *Fortschritte der Chemie Organischer Naturstoffe/Progress in the Chemistry of Organic Natural Products*; Springer: New York, NY, USA, 1995; pp. 1–117.

178. Chieli, E.; Romiti, N.; Rodeiro, I.; Garrido, G. In vitro modulation of abcb1/p-glycoprotein expression by polyphenols from mangifera indica. *Chem. Boil. Interact.* **2010**, *186*, 287–294. [CrossRef] [PubMed]

179. Basheer, L.; Kerem, Z. Interactions between cyp3a4 and dietary polyphenols. *Oxidative Med. Cell. Longev.* **2015**, *2015*. [CrossRef]

180. Athukuri, B.L.; Neerati, P. Enhanced oral bioavailability of diltiazem by the influence of gallic acid and ellagic acid in male wistar rats: Involvement of cyp3a and p-gp inhibition. *Phytother. Res.* **2017**, *31*, 1441–1448. [CrossRef]

181. Athukuri, B.L.; Neerati, P. Enhanced oral bioavailability of metoprolol with gallic acid and ellagic acid in male wistar rats: Involvement of cyp2d6 inhibition. *Drug Metab. Pers. Ther.* **2016**, *31*, 229–234. [CrossRef]

182. Kesarwani, K.; Gupta, R. Bioavailability enhancers of herbal origin: An overview. *Asian Pac. J. Trop. Biomed.* **2013**, *3*, 253–266. [CrossRef]
183. Bhadoriya, S.S.; Mangal, A.; Madoriya, N.; Dixit, P. Bioavailability and bioactivity enhancement of herbal drugs by "nanotechnology": A review. *J. Curr. Pharm. Res.* **2011**, *8*, 1–7.
184. Hayeshi, R.; Masimirembwa, C.; Mukanganyama, S.; Ungell, A.-L.B. The potential inhibitory effect of antiparasitic drugs and natural products on p-glycoprotein mediated efflux. *Eur. J. Pharm. Sci.* **2006**, *29*, 70–81. [CrossRef]
185. Limtrakul, P.; Khantamat, O.; Pintha, K. Inhibition of p-glycoprotein function and expression by kaempferol and quercetin. *J. Chemother.* **2005**, *17*, 86–95. [CrossRef]
186. Bobrowska-Hägerstrand, M.; Wróbel, A.; Rychlik, B.; Bartosz, G.; Söderström, T.; Shirataki, Y.; Motohashi, N.; Molnár, J.; Michalak, K.; Hägerstrand, H. Monitoring of mrp-like activity in human erythrocytes: Inhibitory effect of isoflavones. *Blood Cells Mol. Dis.* **2001**, *27*, 894–900. [CrossRef] [PubMed]
187. Dube, A.; Nicolazzo, J.A.; Larson, I. Chitosan nanoparticles enhance the plasma exposure of (−)-epigallocatechin gallate in mice through an enhancement in intestinal stability. *Eur. J. Pharm. Sci.* **2011**, *44*, 422–426. [CrossRef] [PubMed]
188. Perez, M.; Otero, J.A.; Barrera, B.; Prieto, J.G.; Merino, G.; Alvarez, A.I. Inhibition of abcg2/bcrp transporter by soy isoflavones genistein and daidzein: Effect on plasma and milk levels of danofloxacin in sheep. *Vet. J.* **2013**, *196*, 203–208. [CrossRef] [PubMed]
189. Chen, Y.; Huang, C.; Zhou, T.; Chen, G. Genistein induction of human sulfotransferases in hepg2 and caco-2 cells. *Basic Clin. Pharmacol. Toxicol.* **2008**, *103*, 553–559. [CrossRef] [PubMed]
190. Eaton, E.A.; Walle, U.K.; Lewis, A.J.; Hudson, T.; Wilson, A.A.; Walle, T. Flavonoids, potent inhibitors of the human p-form phenolsulfotransferase. Potential role in drug metabolism and chemoprevention. *Drug Metab. Dispos.* **1996**, *24*, 232–237. [PubMed]
191. Reddy, S.A.; Sen, S.; Chakraborty, R.; Parameshappa, B. Effect of gokhru plant extract on intestinal absorption of aspirin using everted sac technique. *Int. J. Pharm. Boil. Arch.* **2011**, *2*, 549–553.
192. Bailey, D.G.; Malcolm, J.; Arnold, O.; Spence, J.D. Grapefruit juice–drug interactions. *Br. J. Clin. Pharmacol.* **1998**, *46*, 101–110. [CrossRef]
193. Mouly, S.; Lloret-Linares, C.; Sellier, P.-O.; Sene, D.; Bergmann, J.-F. Is the clinical relevance of drug-food and drug-herb interactions limited to grapefruit juice and saint-john's wort? *Pharmacol. Res.* **2017**, *118*, 82–92. [CrossRef]
194. Bailey, D.; Spence, J.; Munoz, C.; Arnold, J. Interaction of citrus juices with felodipine and nifedipine. *Lancet* **1991**, *337*, 268–269. [CrossRef]
195. Mertens-Talcott, S.; Zadezensky, I.; Castro, W.; Derendorf, H.; Butterweck, V. Grapefruit-drug interactions: Can interactions with drugs be avoided? *J. Clin. Pharmacol.* **2006**, *46*, 1390–1416. [CrossRef]
196. Ahmed, I.S.; Hassan, M.A.; Kondo, T. Effect of lyophilized grapefruit juice on p-glycoprotein-mediated drug transport in-vitro and in-vivo. *Drug Dev. Ind. Pharm.* **2015**, *41*, 375–381. [CrossRef] [PubMed]
197. Butterweck, V.; Zdrojewski, I.; Galloway, C.; Frye, R.; Derendorf, H. Toxicological and pharmacokinetic evaluation of concomitant intake of grapefruit juice and simvastatin in rats after repeated treatment over 28 days. *Planta Med.* **2009**, *75*, 1196. [CrossRef] [PubMed]
198. Shirasaka, Y.; Shichiri, M.; Mori, T.; Nakanishi, T.; Tamai, I. Major active components in grapefruit, orange, and apple juices responsible for oatp2b1-mediated drug interactions. *J. Pharm. Sci.* **2013**, *102*, 280–288. [CrossRef] [PubMed]
199. Spahn-Langguth, H.; Langguth, P. Grapefruit juice enhances intestinal absorption of the p-glycoprotein substrate talinolol. *Eur. J. Pharm. Sci.* **2001**, *12*, 361–367. [CrossRef]
200. Tian, R.; Koyabu, N.; Takanaga, H.; Matsuo, H.; Ohtani, H.; Sawada, Y. Effects of grapefruit juice and orange juice on the intestinal efflux of p-glycoprotein substrates. *Pharm. Res.* **2002**, *19*, 802–809. [CrossRef] [PubMed]
201. Lown, K.S.; Bailey, D.G.; Fontana, R.J.; Janardan, S.K.; Adair, C.H.; Fortlage, L.A.; Brown, M.B.; Guo, W.; Watkins, P.B. Grapefruit juice increases felodipine oral availability in humans by decreasing intestinal cyp3a protein expression. *J. Clin. Investig.* **1997**, *99*, 2545–2553. [CrossRef]
202. Dresser, G.K.; Kim, R.B.; Bailey, D.G. Effect of grapefruit juice volume on the reduction of fexofenadine bioavailability: Possible role of organic anion transporting polypeptides. *Clin. Pharmacol. Ther.* **2005**, *77*, 170–177. [CrossRef]

203. Tamai, I.; Nakanishi, T. Oatp transporter-mediated drug absorption and interaction. *Curr. Opin. Pharmacol.* **2013**, *13*, 859–863. [CrossRef]

204. Khanuja, S.; Arya, J.; Srivastava, S.; Shasany, A.; Kumar, T.S.; Darokar, M.; Kumar, S. Antibiotic Pharmaceutical Composition with Lysergol as Bio-Enhancer and Method of Treatment. U.S. Patent 11/395,527, 15 March 2007.

205. Alexander, A.; Qureshi, A.; Kumari, L.; Vaishnav, P.; Sharma, M.; Saraf, S.; Saraf, S. Role of herbal bioactives as a potential bioavailability enhancer for active pharmaceutical ingredients. *Fitoterapia* **2014**, *97*, 1–14. [CrossRef]

206. Paine, M.F.; Criss, A.B.; Watkins, P.B. Two major grapefruit juice components differ in intestinal cyp3a4 inhibition kinetic and binding properties. *Drug Metab. Dispos.* **2004**. [CrossRef]

207. Hochman, J.H.; Fix, J.A.; LeCluyse, E.L. In vitro and in vivo analysis of the mechanism of absorption enhancement by palmitoylcarnitine. *J. Pharmacol. Exp. Ther.* **1994**, *269*, 813–822. [PubMed]

208. LeCluyse, E.L.; Appel, L.E.; Sutton, S.C. Relationship between drug absorption enhancing activity and membrane perturbing effects of acylcarnitines. *Pharm. Res.* **1991**, *8*, 84–87. [CrossRef] [PubMed]

209. Duizer, E.; Van Der Wulp, C.; Versantvoort, C.H.; Groten, J.P. Absorption enhancement, structural changes in tight junctions and cytotoxicity caused by palmitoyl carnitine in caco-2 and iec-18 cells. *J. Pharmacol. Exp. Ther.* **1998**, *287*, 395–402. [PubMed]

210. Bhardwaj, R.K.; Glaeser, H.; Becquemont, L.; Klotz, U.; Gupta, S.K.; Fromm, M.F. Piperine, a major constituent of black pepper, inhibits human p-glycoprotein and cyp3a4. *J. Pharmacol. Exp. Ther.* **2002**, *302*, 645–650. [CrossRef] [PubMed]

211. Ahmad, N.; Fazal, H.; Abbasi, B.H.; Farooq, S.; Ali, M.; Khan, M.A. Biological role of piper nigrum l.(black pepper): A review. *Asian Pac. J. Trop. Biomed.* **2012**, *2*, S1945–S1953. [CrossRef]

212. Riedmaier, A.E.; Nies, A.T.; Schaeffeler, E.; Schwab, M. Organic anion transporters and their implications in pharmacotherapy. *Pharmacol. Rev.* **2012**, *64*, 421–449. [CrossRef]

213. Fukuhara, K.; Ikawa, K.; Morikawa, N.; Kumagai, K. Population pharmacokinetics of high-dose methotrexate in japanese adult patients with malignancies: A concurrent analysis of the serum and urine concentration data. *J. Clin. Pharm. Ther.* **2008**, *33*, 677–684. [CrossRef]

214. Li, J.; Liu, Y.; Zhang, J.; Yu, X.; Wang, X.; Zhao, L. Effects of resveratrol on p-glycoprotein and cytochrome p450 3a in vitro and on pharmacokinetics of oral saquinavir in rats. *Drug Des. Dev. Ther.* **2016**, *10*, 3699. [CrossRef]

215. Sharma, P.; Varma, M.V.; Chawla, H.P.; Panchagnula, R. In situ and in vivo efficacy of peroral absorption enhancers in rats and correlation to in vitro mechanistic studies. *IL Farmaco* **2005**, *60*, 874–883. [CrossRef]

216. Fasano, A.; Fiorentini, C.; Donelli, G.; Uzzau, S.; Kaper, J.B.; Margaretten, K.; Ding, X.; Guandalini, S.; Comstock, L.; Goldblum, S.E. Zonula occludens toxin modulates tight junctions through protein kinase c-dependent actin reorganization, in vitro. *J. Clin. Investig.* **1995**, *96*, 710–720. [CrossRef]

217. Yang, T.; Hussain, A.; Paulson, J.; Abbruscato, T.J.; Ahsan, F. Cyclodextrins in nasal delivery of low-molecular-weight heparins: In vivo and in vitro studies. *Pharm. Res.* **2004**, *21*, 1127–1136. [CrossRef] [PubMed]

218. Cheng, Y.; Yao, H.; Lin, H.; Lu, J.; Li, R.; Wang, K. The events relating to lanthanide ions enhanced permeability of human erythrocyte membrane: Binding, conformational change, phase transition, perforation and ion transport. *Chem. Boil. Interact.* **1999**, *121*, 267–289. [CrossRef]

219. Cheng, Y.; Liu, M.; Li, R.; Wang, C.; Bai, C.; Wang, K. Gadolinium induces domain and pore formation of human erythrocyte membrane: An atomic force microscopic study. *Biochim. Biophys. Acta* **1999**, *1421*, 249–260. [CrossRef]

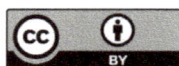

pharmaceutics

MDPI

Review

Application of Permeation Enhancers in Oral Delivery of Macromolecules: An Update

Sam Maher [1,*], David J. Brayden [2], Luca Casettari [3] and Lisbeth Illum [4]

[1]   School of Pharmacy, Royal College of Surgeons in Ireland, St. Stephens Green, Dublin 2, Ireland
[2]   School of Veterinary Medicine and UCD Conway Institute, University College Dublin,
      Belfield, Dublin 4, Ireland; david.brayden@ucd.ie
[3]   Department of Biomolecular Sciences, University of Urbino Carlo Bo, Piazza del Rinascimento 6,
      61029 Urbino (PU), Italy; luca.casettari@uniurb.it
[4]   IDentity, 19 Cavendish Crescent North, The Park, Nottingham NG7 1BA, UK; lisbeth.illum@illumdavis.com
*   Correspondence: sammaher@rcsi.com; Tel.: +353-1-402-2362

Received: 21 December 2018; Accepted: 14 January 2019; Published: 19 January 2019

Abstract: The application of permeation enhancers (PEs) to improve transport of poorly absorbed active pharmaceutical ingredients across the intestinal epithelium is a widely tested approach. Several hundred compounds have been shown to alter the epithelial barrier, and although the research emphasis has broadened to encompass a role for nanoparticle approaches, PEs represent a key constituent of conventional oral formulations that have progressed to clinical testing. In this review, we highlight promising PEs in early development, summarize the current state of the art, and highlight challenges to the translation of PE-based delivery systems into safe and effective oral dosage forms for patients.

Keywords: permeation enhancer; oral delivery; formulation; permeability; safety; simulated intestinal fluid; hydrophobization; epithelium

---

1. Introduction

Since the early 1990s, the pharmaceutical industry has gradually reduced attrition related to non-optimal pharmacokinetics (PK) and low bioavailability (BA) of drugs in development [1]. A combination of tools that predict sub-optimal physicochemical properties, as well as technologies that address impediments to translation from in vitro/preclinical studies to successful clinical trials (e.g., low aqueous solubility, short plasma half-life ($t_{1/2}$)) has led to a shift in overall attrition from PK to safety. Despite this, non-optimal PK characteristics continue to rank amongst the most common cause of attrition [2]. The shift towards the development of more lipophilic compounds that are less likely to suffer from sub-optimal PK has however been associated with low solubility and increased toxicity [3,4]. A cohort of macromolecules that can exhibit desirable safety and efficacy are large hydrophilic compounds with greater molecular complexity (e.g., oligomeric peptide backbones), but such properties inevitably confer low intestinal epithelial permeability. In theory, poorly permeable drugs may be administered orally at higher doses to offset low absorption, but this is usually impractical for formulation and cost reasons. Low permeability might be acceptable if a safe and consistent therapeutic effect can be achieved with a molecule that has a long $t_{1/2}$, even in the context of high variability in BA, otherwise poorly permeable drugs are typically formulated in injectable dosage forms or in dosage forms using other routes of delivery with higher membrane permeability than the intestine, such as the nasal route.

A paucity of delivery technologies that address low intestinal epithelial permeability for macromolecules has left pharmaceutical manufacturers with little option but to limit screening of these complex hydrophilic macromolecules or default to parenteral formulation. Delivery systems that enable poorly permeable molecules to be efficiently delivered across the intestine may diversity the type of compounds screened in discovery and may permit reformulation of selected injectable macromolecules. There is debate as to whether medicinal chemists in the discovery field should solely focus on safety and efficacy of the active, and rely on formulation and delivery scientists to address sub-optimal solubility, ADME (absorption, distribution, metabolism and excretion), and stability characteristics—or whether medicinal chemists should focus on all of the aforementioned properties to rely less on delivery and formulation scientists [5]. Recent advances highlight the importance of dual focus early in development: optimizing the molecule and the formulation [6,7]. The key challenge with focusing on delivery platforms is the current lack of proven technologies that can significantly improve intestinal permeability in humans.

2. Permeation Enhancer (PE) Categories

The potential of improving the oral BA of macromolecules has been extensively researched, but the majority of delivery systems have failed to progress beyond preliminary animal model evaluation. The inclusion of an excipient that facilitates transport across the intestinal epithelial barrier is a desirable approach. Proprietary formulations that attempt to improve oral absorption of macromolecules in humans usually include permeation enhancers (PEs). However, failure of these PE-based formulations to translate into commercial products has led academic investigators to prioritize development of more technologically advanced drug delivery systems rather than address impediments to translation of PEs. Several hundred compounds have been shown to alter permeability in oral, nasal, buccal, pulmonary, vaginal, and corneal delivery models. These compounds are broadly categorized as paracellular or transcellular PEs.

Paracellular PEs can be sub-categorized into first and second generation [8]. The older first generation paracellular PEs open tight junctions (TJs) through intracellular signaling mechanisms, while the second sub-category act via direct disruption of homophilic interactions at cell adhesion recognition (CAR) sequences. Major targets to afford TJ opening include: the cytoskeleton, claudins, occludin, and E-cadherin and Ca^{2+} [9]. Toxins and their derivatives are one of the largest sources of paracellular PEs, irrespective of sub-category (e.g., *zonula occludins* toxin, *clostridium perfringens* enterotoxin (CPE) [10]). Despite extensive preclinical assessment of microbial toxins and derived motifs, clinical trials with paracellular PEs are dominated by older agents with broader mechanisms of action, one example being ethylenediaminetetraacetic acid (EDTA) (POD^{TM}, Oramed, Israel [11]).

Transcellular PEs alter epithelial permeability by two contrasting mechanisms, (i) reversible perturbation of the epithelial plasma membrane [9], or (ii) physical interaction with the active to improve passive transcellular permeation (e.g., hydrophobization [12]). Surfactant-based PEs are a widely tested category that alter membrane integrity. Included in this category are medium chain fatty acids, acylcarnitines, acylated amino acids, bile salts, and a variety of non-ionic surfactants (e.g., polyoxyethylene-8 lauryl ether ($C_{12}E_8$), sucrose laurate, macrogol-8 glycerides [13,14]). A number of surfactants have been evaluated clinically in oral delivery systems for macromolecules: lauroylcarnitine chloride (Peptilligence^{TM}, Enteris Biopharma, Boonton, NJ, USA [15]) sodium caprate (C_{10}) (GIPET^{TM}, Merrion Pharma, Dublin, Ireland [16]), sodium caprylate (TPE^{TM} Chiasma, Ness Ziona, Israel [17]), and sodium cholate (Biocon, Bangalore, India [18]). Soluble and insoluble surfactants are also constituents of complex lipoidal systems including oily suspensions [17] and emulsions [19]. At low test concentrations in reductionist cell and tissue based delivery models, transcellular perturbants (i) activate plasma membrane receptors and enzymes, (ii) modulate intracellular mediators, (iii) selectively remove TJ proteins from fluidic regions of the membrane, and (iv) initiate repair mechanisms related to opening of TJs [20]. In some cases, these actions are uncoupled from membrane perturbation [21]. This has led investigators to suggest that some perturbants may in part act indirectly via a paracellular mode of action. However, low concentrations of such agents that do not induce transcellular perturbation cause only modest increases on permeability in vitro [21].

Transcellular permeation may also be improved by physical complexation, either by hydrophobic ion pairing (HIP) or dipole–dipole interaction [9]. HIP involves electrostatic-based complexation of an ionizable lead (usually a peptide) with an amphiphilic counterion. The hydrophobic moiety of the counter ion confers a lower capacity for solvation than conventional counterions typically used in the preparation of pharmaceutical salts to address low aqueous solubility. HIP reduces the solubility of several peptides including insulin [22], desmopressin [23], octreotide [24], and exenatide [25]. Hydrophobization via dipole–dipole interactions between the poorly permeable macromolecule and acylated amino acids (the so-called Eligen® carriers of Emisphere, Roseland, NJ, USA [26]) is a more widely studied approach than HIP, although the less well understood. Emisphere have assessed the clinical potential of Eligen carriers most notably SNAC (sodium salcaprozate) and 5-CNAC (N-(5-chlorosalicyloyl)-8-aminocaprylic acid) over a 20-year period. In that time, Emisphere discontinued development of SNAC for oral delivery of heparin and insulin. SNAC has however been successfully used in a marketed oral vitamin B_{12} supplement (Eligen B_{12}) [27], and more recently was shown to improve oral absorption of semaglutide in Phase II trials [28]. Development of an oral salmon calcitonin (sCT) using 5-CNAC failed to meet primary endpoints in two Phase III trials [29].

Several non-surfactant PEs have also been tested in pre-clinical studies. These include chitosan and its derivatives, cell penetrating peptides (CPPs), solvents (e.g., ethanol), salicylates, and enamines. CPPs such as penetratin and its analog, PentraMax™, continue to be researched for oral peptide delivery. There is evidence that these CPPs act by altering membrane barrier integrity [30], endocytosis [30], and physical complexation [31]. Although a few CPPs have progressed to clinical evaluation, the majority relate to the intracellular delivery of small molecules and not to oral delivery of macromolecules [32]. It remains to be seen if CPPs will eventually advance to clinical testing in oral delivery of anti-diabetic peptides [33].

3. Targets for Intestinal Permeation Enhancement: Beyond Insulin

Development of delivery platforms that improve epithelial permeability was historically associated with creating non-invasive formulations of insulin. Insulin represents an inexpensive and available prototype peptide with established analytical methods for PK and pharmacodynamic assays. In justifying the use of insulin, it can be argued that a prototype that can improve permeation of this large peptide (5.8 kDa) could be even more effective with smaller peptides (1–4 kDa), so it is a high bar. While there is some merit to the development of an oral insulin dosage, the focus on insulin has restricted effort to develop oral delivery systems for other macromolecules with more favourable physicochemical properties. Additionally, the emphasis on oral delivery of insulin and the lack of success in that pursuit during the hype of the 1990s has led to a largely negative view in the pharmaceutical industry and with journal editors of novel strategies to improve intestinal permeability.

Table 1 shows a selection of licensed peptides marketed via oral or injectable routes. This table shows that dose (potency), $t_{1/2}$, Mw, lipophilicity (LogP) and target action site are important factors that influence whether a peptide is commercially successful via oral or injectable routes. There are currently nine peptides on the market as oral products [34], although only two desmopressin and cyclosporin are intended to act on systemic targets; the properties of which are shown in Table 1. All other peptides in Table 1, except the regionally acting vancomycin, are marketed in injectable formulations and BA values are considered negligible (<0.1%).

All peptides marketed via the oral route are assigned low permeability within the Biopharmaceutics Classification System (BCS). Marketed injectable peptides are not formally assigned a BCS Class, although all peptides in Table 1 are considered BCS Class III. It is evident from Table 1 that while peptides exhibit low and variable BA (apart from cyclosporin), an optimal balance between potency, size/complexity, and apparent plasma $t_{1/2}$ can facilitate the development of a successful oral form (e.g., desmopressin) (Table 1). The extent to which chemical modification and the delivery system can compensate for peptides that do not exhibit an optimal balance between potency, size/complexity, and apparent plasma half-life is not clear. Structural modifications can reduce demand on delivery systems for peptides that are larger and more complex. A recent example being the very long $t_{1/2}$ GLP-1 analog, semaglutide [35], which has demonstrated promising results in clinical trials in an oral formulation containing SNAC, a PE that failed with macromolecules that did not have such favorable features.

In atypical cases where peptides are lipophilic and stable to proteolytic degradation, oral BA can be significantly higher than equivalent hydrophilic peptides (e.g., cyclosporin). The downside of high lipophilicity is low aqueous solubility, which has been addressed using lipid-based formulations [36]. Clinical evaluation of the cyclosporin (Sandimmune® Neoral, Novartis) has shown that 86% of the intact peptide permeates the intestinal epithelium [37]. While brush border and hepatic metabolism reduce BA of cyclosporin to 27%, oral BA is far higher than equivalent hydrophilic peptides such as desmopressin and octreotide. Chemical modification has been less successful in addressing low permeability, for example, in the case of insulin [38], although there is emerging evidence that physical modification of peptides using hydrophobizing agents may improve passive permeation (Section 4.7) [9,12,39]. A key area of development, therefore, is the combined development of hydrophobized peptides with a suitable lipid-based delivery system.

Table 1. Properties of selected approved peptides and their routes of delivery (source of information: Health Products Regulatory Authority (HPRA) summary of product characteristics (SPC), Drugbank, PubChem, and Welcome Compound Report Card).

Active	Mw	Dose	Frequency	Route	$t_{1/2}$	LogP [†]	BCS	Oral BA
Desmopressin	1069 Da	1–4 mcg	Daily	sc	~2.8 h	−4	III	0.17%
Octreotide	1019 Da	200 mcg	Thrice daily	sc	~1.7 h	−1.4	—	Phase 3
Cyclosporin	1203 Da	280 mg	Daily	iv inf.	~8.4 h	7.5	II	27%
Vancomycin	1449 Da	1500 mg	Twice daily	iv inf.	~7.2 h	−2.6	III	Local
Salmon calcitonin	3432 Da	16.7 mcg	Daily	sc	~1.3 h	−16.6	—	Phase 3
Semaglutide	4114 Da	500 mcg *	Weekly	sc	~168 h	−5.8	—	Phase 3
Exenatide	4186 Da	10 mcg	Daily	sc	~2.4 h	−21	—	Phase 1
Insulin degludec	6108 Da	350 mcg	Daily	sc	~25 h	−4.9	—	—
Insulin aspart	5832 Da	1.8 mg **	—	sc	~1.4 h	—	—	—

* oral dose in clinical testing [28]; ** estimated daily dose; [†] estimated logP (XLogP3-AA [40]); BCS: Biopharmaceutics classification system; $t_{1/2}$: plasma half-life; LogP: octanol water partition coefficient.

4. Recent Highlights

4.1. Oral Semaglutide Reduces HBA1c in Type 2 Diabetics by over 1.5% in Phase II Trials

Novo Nordisk (Bagsværd, Denmark) has adopted an integrated approach to enabling oral peptide delivery, combining structural engineering and formulation optimization [6]. Semaglutide is a long-acting acylated GLP-1 agonist (Ozempic® once weekly, s.c.) that also has greater stability to enzymatic degradation in the gastrointestinal (GI) tract. A once-a-day oral formulation of semaglutide in an immediate release formulation with SNAC is likely to have a significant effect on the management of diabetes. In a Phase II randomised controlled trial of 632 patients, daily administration of oral semaglutide (2.5–40 mg) lowered HbA1c by 0.7% to 1.9% [28]. Although there was a 280-fold difference in the cumulative dose relative to the once weekly sub-cutaneous (sc) injection (1 mg), the long plasma $t_{1/2}$, high potency, and improved stability reduces the need for a high-performing PE. Induction of high local pH in the immediate vicinity of the semaglutide/SNAC tablet in the stomach to increase solubility is considered a central aspect of the technology [41], where the contemporaneous release of SNAC and semaglutide to fasting patients enables co-localisation in high concentration at the site of enhancement. In gamma scintigraphy studies in healthy volunteers, the anatomical location for tablet erosion was confirmed as the stomach irrespective of whether participants ingested the formulation with 50 mL or 240 mL water [42]. The time to complete tablet erosion was 95 min (50 mL water) and 66.2 min (240 mL). Slow erosion of tablets (<54% in 1 h) was associated with higher plasma semaglutide levels and a longer T_{max} compared to fast eroding tablets. It is unclear why gastric emptying does not occur in patients receiving oral semaglutide, although it is possible that the peptide could slow gastric emptying [43]. It is not clear if the slow progressive release of semaglutide in the stomach may necessitate a longer delay before ingestion of a meal. The unusual gastric pH mechanism advocated for semaglutide/SNAC seems to be highly specific for this peptide. This topic is discussed in detail in the current special issue review by Twarog et al.

4.2. The Ionic Liquid Choline Geranate (CAGE) Has a Major Effect on Oral BA of Insulin

Ionic liquids are salt-like materials that are liquids below 100 °C. There has been renewed interest in the use of ionic liquids primarily due to their solvent properties. A recent study showed that intestinal co-instillation of a relatively low dose of insulin with choline geranate (CAGE) led to a dramatic lowering in blood sugar levels in non-diabetic rats [44]. The decrease in blood sugar compared favourably with the s.c. delivered insulin. The oral BA of insulin (10 IU) in rats was 45% following delivery with CAGE (80 mg) in enteric coated capsules in rodents, one of the highest values ever recorded for an insulin formulation in a rat PK study, albeit relative to 2 IU (s.c.) as against 1IU (s.c.) in most studies. CAGE increased the fluidity of mucous, reduced epithelial barrier integrity and protected insulin from degradation by trypsin. There was no apparent histological damage to the intestinal mucosa of rats. However, CAGE caused a partial reduction in Caco-2 cell viability, a decrease in transepithelial electrical resistance (TEER) and evidence of intracellular insulin-fluorescein isothiocyanate (FITC) in fluorescence microscopy, suggesting some transcellular perturbation. It is noteworthy that choline-based ionic liquids were amongst the least cytotoxic in a screen assessing the effect of a panel on the viability of Caco-2 and HT29 cells [45]. Moreover, insulin was stable in CAGE for four months at 4 °C. It is noteworthy that peptide stability concerns have been overcome in non-aqueous polyprotic solvents [46]. It will be interesting to see if these results translate to large animal models with a dosage form that can translate to human trials.

4.3. Mode of Action Studies on the PE, PIP 640

Permeant inhibitor of phosphatase (PIP) peptide 640 (PIP 640) is a decapeptide that transiently opens TJs. PIP640 inhibits myosin light chain phosphatase (MLCP), which in turn inhibits dephosphorylation of myosin light chain (MLC) [47]. This is achieved by binding to a subunit complex of protein phosphatase 1 (PP1) and MYPT1 (myosin phosphatase target subunit) in the same manner as CPI-17 (C-kinase-activated protein phosphatase-1 (PP1) inhibitor-17kDa). PIP-640 increased fluorescein isothiocyanate dextran 4 kDa (FD4) permeation across Caco-2 monolayers and improved BA of insulin to 4% in rat intestinal instillations [47]. More recently, a structure–activity assessment of PIP 640 showed that residues of glutamic acid and tyrosine are requisite for binding to MYPT1 subunit of the MLCP complex, while substitution of aspartic acid for arginine led to more specific targeting of PP1 subunit, which was associated with greater cytotoxicity [48]. In a follow-on study, PIP 640 was shown to selectively increase total levels of claudin 2 (both the cytoplasm and at the membrane) [49]. This increment was attributed to the preserved stability of existing claudin 2 rather than increased expression. Alteration of Caco-2 monolayer permeability by PIP 640 was biased towards paracellular transport of positively-charged diethylaminoethyl dextran compared to neutral dextran or carboxymethyl dextran, in keeping with data showing that claudin-2 is responsible for the formation of a channel that is selective for cations. A similar effect was observed in the comparison of sCT (cationic at the pH in the small intestine) and exenatide (anionic at the pH in the small intestine). PIP640 caused a greater increase on permeation of sCT over exenatide in both Caco-2 monolayers and rat intestinal instillations. Together these data highlight a potential for development of new chemical entity PEs that show bias towards permeation of cationic actives. These studies are noteworthy due the molecular biology and rational screening approaches taken to produce a PE molecule. Increasing the potency of PIP 640 is however likely to be required in order to allow a translatable oral dosage formulation to be developed.

4.4. Application of Nanoparticles to Co-Localise Active and PE

Nanotechnology has several potential applications in the science of oral delivery including protecting payload, targeting epithelial receptors in GI regions, and improving permeability [50]. The original working hypothesis for application in oral delivery of peptides was that nanoencapsulation would protect labile actives from pre-systemic degradation and shuttle cargo across the intestinal epithelium [51]. While this is the desired outcome, low and variable transmucosal uptake of nanoparticles and formulation complexity continue to impede progression. Investigators have attempted to improve transmucosal flux of drug-loaded nanoparticles using PEs, but it is difficult to envisage a PE improving uptake of colloids when uptake of peptides is inherently low and variable. An evolving view of nanoencapsulation is their potential to permeate mucus and to co-localise release of the macromolecule and PE at the intestinal epithelial wall, a key requirement for effective permeation enhancement [52,53]. It remains to be seen whether PE-macromolecule loaded nanoparticles, either passive or receptor-targeted, can be an effective strategy for delivering payloads across the intestine.

4.5. Application of PEs in Delivery of Nutraceuticals

Bioactive molecules in foodstuffs may have potential health benefits beyond their basic nutritional value. Many of these are complex natural substances that have low aqueous solubility and/or low intestinal permeability. These include peptides, carbohydrates, lipids, and complex organic phytochemicals. There is considerable overlap in the approaches to enable oral delivery of pharmaceutical and nutraceutical products [54], although development considerations related to safety, efficacy, and cost-effectiveness vary between the two.

Application of PEs to improve the oral BA of nutraceuticals is an emerging area. Safety concerns related to additives that might alter intestinal barrier integrity may outweigh any health benefits derived from selected nutraceuticals. PEs that are likely to be useful in oral delivery of nutraceuticals are substances that have food additive status, GRAS status, or can be made to food grade, so this limits the range for selection. These include medium and long chain fatty acids, bile salts (e.g., sodium chloeate [13]), chitosan and its derivatives [55] and certain non-ionic surfactants (e.g., sucrose esters [56], lactose esters [57], polysorbates [58]). Although most PEs are tested with transport markers of poorly permeable drugs, recent studies have evaluated oral delivery of antihypertensive tripeptides derived from milk and chicken muscle. Co-delivery of C_{10} (180 mM) with isoleucine-proline-proline (IPP) and leucine-lysine-proline (LKP) from milk did not improve oral absorption any further in rats in part because basal permeability seemed to be already high [59]. C_{10} reversed the effect of the Pep-T1 inhibitor (glycyl sarcosine) on oral absorption of these tripeptides. Other PEs have been shown to act in part via solubilization (bile salts [60]), inhibition of transporters (piperine [61]), or alteration to pre-systemic metabolism (genistein [62]). There are questions as to whether PEs can be effective as part of food matrices, and it may, therefore, be necessary to deliver bioactives as nutritional supplements in capsules or tablets. The relatively lower potency of nutraceutical versus therapeutic peptides is a challenge to the use of PEs. On the other hand, bioactive nutraceutical peptides are likely to be cheap to manufacture and exhibit intrinsically low toxicity. Thus it may be possible to offset lower potency with a higher amount of peptide and PE.

4.6. Can Non-Ionic Surfactants be More Effective than Ionizable Surfactants?

Surfactant-based PEs have long been the leading candidates to improve oral absorption of poorly permeable actives. The most prominent surfactant categories include medium chain fatty acids (anionic), acylcarnitines (amphoteric), alkyl sulfates (anionic), and bile salts (anionic). A structurally diverse group of non-ionic surfactants have been shown to alter epithelial barrier integrity including fatty alcohol ethoxylates, ethoxylated sugar esters, alkylphenol ethoxylates, alkyl maltosides/glucosides, macrogol glycerides, and sucrose/lactose esters. Most non-ionic surfactants in this category are liquid or unctuous semi-solids at room temperature, which limits their formulation potential. Small quantities of liquid PE can be incorporated into solid dosage forms using adsorbent. However, it is more challenging to prepare powders that have acceptable properties for capsule filling or compaction into tablets (such as flowability, disintegration, dissolution, desorption). For example, solidification of Labrasol® (Gattefosse, Saint Priest, Lyon, France) was achieved using relatively low quantities of silica (e.g., Neusilin® US2, Fuji Chemicals, Nakaniikawa-gun, Toyama, Japan) (Figure 1). Tablets prepared using a Labrasol® (50%), and Neusilin® US2 had poor disintegration times, but this was corrected by inclusion of a disintegrant (Table 2). Use of additional excipients lowers the quantity by weight of PE that can be incorporated into the formulation. This approach is more therefore likely to be only useful for the most potent non-ionic surfactants (e.g., $C_{12}E_8$), where less PE is required to improve permeation.

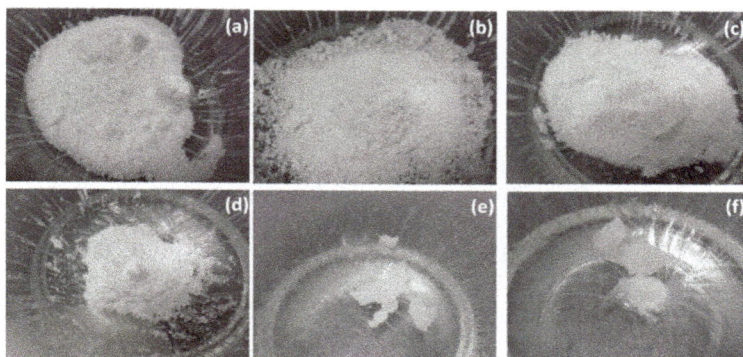

Figure 1. Visual effect of Neusilin® US2 on physical state of Labrasol®. Ratio of Neusilin® US2 to Labrasol® are (**a**) 1:0, (**b**) 0.75:0.25, (**c**) 0.67:0.33, (**d**) 0.5:0.5, (**e**) 0.33:0.67, (**f**) 0.25:0.75 (Maher unpublished).

Table 2. Disintegration times and break strength values for a panel of formulations containing Labrasol®, Neusilin® US2 and a disintegrant (Croscarmellose Sodium).

Formulation Additives	Disintegrant (% w/w)	Tableting Pressure (psi)	Disintegration Time (min)	Break Strength (N)
Labrasol and Neusilin® US2 (1:1)	0	1000	>60	29.1 ± 2.9
Labrasol and Neusilin® US2 (1:1)	0	2000	>60	68.8 ± 3.2
Labrasol and Neusilin® US2 (1:1)	5	1000	5.5 ± 0.2	49.8 ± 6.2
Labrasol and Neusilin® US2 (1:1)	5	2000	4.9 ± 0.3	72.4 ± 2.7

Some non-ionic surfactants are solids at room temperature (e.g., sucrose and lactose esters) although a low melting point makes it challenging to incorporate into tablets. Growth in the number of poorly soluble drugs administered in lipid-based formulations (LBFs) has led investigators to assess delivery of macromolecules in non-aqueous vehicles in soft or hard gelatin capsules. An underpinning question is what are the advantages of non-ionic surfactants versus ionizable surfactants, salts of which are easier to formulate into solid dosage forms? In general, non-ionic surfactants are safer and more widely used as excipients and food additives, primarily as emulsifiers. Sucrose laurate is an excipient included in some marketed formulations, and, although it is present in low amounts, its status as an excipient reduces risks in development. In a recent head-to-head, sucrose laurate and Labrasol® (Gattefosse, France) improved the flux of transmucosal marker molecules to a similar level to C_{10} and sodium undecylenate ($C_{11:1}$) at comparable concentrations across isolated rat intestinal tissue mucosae [13]. Sucrose laurate caused less damage to isolated rat colonic mucosae compared with C_{10} at similar concentrations [63]. In intestinal instillations, sucrose laurate improved permeation of insulin in the absence of histological damage [64]. It is noteworthy that other sugar esters have recently been shown to exhibit permeation enhancement. For example, the enhancement action of lactose laurate was comparable to sucrose laurate [65]. Although sucrose laurate and other sucrose esters can be synthesized as monoesters and have demonstrated enhancement action in their pure forms, food and excipient grades are typically supplied as mixtures containing the soluble mono-ester assigned a hydrophilic lipophilic balance (HLB) of 15 and a significant proportion of insoluble di-, tri-, and polyesters (HLB < 5). Thus, dispersions formed by mixed sucrose esters are not simple micellar systems; they comprise mixed micelles and/or micro/nanoemulsions. There is a requirement for safe and selective methods for production and material separation.

Labrasol® is another example of a complex blend of soluble and insoluble surfactants containing a large proportion of macrogol glycerides and 10% medium chain glycerides. Although Labrasol® caused perturbation of isolated rat intestinal mucosae, there was a degree of separation between the enhancement action and the histology damage score [13]. The effect of the difference in dispersion properties has not yet been fully elucidated, although there is emerging evidence that the extent of the monomeric surfactant that is free to interact with the mucosal surface plays a role in permeation enhancement [66,67]. The effect of free surfactant on enhancement action is discussed further in Section 4.9.

4.7. Can Physical Hydrophobization Improve Passive Intestinal Flux?

The majority of PEs act by altering epithelial barrier integrity. In recent years, investigators have attempted to improve the lipophilicity of the active to facilitate passive intestinal permeation. Hydrophobisation can be achieved by chemical conjugation (prodrugs [68]) or physical complexation [9] (Section 2). Chemical modification is not ideal for large ionizable peptides as it is not practical to mask several amino acid side chains within a macromolecule. The reversible formation of a salt between the peptide and a complexing agent can lead to a more dramatic increase in lipophilicity. This occurs through a combination of charge neutralization, exposure of hydrophobic domains within the peptide and/or the introduction of lipophilic moieties via the counterion. The process of HIP, therefore, leads to extensive lowering of aqueous solubility, which can be addressed through encapsulation in nanoparticles (e.g., poly(lactic-co-glycolic acid [69]), solubilization in lipid-based formulations [70], and non-aqueous solvents [22,71]. Incorporation of HIP complexes in the non-aqueous vehicle may prevent enzymatic degradation, limit pH dependent complex destabilization, and counterions may also perform as PEs [72]. Given the successful application of lipoidal vehicles in oral delivery of cyclosporin, there is research effort assessing the factors that impact loading in LBFs [70]. There are cases where HIP does not result in loss of aqueous solubility [73] and do not immediately breakdown at high pH values where deprotonation of cationic functional groups is known to occur [74]. However, further investigation is required to understand the permeability of soluble HIP complexes. Other considerations require kinetic and thermodynamic assessment of the dissociation of the hydrophobized peptide complex during permeation.

4.8. Mode of Action Studies are Required to Provide Evidence for a Paracellular Effect

The mechanism by which PEs alter the intestinal barrier has implications for safety and approval of PE-containing oral macromolecule formulations. In general, few PEs solely act via a paracellular mode of action, and it is necessary to distinguish paracellular and transcellular pathways across intestinal epithelia. Reduction in TEER for example or an increase in flux of paracellular transport markers is not direct proof of a paracellular mode of action, as transcellular perturbation can also reduce TEER and increase such fluxes. The absence of cytotoxicity in common cell viability assays (e.g., MTT) at concentrations that cause alteration to TEER and marker transport favour an interpretation relating to paracellular pathways. However, cytotoxicity assays based on mitochondrial enzymes may not represent the first sign of membrane perturbation. In this case, it may be appropriate to combine the use of MTT assay and techniques that directly evaluate membrane perturbation (e.g., lactate dehydrogenase (LDH) release assay). Two-path impedance spectroscopy has been used to show that C_{10} acts via a paracellular mode of action in vitro at low concentrations [75]. However, this method requires strict verification that the PE does not cause intracellular uptake of a paracellular dye [76], and applications that do not assess membrane integrity can overestimate the contribution of the paracellular route [75]. A recent study showed restoration of barrier integrity and a parallel decrease in absorption of a model peptide following cessation of intra-duodenal perfusion of C_{10} in rats [77]. This reversible action was equated to a paracellular mode of action, the rationale being that, had the effect been related to mucosal perturbation, the absorption of peptide would have continued to remain high. This conclusion does not, however, take into account the capacity of the GI tract to undergo rapid repair following perturbation [78]. Overall, more direct mode of action studies are required to confirm a paracellular mode of action.

4.9. Growing Need for Simulated Intestinal Fluid in PE Experiments

Over the last 30 years, there has been extensive effort to predict the behaviour of oral formulations in humans from solubility and release characteristics in vitro. This has given rise to important topics in biopharmaceutics including bioequivalence testing and in vitro/in vivo correlations. Solubility enhancement strategies highlighted the importance of replicating in vivo fasted and fed state conditions in order to predict release characteristics in humans, however there has not been the same emphasis on how constituents of intestinal luminal fluids affect intestinal permeability and in vivo absorption in preclinical models (including cell culture monolayers grown on Transwell® supports, isolated tissues mounted in Ussing chambers, everted and non-everted intestinal sacs, open/closed loop instillations, tablet insertion into gut loop, single-pass intestinal perfusion, infusion via intubation, oral administration as liquid or solid dosage forms).

Gastrointestinal fluid contains a complex mixture of endogenous secretions (including gastric, pancreatic, luminal, and biliary secretions, sloughed cells) and dietary substances (nutrients, drugs, microorganisms). This heterogeneous milieu consists of a cocktail of ions, bicarbonate, enzymes, mucin, bile acids, phospholipids, carbohydrates, proteins, amino acids, lipids, fatty acids, indigestible solid particles, and lysates from sloughed epithelial cells and non-viable microorganisms. In principle, the luminal milieu can modulate enhancement action of PEs. In the simplest example, PEs that are peptides/proteins may be degraded by proteolytic enzymes. Not all protein-based PEs are inactivated by luminal fluid as evident from the fact that many protein-based toxins stimulate electrogenic chloride secretion and TJ openings [79]. It remains to be seen whether peptide-based PEs can consistently modulate epithelial permeability or whether these additives must be chemically-modified to increase stability (e.g., cyclisation, synthesis of all D-forms, amino acid substitutions) or mixed with excipients that prevent enzymatic degradation of the therapeutic peptide (e.g., citric acid, soybean trypsin inhibitor). Other structural PEs categories can also be enzymatically degraded in the small intestine. Macrogol glycerides (e.g., Labrasol®, Gattefosse, France) are substrates of digestive lipase [80], although the degradation products in this instance are free medium chain fatty acids which may contribute to permeation enhancement [81].

It is not only chemical degradation that can attenuate the enhancement action. PEs that have demonstrated the most significant effect on epithelial permeability are soluble surfactants. This surfactant type exists in the monomeric form up to threshold concentration above which they form micelles. This critical micelle concentration (CMC) is both a measure of the solubility of the monomeric surfactant form and a direct measure of when surfactants begin to form micelles. Ionic surfactants with high CMC values are generally good detergents because it is the monomeric form of the surfactant that is responsible. As detergent-like membrane perturbation caused by surfactants is largely driven by the monomeric form of the surfactant, any physiological factor that reduces the CMC can potentially reduce efficacy. The CMC of ionizable surfactants such as medium chain fatty acids, acylcarnitines, and alkyl sulfates can be decreased by increasing the ionic strength of the medium, as the addition of counterions reduces repulsion between anionic hydrophilic head groups, which makes micellization favorable at low concentrations [82]. Recently, enhancement action of C_{10} and sodium dodecyl sulphate (SDS) was increased in hypotonic conditions (achieved with NaCl) in a single-pass intestinal perfusion in rats [83], an effect that could relate to a reduction in the CMC. In the case of ionizable surfactants that contain weakly acidic or weakly basic hydrophilic head groups, alteration to pH can transform a surfactant from its soluble form to its insoluble form, which although still capable of lowering surface tension, has reduced capacity to act as a detergent.

Divalent cations such as calcium found in milk can decrease the permeation enhancement of anionic surfactants through precipitation of inactive salts [84]. On the other hand, alteration to pH may increase permeation enhancement. For example, reduction in the regional pH with an amphoteric surfactant may increase the proportion of the surfactant in the cationic form, which is likely to have a greater affect. Additionally, it has been proposed that co-solvents that increase the solubility of insoluble surfactants can improve aqueous solubility and enable greater interaction with the cell membrane [66]. Several other factors may modulate the free surfactant concentration within the small intestine. These include adsorption to undigested solid particles and oil droplets and incorporation into colloidal structures (e.g., mixed micelles with free fatty acids and bile salts). Depending on the quantity and type of materials within the GI tract, free surfactant monomers may be efficiently replenished from micelles, but as the window for efficient enhancement can be shortened by dilution, spreading, and absorption of the PE itself, the availability of surfactant within that window may be quickly diluted. Phospholipid and bile salt constituents of simulated intestinal media can attenuate the effects of alkyl maltopyranosides through the formation of mixed micelles [67]. Fasted state simulated intestinal media (FaSSIF) containing taurocholate, phosphatidylcholine in buffered isosmotic buffer salt solution (pH 7.1) also attenuated the permeation enhancement of palmitoylcarnitine and hexyphosphocholine surfactants in Caco-2 monolayers [85]. In the same study, FaSSIF did not affect the enhancement action of non-surfactant PEs, EDTA and 3-nitrocoumarin. In some cases, mixing surfactants can increase enhancement action still further [86]. Combinations of medium chain fatty acids with PEG-8 glycerides increased permeation of FD4 across isolated rat intestinal tissue by 10-fold over the respective individual agents [87].

A recent study assessed the effect of FaSSIF and fed state simulated intestinal fluid (FeSSIF on the absorption of BCS Class I, II and III drugs in a single pass intestinal perfusion (Roos et al., submitted). Even in the absence of PEs, there was a significant difference in the absorption of atenolol, enalaprilat, ketoprofen, and metoprolol between FaSSIF and FeSSIF. This result was not surprising as an analysis of 92 clinical datasets found that 67% of BCS Class I drugs had no food effect, 71% of Class II had a positive food effect, and 61% of BCS Class III had an adverse food effect [88]. Additionally, there is evidence of reduced drug absorption in rats when metoprolol was perfused in aspirated fed state intestinal fluids compared to fasted state aspirates [89]. Absorption of selected PE active combinations were reduced in FeSSIF, which the authors attributed to the presence of colloidal structures formed by lecithin and bile acids in FeSSIF (Roos et al., submitted). Surfactant PEs have potential to emulsify dietary lipids and can form mixed micelles with both soluble (e.g., bile salts, ionized free fatty acids) and insoluble surfactant (glycerides, phospholipids), and as the CMC of these mixed micelles is typically lower than the native surfactant, these structures are capable of lowering the sufficient quantity of free monomeric surfactant that is available to perturb membranes. A conclusion is that luminal surfactants can exert a protective effect against mucosal perturbation by ionizable surfactants. It is noteworthy that the presence of a luminal surfactant does not change the CMC of the PE, so if there is a large excess of PE over the luminal surfactants, it will exist in the molecular form at its CMC and will therefore be available to exhibit transcellular perturbation.

Further work is required to determine the effect of luminal composition on the absorption of soluble macromolecules and the enhancement action of PEs. A question arising from studies showing the effect of luminal constituents on PE actions is what constitutes the typical composition within the GI tract? Given the variability in free fatty acid, lipids, and bile salts in human intestinal fluid [90], it may be difficult to precisely identify the type and amount of substances that must be included in the SIF for permeability studies. Additionally, it remains unclear whether there is a substantial difference in the concentration and type of constituents in bulk luminal fluid and local extrinsic mucus gel layer.

Therefore, it is also unclear if SIF for permeability testing should represent bulk luminal fluid (and hence mirror dissolution media), or whether it should mirror the composition of the extrinsic mucus gel layer. In addition, it is difficult to use SIFs designed for dissolution testing [91] in cell- or tissue-based in vitro assays, as several constituents of intestinal fluid (e.g., bile acids, phospholipids, and free fatty acids) are themselves capable of altering permeability and causing local perturbation. There have been efforts to develop biorelevant media that do not alter the viability or barrier integrity of Caco-2 monolayers over short periods [92]. By necessity there are reductions in the concentrations of bile salts in the SIF used in vitro compared to intestinal aspirates (e.g., free fatty acids). Other investigators have opted to use full biorelevant media and overcome damage to Caco-2 monolayers using overlying biosimilar mucus [93,94]. It may be that studies with SIF should begin with more robust in situ models such as the rat single pass intestinal perfusion [83,95,96]. More research assessing the effect of PEs in SIF would also help investigators understand how a growing number of lipoidal dispersions improve intestinal permeability (e.g., TPE^{TM}, Chiasma, Ness Ziona, Israel [17]).

4.10. Improving PE Action in the Dynamic GI Tract

Of those PE that have been assessed in oral formulation of macromolecules in clinical trials, only a modest single digit increase in oral BA has ever been observed. The majority of PEs are effective in static delivery models, where the PE and active are co-delivered in liquid dosage forms to cells, isolated tissues or tied intestinal loops for extended periods. In these models, the PE and active are typically presented to the epithelial surface above a threshold concentration for an extended period of several hours. This provides the PE sufficient time to alter barrier integrity in the presence of a high concentration gradient of both macromolecule and PE. These optimal conditions do not prevail in the human GI tract following oral delivery of a solid dosage form (Figure 2).

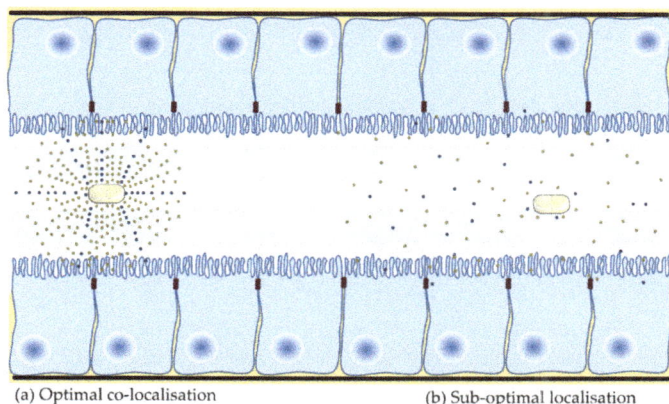

(a) Optimal co-localisation   (b) Sub-optimal localisation

Figure 2. Presentation of PE and active at the small intestinal mucosa. (**a**) Co-localization of PE and active at the intestinal epithelium ensures that the PE is present at a high concentration and is present for long enough to alter barrier integrity. (**b**) A high local concentration of active provides the drive force for intestinal flux. A low release rate and more gradual dissolution of PE dosage forms, fast transit, spreading and dilution in luminal fluid and interaction with constituents of luminal fluid will impede optimal co-localization because the concentration of both are ultimately not high enough.

Few published studies assess the effect of PEs in oral dosage forms. The majority of oral peptide dosage forms in clinical development are enteric coated, and so that active and PE are co-released in the small intestine. Relatively quick transit along the small intestine attenuates enhancement in the GI lumen as the PE requires time at a focal point within the lumen to alter integrity and facilitate permeation of the macromolecule, while not being too rapidly absorbed itself (as is the case with C_{10}

and SNAC). This is problematic for all PEs, in particular, those that do not cause a rapid decrease in barrier integrity. Investigators have shown that confining PE and macromolecule over a focussed area [97] and the synchronous co-release of both in high concentration in a short period [78,98,99] can improve enhancement. The fluid volume within the stomach and small intestine is another potential variable. Intestinal fluid is not homogeneously spread across the small intestine, it forms fluid-filled pockets of varying number and volume [100], which may give rise to variable absorption. This is because dissolution of PE in a small volume will lead to greater enhancement action than if the PE is dissolved in a larger fluid volume. As there has been little research assessing the effect of release metrics on permeability, it follows that few delivery technologies have been developed to improve localization of PE and active at the intestinal epithelium. Initial experimental strategies tested include mucoadhesives, superporous hydrogels [101], electronic capsules (e.g., IntelliCap^{TM} [102]), controlled release of PE [98,103,104], intestinal patches (Section 4.11) and pharmacological motility (e.g., loperamide). Overall, the goal of optimizing co-presentation aims to create a diffusion gradient to improve the rate and extent of enhancement action and all PEs to reach and sustain a threshold concentration required to improve intestinal flux.

Dissolution of the PE and active is another factor that must be considered for effective translation. Peptides often exhibit their lowest solubility at the isoelectric point (pI) and greatest solubility at pH values below the pI owing to ionization of basic side chains in acidic conditions. Insulin (pI 5.5) for example, dissolves well in acidic media, but has low solubility at neutral pH. Peptides with low potency and low intrinsic solubility may dissolve more slowly in the small intestine, which may lower the concentration gradient that drives flux. Gradual dissolution may prevent a PE from reaching and sustaining a threshold local concentration for enhancement (e.g., chitosan [105], medium chain fatty acids [106]). Investigators have attempted to improve release through the inclusion of disintegrants [97], or via formulation as liquids [46].

4.11. Intestinal Patches to Co-Localise PE and Active

Intestinal patches are a more recent strategy for localization of poorly permeable solutes at the small intestinal epithelium. Some of the earliest patches did not include PEs [107], but their inclusion in more recent iterations suggests they may be required for optimal patch performance. Assessment of a 13 mm patches (coated on one side with ethyl cellulose backing) in Caco-2 monolayers showed a modest two-fold enhancement of insulin and exenatide flux [108]. In the same study, there was significant absorption of insulin in patches, especially those that contained the PE, dimethyl palmitoyl ammonio propanesulfonate (PPS) (0.5% w/v). Other PEs incorporated into patches include SDS, polyoxyethylene hydrogenated castor oil 60 [109], thiolated polycarbophils [110] and Labrasol® [111]. Patches are delivered in enteric-coated capsules, so there are no compaction forces associated with tableting. More recently, patches have been miniaturized into micropatch formats, which offer a large surface area for absorption. Oral delivery of capsules containing micropatches (50 U/kg insulin and 0.2 mg PPS) admixed with citric acid (15 mg) decreased plasma glucose in rats by 22% compared to a drop of 54% with free insulin (1 U/kg, s.c.) [112]. Further optimization is required to ensure adequate adhesion within the GI tract and optimal retention at the mucosal surface.

4.12. Is Safety of PEs a Real Impediment to Translation?

Safety is a widely held concern to the application of PEs in oral delivery (reviewed in [113]). This concern can be sub-categorized into those related to individual or sub-classes of compounds and concerns relating to modulation of intestinal barrier integrity on a chronic basis. Over 250 compounds have been shown to alter intestinal permeability, but only about a dozen of these are realistic candidate PEs for clinical trials. The reversible modulation of TJ opening might be viewed as a safer approach to improving permeation relative to transcellular membrane perturbation.

The first-generation TJ modulators acted via intracellular cell signaling pathways which alter TJ architecture from within epithelial cells. There are risks related to PEs that alter permeability through ubiquitous cell signaling processes such as protein kinase C [114]. Although additional pharmacological effects observed with currently 'allowed' excipients, this is secondary to a primary action, examples including depression of the CNS (e.g., ethyl alcohol), inhibition of metabolic enzymes and transporters (D-alpha-tocopherol polyethylene glycol 1000 succinate [115], and Cremophor EL [116]) and interference with metabolic enzymes [116]. Most second-generation paracellular PEs selectively disrupt the interaction between TJ proteins in adjacent cells [8], although the consequences of modulating TJ at other barriers is not yet entirely clear [9].

The alternative is to use surfactant-based PEs that increase permeation via transcellular perturbation. High concentrations of these additives often cause temporary mild local mucosal injury, but when diluted are less likely to reach the high concentrations required for cell perturbation at other sites within the body even if absorbed. Additionally, some leading candidates in this category have food additive (e.g., C_{10}) or GRAS status (e.g., SNAC) or are pharmaceutical excipients (e.g., sucrose esters). There may be a relatively low risk of systemic toxicity for such surfactants, although there are ongoing concerns related to local mucosal perturbation. The majority of evidence to date suggests that surfactant PEs do not possess a discrete mechanism of action; instead they act by directly compromising the integrity of enterocyte plasma membranes. This category of PE has been assessed extensively in clinical trials over the last 20 years, and while there have been no major adverse events reported, there has also been only a modest effect on oral BA in most trials. It remains to be seen if new technologies designed to improve residence of PE and active at a focal point within the intestinal lumen may result in more histological damage. It is difficult to determine if PEs cause histological damage at the site of release in the human GI tract, owing to difficulty pinpointing the site of release and performing a biopsy within the enhancement window and before epithelial repair. In one of the few clinical trials assessing the effect of PEs on histology score within the GI tract, administration of Doktacillin™ suppositories (ampicillin (250 mg), C_{10} (25 mg) and hard fat (950 mg, Pharmasol™ B-105, NOF Corp. Shibuya-ku, Tokyo, Japan)) improved rectal BA of ampicillin from 13 to 23% [117]. Doktacillin™ suppositories caused a significant increase in the average histology score from 0.62 in the control group (before administration) to a score of 1.94 after administration of the suppository (25 min). The average histology score measured three hours after administration of Doktacillin™ was 0.96, suggesting the barrier can repair from mucosal perturbation. The authors note that C_{10} itself and hyperosmolarity of the rectal fluid contribute to the histological damage score. Irrespective of whether C_{10} causes hyperosmolarity, exposure time in the rectum is longer than any equivalent segment of the small intestine owing to longer residence time. There is also a higher concentration of PE due to a lower amount of rectal fluid than in other intestinal segments. To allay fears over chronic daily use of PEs, some may be confined to administrations with a different dosing regimen. Some PE formulations tested in trials include for example, a once-weekly tablet zoledronic acid with C_{10} (Orazol®, Merrion Pharma, Ireland [118]), which would provide time for recovery of barrier integrity. Nonetheless, time to recovery from PEs that cause mild mucosal perturbation does not seem to be a problem in clinical trials so far (e.g., daily administration of semaglutide with SNAC [28]). To date, there has been no evidence of intestinal problems that are unrelated to the GLP-1 class in any oral semaglutide trials performed.

It is tempting to justify the use of PEs that cause mild reversible mucosal damage by citing precedence for the use of substances that cause GI disturbances. Regarding medicines approval, it is not possible to justify the use of PEs that act to improve flux via transcellular perturbation by citing the side effects of drugs, excipients or food additives. However, a PE may not be listed as such in any given formulation, and therefore their use may be more comparable to other additives that have been shown to cause membrane perturbation in vitro (e.g., surfactants [119]). Comparison of PEs to established excipients does help to show that mild mucosal perturbation may be common.

There is concern that altering the integrity of the intestinal epithelium, irrespective of mode of action, may facilitate colonization of epithelial cells and invasion of deeper tissues by opportunistic pathogens. While there is no evidence to date that oral PE-macromolecule dosage forms cause infections in clinical trials, it is important to mention that if this is true risk, then potential clinical manifestations range from asymptomatic infection to diarrhea, to more serious infections depending on the micro-organism and host genetic variability [120]. This concern would seem to be more plausible for PEs that cause reversible mucosal damage, and not TJ modulators, because the maximum opening of the TJ is far smaller than the diameter of a bacterium [121]. Compromising the integrity of the intestinal mucosae is more likely to facilitate the translation of microorganisms. In Caco-2 monolayers, co-incubation of octyl phenol ethoxylate (Triton X-100) with *E. coli* increased translocation, although whether such translocation occurs in vivo has not been assessed [118].

There is the additional concern that other luminal bystanders may be translocated within the enhancement window. There is evidence that ischemia can increase levels of plasma lipopolysaccharide (LPS) [122] which may contribute to septic shock [123]. Given that PEs cause only a modest uptake of small peptides co-localised in the formulation, it seems unlikely that large luminal xenobiotics (such as LPS or LPS fragments) that are spread diffusely across the GI lumen would be appreciably absorbed. Again, this potential issue may be less likely for PEs that act via the opening of TJs, as the diameter of an open junction within the small intestine is estimated to be 10 nm [84]. It is noteworthy however, that altered expression of the TJ protein claudin is associated with intestinal bowel disorders [124]. The surfactants hexadecylphosphocholine and octylphenol ethoxylate increase permeation of LPS across Caco-2 monolayers [125]. Co-delivery of C_{10} (154 mM) or penetratin (2 mM) with LPS to mice for seven consecutive days did not cause LPS induced hepatic damage, as measured by plasma levels of alanine aminotransferase (ALT) and aspartate aminotransferase (AST) which are both released during hepatic necrosis [126]. A significant elevation in those enzymes was observed when LPS was co-delivered with taurodeoxycholate (96 mM) in the same study. However, as there was no control treatment in the absence of LPS it remains unclear whether elevated levels of hepatic necrosis markers relate to LPS or PE only. There is also evidence from a controversial study that prolonged exposure of two common emulsifiers (polysorbate 80 and carboxymethyl cellulose) causes low-grade inflammation in healthy mice and colitis in predisposed mice via altering the microbiome [127]. It is not known if these findings have any relevance for human exposure to excipients.

4.13. Convergence between Delivery Concepts, Intestinal Physiology, and Formulation Science

In order to address the hurdles to translation, there must be convergence between delivery concepts, intestinal physiology, and formulation. The material and physicochemical properties of the PE must be considered more; especially as PEs can be a significant proportion of the formulations. As noted in Section 4.6, it can be challenging to incorporate liquid or semi-solid PEs into oral dosage forms. Salts of ionizable surfactants are more readily incorporated into tablets. However, there remains the likely requirement for other excipients in the formulation, which in some instances may require a reduction in the quantity of PE to accommodate these additives. The type of formulation and process additives and their quantity in the final manufacturable scalable dosage form are important considerations as delivery researchers begin to assess optimal luminal presentation, be it for immediate release or controlled release. There are also practical considerations in the progression of PEs to clinical testing, such as availability of GMP grade material or a specification. There is the requirement for extensive information in any regulatory submission, including details of manufacture and purification procedures, extensive physical and chemical properties of any new PE and provision of supporting safety data (non-clinical/clinical).

Reliable animal models are prerequisite for identification of promising macromolecule drug delivery systems that have potential to translate to humans. There is variability between key anatomical and physiological parameters in humans and those observed in rats, pigs and dogs (Table 3). These include differences in gastric emptying time, gastric retention time, absolute water content, transit time, local pH, gut length, mucous thickness, and average stomach capacity [128,129]. It is possible to purchase minicapsules and manufacture minitablets for oral delivery to rats, but there are additional challenges. In the case of minicapsules it can be difficult to load sufficient levels of PE into the capsule shell without prior granulation (e.g., by roll compaction) and these formulations are difficult to enteric coat by manual dip coating (thus necessitating the use of specialist coating equipment). It is possible to purchase single- or multi-tip tooling for the preparation of minitablets, although this requires specialist tableting equipment (granulator, spray coater, and tablet press) and expertise in formulation and process development. There are very few studies where complete dosage forms are administered to rodents, and therefore the formulation factors that impact translation are rarely assessed in this widely used animal model. There is the argument that formulations administered to rats have little relevance to formats tested in larger animals and humans, and there is therefore a need for studies in more representative animals and humans. Nevertheless, if the impediments to translation of PE dosage forms can be partially optimized in rodent models, this could better inform development of formulations in humans. Oral peptide research in rodents typically involves oral gavage of liquid mixtures and not dosage forms tested in humans. This is the same for rat in situ static intestinal instillations, which help identify PEs in ad-mixtures with payloads, but do not offer information on transit time, fluid volume, pH conditions within the small intestine nor do they adequately model dissolution of PE dosage forms. Hence, translation of results from rats to humans is limited by fundamental anatomical and physiological differences in intestinal length (1.8 m versus 5.9 m [128]), transit time in the fed (20 h versus 4 h [130]) and water volume (0.06 g/cm gut length versus 0.58 g/cm [130]).

Dosage forms of similar dimensions to those used in humans are amenable to administration in dogs and pigs. However, as there are longer gastric emptying times in these animals, immediate release PE dosage forms intended to increase flux within the stomach (e.g., semaglutide) could be more effective in dogs and pigs owing to greater residence time (localization of PE and active), although such data may not be replicated in humans due to shorter residence times. In the case of enteric coated macromolecule formulations, longer gastric emptying times in pigs and dogs may result in a longer delay to onset of drug absorption compared to humans. The pH in the stomach of healthy fasted dogs is highly variable (pH 1–8) [129,131], leading some investigators to pre-administer an acidic solution containing 0.1 M HCl and 0.1 M KCl [132] or the hormone pentagastrin to stimulate endogenous acid secretion [133]. Both approaches aim to standardize the pH prior to oral administration to animals. In the absence of pH adjustment, the stomach of dogs may not adequately model release of enteric-coated oral peptide formulations. In the small intestine, transit time is shorter by half in dogs compared to humans and pigs. Faster transit reduces the absorption window for drugs, which gives rise to differences in oral BA. As the importance of local GI retention of PE and macromolecule is requisite for efficient enhancement, study of PEs in dogs may underestimate the action of these additives. Further interspecies divergence is observed at the intestinal epithelium, where mucous thickness is appreciably larger in dogs compared to humans. The anatomy physiology and diet of pigs closely aligns to humans [134], and in some aspects (but not all aspects, e.g., gastric residence time) pigs are considered an appropriate model to assess GI permeability [133]. The composition of enterocyte membranes in different animal models [128] could also play a role in different susceptibility to surfactant PEs [9]. It is also worth emphasizing that there can be differences in GI physiology in different disease states [135], which could also influence the action of PEs.

Interspecies differences highlight that the best model of human is human [136], nevertheless combinations of animal models are still relevant for optimization of oral PE macromolecule formulations and ultimately translation into effective dosage forms in man. Although most oral peptide formulations fail to progress to clinical evaluation, poor translation between animal models and humans is likely to be one of many reasons. There is nearly always higher BA in open- and closed-loop instillations and single pass intestinal perfusion compared to oral dosage forms, but these models still provide a necessary first hurdle with a relatively low bar; it is then the challenge for formulation and delivery researchers to develop technologies that recreate such presentation in appropriate oral dosage forms.

Table 3. Potential effects of GI physiology in different animals on the action of PEs.

Anatomical/Physiological Property	Species	Influence on PE Action
Gastric emptying time (h)	Human: 1 h [130] Rat: 0.7–2.1 h [130] Dog: 3.9–5.3 h [130] Pig: 1.5–6 h [130]	For immediate release dosage forms, slower gastric emptying in pig and dog than in humans may increase gastric residence time of PE and payload, thus overestimating enhancement. For enteric dosage forms, slower gastric emptying, may delay dissolution in the GI tract and ultimately increase Tmax in these species versus humans.
Gastric fluid volume (mL)	Human: 118 mL [137] Rat: 2.29 [137] Dog: 500–1000 mL [137] Pig: 278 mL [137]	For immediate release dosage forms, the larger volume in dogs may result in greater dilution of PE to below a threshold for enhancement action, thereby underestimating enhancement.
Stomach pH	Human: 1.7 [128] Rat: 3.9 [138] Dog: 1.5 [128] Pig: 1.7 [128]	As many PEs that have progressed to clinical testing in oral formulations are weak acid surfactants, differences in solubility can be observed if there is variation in gastric pH. This gives rise to differences in enhancement as acidic surfactants are more effective in their ionizable form at high pH.
Small intestine transit time (Fasted state) (time (h) and length (m))	Human: 3–4 h [139] Human: 6.25 m [137] Rat: 4–5 h [128] Rat: 0.34 m [137] Dog: 1.5 h [137] Dog: 2.48 m [137] Pig: 3–4 h [137] Pig: 14.2 m [137]	Faster transit may reduce the exposure of PE and payload at the epithelium, thereby reducing enhancement, and potentially underestimating the effects of the PE. A short transit time does not strictly mean faster movement, as length of the small intestine is different in different species.
Small intestine fluid volume (total and g/cm)	Human: 212 mL [137] Human: 0.6 g/cm [130] Rat: 3.9 mL [137] Rat: 0.06 g/cm [130] Dog: 300 mL [137] Dog: 0.9 [130] Pig: 476 mL [137] Pig: 0.62 [130]	Differences in fluid volume, or more specifically the volume and number of intestinal fluid pockets in the small intestine could lead to differences in the regional concentration of PE and payload, as well as differences in dissolution rate. This could lead to under- or overestimation of enhancement.
Duodenal mucus thickness (μm)	Human: 15.5 μm [137] Rat: 30.6 μm [137] Dog: — Pig: 25.6 μm [137]	Difference in the thickness of the protective mucus gel layer overlying the epithelium has potential to modulate enhancement.
Small intestine diameter	Human: 5 cm [137] Rat: 2.5–3 mm [137] Dog: — Pig: —	The diameter of the intestinal lumen may impact the proximity of enteric formulations to the epithelium and ultimately impact co-localization of PE and payload.
Plasma membrane phospholipid composition of intestinal epithelium	Human: — Rat: — Dog: — Pig: —	There are differences in phospholipid composition in different species [128], which may impact sensitivity to perturbation by surfactant PEs

5. Conclusions

Discovery of safe, effective, and formulation-compatible PEs for oral delivery of macromolecules has been a priority for investigators. Research on PEs has branched into the discovery of agents that target opening of TJs [47] or using substances with established use in humans [106]. Recent studies have examined (i) the behavior of PEs and acidifiers in the intestinal lumen, (ii) factors that impact enhancement within the dynamic environment in the GI tract in vivo (e.g., intestinal fluid, tonicity, exposure time), (iii) physiochemical properties of PEs that give rise to enhancement, (iv) effect of PE combinations, and (v) learnings from clinical investigations [140,141]. These studies have highlighted the need for greater emphasis on the hurdles to translation, in particular, development of concepts to optimize the co-presentation of PE and macromolecule payload in high concentration for as long as possible at the intestinal wall. Greater focus on this area may improve the likelihood of translation.

Funding: This research received no external funding. Work by DB relating to the subject matter is part-funded Science Foundation Ireland Centre for Medical Devices (CURAM) under grant agreement 13/RC/20173.

Acknowledgments: The research performed in Figure 1 and Table 2 was performed by an Erasmus Exchange student (Ninon Chardon).

Conflicts of Interest: D.J.B. declares consultancies in the past 5 years to the following companies relating to the subject matter: Sanofi, Lilly, MedImmune, Astra-Zeneca, Boehringer-Ingelheim, Chiasma, and Merck. S.M. declares consultancy for Entrega. The other authors declare no conflict of interest.

References

1. Kola, I.; Landis, J. Can the pharmaceutical industry reduce attrition rates? *Nat. Rev. Drug Discov.* **2004**, *3*, 711. [CrossRef] [PubMed]
2. Waring, M.J.; Arrowsmith, J.; Leach, A.R.; Leeson, P.D.; Mandrell, S.; Owen, R.M.; Pairaudeau, G.; Pennie, W.D.; Pickett, S.D.; Wang, J.; et al. An analysis of the attrition of drug candidates from four major pharmaceutical companies. *Nat. Rev. Drug Discov.* **2015**, *14*, 475–486. [CrossRef] [PubMed]
3. Barton, P.; Riley, R.J. A new paradigm for navigating compound property related drug attrition. *Drug Discov. Today* **2016**, *21*, 72–81. [CrossRef]
4. Leeson, P.D. Molecular inflation, attrition and the rule of five. *Adv. Drug Deliv. Rev.* **2016**, *101*, 22–33. [CrossRef] [PubMed]
5. Crew, M.; Lipinski, C. Where to Invest? The Drug or the Delivery System? American Association of Pharmaceutical Scientists Blog. 2016. Available online: https://aapsblog.aaps.org/2016/11/05/where-to-invest-the-drug-or-the-delivery-system/#more-9226 (accessed on 17 January 2019).
6. Buckley, S. Oral Semaglutide: Delivering new possibilities in the treatment of diabetes. In Proceedings of the Annual Meeting and Exposition of the Controlled Release Society (Oral Peptide Workshop), New York, NY, USA, 22–24 July 2018.
7. Maher, S. An Outlook on Oral Peptide Delivery. AAPS Blog. 2017. Available online: https://aapsblog.aaps.org/2017/02/08/an-outlook-on-oral-peptide-delivery/#more-9531 (accessed on 17 January 2019).
8. Kondoh, M.; Yoshida, T.; Kakutani, H.; Yagi, K. Targeting tight junction proteins-significance for drug development. *Drug Discov. Today* **2008**, *13*, 180–186. [CrossRef] [PubMed]
9. Maher, S.; Mrsny, R.J.; Brayden, D.J. Intestinal Permeation Enhancers for Oral Peptide Delivery. *Adv. Drug Deliv. Rev.* **2016**, *106*, 277–319. [CrossRef] [PubMed]
10. Eichner, M.; Protze, J.; Piontek, A.; Krause, G.; Piontek, J. Targeting and alteration of tight junctions by bacteria and their virulence factors such as Clostridium perfringens enterotoxin. *Pflügers Arch. Eur. J. Physiol.* **2017**, *469*, 77–90. [CrossRef] [PubMed]
11. Eldor, R.; Arbit, E.; Corcos, A.; Kidron, M. Glucose-reducing effect of the ORMD-0801 oral insulin preparation in patients with uncontrolled type 1 diabetes: A pilot study. *PLoS ONE* **2013**, *8*, e59524. [CrossRef]
12. Zupančič, O.; Bernkop-Schnürch, A. Lipophilic peptide character—What oral barriers fear the most. *J. Control. Release* **2017**, *255*, 242–257. [CrossRef]
13. Maher, S.; Heade, J.; McCartney, F.; Waters, S.; Bleiel, S.B.; Brayden, D.J. Effects of surfactant-based permeation enhancers on mannitol permeability, histology, and electrogenic ion transport responses in excised rat colonic mucosae. *Int. J. Pharm.* **2018**, *539*, 11–22. [CrossRef]
14. Perinelli, D.R.; Cespi, M.; Casettari, L.; Vllasaliu, D.; Cangiotti, M.; Ottaviani, M.F.; Giorgioni, G.; Bonacucina, G.; Palmieri, G.F. Correlation among chemical structure, surface properties and cytotoxicity of N-acyl alanine and serine surfactants. *Eur. J. Pharm. Biopharm.* **2016**, *109*, 93–102. [CrossRef] [PubMed]
15. Lee, Y.-H.; Sinko, P.J. Oral delivery of salmon calcitonin. *Adv. Drug Deliv. Rev.* **2000**, *42*, 225–238. [CrossRef]
16. Leonard, T.W.; Lynch, J.; McKenna, M.J.; Brayden, D.J. Promoting absorption of drugs in humans using medium-chain fatty acid-based solid dosage forms: GIPET. *Expert Opin. Drug Deliv.* **2006**, *3*, 685–692. [CrossRef]
17. Tuvia, S.; Pelled, D.; Marom, K.; Salama, P.; Levin-Arama, M.; Karmeli, I.; Idelson, G.H.; Landau, I.; Mamluk, R. A novel suspension formulation enhances intestinal absorption of macromolecules via transient and reversible transport mechanisms. *Pharm. Res.* **2014**, *31*, 2010–2021. [CrossRef] [PubMed]

18. Khedkar, A.; Iyer, H.; Anand, A.; Verma, M.; Krishnamurthy, S.; Savale, S.; Atignal, A. A dose range finding study of novel oral insulin (IN-105) under fed conditions in type 2 diabetes mellitus subjects. *Diabetes Obes. Metab.* **2010**, *12*, 659–664. [CrossRef] [PubMed]
19. Cilek, A.; Celebi, N.; Tirnaksiz, F. Lecithin-based microemulsion of a peptide for oral administration: Preparation, characterization, and physical stability of the formulation. *Drug Deliv.* **2006**, *13*, 19–24. [CrossRef]
20. Blikslager, A.T.; Moeser, A.J.; Gookin, J.L.; Jones, S.L.; Odle, J. Restoration of barrier function in injured intestinal mucosa. *Physiol. Rev.* **2007**, *87*, 545–564. [CrossRef]
21. Brayden, D.J.; Gleeson, J.; Walsh, E.G. A head-to-head multi-parametric high content analysis of a series of medium chain fatty acid intestinal permeation enhancers in Caco-2 cells. *Eur. J. Pharm. Biopharm.* **2014**, *88*, 830–839. [CrossRef]
22. Matsuura, J.; Powers, M.E.; Manning, M.C.; Shefter, E. Structure and stability of insulin dissolved in 1-octanol. *J. Am. Chem. Soc.* **1993**, *115*, 1261–1264. [CrossRef]
23. Zupancic, O.; Leonaviciute, G.; Lam, H.T.; Partenhauser, A.; Podricnik, S.; Bernkop-Schnurch, A. Development and in vitro evaluation of an oral SEDDS for desmopressin. *Drug Deliv.* **2016**, *23*, 2074–2083. [CrossRef]
24. Bonengel, S.; Jelkmann, M.; Abdulkarim, M.; Gumbleton, M.; Reinstadler, V.; Oberacher, H.; Prufert, F.; Bernkop-Schnurch, A. Impact of different hydrophobic ion pairs of octreotide on its oral bioavailability in pigs. *J. Control. Release* **2018**, *273*, 21–29. [CrossRef] [PubMed]
25. Menzel, C.; Holzeisen, T.; Laffleur, F.; Zaichik, S.; Abdulkarim, M.; Gumbleton, M.; Bernkop-Schnurch, A. In vivo evaluation of an oral self-emulsifying drug delivery system (SEDDS) for exenatide. *J. Control. Release* **2018**, *277*, 165–172. [CrossRef] [PubMed]
26. Goldberg, M.; Gomez-Orellana, I. Challenges for the oral delivery of macromolecules. *Nat. Rev. Drug Discov.* **2003**, *2*, 289–295. [CrossRef] [PubMed]
27. Castelli, M.C.; Friedman, K.; Sherry, J.; Brazzillo, K.; Genoble, L.; Bhargava, P.; Riley, M.G.I. Comparing the Efficacy and Tolerability of a New Daily Oral Vitamin B12 Formulation and Intermittent Intramuscular Vitamin B12 in Normalizing Low Cobalamin Levels: A Randomized, Open-Label, Parallel-Group Study. *Clin. Ther.* **2011**, *33*, 358–371. [CrossRef] [PubMed]
28. Davies, M.; Pieber, T.R.; Hartoft-Nielsen, M.L.; Hansen, O.K.H.; Jabbour, S.; Rosenstock, J. Effect of Oral Semaglutide Compared With Placebo and Subcutaneous Semaglutide on Glycemic Control in Patients With Type 2 Diabetes: A Randomized Clinical Trial. *JAMA* **2017**, *318*, 1460–1470. [CrossRef] [PubMed]
29. Karsdal, M.A.; Byrjalsen, I.; Alexandersen, P.; Bihlet, A.; Andersen, J.R.; Riis, B.J.; Bay-Jensen, A.C.; Christiansen, C. Treatment of symptomatic knee osteoarthritis with oral salmon calcitonin: Results from two phase 3 trials. *Osteoarthr. Cartil.* **2015**, *23*, 532–543. [CrossRef] [PubMed]
30. Lindgren, M.E.; Hallbrink, M.M.; Elmquist, A.M.; Langel, U. Passage of cell-penetrating peptides across a human epithelial cell layer in vitro. *Biochem. J.* **2004**, *377*, 69–76. [CrossRef]
31. Kamei, N.; Shigei, C.; Hasegawa, R.; Takeda-Morishita, M. Exploration of the Key Factors for Optimizing the in Vivo Oral Delivery of Insulin by Using a Noncovalent Strategy with Cell-Penetrating Peptides. *Biol. Pharm. Bull.* **2018**, *41*, 239–246. [CrossRef]
32. Guidotti, G.; Brambilla, L.; Rossi, D. Cell-Penetrating Peptides: From Basic Research to Clinics. *Trends Pharmacol. Sci.* **2017**, *38*, 406–424. [CrossRef]
33. Rehmani, S.; Dixon, J.E. Oral delivery of anti-diabetes therapeutics using cell penetrating and transcytosing peptide strategies. *Peptides* **2018**, *100*, 24–35. [CrossRef]
34. Lewis, A.L.; Richard, J. Challenges in the delivery of peptide drugs: An industry perspective. *Ther. Deliv.* **2015**, *6*, 149–163. [CrossRef] [PubMed]
35. Dhillon, S. Semaglutide: First Global Approval. *Drugs* **2018**, *78*, 275–284. [CrossRef] [PubMed]
36. Feeney, O.M.; Crum, M.F.; McEvoy, C.L.; Trevaskis, N.L.; Williams, H.D.; Pouton, C.W.; Charman, W.N.; Bergström, C.A.S.; Porter, C.J.H. 50 years of oral lipid-based formulations: Provenance, progress and future perspectives. *Adv. Drug Deliv. Rev.* **2016**, *101*, 167–194. [CrossRef] [PubMed]
37. Benet, L.Z.; Cummins, C.L. The drug efflux-metabolism alliance: Biochemical aspects. *Adv. Drug Deliv. Rev.* **2001**, *50* (Suppl. 1), S3–S11. [CrossRef]
38. Maher, S.; Ryan, B.; Duffy, A.; Brayden, D.J. Formulation strategies to improve oral peptide delivery. *Pharm. Pat. Anal.* **2014**, *3*, 313–336. [CrossRef]

39. Mahmood, A.; Bernkop-Schnurch, A. SEDDS: A game changing approach for the oral administration of hydrophilic macromolecular drugs. *Adv. Drug Deliv. Rev.* **2018**. [CrossRef] [PubMed]

40. Cheng, T.; Zhao, Y.; Li, X.; Lin, F.; Xu, Y.; Zhang, X.; Li, Y.; Wang, R.; Lai, L. Computation of Octanol−Water Partition Coefficients by Guiding an Additive Model with Knowledge. *J. Chem. Inf. Model.* **2007**, *47*, 2140–2148. [CrossRef]

41. Buckley, S.T.; Bækdal, T.A.; Vegge, A.; Maarbjerg, S.J.; Pyke, C.; Ahnfelt-Rønne, J.; Madsen, K.G.; Schéele, S.G.; Alanentalo, T.; Kirk, R.K.; et al. Transcellular stomach absorption of a derivatized glucagon-like peptide-1 receptor agonist. *Sci. Transl. Med.* **2018**, *10*, eaar7047. [CrossRef]

42. Novo Nordisk AS. Tablet Formulation Comprising Semaglutide and a Delivery Agent. U.S. Patent US9993430B2, 12 June 2018.

43. Hjerpsted, J.B.; Flint, A.; Brooks, A.; Axelsen, M.B.; Kvist, T.; Blundell, J. Semaglutide improves postprandial glucose and lipid metabolism, and delays first-hour gastric emptying in subjects with obesity. *Diabetes Obes. Metab.* **2018**, *20*, 610–619. [CrossRef]

44. Banerjee, A.; Ibsen, K.; Brown, T.; Chen, R.; Agatemor, C.; Mitragotri, S. Ionic liquids for oral insulin delivery. *Proc. Natl. Acad. Sci. USA* **2018**, *115*, 7296–7301. [CrossRef]

45. Frade, R.F.M.; Matias, A.; Branco, L.C.; Afonso, C.A.M.; Duarte, C.M.M. Effect of ionic liquids on human colon carcinoma HT-29 and CaCo-2 cell lines. *Green Chem.* **2007**, *9*, 873–877. [CrossRef]

46. Novo Nordisk AS. Stable Non-Aqueous Pharmaceutical Compositions. U.S. Patent US20100190706, 29 July 2010.

47. Taverner, A.; Dondi, R.; Almansour, K.; Laurent, F.; Owens, S.E.; Eggleston, I.M.; Fotaki, N.; Mrsny, R.J. Enhanced paracellular transport of insulin can be achieved via transient induction of myosin light chain phosphorylation. *J. Control. Release* **2015**, *210*, 189–197. [CrossRef]

48. Almansour, K.; Taverner, A.; Eggleston, I.M.; Mrsny, R.J. Mechanistic studies of a cell-permeant peptide designed to enhance myosin light chain phosphorylation in polarized intestinal epithelia. *J. Control. Release* **2018**, *279*, 208–219. [CrossRef] [PubMed]

49. Almansour, K.; Taverner, A.; Turner, J.R.; Eggleston, I.M.; Mrsny, R.J. An intestinal paracellular pathway biased toward positively-charged macromolecules. *J. Control. Release* **2018**, *288*, 111–125. [CrossRef] [PubMed]

50. Date, A.A.; Hanes, J.; Ensign, L.M. Nanoparticles for oral delivery: Design, evaluation and state-of-the-art. *J. Control. Release* **2016**, *240*, 504–526. [CrossRef] [PubMed]

51. Maher, S.; Ryan, K.B.; Ahmad, T.; O'Driscoll, C.M.; Brayden, D.J. Chapter 2.1 Nanostructures Overcoming the Intestinal Barrier: Physiological Considerations and Mechanistic Issues. In *Nanostructured Biomaterials for Overcoming Biological Barriers*; The Royal Society of Chemistry: London, UK, 2012; pp. 39–62. [CrossRef]

52. Brayden, S. Oral Peptide Delivery: The Potential of Combining Nanoparticle Constructs with Permeation Enhancers. In Proceedings of the Annual Meeting and Exposition of the Controlled Release Society, New York City, NY, USA, 22–24 July 2018.

53. Alonso, J.M. Learning from the EU TRANS-INT consortium: Oral peptide formulations using nanotechnologies. In Proceedings of the Annual Meeting and Exposition of the Controlled Release Society, New York City, NY, USA, 22–24 July 2018.

54. Gonçalves, R.F.S.; Martins, J.T.; Duarte, C.M.M.; Vicente, A.A.; Pinheiro, A.C. Advances in nutraceutical delivery systems: From formulation design for bioavailability enhancement to efficacy and safety evaluation. *Trends Food Sci. Technol.* **2018**, *78*, 270–291. [CrossRef]

55. Thanou, M.; Verhoef, J.C.; Junginger, H.E. Chitosan and its derivatives as intestinal absorption enhancers. *Adv. Drug Deliv. Rev.* **2001**, *50* (Suppl. 1), S91–S101. [CrossRef]

56. Onishi, H.; Imura, Y.; Uchida, M.; Machida, Y. Enhancement potential of sucrose laurate (L-1695) on intestinal absorption of water-soluble high molecular weight compounds. *Curr. Drug Deliv.* **2012**, *9*, 487–494. [CrossRef]

57. Lucarini, S.; Fagioli, L.; Campana, R.; Cole, H.; Duranti, A.; Baffone, W.; Vllasaliu, D.; Casettari, L. Unsaturated fatty acids lactose esters: Cytotoxicity, permeability enhancement and antimicrobial activity. *Eur. J. Pharm. Biopharm.* **2016**, *107*, 88–96. [CrossRef]

58. Dimitrijevic, D.; Shaw, A.J.; Florence, A.T. Effects of some non-ionic surfactants on transepithelial permeability in Caco-2 cells. *J. Pharm. Pharmacol.* **2000**, *52*, 157–162. [CrossRef]

59. Gleeson, J.P.; Frías, J.M.; Ryan, S.M.; Brayden, D.J. Sodium caprate enables the blood pressure-lowering effect of Ile-Pro-Pro and Leu-Lys-Pro in spontaneously hypertensive rats by indirectly overcoming PepT1 inhibition. *Eur. J. Pharm. Biopharm.* **2018**, *128*, 179–187. [CrossRef] [PubMed]

60. Moghimipour, E.; Ameri, A.; Handali, S. Absorption-Enhancing Effects of Bile Salts. *Molecules* **2015**, *20*, 14451–14473. [CrossRef] [PubMed]

61. Shoba, G.; Joy, D.; Joseph, T.; Majeed, M.; Rajendran, R.; Srinivas, P.S. Influence of piperine on the pharmacokinetics of curcumin in animals and human volunteers. *Planta Med.* **1998**, *64*, 353–356. [CrossRef] [PubMed]

62. Lambert, J.D.; Kwon, S.J.; Ju, J.; Bose, M.; Lee, M.J.; Hong, J.; Hao, X.; Yang, C.S. Effect of genistein on the bioavailability and intestinal cancer chemopreventive activity of (−)-epigallocatechin-3-gallate. *Carcinogenesis* **2008**, *29*, 2019–2024. [CrossRef] [PubMed]

63. McCartney, F.; Rosa, M.; Coulter, I.; Brayden, D.J. A sucrose ester is a novel permeation enhancer using isolated rat colonic mucosae mounted in Ussing chambers. In Proceedings of the Annual Meeting and Exposition of the American Association of Pharmaceutical Scientists (Poster Presentation), San Antonio, TX, USA, 10–14 November 2013.

64. McCartney, F.; Rosa, M.; Coulter, I.; Brayden, D.J. Sucrose laurate is an effective permeation enhancer for insulin: Rat intestinal instillations. In Proceedings of the Annual meeting and Exposition of the Controlled Release Society (Oral Presentation), Boston, MA, USA, 16–19 July 2017.

65. Casettari, L. Ex-vivo evaluation of intestinal permeability-enhancing effects of mono-esterified sugar based surfactants. In Proceedings of the 11th World Meeting on Pharmaceutics, Biopharmaceutics, and Pharmaceutical Technology (Oral Presentation), Granada, Spain, 19–22 March 2017.

66. Maher, S.; Medani, M.; Carballeira, N.N.; Winter, D.C.; Baird, A.W.; Brayden, D.J. Development of a Non-Aqueous Dispersion to Improve Intestinal Epithelial Flux of Poorly Permeable Macromolecules. *AAPS J.* **2017**, *19*, 244–253. [CrossRef] [PubMed]

67. Gradauer, K.; Nishiumi, A.; Unrinin, K.; Higashino, H.; Kataoka, M.; Pedersen, B.L.; Buckley, S.T.; Yamashita, S. Interaction with Mixed Micelles in the Intestine Attenuates the Permeation Enhancing Potential of Alkyl-Maltosides. *Mol. Pharm.* **2015**, *12*, 2245–2253. [CrossRef] [PubMed]

68. Rautio, J.; Kumpulainen, H.; Heimbach, T.; Oliyai, R.; Oh, D.; Jarvinen, T.; Savolainen, J. Prodrugs: Design and clinical applications. *Nat. Rev. Drug Discov.* **2008**, *7*, 255–270. [CrossRef] [PubMed]

69. Sun, S.; Liang, N.; Kawashima, Y.; Xia, D.; Cui, F. Hydrophobic ion pairing of an insulin-sodium deoxycholate complex for oral delivery of insulin. *Int. J. Nanomed.* **2011**, *6*, 3049–3056. [CrossRef]

70. Griesser, J.; Hetenyi, G.; Moser, M.; Demarne, F.; Jannin, V.; Bernkop-Schnurch, A. Hydrophobic ion pairing: Key to highly payloaded self-emulsifying peptide drug delivery systems. *Int. J. Pharm.* **2017**, *520*, 267–274. [CrossRef]

71. Li, P.; Nielsen, H.M.; Fano, M.; Mullertz, A. Preparation and characterization of insulin-surfactant complexes for loading into lipid-based drug delivery systems. *J. Pharm. Sci* **2013**, *102*, 2689–2698. [CrossRef]

72. Hintzen, F.; Laffleur, F.; Sarti, F.; Müller, C.; Bernkop-Schnürch, A. In vitro and ex vivo evaluation of an intestinal permeation enhancing self-microemulsifying drug delivery system (SMEDDS). *J. Drug Deliv. Sci. Technol.* **2013**, *23*, 261–267. [CrossRef]

73. Meyer, J.D.; Manning, M.C. Hydrophobic Ion Pairing: Altering the Solubility Properties of Biomolecules. *Pharm. Res.* **1998**, *15*, 188–193. [CrossRef] [PubMed]

74. Günday Türeli, N.; Türeli, A.E.; Schneider, M. Counter-ion complexes for enhanced drug loading in nanocarriers: Proof-of-concept and beyond. *Int. J. Pharm.* **2016**, *511*, 994–1001. [CrossRef] [PubMed]

75. Krug, S.M.; Amasheh, M.; Dittmann, I.; Christoffel, I.; Fromm, M.; Amasheh, S. Sodium caprate as an enhancer of macromolecule permeation across tricellular tight junctions of intestinal cells. *Biomaterials* **2013**, *34*, 275–282. [CrossRef] [PubMed]

76. Krug, S.M.; Fromm, M.; Günzel, D. Two-Path Impedance Spectroscopy for Measuring Paracellular and Transcellular Epithelial Resistance. *Biophys. J.* **2009**, *97*, 2202–2211. [CrossRef] [PubMed]

77. Koeplinger, K.A. Oral peptide-protein interaction inhibitors (PPI): Excited about cycling. In Proceedings of the Annual meeting and Exposition of the Controlled Release Society (Oral Presentation, Oral Peptide Workshop), New York, NY, USA, 22–24 July 2018.

78. Wang, X.; Maher, S.; Brayden, D.J. Restoration of rat colonic epithelium after in situ intestinal instillation of the absorption promoter, sodium caprate. *Ther. Deliv.* **2010**, *1*, 75–82. [CrossRef] [PubMed]

79. Fasano, A.; Nataro, J.P. Intestinal epithelial tight junctions as targets for enteric bacteria-derived toxins. *Adv. Drug Deliv. Rev.* **2004**, *56*, 795–807. [CrossRef] [PubMed]
80. Fernandez, S.; Jannin, V.; Rodier, J.D.; Ritter, N.; Mahler, B.; Carriere, F. Comparative study on digestive lipase activities on the self emulsifying excipient Labrasol, medium chain glycerides and PEG esters. *Biochim. Biophys. Acta* **2007**, *1771*, 633–640. [CrossRef]
81. Sadhukha, T.; Layek, B.; Prabha, S. Incorporation of lipolysis in monolayer permeability studies of lipid-based oral drug delivery systems. *Drug Deliv. Transl. Res.* **2018**, *8*, 375–386. [CrossRef]
82. Shaw, D.J. *Introduction to Colloid and Surface Chemistry*; Butterworth-Heinemann: Oxford, UK, 1992.
83. Dahlgren, D.; Roos, C.; Lundqvist, A.; Tannergren, C.; Sjoblom, M.; Sjogren, E.; Lennernas, H. Effect of absorption-modifying excipients, hypotonicity, and enteric neural activity in an in vivo model for small intestinal transport. *Int. J. Pharm.* **2018**, *549*, 239–248. [CrossRef]
84. Anderberg, E.K.; Lindmark, T.; Artursson, P. Sodium Caprate Elicits Dilatations in Human Intestinal Tight Junctions and Enhances Drug Absorption by the Paracellular Route. *Pharm. Res.* **1993**, *10*, 857–864. [CrossRef]
85. Tippin, T.K.; Thakker, D.R. Biorelevant refinement of the Caco-2 cell culture model to assess efficacy of paracellular permeability enhancers. *J. Pharm. Sci.* **2008**, *97*, 1977–1992. [CrossRef] [PubMed]
86. Whitehead, K.; Karr, N.; Mitragotri, S. Discovery of synergistic permeation enhancers for oral drug delivery. *J. Control. Release* **2008**, *128*, 128–133. [CrossRef] [PubMed]
87. Heade, J.; Maher, S.; Bleiel, S.B.; Brayden, D.J. Labrasol((R)) and Salts of Medium-Chain Fatty Acids Can Be Combined in Low Concentrations to Increase the Permeability of a Macromolecule Marker Across Isolated Rat Intestinal Mucosae. *J. Pharm. Sci.* **2018**, *107*, 1648–1655. [CrossRef] [PubMed]
88. Gu, C.-H.; Li, H.; Levons, J.; Lentz, K.; Gandhi, R.B.; Raghavan, K.; Smith, R.L. Predicting Effect of Food on Extent of Drug Absorption Based on Physicochemical Properties. *Pharm. Res.* **2007**, *24*, 1118–1130. [CrossRef] [PubMed]
89. Stappaerts, J.; Wuyts, B.; Tack, J.; Annaert, P.; Augustijns, P. Human and simulated intestinal fluids as solvent systems to explore food effects on intestinal solubility and permeability. *Eur. J. Pharm. Sci.* **2014**, *63*, 178–186. [CrossRef] [PubMed]
90. Riethorst, D.; Mols, R.; Duchateau, G.; Tack, J.; Brouwers, J.; Augustijns, P. Characterization of Human Duodenal Fluids in Fasted and Fed State Conditions. *J. Pharm. Sci.* **2016**, *105*, 673–681. [CrossRef]
91. Jantratid, E.; Janssen, N.; Reppas, C.; Dressman, J.B. Dissolution media simulating conditions in the proximal human gastrointestinal tract: An update. *Pharm. Res.* **2008**, *25*, 1663–1676. [CrossRef]
92. Markopoulos, C.; Thoenen, F.; Preisig, D.; Symillides, M.; Vertzoni, M.; Parrott, N.; Reppas, C.; Imanidis, G. Biorelevant media for transport experiments in the Caco-2 model to evaluate drug absorption in the fasted and the fed state and their usefulness. *Eur. J. Pharm. Biopharm.* **2014**, *86*, 438–448. [CrossRef]
93. Birch, D.; Diedrichsen, R.G.; Christophersen, P.C.; Mu, H.; Nielsen, H.M. Evaluation of drug permeation under fed state conditions using mucus-covered Caco-2 cell epithelium. *Eur. J. Pharm. Sci.* **2018**, *118*, 144–153. [CrossRef]
94. Wuyts, B.; Riethorst, D.; Brouwers, J.; Tack, J.; Annaert, P.; Augustijns, P. Evaluation of fasted state human intestinal fluid as apical solvent system in the Caco-2 absorption model and comparison with FaSSIF. *Eur. J. Pharm. Sci.* **2015**, *67*, 126–135. [CrossRef] [PubMed]
95. Dahlgren, D.; Roos, C.; Lundqvist, A.; Tannergren, C.; Sjoblom, M.; Sjogren, E.; Lennernas, H. Time-dependent effects on small intestinal transport by absorption-modifying excipients. *Eur. J. Pharm. Biopharm.* **2018**, *132*, 19–28. [CrossRef] [PubMed]
96. Roos, C.; Dahlgren, D.; Sjogren, E.; Tannergren, C.; Abrahamsson, B.; Lennernas, H. Regional Intestinal Permeability in Rats: A Comparison of Methods. *Mol. Pharm.* **2017**, *14*, 4252–4261. [CrossRef] [PubMed]
97. Thanou, M.; Verhoef, J.C.; Verheijden, J.H.M.; Junginger, H.E. Intestinal Absorption of Octreotide Using Trimethyl Chitosan Chloride: Studies in Pigs. *Pharm. Res.* **2001**, *18*, 823–828. [CrossRef] [PubMed]
98. Baluom, M.; Friedman, M.; Assaf, P.; Haj-Yehia, A.I.; Rubinstein, A. Synchronized release of sulpiride and sodium decanoate from HPMC matrices: A rational approach to enhance sulpiride absorption in the rat intestine. *Pharm. Res.* **2000**, *17*, 1071–1076. [CrossRef] [PubMed]
99. Sutton, S.C.; LeCluyse, E.L.; Engle, K.; Pipkin, J.D.; Fix, J.A. Enhanced Bioavailability of Cefoxitin Using Palmitoylcarnitine. II. Use of Directly Compressed Tablet Formulations in the Rat and Dog. *Pharm. Res.* **1993**, *10*, 1516–1520. [CrossRef] [PubMed]

100. Schiller, C.; Fröhlich, C.-P.; Giessmann, T.; Siegmund, W.; Mönnikes, H.; Hosten, N.; Weitschies, W. Intestinal fluid volumes and transit of dosage forms as assessed by magnetic resonance imaging. *Aliment. Pharmacol. Ther.* **2005**, *22*, 971–979. [CrossRef]

101. Dorkoosh, F.A.; Verhoef, J.C.; Verheijden, J.H.M.; Rafiee-Tehrani, M.; Borchard, G.; Junginger, H.E. Peroral Absorption of Octreotide in Pigs Formulated in Delivery Systems on the Basis of Superporous Hydrogel Polymers. *Pharm. Res.* **2002**, *19*, 1532–1536. [CrossRef]

102. Koziolek, M.; Grimm, M.; Becker, D.; Iordanov, V.; Zou, H.; Shimizu, J.; Wanke, C.; Garbacz, G.; Weitschies, W. Investigation of pH and Temperature Profiles in the GI Tract of Fasted Human Subjects Using the Intellicap® System. *J. Pharm. Sci.* **2015**, *104*, 2855–2863. [CrossRef]

103. Baluom, M.; Friedman, M.; Rubinstein, A. The importance of intestinal residence time of absorption enhancer on drug absorption and implication on formulative considerations. *Int. J. Pharm.* **1998**, *176*, 21–30. [CrossRef]

104. Tillman, L.G.; Geary, R.S.; Hardee, G.E. Oral delivery of antisense oligonucleotides in man. *J. Pharm. Sci.* **2008**, *97*, 225–236. [CrossRef] [PubMed]

105. Junginger, H. Excipients as Absorption Enhancers. In *Biopharmaceutics Applications in Drug Development*; Krishna, R., Yu, L., Eds.; Springer: New York, NY, USA, 2008; pp. 139–174. [CrossRef]

106. Brayden, D.J.; Walsh, E. Efficacious intestinal permeation enhancement induced by the sodium salt of 10-undecylenic acid, a medium chain fatty acid derivative. *AAPS J.* **2014**, *16*, 1064–1076. [CrossRef] [PubMed]

107. Whitehead, K.; Shen, Z.; Mitragotri, S. Oral delivery of macromolecules using intestinal patches: Applications for insulin delivery. *J. Control. Release* **2004**, *98*, 37–45. [CrossRef] [PubMed]

108. Gupta, V.; Hwang, B.H.; Doshi, N.; Banerjee, A.; Anselmo, A.C.; Mitragotri, S. Delivery of Exenatide and Insulin Using Mucoadhesive Intestinal Devices. *Ann. Biomed. Eng.* **2016**, *44*, 1993–2007. [CrossRef] [PubMed]

109. Eiamtrakarn, S.; Itoh, Y.; Kishimoto, J.; Yoshikawa, Y.; Shibata, N.; Murakami, M.; Takada, K. Gastrointestinal mucoadhesive patch system (GI-MAPS) for oral administration of G-CSF, a model protein. *Biomaterials* **2002**, *23*, 145–152. [CrossRef]

110. Grabovac, V.; Foger, F.; Bernkop-Schnurch, A. Design and in vivo evaluation of a patch delivery system for insulin based on thiolated polymers. *Int. J. Pharm.* **2008**, *348*, 169–174. [CrossRef] [PubMed]

111. Venkatesan, N.; Uchino, K.; Amagase, K.; Ito, Y.; Shibata, N.; Takada, K. Gastro-intestinal patch system for the delivery of erythropoietin. *J. Control. Release* **2006**, *111*, 19–26. [CrossRef]

112. Banerjee, A.; Wong, J.; Gogoi, R.; Brown, T.; Mitragotri, S. Intestinal micropatches for oral insulin delivery. *J. Drug Target.* **2017**, *25*, 608–615. [CrossRef]

113. McCartney, F.; Gleeson, J.P.; Brayden, D.J. Safety concerns over the use of intestinal permeation enhancers: A mini-review. *Tissue Barriers* **2016**, *4*, e1176822. [CrossRef]

114. Fasano, A.; Fiorentini, C.; Donelli, G.; Uzzau, S.; Kaper, J.B.; Margaretten, K.; Ding, X.; Guandalini, S.; Comstock, L.; Goldblum, S.E. Zonula occludens toxin modulates tight junctions through protein kinase C-dependent actin reorganization, in vitro. *J. Clin. Investig.* **1995**, *96*, 710–720. [CrossRef]

115. Bogman, K.; Zysset, Y.; Degen, L.; Hopfgartner, G.; Gutmann, H.; Alsenz, J.; Drewe, J. P-glycoprotein and surfactants: Effect on intestinal talinolol absorption. *Clin. Pharmacol. Ther.* **2005**, *77*, 24–32. [CrossRef] [PubMed]

116. Tomaru, A.; Takeda-Morishita, M.; Maeda, K.; Banba, H.; Takayama, K.; Kumagai, Y.; Kusuhara, H.; Sugiyama, Y. Effects of Cremophor EL on the absorption of orally administered saquinavir and fexofenadine in healthy subjects. *Drug Metab. Pharmacokinet.* **2015**, *30*, 221–226. [CrossRef] [PubMed]

117. Lindmark, T.; Soderholm, J.D.; Olaison, G.; Alvan, G.; Ocklind, G.; Artursson, P. Mechanism of absorption enhancement in humans after rectal administration of ampicillin in suppositories containing sodium caprate. *Pharm. Res.* **1997**, *14*, 930–935. [CrossRef] [PubMed]

118. Maher, S.; Leonard, T.W.; Jacobsen, J.; Brayden, D.J. Safety and efficacy of sodium caprate in promoting oral drug absorption: From in vitro to the clinic. *Adv. Drug Deliv. Rev.* **2009**, *61*, 1427–1449. [CrossRef]

119. Kiss, L.; Walter, F.R.; Bocsik, A.; Veszelka, S.; Ozsvari, B.; Puskas, L.G.; Szabo-Revesz, P.; Deli, M.A. Kinetic analysis of the toxicity of pharmaceutical excipients Cremophor EL and RH40 on endothelial and epithelial cells. *J. Pharm. Sci.* **2013**, *102*, 1173–1181. [CrossRef] [PubMed]

120. Ribet, D.; Cossart, P. How bacterial pathogens colonize their hosts and invade deeper tissues. *Microbes Infect.* **2015**, *17*, 173–183. [CrossRef] [PubMed]

121. Gunzel, D.; Yu, A.S. Claudins and the modulation of tight junction permeability. *Physiol. Rev.* **2013**, *93*, 525–569. [CrossRef] [PubMed]

122. Drewe, J.; Beglinger, C.; Fricker, G. Effect of ischemia on intestinal permeability of lipopolysaccharides. *Eur. J. Clin. Investig.* **2001**, *31*, 138–144. [CrossRef]

123. Tomlinson, J.E.; Blikslager, A.T. Interactions between lipopolysaccharide and the intestinal epithelium. *J. Am. Vet. Med Assoc.* **2004**, *224*, 1446–1452. [CrossRef]

124. Barmeyer, C.; Schulzke, J.D.; Fromm, M. Claudin-related intestinal diseases. *Semin. Cell Dev. Boil.* **2015**, *42*, 30–38. [CrossRef]

125. Tippin, T.K.; Thakker, D.R. Novel Approaches to Assess the Efficacy and Toxicity of Intestinal Absorption Enhancers. Ph.D. Thesis, ProQuest, Ann Arbor, MI, USA, 2006.

126. Nielsen, E.J.; Kamei, N.; Takeda-Morishita, M. Safety of the cell-penetrating peptide penetratin as an oral absorption enhancer. *Boil. Pharm. Bull.* **2015**, *38*, 144–146. [CrossRef] [PubMed]

127. Chassaing, B.; Koren, O.; Goodrich, J.K.; Poole, A.C.; Srinivasan, S.; Ley, R.E.; Gewirtz, A.T. Dietary emulsifiers impact the mouse gut microbiota promoting colitis and metabolic syndrome. *Nature* **2015**, *519*, 92–96. [CrossRef]

128. Kararli, T.T. Comparison of the gastrointestinal anatomy, physiology, and biochemistry of humans and commonly used laboratory animals. *Biopharm. Drug Dispos.* **1995**, *16*, 351–380. [CrossRef] [PubMed]

129. Dressman, J.B. Comparison of canine and human gastrointestinal physiology. *Pharm. Res.* **1986**, *3*, 123–131. [CrossRef] [PubMed]

130. Tyagi, P.; Pechenov, S.; Anand Subramony, J. Oral peptide delivery: Translational challenges due to physiological effects. *J. Control. Release* **2018**, *287*, 167–176. [CrossRef] [PubMed]

131. Lui, C.Y.; Amidon, G.L.; Berardi, R.R.; Fleisher, D.; Youngberg, C.; Dressman, J.B. Comparison of gastrointestinal pH in dogs and humans: Implications on the use of the beagle dog as a model for oral absorption in humans. *J. Pharm. Sci.* **1986**, *75*, 271–274. [CrossRef]

132. Polentarutti, B.; Albery, T.; Dressman, J.; Abrahamsson, B. Modification of gastric pH in the fasted dog. *J. Pharm. Pharmacol.* **2010**, *62*, 462–469. [CrossRef] [PubMed]

133. Henze, L.J.; Koehl, N.J.; O'Shea, J.P.; Kostewicz, E.S.; Holm, R.; Griffin, B.T. The pig as a preclinical model for predicting oral bioavailability and in vivo performance of pharmaceutical oral dosage forms: A PEARRL review. *J. Pharm. Pharmacol.* **2018**. [CrossRef]

134. Sjogren, E.; Abrahamsson, B.; Augustijns, P.; Becker, D.; Bolger, M.B.; Brewster, M.; Brouwers, J.; Flanagan, T.; Harwood, M.; Heinen, C.; et al. In vivo methods for drug absorption—Comparative physiologies, model selection, correlations with in vitro methods (IVIVC), and applications for formulation/API/excipient characterization including food effects. *Eur. J. Pharm. Sci.* **2014**, *57*, 99–151. [CrossRef]

135. Hatton, G.B.; Madla, C.M.; Rabbie, S.C.; Basit, A.W. Gut reaction: Impact of systemic diseases on gastrointestinal physiology and drug absorption. *Drug Discov. Today* **2018**. [CrossRef]

136. Davis, S.S.; Wilding, I.R. Oral drug absorption studies: The best model for man is man! *Drug Discov. Today* **2001**, *6*, 127–130. [CrossRef]

137. Hatton, G.B.; Yadav, V.; Basit, A.W.; Merchant, H.A. Animal Farm: Considerations in Animal Gastrointestinal Physiology and Relevance to Drug Delivery in Humans. *J. Pharm. Sci.* **2015**, *104*, 2747–2776. [CrossRef] [PubMed]

138. McConnell, E.L.; Basit, A.W.; Murdan, S. Measurements of rat and mouse gastrointestinal pH, fluid and lymphoid tissue, and implications for in-vivo experiments. *J. Pharm. Pharmacol.* **2008**, *60*, 63–70. [CrossRef]

139. Bak, A.; Ashford, M.; Brayden, D.J. Local delivery of macromolecules to treat diseases associated with the colon. *Adv. Drug Deliv. Rev.* **2018**, *136–137*, 2–27. [CrossRef]

140. Karsdal, M.A.; Henriksen, K.; Bay-Jensen, A.C.; Molloy, B.; Arnold, M.; John, M.R.; Byrjalsen, I.; Azria, M.; Riis, B.J.; Qvist, P.; et al. Lessons learned from the development of oral calcitonin: The first tablet formulation of a protein in phase III clinical trials. *J. Clin. Pharmacol.* **2011**, *51*, 460–471. [CrossRef] [PubMed]

141. Karsdal, M.A.; Riis, B.J.; Mehta, N.; Stern, W.; Arbit, E.; Christiansen, C.; Henriksen, K. Lessons learned from the clinical development of oral peptides. *Br. J. Clin. Pharmacol.* **2015**, *79*, 720–732. [CrossRef] [PubMed]

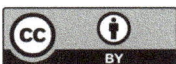

pharmaceutics

MDPI

Review

Penetration Enhancers in Ocular Drug Delivery

Roman V. Moiseev [1], Peter W. J. Morrison [1], Fraser Steele [2] and Vitaliy V. Khutoryanskiy [1,*]

[1] Reading School of Pharmacy, University of Reading, Whiteknights, P.O. Box 224, Reading RG66AD, UK
[2] MC2 Therapeutics, James House, Emlyn Lane, Leatherhead KT22 7EP, UK
[*] Correspondence: v.khutoryanskiy@reading.ac.uk; Tel.: +44-(0)-118-378-6119

Received: 30 May 2019; Accepted: 3 July 2019; Published: 9 July 2019

Abstract: There are more than 100 recognized disorders of the eye. This makes the development of advanced ocular formulations an important topic in pharmaceutical science. One of the ways to improve drug delivery to the eye is the use of penetration enhancers. These are defined as compounds capable of enhancing drug permeability across ocular membranes. This review paper provides an overview of anatomical and physiological features of the eye and discusses some common ophthalmological conditions and permeability of ocular membranes. The review also presents the analysis of literature on the use of penetration-enhancing compounds (cyclodextrins, chelating agents, crown ethers, bile acids and bile salts, cell-penetrating peptides, and other amphiphilic compounds) in ocular drug delivery, describing their properties and modes of action.

Keywords: ocular drug delivery; cornea; penetration enhancers; ocular conditions; ophthalmology

1. Introduction

According to the World Health Organization, the number of people who live with some form of distance or near vision impairment is about 1.3 billion worldwide [1]. This problem is very important because approximately 80% of external input of information delivered to the brain is processed by the visual pathway [2]. There were many methods and improvements of ocular drug delivery developed over the last decades exploring more effective treatments for different ocular diseases. Nevertheless, this field of medicine remains one of the most challenging.

The preferred method of ocular drug delivery is via topical application due to ease of access to the eye and the non-invasive nature of this administration route [3]. Self-medication by this means is achievable by most people that are not limited by dexterity issues or conditions affecting mental ability. Administration by a helper eliminates these potential difficulties. Ocular drug penetration is possible via the transcellular pathway, i.e., into and through cells, or the paracellular route, i.e., between cells, or a combination of both pathways [4].

Drug penetration enhancement can be achieved by inclusion of agents capable of modifying the tear film, mucous layer, and ocular membranes in a drug formulation [5]. A further strategy for enhancing drug penetration into the eye can be achieved by energy-driven means, where a small electrical current is used (iontophoresis) [6] or ultrasound is employed to drive the drug to enter the ocular tissues [7–9]. The use of microneedles for enhanced ocular drug delivery is another emerging area of research; however, this could be considered somewhat invasive and inconvenient [10–12].

Penetration enhancers are compounds that are able to enhance drug delivery across otherwise impermeable or limited permeability membranes such as the cornea, acting predominantly on the epithelia [5]. The use of penetration enhancers in transdermal applications is a well-established approach to facilitate drug delivery across the skin and this topic was covered in a number of excellent reviews [13,14]. Ocular drug delivery is still lacking good understanding and analysis of the effects of various penetration enhancers. It is, however, already established that penetration enhancers in ocular drug delivery facilitate delivery of active pharmaceutical ingredients through three main mechanisms or their combination [15,16]:

1. Altering tear film stability and the mucous layer at the ocular surface [17,18];
2. Modifying membrane components such as lipid bilayers of associated epithelial cells [19];
3. Loosening epithelial tight junctions [4,17].

Penetration-enhancing excipients for use in ocular formulations should ideally have the following characteristics: they should be non-toxic and non-irritating, efficacious at low concentrations, fast-acting, and their effect should be reversible [20,21].

This paper provides an overview of anatomy and physiology of the eye, discusses some common ophthalmological conditions, and presents an analysis of literature on the use of penetration enhancers in ocular drug delivery.

2. Ocular Anatomy and Physiology

The visual system is a sensory unit helping us to understand our environment, comprising a receptor (retina), sensory pathway (optic tract), and brain center (primary visual cortex). Each eyeball is embedded within the orbit, which is a pear-shaped cavity physically protecting the eye [1,22]. Adipose tissue surrounds the eye within the orbital cavity and helps to cushion the eye. Other accessory organs include lacrimal glands, eyebrows, eyelids, eyelashes, and muscles of the eye. The human eye is a complex organ comprising three different coats or layers, enclosing various anatomical structures as shown in Figure 1. Below, we briefly consider some specific tissues in the eye.

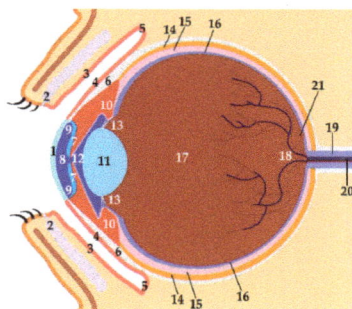

Figure 1. Anatomy of the human eye: 1—cornea; 2—meibomian glands; 3—palpebral conjunctiva; 4—bulbar conjunctiva; 5—conjunctival fornix; 6—sclera; 7—iris; 8—anterior chamber; 9—iridocorneal angle; 10—ciliary body; 11—lens; 12—posterior chamber; 13—suspensory ligament; 14—choroid; 15—retinal pigmented epithelium; 16—retina; 17—vitreous body; 18—optic disc; 19—optic nerve; 20—central artery and vein of the retina; 21—fovea.

2.1. The Outermost Layer (Tunica Fibrosa Oculi)

The fibrous tunic helps maintain the spherical shape of the eyeball and consists of the cornea and sclera. It is well known that less than 5% of the topically applied drug penetrates through the cornea [23]. However, the most accessible regions for drug application are the conjunctiva, sclera, and cornea. The cornea is an avascular, transparent, highly innervated structure, whose average diameter is ~11.5 mm vertically and ~12 mm horizontally. The average thickness of this structure is ~540 μm in the central part, and it is thicker toward the periphery [22]. The refractive power of this structure in the eye is roughly 42 diopters. The cornea is covered with the tear fluid, forming a film that protects its surface from dust and other particles. This film consists of three layers as shown in Figure 2: the outer lipid layer (delivered to the lid margins from the meibomian glands located within the tarsal plate) [24], middle aqueous layer (produced by the lacrimal gland, containing free lipid and soluble mucin), and mucous layer (which is mainly secreted by the goblet cells located within the conjunctiva as single cells with the highest density of those in the conjunctiva of the inferior eyelid) [25].

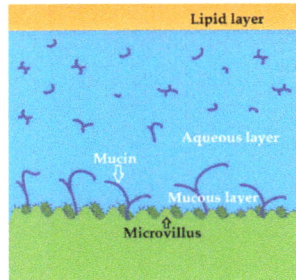

Figure 2. The tear film consists of the outer lipid layer, middle aqueous layer, and mucous layer.

The mucous layer is in contact with the corneal epithelium and is anchored via microvilli of the superficial epithelium cells. Apart from the tear film, there is another factor hampering ocular drug delivery—the structure of the cornea (Figure 3). The cornea consists of six different layers (epithelium, Bowman's membrane, stroma, Dua's layer, Descemet's membrane, and endothelium). The external layer of the cornea is the epithelium. It is relatively thin and is about 100 μm in the periphery of the cornea and approximately 50 μm in its center.

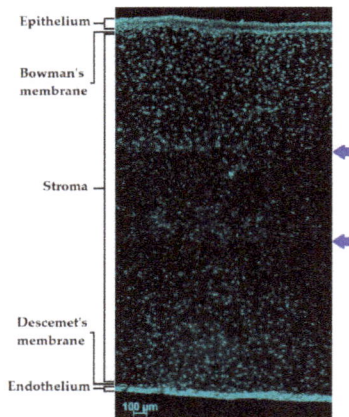

Figure 3. Micrograph demonstrating a cross-section of the multilayered structure of porcine cornea. Scale bar = 100 μm. Please note that this micrograph is a combination of three images stitched together using Inkscape 0.92.4 software due to the restrictions of the microscope camera field of view posing restrictions to the image in view. The arrows indicate stitches between images.

The main feature of this layer is the ability to regenerate non-keratinized stratified squamous epithelium. The high lipophilicity of the epithelium allows permeability to up to 90% of lipophilic small drug molecules and only about 10% of hydrophilic molecules. The cells of this layer have Ca^{2+}-dependent membrane adherent regions; tight junctions are formed between the zonula occludens, zonula adherens, and desmosomes [5]. The epithelium protects the eye against ultraviolet radiation (UVR) by means of a high concentration of tryptophan residues and ascorbate that absorb UVR [26]. The next layer that is placed right underneath the epithelium is the Bowman's membrane that is also called the anterior limiting membrane. Bowman's layer is acellular and composed primarily of collagen. The anterior limiting membrane reaches from 8 μm to 14 μm in thickness. The middle corneal layer is the stroma, also known as substantia propria due to the fact that it makes up to 90% of the total thickness of the cornea. It is composed of about 80% of water and collagen, proteins, mucopolysaccharides, and proteoglycans [5]. In 2013, Dua et al. reported a discovery of an additional corneal layer that was not detected previously [27]. According to Dua et al., this layer is about 15 μm in thickness and is located between the corneal stroma and the fifth corneal layer, Descemet's membrane. This is also the posterior limiting membrane of the cornea. This membrane is a ~6-μm-thick basement of the endothelium cells. The innermost layer of the cornea is known as the endothelium and plays the role of a pump, providing the cornea with the correct hydration to ensure transparency of this tissue. The clarity of the cornea depends on an ordered lamellar collagen structure and relative dehydration which requires endothelial cell density of at least 1000 cells/mm^2. According to the literature, there is a loss of the human cornea mean endothelial cell density in normal eye by approximately 0.6% per year [28]. The endothelium is ~5 μm in thickness and consists of a monolayer of squamous or low cuboidal cells [5].

Another layer providing the eyeball with protection is called the conjunctiva, of which all three portions are shown in Figure 4. The palpebral conjunctiva has blood vessels and covers the posterior surface of the upper and lower lids. The conjunctiva comprises two or more layers of isoprismatic to highly prismatic epithelial cells. The bulbar conjunctiva is an avascular slightly mobile layer that starts from the upper and lower fornices and lies over the sclera up to the cornea region. This anatomical coat consists of stratified non-keratinized epithelial cells [29]. The superior and inferior fornices form the conjunctival sac, which can act as a reservoir for instilled medicine or the placement of a drug-loaded ocular insert [30,31]. According to the literature, the estimated total area of the human conjunctival sac is approximately 16 cm^2 [24]. Figure 4 clearly demonstrates all three portions of the conjunctiva.

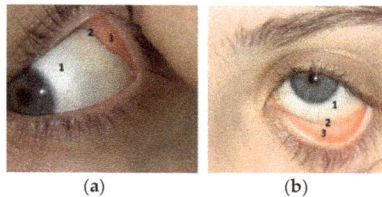

(a)   (b)

Figure 4. Three portions of conjunctiva: (**a**) 1—bulbar conjunctiva; 2—superior conjunctival fornix; 3—palpebral conjunctiva of the upper lid; (**b**) 1—bulbar conjunctiva; 2—inferior conjunctival fornix; 3—palpebral conjunctiva of the lower lid.

The tough outer layer of the eye globe is called the sclera. This is covered by the episcleral, a loose connective tissue layer. In the anterior part of the eye, the sclera lies up to the corneal limbus, and posteriorly to the optic nerve. This layer comprises collagen, proteoglycans, elastin, and glycoproteins. These collagen bundles are not uniformly oriented, which results in the opaque but mechanically strong nature of the sclera. The sclera itself is pierced by a number of blood vessels, while being effectively avascular itself [32].

2.2. Eye Chambers, Iris, Ciliary Body, and Lens

One of the first intraocular structures that can be partially seen, due to the corneal transparency, is the anterior chamber of the eye. This is a space between the cornea's endothelium and anterior surface of the iris that is filled with aqueous humor. The latter is an optically clear fluid resembling blood plasma. The aqueous humor helps maintain appropriate intraocular pressure (IOP), and provides the cornea, trabecular meshwork, and lens with nutrition and oxygen, while removing metabolic wastes, as well as delivering molecules of neurotransmitters [33].

This fluid is formed and delivered to the posterior chamber by nonpigmented cells of the epithelia via ciliary processes [34]. Then, it flows through the pupil into the anterior chamber where two ways of outflow are found (Figure 5): (1) the conventional route is the primary outflow, where the aqueous humor is drained through the trabecular meshwork located at the anterior chamber angle (iridocorneal angle) to the Schlemm's canal (circular tube located in the limbus, 1-mm-wide region of merging epithelium of cornea and sclera), which delivers it directly into aqueous veins [35]; (2) uveoscleral outflow is provided by means of the iris root and the ciliary body face, where the aqueous humor crosses between fibers of the muscle into the supraciliary and suprachoroidal spaces and is collected by the choroidal blood circulation. The proportion of aqueous outflow via each route could be different according to the age and disease [36]. The aqueous humor consists of inorganic and organic ions, carbohydrates, glutathione, urea, amino acids, proteins, oxygen, carbon dioxide, and water. According to the literature, the concentration of Na^+ in the aqueous humor is almost the same as in the blood plasma, while the concentration of proteins is 200 times lower compared to plasma levels, and ascorbate's concentration is 20 to 50 times higher [33].

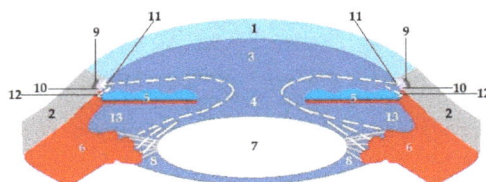

Figure 5. Pathways of aqueous humor outflow are indicated with arrows. 1—cornea; 2—sclera; 3—anterior chamber; 4—pupil; 5—iris; 6—ciliary body; 7—lens; 8—suspensory ligament; 9—Schlemm's canal; 10—trabecular meshwork; 11—trabecular route; 12—uveoscleral route; 13—posterior chamber.

The anterior chamber houses the iris, which separates anterior and posterior segments. Being attached to the anterior part of the ciliary body from the periphery, this anatomical structure has an aperture in its center that is called the pupil, the diameter of which can be regulated by the sphincter and dilator muscles located within the iris stroma (vascular connective tissue) to control the amount of light transmitting into the eye. At the posterior part of the iris, there are two epithelial layers—the anterior layer is slightly pigmented, while the posterior one has a high density of pigmentation and faces the posterior chamber. Just behind the iris lies another part of the uveal tract called the ciliary body. As already mentioned, production of the aqueous humor and uveoscleral outflow are among its functions. Additionally, the ciliary body is responsible for hyaluronate production and its release into the vitreous body, as well as for being a part of the accommodation mechanism due to the circular muscle fibers within the ciliary body. Also, this structure of the eye plays an important role in maintaining the blood–aqueous barrier [37].

The capsular bag is situated between the iris and the vitreous body and encapsulates the crystalline lens, which is a transparent biconvex avascular structure enclosed in the elastic capsule composed of collagen and that is attached to the ciliary body with the help of zonular fibers (the zonule of Zinn). Interestingly, the thickness of the anterior part of the capsular bag grows from 12–15 μm to 21 μm throughout life. Conversely, the thickness of the posterior part remains at about 2 μm. It is well known that the lens is the second most powerful refractive structure of the eye (after the cornea). It helps refract incoming light and focuses it onto the retina. When light is focused at a short focal distance, the suspensory ligaments are not under tension due to contraction of the ciliary muscle; thus, the lens thickens and results in higher refractive power. At the same time, distance vision requires the ciliary muscle to relax and, hence, to tense the lens-supportive apparatus which flattens the lens. Regarding the microscopic structure of the lens, it is composed of two types of cells. The cuboidal lens epithelial cells form a single layer that lines the anterior hemisphere, enlarging in the equator region and forming the lens "bow". The cells in this region function as stem cells for the lens. The bulk of the lens consists of lens fibers that differentiate to the point where no lens nucleus remains. These fiber cells extend in concentric layers from the anterior lens pole to the posterior one, where junctions at the terminus of the cells form the lens sutures [38]. The transparency and refractive properties of the lens are due to the uniform concentration gradient of the crystallins (α-, β-, γ-crystallins) that represent about 90% of the water-soluble proteins [39].

The third chamber of the eye is called the vitreous body, which is positioned at the back of the eyeball between the lens and the retina. It is a clear, gel-like substance occupying the main volume of the eye and is composed of long fine collagen fibers, proteins (over 80% of those are albumin and immunoglobulins), fibrillins, fibulins, agrin, opticin, pigment epithelium-derived factor, leucine-rich alpha-2 glycoprotein, thrombospondins, hyaluronic acid, polysaccharides, ascorbic acid, and water (about 98% of the whole volume). The vitreous body has no circulatory flow; hence, molecular movements are driven mostly by diffusion. Although the vitreous body is a remarkably stable structure, there is a gradual tendency for the gel to collapse in the course of a lifetime. This is commonly believed to be a result of degradation or alteration of the collagen fiber network. Moreover, the volume of the vitreous gel is about 4 mL at the age of 20 years, starting to gradually decrease after 40 years to less than 2.5 mL at 80 years [40–42].

2.3. Choroidea and Retina

The choroid is a vascular layer located between the sclera and Bruch's membrane (BM) extending from the ora serrata (region of the anterior edge of the retina) to the optic nerve. The choroid coat includes five distinct regions: (1) BM—thin, acellular extracellular matrix positioned right under the retina which acts like a filter to the retina; (2) the choriocapillaris (provides the outer retina with oxygen and nutrients); (3) layer with small and medium-sized vessels; (4) layer with large vessels; and (5) the suprachoroid. Apart from BM and the layer with choriocapillaris, the remainder of the choroidea, the stroma, is populated with melanocytes, connective tissue elements (including fibroblasts, mastocytes, elastic, and collagen fibrils), blood vessels, macrophages, dendritic cells, lymphocytes, nonvascular smooth muscle cells, intrinsic neurons, and nerve fibers associated with vessels [43–45].

The retina is a complex transparent tissue of ~0.55 mm at the edges of the fovea and of ~0.13 mm at the center (umbo). This innermost layer of the eye includes a nonsensory part and an optic part that are divided by the ora serrata. The anterior part does not provide any sensory function and covers the ciliary body and iris with bilaminar epithelium. The posterior portion of the retina lies from the ora serrata to the optic disc being attached only at these two locations. Interestingly, there is an area on the optic retina, roughly 5.5 mm in diameter, which is centered about 4 mm temporal to and 0.8 mm inferior to the center of the optic disc that is called macula (macula lutea or central retina) and which has xanthophyll and two or more layers of ganglion cells. Moreover, few regions can be distinguished within this part of the retina: (1) the fovea (fovea centralis) is a depression in the center of the macular area (~1.5 mm in diameter); (2) the foveola is a central floor of the fovea, which is approximately 0.35 mm in diameter; and (3) the umbo (central depression of the foveola). The optic part of the retina is composed of the retinal pigmented epithelium (RPE; the outer layer) and the cerebral layer (inner). RPE supplies the neurosensory layer with nutrition, as well as removes metabolic products. Additionally, it plays a key role in maintaining the blood–retina barrier (BRB) separating the neurosensory retina from the circulating blood. The inner retina comprises photoreceptors (approximately 120 million rods and 6–7 million cones that constitute the first neuron), bipolar cells (the second neuron), and multipolar ganglion cells (the third neuron), along with horizontal and amacrine cells. Interestingly, rod cells are responsible for peripheral vision acting at low light levels using the photosensitive molecule (rhodopsin) in visual phototransduction. In contrast, three types of cone cells (according to the color perception: red, blue, and green) are located only within the fovea area and are 30- to 100-fold less sensitive compared to rod cells, requiring the simultaneous activation of tens to hundreds of visual pigment molecules (that are homologous or even identical to those found in rods) to generate a detectable response resulting in their activity at relatively high light levels, thereby providing central vision and the ability to distinguish colors. Therefore, the retina is the site of transformation of light energy into a neural signal that is transmitted via the optic nerve to the visual cortex to be analyzed by the brain helping to "see" the environment [29,46,47].

3. Ocular Conditions

There are more than 100 recognized disorders of the eye [22]. Therefore, only some of the most common disorders or the conditions that could potentially benefit from the development of advanced topical formulations with enhanced drug permeability are briefly discussed here. Most frequent diseases of the cornea include keratitis, keratoconus, and dry eye syndrome.

Keratitis is a condition when the patient's cornea becomes inflamed. A wide range of germs could lead to this inflammatory condition, but the most common are *Staphylococcus aureus*, *Staphylococcus epidermidis*, *Streptococcus pneumoniae*, *Pseudomonas aeruginosa*, *Neisseria gonorrhoeae*, *Haemophilus*, herpes simplex and varicella zoster viruses, *Fusarium*, *Aspergillus*, *Candida*, and acanthamoeba. Patients typically complain of pain, foreign body sensation, photophobia, redness of the eye, tearing, discharge (sometimes purulent), and decreased visual acuity. Although this condition is mostly quite painful for the patient and requires urgent treatment, sometimes it can be almost asymptomatic (for instance, if caused by acanthamoeba).

Antibacterial drops combined with subconjunctival injections in severe cases are the choices of therapy in patients with keratitis. According to the most recent clinical recommendations [48], two main schemes are used to treat bacterial keratitis depending on the pathogen and the response to its therapy. The monotherapy includes the use of antibacterial eye drops consisting of fluoroquinolones (levofloxacin, moxifloxacin, gatifloxacin, besifloxacin, ofloxacin, or ciprofloxacin) that cover both Gram-positive (*Staphylococcus aureus*, *Staphylococcus epidermidis*, *Streptococcus pneumoniae*) and Gram-negative (*Pseudomonas aeruginosa*, *Neisseria gonorrhoeae*, *Haemophilus*) bacteria. However, these medications should be used with caution due to the possible resistance of some organisms, which can be noticed by controlling the clinical response. Therefore, there is a second treatment scheme, which combines fluoroquinolone eye drops and solutions for a topical or subconjunctival route that comprise other groups of antibiotics including cephalosporin (cefazolin, ceftazidime), aminoglycosides (gentamicin or tobramycin), penicillins (penicillin G, methicillin, or piperacillin), and glycopeptide antibiotics (vancomycin). For instance, cefazolin is commonly used for *Pseudomonas aeruginosa* infection. On the other hand, ceftazidime is effective against resistant forms of *Pseudomonas aeruginosa*. Vancomycin has efficacy against methicillin-resistant staphylococci, as well as against other Gram-positives. Additionally, corticosteroids (dexamethasone, prednisolone) can be used topically in terms of reducing pain and inflammation in bacterial keratitis but with caution, keeping in mind they inhibit re-epithelialization of the cornea [49,50]. Treatment with steroids should be avoided, when keratitis is induced by fungi or acanthamoeba, as well as in cases of any doubts regarding the effectiveness of the antimicrobial regimen.

Nonsteroidal anti-inflammatory drugs (NSAIDs) also may be recommended for reducing symptoms of inflammation only in the case of efficient antimicrobial therapy. In addition, preservative-free lubricants may be used for promoting healing and cycloplegic agents (cyclopentolate) to reduce discomfort associated with spasm of the ciliary body, as well as for decreasing formation of synechiae [48].

Topical usage of antiviral eye drops (acyclovir) is the core of treatment in cases of herpes simplex keratitis. Eye drops with trifluorothymidine or ganciclovir can be prescribed instead of acyclovir in cases of resistance to therapy. Also, prednisolone acetate- or dexamethasone-including eye drops are used to reduce the inflammation, albeit with the caveat regarding epithelial damage discussed above. In terms of preventing virus reactivation, the administration of oral antiviral agents is preferred. Conversely, in patients with keratitis induced by varicella zoster virus (herpes zoster ophthalmicus), Dworkin et al. [51] reported that topical antiviral therapy is ineffective. Hence, systemic usage of antiviral drugs is the choice of treatment. Additionally, cycloplegic eye drops (cyclopentolate) are used for preventing ciliary spasm that can be associated with this pathological condition. Topical preservative-free lubricants such as hydroxypropyl methylcellulose (and others) can also be added to the treatment [48].

Fungal keratitis should be generally treated with topical antifungal formulations that can be divided into a few groups depending on their mode of action: polyenes (amphotericin B, natamycin), imidazoles (clotrimazole, miconazole, econazole, ketoconazole), triazoles (itraconazole, fluconazole, voriconazole), pyrimidines (flucytosine), and echinocandins (micafungin, caspofungin) [49]. Systemic antifungal drugs can be recommended in severe cases involving deep stromal layers with a high risk of perforation of the cornea. Additionally, topical cycloplegic drugs can be used. The keratitis caused by acanthamoeba should be treated with topical anti-amoebic formulations [48]. Of note, the aim of this treatment is to eradicate amoebic cysts from the cornea. The first-line therapy includes biguanide agents (polyhexamethylene biguanide (PHMB), chlorhexidine) that are cystidical (active against cysts). The aromatic diamidines (propamidine, hexamidine) belong to the second-line medications providing more variable activity, along with being cystidical. In contrast, aminoglycosides (neomycin, paromomycin) or azole agents (clotrimazole, fluconazole, ketoconazole, miconazole) are almost not cystidical, being active against trophozoites [49]. However, they can be used in addition to first- or second-line therapy. According to the literature, adenylate cyclase can be administered topically to promote the conversion of cysts into a protozoal state [48].

Keratoconus is defined by Kanski and Bowling as a progressive disorder in which thinning of the central or paracentral stroma of the cornea occurs, accompanied by apical protrusion and irregular astigmatism [22]. It affects 0.05–5% of the population [48]. Patient complaints include blurred vision, mild photophobia, and increased vision impairment due to progressive myopia and astigmatism. The cause of this condition is still unknown, but some authors refer to such factors as combination of repeated trauma and existing abnormalities of the stroma. Additionally, in some cases, keratoconus presents in patients with other ocular and systemic conditions including, for example, disorders of the connective tissue. One widely used method for treatment of this condition is a corneal collagen cross-linking, which leads to stabilization of ectasia by using riboflavin eye drops and subsequent exposure to ultraviolet-A light. Also, implantation of the ring segment within the cornea can be used as an addition to the cross-linking procedure. In severe cases, keratoplasty (corneal transplantation) is a choice of treatment [22].

Dry eye disease (keratoconjunctivitis sicca) occurs in cases of inadequate tear volume or function, which results in an unstable tear film with disease of the surface of the eye. The prevalence of dry eye syndrome in American and Australian population is estimated to be around 5–16%, while in Asia it is higher and could reach up to 27–33% [49]. Severity of the symptoms may highly vary from patient to patient, but they mostly include a feeling of burning and blurred vision. Pathologies affecting the lacrimal gland and dysfunction of the Meibomian glands, as well as neurological diseases, can lead to the keratoconjunctivitis sicca [22,32]. The aim of therapy is to restore the normal surface of the eye by using tear supplementation along with inhibiting the aberrant inflammation observed in patients with chronic dry eye syndrome. Treatment of this condition is complex, but only the most common topical ocular formulations are discussed in this paper. The following groups of medicines are recommended: lubricants (carboxymethylcellulose, hydroxypropyl methylcellulose, and carbomer gels), hydroxypropyl guar/sodium hyaluronate or combinations (carboxymethylcellulose, polysaccharides or disaccharide), xanthan gum, phospholipids and soybean), artificial tears (with various electrolyte compositions, viscosity, and presence of preservatives), and eye drops with cyclosporine A (increasing tear production by reducing the inflammation of the lacrimal gland). However, lifitegrast is a topical anti-inflammatory medicine which is, at the moment, the only drug approved by the Food and Drug Administration for treating both symptoms and signs in patients with dry eye disease [48,49].

Cataract is a condition in which opacification of the crystalline lens occurs principally as a result of protein aggregation. According to some studies, the number of people in the world who become blind due to cataract is estimated as 20 million [52]. The Vision Loss Expert Group funded by the Bill and Melinda Gates Foundation, Fight for Sight, and others calculated that cataracts led to blindness in 10.6 million people and moderate to severe visual impairment in 34.4 million people [49]. A few classifications are used (depending on morphology, etiology, and maturity) but, in general, all cataracts can be divided into two groups: congenital and acquired. Among the latter group, one of the common types is the age-related cataract induced by metabolic processes of aging (including oxidative stress) of the human lens. Clinicians can hear from patients such symptoms as decreased visual acuity, changing of the contrast sensitivity, color perception, glare, monocular diplopia, and ghosting [48]. Surgical removal of the natural lens and its replacement with an intraocular lens (IOL) is currently the only solution for patients with this condition. However, scientists are actively searching for a potential topical treatment. Thus, it was found that pyruvate eye drops can effectively penetrate ocular membranes and potentially provide protection against oxidative stress [53], while Zhao et al. reported that using lanosterol-loaded nanoparticles can reverse protein aggregation in the lens [54].

Glaucoma is a progressive optic neuropathy that is accompanied by the excavation of the optic nerve head and a loss of visual sensitivity in the sequence beginning in the mid-peripheral visual field. Types of glaucoma are classified as open-angle, angle-closure, glaucoma due to another disease, and childhood onset glaucoma [55,56]. It is worth noting that the leading cause of irreversible blindness worldwide is glaucoma. The following indicators are considered as risk factors for developing glaucoma: increasing age (mostly after 40 years), race, family history, and using steroids. One of the major risks for the development and progression of glaucoma is intraocular pressure (IOP). The prevalence of this condition is 3.54% for people aged 40–80 years worldwide [56]. Even in normal-tension glaucoma with IOP not exceeding 21 mmHg, IOP remains a risk factor for progressive damage of the optic nerve [49]. One of the reasons why patients may not ask for medical help until developed stages of the disease occur is that it is usually asymptomatic. In some cases, patients may complain of halos, pain in the eye, headache, precipitants, and subjective loss of vision field [32]. Pharmacological treatment of glaucoma includes five main groups of topical formulations (prostaglandin analogues, beta-blockers, sympathomimetics (alpha-2-agonists), carbonic anhydrase inhibitors, and miotics). Eye drops with prostaglandin analogues (latanoprost, travoprost, bimatoprost, tafluprost) are considered to be a first-line therapy in open-angle glaucoma patients to reduce the IOP primarily by increasing uveoscleral outflow. A number of side effects (conjunctival hyperemia, irreversible hyperpigmentation of iris, reversible increasing pigmentation of the lid skin, lengthening along with thickening of eyelashes, and orbital fat loss), as well as limitations of using these therapies in inflamed eyes and in patients with herpetic keratitis in their anamnesis, may lead to replacing prostaglandin derivatives with beta-blockers. The latter IOP-lowering class of drugs reduces aqueous production and can be divided into two kinds of beta-blockers depending on the involved receptors: non-selective (timolol, carteolol, levobunolol) and β1-selective (betaxolol). However, the use of beta-blockers is relatively restricted in patients with asthma and cardiovascular diseases due to the potential bronchospasm, hypotension, heart block, and bradycardia. The carbonic anhydrase inhibitors (brinzolamide, dorzolamide) represent another type of topical formulations, which also lower levels of aqueous humor production, being contraindicated in patients with an allergy to sulfonamide antibiotics and patients with renal or liver failure. The mode of action of sympathomimetics (brimonidine and apraclonidine) is based on the stimulation of alpha-2-receptors, resulting in both the decrease of the aqueous secretion and enhancement of the uveoscleral outflow. On the other hand, bradycardia and heart block are among the contraindications for the use of these sympathomimetics. Alpha-2 agonists are mostly prescribed for short-term use (for instance, after laser iridotomy). The treatment of angle-closure glaucoma includes the use of miotics (pilocarpine and carbachol) that increase the outflow through the trabecular meshwork. Currently, numerous combined preparations are commercially available on the market (timolol and dorzolamide/brinzolamide/travoprost/bimatoprost/brimonidine/pilocarpine or brimonidine and brinzolamide). Regardless of the number of available options for topical treatment of glaucoma, there is still a demand of using systemic drugs, and laser and surgical procedures in some clinical cases [22,48].

Age-related macular degeneration (AMD) is a degenerative disorder affecting people over the age of 50 years. An estimated number of people affected by AMD is approximately 30–50 million worldwide [49]. There are two known forms of AMD. The majority of patients have so-called "dry" AMD that is usually asymptomatic, except for gradual central visual loss of night vision. Also, it may be accompanied by metamorphopsia and prolonged afterimages [57]. This stage is defined by formation of drusen (amorphous deposits located between the retinal pigmented epithelium (RPE) and the Bruch's membrane) and abnormalities of RPE including hyperpigmentation and atrophy. In a relatively small share of patients, this form progresses to the neovascular ("exudative" or "wet") AMD. This condition is characterized by the growth of new abnormal capillaries from the choriocapillaris (choroidal neovascularization) that penetrate the Bruch's membrane, resulting in hemorrhages or exudation, producing scar, retina, or RPE detachment. At this stage, patients complain of a rapid onset of visual loss, a central blind spot, or metamorphopsia. The treatment of "dry" AMD is mostly based on changing lifestyle and using oral vitamin supplements (ascorbic acid, vitamin E, alpha-carotene, and zinc), which are thought to delay its progression. On the other hand, the treatment of the neovascular ("wet") AMD should be started with intravitreal injections of anti-vascular endothelial growth factor agents (anti-vascular endothelial growth factor (VEGF) treatment: ranibizumab, aflibercept, pegaptanib, bevacizumab), which is an invasive procedure posing concern and discomfort for the patient. Moreover, there are some potential vision-threatening complications associated with intravitreal injections: infectious endophthalmitis, retinal tears, sterile inflammation, vitreous hemorrhage, cataract, elevation of the IOP, etc. [49]. The intravitreal injection still remains a primary delivery route of anti-VEGF agents. A serious limitation of this therapy is a relatively short half-life of VEGF following intravitreous injections [58], which implies the need for frequent administrations. Some approaches were recently reported to develop less invasive methods of delivery, for example, subconjunctival administration of lyophilized matrices containing bevacizumab [59].

The development of formulations capable of delivering anti-VEGF agents into the eye, when administered topically, will be of great advantage and could revolutionize the therapy of this condition. Davis et al. [60] reported the successful topical delivery of Avastin using annexin A5-associated liposomal formulations to the posterior segment of the eye in vivo (rats and rabbits) at physiologically significant levels. This could be considered as a major advancement that should attract further research and perhaps some studies into the use of penetration enhancers. Some advances in the development of topical formulations to the delivery of biopharmaceuticals to the posterior segment of the eye were recently discussed in several reviews [61].

Photodynamic therapy (PDT) is an option if patients have any contraindications for anti-VEGF therapy. Focal laser photocoagulation is the third solution that can be offered to a patient, which is uncommon due to common recurrence and presence of localized scotoma after the procedure [48].

Diabetic retinopathy (DR) also belongs to one of the leading causes of vision impairment, as prevalence of diabetes mellitus is increasing dramatically worldwide [62]. In fact, this is the most frequent microvascular complication of diabetes. According to Duh et al. [63], almost 100 million individuals were diagnosed with diabetic retinopathy. DR is divided into two groups: (1) the earlier stage of non-proliferative diabetic retinopathy (NPDR), which is characterized by microaneurysms, retinal hemorrhages, intraretinal microvascular abnormalities, and venous caliber changes; and (2) proliferative diabetic retinopathy (PDR) with pathologic pre-retinal neovascularization. Additionally, diabetic macular edema may occur during both NPDR and PDR, representing the most common cause of vision loss in patients with DR. This edema arises from diabetes-induced breakdown of the blood–retinal barrier, with consequent leakage of fluid and circulating proteins from the vessels into the neurosensory retina [63]. As a matter of priority, assessment of patients with DR relies on the control of glucose concentration in the patient's blood. The treatment of this condition involves laser photocoagulation (panretinal, focal, and grid), intravitreal anti-VEGF agents (aflibercept and ranibizumab), corticosteroids (dexamethasone and fluocinolone acetonide intravitreal implants), and vitrectomy in the case of vitreous hemorrhage [48]. Some of these therapeutic approaches could potentially benefit from the development of formulations that could deliver drugs to the eye topically.

4. Permeability of Ocular Membranes

The analysis of the physicochemical properties of various chemical compounds that cross membranes in the eye could be key in understanding the opportunities and obstacles in ocular drug delivery. Thus, according to Prausnitz and Noonan [64], the octanol–water partitioning coefficient (logP), which helps characterize the drug's hydrophilic–lipophilic properties, determines the ability of molecules to pass through cells of the epithelial and endothelial layers of the cornea and conjunctiva. The epithelium permeability accounts up to 90% for the lipophilic substances as a result of the high dependence on logP, while almost totally excluding macromolecules (with radius larger than 10 Å) [64]. Hence, the epithelium is the main limitation for intracorneal drug delivery. In contrast, stromal drug permeability is less dependent on logP but highly dependent on the radius of the molecules, providing a great barrier for lipophilic compounds of a small size (radius < 10 Å). Interestingly, the permeation across the endothelium layer relies on both logP and the size of the molecule (paracellular penetration route) and is slightly more impermeable for lipophilic small molecules in comparison to the corneal stroma. However, macromolecules cross the endothelium more easily than the stroma. The permeability of another ocular membrane, sclera, is relatively close to that of the corneal stroma. The data on conjunctival permeation are limited; however, according to some reports, it demonstrates a higher permeability compared to the cornea [64].

Edwards and Prausnitz [65] reported the development of a theoretical model that can help in predicting the permeability of the cornea for different solutes, which can be calculated using only two parameters: radius of the molecule and logP. This could be a very useful model in ocular drug delivery, but there are a few factors that were not taken into account by the authors: simplification of the structure of openings between the cells, as well as tight junctions in epithelial and endothelial layers, various permeability of cells within the epithelium layer, possible intracorneal binding of compounds, and different shape of molecules (assuming all of them to be solid spheres).

Recently, a few in vitro and ex vivo models were used to evaluate permeability and drug absorption by the cornea. Thus, according to Agarwal and Rupenthal [66], cell-based models are commonly used for studies of penetration. Advantages of these models include relatively lower cost compared to the use of laboratory animals, as well as minimizing the number of animal studies. However, this type of model is more suitable to evaluate the cytotoxicity of the compounds rather than their permeability and absorption by the cornea. This is because cell-based models are, in simple terms, five to six layers of the epithelial cells of the cornea (usually, corneal culture of the rabbit) but not the entire structure of the cornea. Additionally, these cell cultures neither have transporter molecules nor enzymes responsible for drugs metabolism. One of the closest models to the real cornea involves reconstructed tissue cultures which comprise different types of cells that help mimic the three-layer structure including the epithelium, stroma, and endothelium. For example, Kaluzhny et al. [67] recently developed an in vitro human three-dimensional corneal epithelial tissue model and demonstrated the applicability of this membrane for studies of drug permeability using several fluorescent markers, as well as latanoprost and bimatoprost.

Ex vivo corneas of various animals (rabbit, porcine, bovine) are also commonly used for evaluating corneal permeability and absorption; however, this model is not ideal due to the differences in the anatomical structure compared to the human cornea, as well as potentially different enzymes and molecules of active transporters. Thus, rabbit eyes are commonly used as ex vivo models, but the rabbit cornea does not have Bowman's layer, which results in higher penetration of substances in comparison with the human cornea. The eyeball size, thickness of the cornea, ratio of length of the cornea to eye-globe diameter, and histological structure (including Bowman's membrane) in porcine eyes are the closest to the human eye. Bovine eyes are also used in the studies of ocular tissue drug permeability despite the fact that these are larger than human eyes and their corneal epithelium is almost twice the thickness [66]. Loch et al. [21] conducted a comparative study of the permeation of three different drugs (ciprofloxacin hydrochloride, lidocaine hydrochloride, and timolol maleate) through porcine, rabbit, and bovine ocular tissues. They observed substantial differences between the apparent permeability coefficients (P_{app}) for different animal species.

$$P_{app} = \frac{Q}{A \times C_0},$$ (1)

where Q is the steady-state appearance rate of the investigated substance on the acceptor side of the tissue (mol/s), C_0 is the initial concentration of the drug in the donor chamber (mol/L), and A is the surface area of the tissue (cm^2). In order to take into account the differences in the thicknesses of porcine, rabbit, and bovine tissues, they calculated effective diffusion coefficients using the following equation:

$$D_{eff} = P_{app} \times l,$$ (2)

where l is the tissue thickness (cm). The results of D_{eff} determination are presented in Figure 6. These results clearly show that the chemical nature of the drug has great influence on the tissue permeability. The authors also hypothesized that protein binding, tissue hydration, or transporters may play some role in the differences between different species.

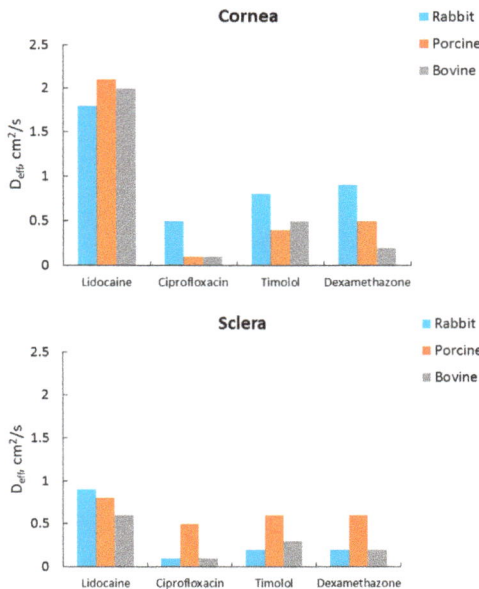

Figure 6. Effective diffusion coefficients D_{eff} (cm^2/s) of several drugs for rabbit, porcine, and bovine cornea and sclera. Data taken from Reference [21] with permission from Elsevier, 2012.

5. Penetration Enhancers

Anatomical and physiological features of the eye, ocular conditions, and permeability of ocular membranes were discussed above, and the review now moves to consider some of the different classes of penetration-enhancing compounds, describing their properties and modes of action.

5.1. Cyclodextrins

Cyclodextrins (CD) are water-soluble cyclic oligosaccharides shaped like a truncated cone. Native cyclodextrins include α-CD, β-CD, and γ-CD, which differ in the number of α-(1-4)-linked glucopyranose subunits (six, seven, and eight, respectively, Figure 7) [68]. There were many derivatives of CDs developed over the last decades, each bringing some improved properties such as enhanced aqueous solubility. The most common derivatives of CDs include hydroxypropyl-β- and γ-CD, the randomly methylated β-CD, and sulfobutylether β-CD [69]. Cyclodextrins have lipophilic cavities and hydrophilic hydroxyl groups associated with the external surfaces of their molecule [70]. They are capable of forming guest–host inclusion complexes, whereby lipophilic drugs with poor aqueous solubility reside within the hydrophobic cavity, where they are protected, but not covalently bound. The drug–CD complexes usually have improved aqueous solubility due to the hydrophilic properties of the external surface of the cyclodextrin molecule [71]. It is generally established that only free drug molecules from topical formulations with cyclodextrins are able to penetrate ocular membranes [72]. Since cyclodextrins are relatively large molecules, they are unable to permeate through intact lipophilic membranes, for example, the corneal epithelium; however, they allow drugs to interact with the epithelial surface. They have uses in pharmaceutical applications due to their drug solubility-enhancing properties, improved bioavailability, and improved formulation stability, capable of masking a drug's irritation effects; they are generally regarded as safe (GRAS) [73]. Drug–CD inclusion complex formation/dissociation is a dynamic process, where drug molecules are released and taken up spontaneously in the aqueous environment [74,75]. Lipophilic compounds are able to reside within the cyclodextrin molecule cavity through weak hydrophobic interactions. In the aqueous environment of the tear film, drugs can be released from drug–CD complexes by preferential take-up of cell-membrane lipids, such as cholesterol and phospholipids, and simultaneous ejection of the drug guest. There remains an opportunity for the drug to enter the epithelium membrane via the temporary disruption caused by lipid extraction during membrane–cyclodextrin interaction [68,76].

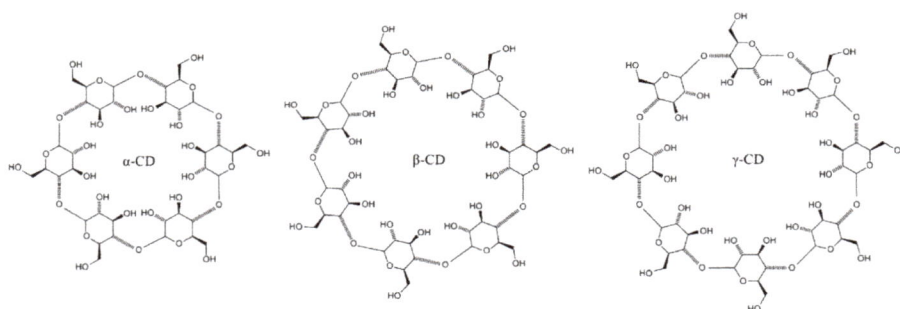

Figure 7. Structures of α-cyclodextrin, β-cyclodextrin, and γ-cyclodextrin. The image was reproduced under the Creative Commons Attribution Share Alike 3.0 Unported license [77].

The ability of α-CD to enhance corneal penetration for cysteamine (β-mercaptoethylamine; medication used to treat cystinosis, which is a rare, genetic disorder with abnormal accumulation of cystine within the corneal stroma resulting in photophobia) [78] was established by Pescina et al. [79] in ex vivo experiments with freshly excised pig corneas. The researchers also demonstrated lack of irritation caused by a 5.5% α-CD solution employing the Hen's Egg Test on the Chorioallantoic Membrane. Moreover, the addition of ethylenediamine-N,N,N′,N′-tetraacetic acid (EDTA) to α-CD established a good stability profile of cysteamine. According to Aktaş et al. [80], the eye drops consisting of pilocarpine nitrate and hydroxypropyl β-cyclodextrin (HP-β-CD) demonstrated a four-fold increase in transcorneal penetration compared to a drug formulation without CD. The researchers used side-by-side diffusion cells and corneas harvested from rabbits. In addition, the pupillary-response pattern was monitored in rabbits in vivo. The constriction of the pupil was remarkably increased due to the addition of the HP-β-CD-containing formulation of pilocarpine nitrate. Loftsson and Stefansson [81] designed low-viscosity eye-drop formulations with drug/γ-CD complexes which were then tested in vivo in rabbits and clinically in patients. The first aqueous eye-drop formulation included dorzolamide/γ-CD complexes and demonstrated high levels of the drug in the aqueous humor of rabbit eyes more than 24 h after a single application. The IOP-lowering effect of this solution in patients was observed after daily use compared to conventional eye drops with dorzolamide that should be given three times a day to provide the same effect. Other eye drops consisted of dexamethasone/γ-CD complexes and showed the ability to deliver dexamethasone to the posterior segment of the rabbit eye. Moreover, there were significant clinical improvements in patients with diabetic macular edema (DME) and intermediate uveitis patients with cystoid macular edema after the topical use of eye drops with dexamethasone/γ-CD. The results for DME patients were clinically similar to those after the intravitreal corticosteroid injection.

Morrison and co-workers [68] studied the penetration of riboflavin through freshly excised bovine corneas using formulations containing various cyclodextrins. They established that β-CD and HP-β-CD facilitate the permeation of riboflavin through the cornea; however, they do not affect the lag time of approximately 90–120 min, where the first portions of the drug begin crossing the cornea. The microscopic examination of the corneas treated with cyclodextrins indicated that these permeability enhancers cause some disruption of the epithelial structure. Further analysis of this disruption allowed the authors to establish the mechanism of permeability enhancement related to the extraction of cholesterol from corneal tissue observed in the case of formulations with β-CD and HP-β-CD. This resulted in a partial disruption of the corneal epithelia, which was evidenced from histological examination of the bovine corneal membranes exposed to solutions of cyclodextrins for different contact times. Figure 8 shows exemplary micrographs of corneas exposed to 30 mg·mL^{-1} solutions of β-CD compared to control non-exposed tissues. Samples of the cornea treated with β-cyclodextrin showed some epithelial disruption, which became more noticeable with longer exposure time. However, no extraction of cholesterol was observed when the corneas were exposed to water or α-CD and γ-CD.

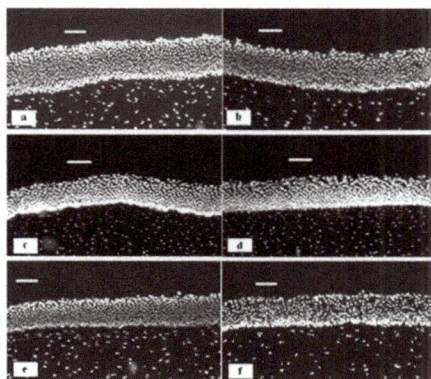

Figure 8. Micrographs of bovine cornea exposed to 1 mL of β-cyclodextrin (30 mg·mL^{-1}) (**b**,**d**,**f**) against non-exposed regions (**a**,**c**,**e**). Exposure time: 15 (**a**,**b**), 45 (**c**,**d**), and 75 min (**e**,**f**). Scale bar = 100 µm. Reproduced from Reference [68] with permission from American Chemical Society, 2013.

5.2. Chelating Agents

The corneal epithelium offers a highly resistant barrier against alien matter due to its lipophilic characteristics, preventing the transcellular transport of many drugs, and the existence of tight junctions, i.e., tightly adherent regions between cells, maintaining intimate cell contact, effectively preventing drug transport via the paracellular route. Tight junction functionality of the superficial epithelial cells depends on an undetermined availability of Ca^{2+} ions [4,82]. Calcium chelating agents are often included in topical ocular drug formulations as stabilizers. They were shown to offer temporary and reversible action when used for enhancement of ocular drug delivery. However, there is evidence that ethylenediamine-*N*,*N*,*N'*,*N'*-tetraacetic acid (EDTA) in topical ocular formulations can bring side effects due to accumulation within the iris and ciliary body, and can affect endothelial cells and capillaries associated with the uveal tract. Caution should be exercised due to toxicity implications, especially when medication is required in the long term [83]. Calcium chelators, a class of polyaminocarboxylic acids, for example, EDTA, ethylene glycol-bis(beta-aminoethyl)-*N*,*N*,*N'*,*N'*-tetraacetic acid (EGTA), 1,2-bis(o-aminophenoxy)ethane-*N*,*N*,*N'*,*N'*-tetraacetic acid (BAPTA) [84], and ethylenediamine-*N*,*N'*-disuccinic acid (EDDS) (Figure 9), are capable of reversibly enhancing drug penetration across otherwise penetration-resistant barriers such as the corneal epithelium [17].

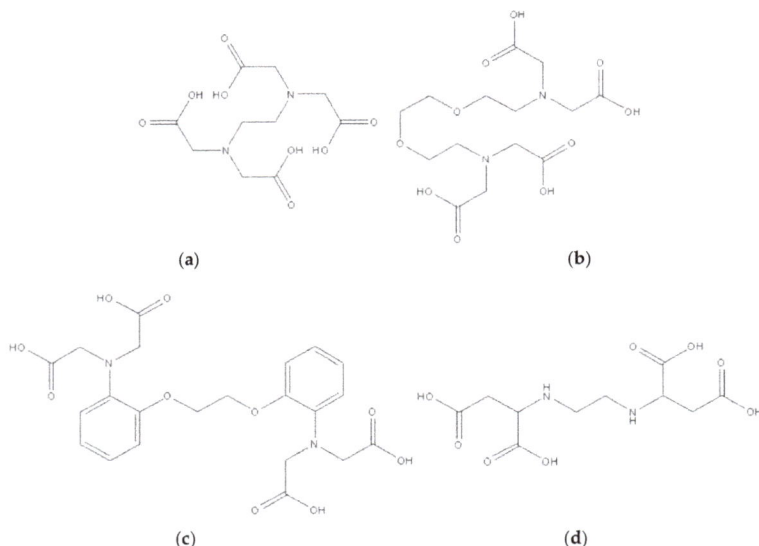

Figure 9. Structures of ethylenediamine-*N*,*N*,*N'*,*N'*-tetraacetic acid (EDTA) (**a**), ethylene glycol-bis(beta-aminoethyl)-*N*,*N*,*N'*,*N'*-tetraacetic acid (EGTA) (**b**), 1,2-bis(o-aminophenoxy)ethane-*N*,*N*,*N'*,*N'*-tetraacetic acid (BAPTA) (**c**), and ethylenediamine-*N*,*N'*-disuccinic acid (EDDS) (**d**).

Their mode of action is achieved via disruption of tight junctions and adherens junctions by sequestration of interstitial Ca^{2+} ions, on which the barrier function is dependent. Research carried out by Morrison and Khutoryanskiy [17] showed that low-concentration aqueous solutions of EDTA, EGTA, and EDDS at 1 mg·mL^{-1} were capable of extracting Ca^{2+} ions from bovine corneas in vitro (Figure 10). The three formulations studied enhanced Ca^{2+} extraction and corneal penetration of riboflavin compared with phosphate-buffered saline. The same researchers investigated permeability enhancement of bovine corneas in vitro using transepithelial electrical resistance analysis (TEER), finding that all polyaminocarboxylic acid formulations investigated lowered TEER values, correlating with enhanced penetration of riboflavin across bovine epithelia into the corneal stroma. EGTA showed the best performance for Ca^{2+} extraction and penetration enhancement from the formulations explored.

Kikuchi et al. [85] investigated a synergistic relationship for enhancing ocular drug penetration when using a combination of EDTA and boric acid in various proportions. The researchers found that the co-formulation brought an improvement in drug penetration across the highly resistant epithelial membrane, but no enhancement to the already efficient permeation across de-epithelialized rabbit corneas. They concluded that the synergistic effects observed were due to improved transcellular permeability when compared to formulations with either EDTA or boric acid alone [85]. Topical aqueous ocular drug formulations incorporating polyaminocarboxylic acid penetration-enhancing agents induce disruption to the corneal epithelium, even at concentrations as low as 1 mg·mL^{-1}. Although this enhances corneal permeability to drugs, it can also introduce undesirable side effects such as ocular irritation. The use of topical ocular drug formulations incorporating mucoadhesive polymers, i.e., hyaluronic acid, chitosan, and alginate, together with polyaminocarboxylic acid penetration-enhancing agents, gives the benefits from these chelating agents whilst moderating the epithelial disruptive effects, allowing them to give moderate enhancement to ocular drug penetration without inducing irritation. The use of mucoadhesive polymers potentially offers a means to give improved drug efficacy, low dose, and sustained delivery with reduced issues of toxicity and minimal undesired side effects [86,87]. However, Rodriguez et al. [86] demonstrated that the combination of mucoadhesive polymers with permeability enhancers leads to the inhibition of permeability-enhancing effects.

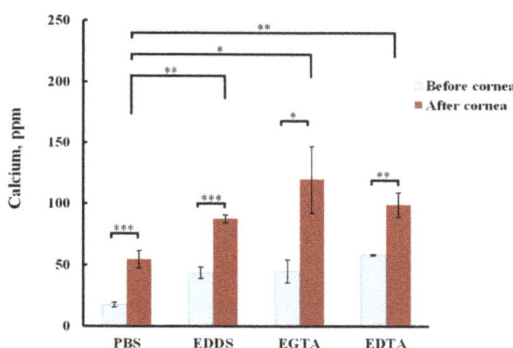

Figure 10. Calcium concentration in solutions containing phosphate-buffered saline (PBS), EDDS, EGTA, and EDTA (1 mg·mL^{-1}) before and after 3 h of exposure to bovine cornea. * $p < 0.05$, ** $p < 0.01$, *** $p < 0.001$; one-way ANOVA; $n = 3$. Reproduced from Reference [17] under the terms of the Creative Commons Attribution License (CC BY).

5.3. Crown Ethers

Crown ethers are synthetic cyclic oligomers of ethylene oxide consisting of linked ether groups; they are named this way because the shape of their molecules resembles that of a crown when its structure is viewed at its side elevation. Naming convention follows numbers divided by the letter "C" for "crown", whereby the larger number represents the number of atoms contained in the molecule, and the smaller number represents the number of oxygen atoms. The most common members are 12C4, 15C5, and 18C6, namely, the tetramer ($n = 4$), pentamer ($n = 5$), and hexamer ($n = 6$) (Figure 11).

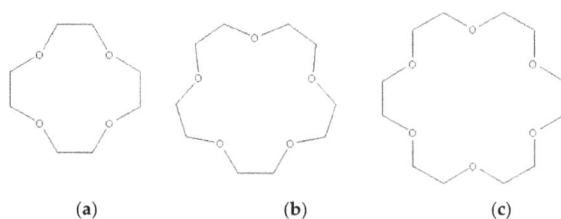

(a)   (b)   (c)

Figure 11. Structures of 12-crown-4 (a), 15-crown-5 (b), and 18-crown-6 (c).

Crown ethers were discovered accidentally by Pedersen whilst researching the development of complexing agents for divalent cations in the 1960s. During his research, Pedersen realized that the cyclic polyether by-products were capable of forming complexes with alkali metals [88]. Since Pedersen's pioneering work, many derivatives were developed [89–91], and these found uses in various fields of science, industry, and pharmacology. Crown ethers are able to form complexes with metal ions, as well as neutral and ionic organic molecules, and their complexes have the ability to traverse biological membranes [92–94]. They are employed for the treatment of tumors [95,96] and drug-loaded vesicular preparations [97,98]. Crown ethers are flexible molecules, allowing them to adapt to the environment they are exposed to. In aqueous solutions, they interact with this medium by exposing their hydrophilic oxygen atoms to water molecules; however, when these molecules encounter a lipophilic solvent, they interact via their lipophilic ethylenic groups [91]. These properties, together with their ionophoric qualities, make them ideal compounds for use in ocular drug delivery, where the formulation has to interact with both aqueous and lipophilic phases. At the time of writing of this review, there was only one published study investigating the use of crown ethers for enhanced ocular drug delivery [99]; Morrison et al. [100] investigated 12C4, 15C5, and 18C6 for use in ocular drug delivery, and they were able to show enhanced aqueous solubility of riboflavin up to 46%, potentially improving bioavailability (Table 1). Furthermore, all crown ether variants studied were capable of significantly enhancing Ca^{2+} extraction from bovine corneas in vitro compared with phosphate-buffered saline. In the same study the researchers were able to show enhanced corneal delivery of riboflavin to bovine corneal stroma in vitro with crown ether concentrations as low as 1 mg·mL^{-1}.

Table 1. Steady-state flux and apparent permeability of riboflavin through bovine cornea in phosphate-buffered saline (PBS) with and without crown ether. Reproduced from Reference [100] with permission from American Chemical Society, 2017.

Solution	Steady-State Flux (µmol·min^{-1})	P_{app} (cm·s^{-1} × 10^{-3})
PBS	0.0478	1.945
12C4 (1 mg·mL^{-1})	0.1208	6.138
15C5 (1 mg·mL^{-1})	0.1074	5.457
18C6 (1 mg·mL^{-1})	0.0753	3.826
12C4 (30 mg·mL^{-1})	0.3410	17.326
15C5 (30 mg·mL^{-1})	0.1961	9.964
18C6 (30 mg·mL^{-1})	0.1811	9.202

Morrison et al. [100] also carried out a toxicological investigation and in vivo penetration studies using the rat model. The toxicological investigation was able to show that crown ethers were no more toxic to ocular tissue than benzalkonium chloride, an excipient often used at low concentrations as a preservative in ocular drug formulations. The in vivo drug penetration study failed to show any statistically significant permeability enhancement compared to enhancer-free formulations, the most probable reason being due to natural clearance mechanisms that protect the eye from foreign material. However, their in vivo study was conducted using a very limited number of animals ($n = 3$) to achieve good levels of statistical significance. They concluded that further in vitro and in vivo investigations are required to better understand crown ethers as penetration enhancers for ocular drug formulations [100].

5.4. Surfactants

Surface active compounds (surfactants) are compounds that have lipophilic and hydrophilic moieties. Acting on a surface, or between aqueous and non-aqueous media interfaces, surfactants are able to reduce interfacial surface tension [101]. In pharmaceutical applications, surfactants are commonly used as excipients to solubilize formulation components, or in the case of permeability enhancement, they alter membrane properties by disrupting tear film and mucin, removing their protective properties, disrupting the integrity of the epithelia by loosening tight junctions or modifying epithelial cell membranes. These compounds are included in formulations in a wide range of pharmaceutical applications including oral, injectable, nasal, ocular, and transdermal, amongst others. The polar group determines the specific properties of surfactants, and they can be classified into four main groups: cationic, anionic, zwitterionic, and non-ionic. Cationic surfactants have a positive charge on the polar head group, anionic surfactants have a negative charge, zwitterionic surfactants have positive and negative charges depending on which environment they are exposed to, and non-ionic surfactants are neutral [102]. Non-ionic surfactants are the compounds of choice for many drug delivery scenarios including ocular drug delivery, bringing enhanced drug solubility, formulation stability, biocompatibility, and low toxicity compared with their anionic, amphoteric, and cationic counterparts [103,104]. Polyoxyethylene-9-lauryl ether, Tween-80 and Span-60 are non-ionic surfactants, and their mode of action is via phospholipid acyl chain perturbation. According to Marsh et al. [105], the 1% solutions of Tween-20 and Brij-35 showed a relatively high effectiveness in enhancing permeability of the cornea by a five-fold increase in penetration of fluorescein through the cornea without detected irritation of the eye. Saettone et al. [106] reported improved permeability of the rabbit cornea for the β-blockers (atenolol, timolol, levobunolol, and betaxolol) combined with Brij-35, -78, and -98. The increased penetration was greater for atenolol and timolol, which are hydrophilic, than for hydrophobic β-blockers (levobunolol and betaxolol), which can be due to the hydrophilic properties of the corneal stroma. The non-ionic surfactant ᴅ-alpha-tocopheryl poly(ethylene glycol) 1000 succinate is also a potential permeability enhancer for ocular drug delivery. Ostacolo et al. [107] showed that this penetration enhancer effectively increased the permeation of riboflavin through porcine corneas. Pharmasolve® (*N*-methyl-2-pyrrolidone) is another permeation enhancer that was studied by Li et al. [108] for transcorneal drug delivery using rabbit eyes. Interestingly, this penetration enhancer increased the apparent corneal permeability coefficients for ribavirin, enoxacin, puerarin, and ibuprofen by 4.04-, 2.76-, 2.67-, and 1.47-fold, respectively. Also, no ocular irritation was observed for formulations with less than 10% *N*-methyl-2-pyrrolidone. Montenegro et al. [109] demonstrated a significant improvement in penetration of acyclovir through the rabbit corneas in the presence of 5% *N*-methyl-2-pyrrolidone, positively charged phospholipid mixture, and sodium taurocholate after 90 min since the drug was administered on the ocular surface; however, after 180 min, only the phospholipid mixture was still effective. The taurocholate, Brij-78, and phospholipid mixture enhanced the permeation of timolol maleate across the cornea after 90 min, but only Brij-78 showed the ability to retain this effect after 180 min.

These are also natural surfactants produced by some plants that could be potentially useful as penetration enhancers. Saponins are a class of amphiphilic glycosides abundantly found in different plants that exhibit good penetration-enhancement properties. For instance, digitonin is a steroidal saponin (Figure 12) isolated from the *Digitalis purpurea* plant; it is capable of solubilizing cellular membrane lipids and cholesterol. Shih and Lee demonstrated that digitonin caused ocular epithelial exfoliation [110–112].

Benzalkonium chloride (BAC) is a cationic surfactant that is commonly used in many formulations for ocular drugs in low concentrations as a preservative. BAC is a known irritant even at low concentration (<0.01%); nevertheless, it acts as a penetration enhancer, which destabilizes the tear film and the protection offered by the mucous layer at the cornea surface. BAC also initiates changes within phospholipid bilayers of cellular membranes [113]. Recently, Johannsdottir et al. [114] reported an in vivo study of benzalkonium chloride's effect on the ocular penetration of dexamethasone in pigmented rabbits. They compared two eye-drop formulations of dexamethasone, where the drug formed a microsuspension with γ-CD in a vehicle containing poloxamer, NaCl, and EDTA with and without 0.02% (*w/v*) benzalkonium chloride. The analysis of the drug concentrations in different ocular tissues 2 h following the eye-drop administration indicated no statistically significant effects of benzalkonium chloride. The authors related the absence of permeability enhancement to the quick removal of benzalkonium chloride with tear fluid and its inability to penetrate into the cornea/conjunctiva and sclera to cause disruption of barrier function.

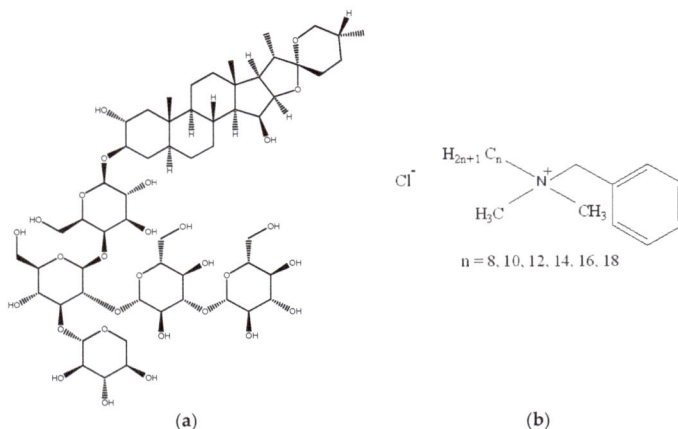

(a)   (b)

Figure 12. Structures of digitonin (**a**) and benzalkonium chloride (**b**).

Sasaki et al. [115] compared the influence of a few penetration enhancers (saponin, EDTA, benzalkonium chloride, and paraben) on improving ocular absorption of thyrotropin-releasing hormone and luteinizing hormone-releasing hormone using diffusion cells with rabbit conjunctiva and cornea. The researchers showed that penetration of both hormones through the conjunctiva was improved by 0.5% saponin, 0.05% benzalkonium chloride, and 0.01% benzalkonium chloride. The permeability coefficient of conjunctiva was significantly improved for luteinizing hormone-releasing hormone using EDTA and paraben. The observed effects of permeation enhancers for conjunctiva were smaller compared to those on corneal penetration with luteinizing hormone-releasing hormone with paraben as the exception. EDTA and saponin increased the ratios of corneal to conjunctival permeation of both hormones. According to van der Bijl et al. [116], 0.01% benzalkonium chloride enhanced the permeation of cyclosporin A through frozen/thawed rabbit cornea.

Transcutol® P is another solubilizer mostly used as a transdermal penetration enhancer. Liu et al. [117] demonstrated that 0.005–0.03% Transcutol® P increased the apparent permeability coefficient by 1.5-, 1.5-, 3.0-, and 3.3-fold for ribavirin, gatifloxacin, levofloxacin hydrochloride, and enoxacin, respectively. Permeation for oxaprozin was inhibited with a maximum decrease by 2.8-fold for 0.03% Transcutol® P. In addition, no irritation was observed with Transcutol® P at concentrations of 0.005–0.03%, with the presence of slight irritation for 0.05% Transcutol® P. A non-ionic oil-in-water surfactant, Labrasol®, is also a potential excipient as a corneal penetration enhancer. It is composed of well-characterized polyethylene glycol (PEG) esters, a small glyceride fraction, and free PEG. Liu et al. [118] observed no ocular surface irritation for 0.5–3.0% Labrasol® and slight irritation for 5.0% Labrasol®. The penetration of baicalin solution through the rabbit cornea was enhanced by 1.69-, 3.14-, and 2.23-fold in the presence of 1.5%, 2.0%, and 3.0% Labrasol®, respectively.

5.5. Bile Acids and Bile Salts

Bile acids are steroid acids, all forms of cholic acid, and their sodium or potassium salts, and there are a number of derivatives that result from cholesterol metabolism in the liver which then undergo further transformations in the intestinal tract. They are soluble in water and are involved in the solubilization of dietary lipids within the gut. In the intestinal tract, they become conjugated with taurine and glycine, where the sodium and potassium salts of these conjugates are termed bile salts [119,120]. Bile acids are amphiphilic compounds naturally produced in the human digestive system; they are able to promote drug penetration across biological membranes. They are employed in drug formulations for enhancement of drug penetration via many mucosal routes including nasal, oral, buccal, ocular, pulmonary, and rectal mucosa. They are capable of forming vesicular drug-carrying systems which are able to promote epithelial drug transport via transcellular and paracellular routes [121]. Bile acids and bile salts have surfactant properties with an ability to form micelles or liposomes in the aqueous environment, otherwise known as "bilosomes"; these vesicular entities offer some interesting and novel properties in drug delivery [122]. Examples of many bile acid/bile salt derivatives include deoxycholate, glycocholate, and taurodeoxycholate (Figure 13). They are able to alter the rheological properties of ocular mucosal membranes [123], and the mucolytic properties of bile salts alter the protective mucus barrier, inducing changes in membrane characteristics allowing for enhanced drug transit into ocular tissue [4,124]. Dai et al. [125] investigated liposomes with bile salts for the ocular delivery of tacrolimus FK506, a calcineurin inhibitor, as a model drug. The liposomes they developed contained cholesterol (control) or bile salts (sodium taurocholate, sodium deoxycholate, and sodium glycocholate), prepared using a thin-membrane dispersion technique, achieving uniform particle size and drug entrapment. These liposomes exhibited controlled release of <5% over 24 h, thus avoiding a "burst release" often seen with some ocular drug delivery systems. They conducted ex vivo corneal permeability and in vivo corneal uptake experiments and demonstrated that liposomes with bile salts offered enhanced transcorneal drug permeability compared to the cholesterol-containing liposomes, enhancing the permeation of tacrolimus across the cornea up to four-fold. Furthermore, cytotoxicity studies showed that the liposomes with sodium taurocholate or sodium glycocholate were well tolerated, whereas those with deoxycholate showed evidence of corneal toxicity to spontaneously derived human corneal epithelial cells and in the rabbit model. The researchers concluded that liposomes incorporating sodium taurocholate and sodium glycocholate offer potential as ocular drug delivery systems for drugs of low aqueous solubility such as tacrolimus, due to their low toxicity and improved ocular permeability [125]. A cautious approach is generally required when employing bile acids and bile salts for enhanced ocular drug delivery; however, given the right choice of cholic acid variant or a derivative therewith, and the right choice of delivery vehicle, bile acids and their salts offer much potential for future ocular drug delivery systems.

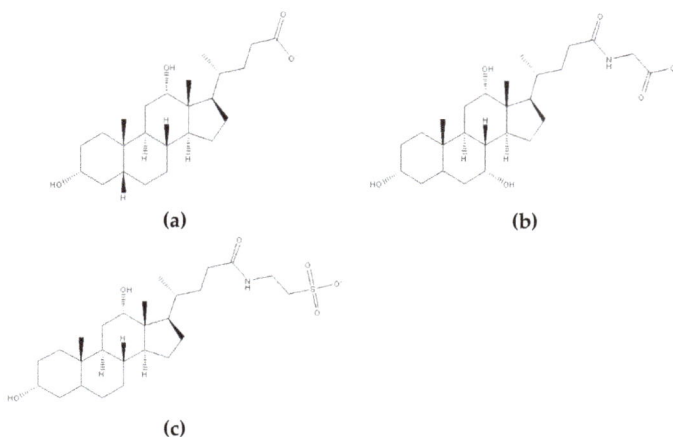

(a)

(b)

(c)

Figure 13. Structures of deoxycholate (**a**), glycocholate (**b**), and taurodeoxycholate (**c**).

Mahaling and Katti [126] recently investigated the effect of different enhancers (benzalkonium chloride, capric acid, EDTA, sodium glycocholate, and sodium taurocholate) on the penetration of polymeric nanoparticles in vivo in pigmented mice. It was established that sodium glycocholate and sodium taurocholate enhanced the permeability of nanoparticles in the conjunctiva. Benzalkonium chloride, sodium glycocholate, and sodium taurocholate enhanced bioavailability of nanoparticles in the iris and ciliary body. They also observed some inhibition effects; the use of EDTA decreased the bioavailability of nanoparticles in the lens and choroid, whereas sodium glycocholate showed a reduction in their presence in the choroid and retina. The authors concluded that a combination of penetration enhancers with a hydrophilic mucoadhesive coating on nanoparticles is a promising approach to enhance their bioavailability.

5.6. Cell-Penetrating Peptides

Cell-penetrating peptides (CPPs) are short chains of amino acids connected by amide bonds (peptide bonds); they form a diverse group of compounds derived from variable combinations of many different natural amino acid residues [127]. CPPs are capable of penetrating cellular membranes and have the ability to transport internalized hydrophilic cargo into cells, for example, drugs [128]. Liu et al. [129] investigated a number of fluorophore-labeled cell-penetrating peptides, namely, trans-activating transcriptional activator (TAT), penetratin, poly(arginine), low-molecular-weight protamine, and poly(serine), for their ocular permeability using side-by-side diffusion cells, ex vivo in a rabbit model. Protamine is a small arginine-rich protein; TAT and penetratin are complex polypeptides consisting of specific sequences of different amino acids, whereas poly(arginine) and poly(serine) represent homopolymers of corresponding amino acids. The structures of poly(arginine) and poly(serine) are shown in Figure 14. They also used human conjunctival epithelial cells to determine cytotoxicity and cellular uptake of CPPs. The researchers found penetratin to have excellent performance in enhancing drug permeability, whilst also showing the lowest cytotoxicity. Penetratin showed cellular uptake more than 25-fold compared with the control peptide poly(serine). This peptide also showed an increased permeation of 87.5 times using the rabbit excised corneas. When fluorophore-labeled penetratin was instilled into the cul-de-sac of rat eyes, it was widely distributed in the anterior and posterior segments and could be measured in the corneal epithelium and retina for at least 6 h. They concluded that penetratin could be a potential permeability enhancer for ophthalmic use; this peptide can be conjugated with bioactive compounds for topical delivery into the eye reaching as far as the retina. Further research on the design and synthesis of new cell-penetrating peptides for topical delivery into different layers of the cornea, with potential application as absorption enhancers for metabolic sensitive ophthalmic drugs, was recently conducted by Pescina et al. [130]. The researchers labeled the synthesized CPPs with 5-carboxyfluorescein and measured their diffusion and distribution within the cornea using an ex vivo porcine model and confocal microscopy. The synthesized peptides were also shown to be safe and well tolerated when tested on human conjunctival cell line. They concluded that the tested CPPs could provide useful ocular therapies, especially when used as transcorneal transporters for some drugs with unfavorable molecular characteristics, examples being the aminoglycoside antibiotic, cysteamine, and antiviral agents. Interestingly, in 2017, de Cogan et al. [131] reported a promising approach for topical delivery of an anti-VEGF agent (bevacizumab) linked to the CPP (5(6)-carboxyfluorescein–RRRRRR–COOH) to the posterior segment of the eye. The toxicity of CPP, assessed using cell cultures, was found to be low. This complex study was done in vivo and included optical coherence tomography (OCT) imaging of the CPP tagged with fluorescent dye passing into the rat's eye anterior segment, as well as assessment of topical delivery of the complex CPP–bevacizumab into the vitreous body with subsequent fixation of the time course of bevacizumab clearance from the vitreous body and retina. Moreover, the in vivo effectiveness of eye drops comprising a complex formulation of CPP with anti-VEGF agent was evaluated in a mouse model with choroidal neovascularization (CNV) which, as mentioned above, is common in patients with neovascular AMD. Mice received different treatment, which included intravitreal injection of the anti-VEGF agent, topical application of CPP with anti-VEGF (twice a day), or dexamethasone gavage (every day) for 10 days. Additionally, ex vivo experiments with topical delivery of anti-VEGF agents (ranibizumab and bevacizumab) into pig eyes were also conducted. As a result, CPP was observed within 6 min in the anterior chamber of the eye in rats. A single application of CPP–bevacizumab complex on the rat's cornea showed drug levels in the posterior segment that could be relevant to clinical concentrations. CPP–ranibizumab and CPP–bevacizumab complex concentrations in the posterior chamber of porcine eyes were also found to be clinically relevant. There was a significant decrease in CNV area in all mice that received intravitreal injection, eye drops with CPP with anti-VEGF drug, and dexamethasone gavage compared to the eyes treated with a laser only.

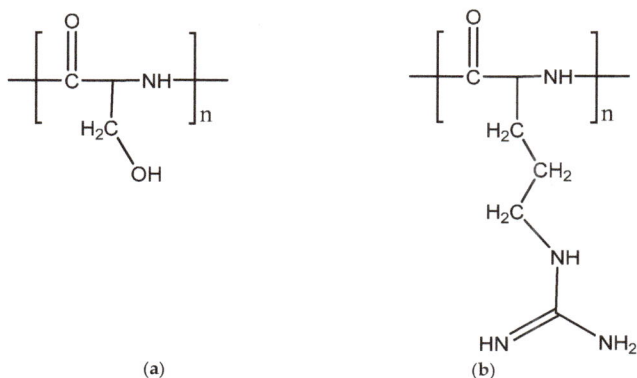

(a)   (b)

Figure 14. Structures of poly-L-serine (**a**) and poly-L-arginine hydrochloride (**b**).

Nemoto et al. [132] demonstrated the permeability-enhancing features of poly-L-arginine hydrochloride for hydrophilic molecules (fluorescein isothiocyanate (FITC)-labeled dextran and pyridoxamine), across ocular membranes taken from Japanese white rabbits. The increase in P_{app} of FITC-labeled dextran in the cornea, conjunctiva, and conjunctiva/sclera composite was observed in the presence of poly-L-arginine (0.1 mg/mL) by 6.81-, 9.78-, and 7.91-fold, respectively. The permeation of pyridoxamine was also improved by adding poly-L-arginine by 7.98-, 4.67-, and 8.31-fold, respectively. The authors suggested that the mechanism of this permeability enhancement lies in the ability of poly-L-arginine to disassemble tight junction-associated proteins present in the cornea and conjunctiva. Thus, this compound can be used as a permeability enhancer for lipophobic compounds without producing significant damage to the epithelium.

Some progress in the application of cell-penetrating peptides in ocular drug delivery was recently reviewed by Pescina et al. [133]. The authors highlighted this topic as an emerging area in ocular therapeutics, which has great potential for the delivery of drugs and biopharmaceuticals both to the anterior and posterior segments of the eye.

5.7. Other Amphiphilic Compounds

Fatty acids facilitate ocular drug permeation by altering cell-membrane properties and loosening tight junctions. These compounds can also induce ion–pair complexation when formulated with cationic drugs. Caprylic acid and capric acid are examples of fatty acids (Figure 15). The former interacts with proteins, whilst the latter can affect both proteins and lipid components of cellular membranes [111]. Capric acid was shown to enhance ocular penetration of β-blockers, bringing moderate enhancement to the penetration of hydrophilic β-blockers, whilst only offering slight enhancement for lipophilic β-blockers [123]. Kato and Iwata attributed the penetration-enhancing effects of fatty acids for bunazosin to ion–pair interactions [134,135].

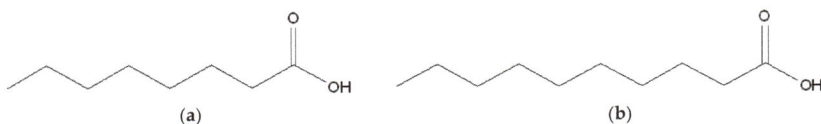

Figure 15. Structures of caprylic acid (**a**) and capric acid (**b**).

Gelucires are glyceride-based compounds with amphiphilic surfactant properties. Gelucires comprise mono-, di-, and triglycerides with mono- and diesters of polyethylene glycol [136]. The numbers 44 and 14 in the name of Gelucire 44/14 indicate the melting temperature of 44 °C and a hydrophilic–lipophilic balance of 14. Known for their drug absorption-enhancing performance, Gelucires have a good safety profile for pharmaceutical formulations and are "generally regarded as safe" (GRAS). Gelucire 44/14 was evaluated as a potential permeability enhancer in vitro and in vivo using different ophthalmic drugs and was shown to enhance transcorneal permeability of drugs with a range of hydrophilicity/lipophilicity whilst remaining safe to use and non-irritating [5,20]. Another potential corneal permeability enhancer is Azone™ (1-dodecylazacycloheptan-2-one), which is currently used mostly for transdermal drug delivery. This formulation is thought to act by partitioning into lipid bilayers of the bio-membrane and, as a result, disrupting its structure. Tang-Liu et al. [137] compared effects of four permeation enhancers (Azone™, hexamethylenelauramide, hexamethyleneoctanamide, and decylmethylsulfoxide (Figure 16)) with lipophobic (acetazolamide, cimetidine, guanethidine, and sulfacetamide), moderately hydrophobic (bunolol and prednisolone), and hydrophobic (flurbiprofen and its amide analogue) drugs through the rabbit cornea.

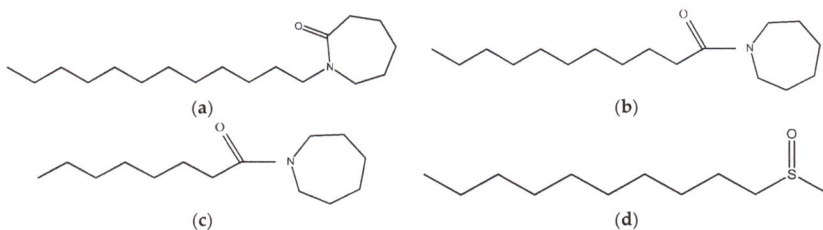

Figure 16. Structures of Azone™ (**a**), hexamethylenelauramide (**b**), hexamethyleneoctanamide (**c**), and decylmethylsulfoxide (**d**).

The researchers demonstrated that 0.1% Azone™ enhanced the permeability of lipophobic formulations 20-fold, while permeation of moderately hydrophobic compounds was enhanced at 0.025–0.1% Azone™ by two- to five-fold. Interestingly, there was inhibition instead of promotion of corneal permeability for flurbiprofen and its amide analogue in the presence of Azone™. Also, all four penetration enhancers used in this study showed similar ability to promote penetration through the cornea for cimetidine. Additionally, the researchers noticed a parabolic relationship between the rate of drug penetration and the lipophilicity of this compound. Afouna et al. [138] also tested gel formulations with Azone™ as a permeability enhancer, Carbopol-974® as a mucoadhesive, and s-timolol maleate as a model drug using rabbits. It was demonstrated that in vivo reduction of intraocular pressure for these formulations lasted roughly 3–4 times longer in comparison with the conventional timolol maleate eye drops. In 2016, Afouna et al. [139] reported the extension of in vitro parameters including release, onset, magnitude, and action duration up to two days for the gel formulations containing Azone™, Carbopol-974®, and latanoprost acid.

Borneol is a terpene derivative that can also be used as ocular penetration enhancer (Figure 17). According to Yang et al. [140], 0.1% synthetic borneol improved the permeability of two hydrophobic compounds (indomethacin and dexamethasone) through rabbit corneas by 1.23-and 2.40-fold, respectively, while the permeation of more hydrophilic drugs (ofloxacin, ribavirin, and tobramycin) was increased by 1.87-, 2.80-, and 3.89-fold, respectively. Natural borneol also enhanced the permeability with the following levels: 1.67, 2.00, 2.15, 2.18, and 3.39, respectively. It was also established that 0.1% borneol did not produce any damage to the cornea. The authors suggested that borneol's ability of promoting corneal permeability might be due to the changes in the arrangement of lipid molecules in the cell membrane of corneal epitheliocytes, increasing the orderliness of the molecular chains of lecithin.

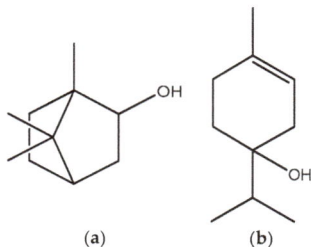

(a)　　　　　(b)

Figure 17. Structures of borneol (**a**) and terpinen-4-ol (**b**).

At the same time, terpinen-4-ol (Figure 17) can also be used as an ocular drug permeability enhancer. Afouna et al. [141] prepared and tested ophthalmic gel formulations with different concentrations of terpinen-4-ol as a penetration enhancer, Carbopol-934 as a mucoadhesive, and dorzolamide hydrochloride as a model drug. They demonstrated that permeation of this IOP-lowering drug across the excised rabbit's cornea was increased significantly with the concentration of terpinen-4-ol. It was shown that the highest concentration of this penetration enhancer (0.5%) demonstrated the best permeation features among tested formulations. The authors suggested that this permeability improvement may result from the thermodynamic activity increase, as well as from the change in the ratio between ionized and unionized dorzolamide hydrochloride species in favor of the latter. The cumulative amount of dorzolamide hydrochloride in the receiver chamber of a vertical Franz diffusion cell from ophthalmic gel formulations with different terpinen-4-ol concentrations and fixed concentration of Carbopol-934 through the excised rabbit's cornea is shown in Figure 18.

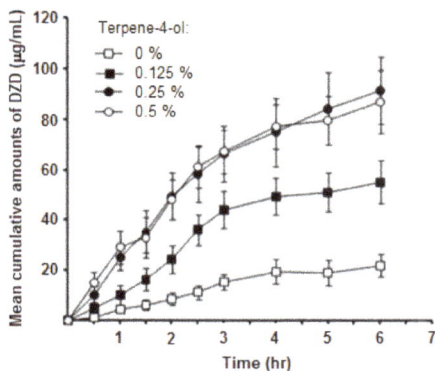

Figure 18. The cumulative amount of dorzolamide hydrochloride in the receiver chamber of a vertical Franz diffusion cell from ophthalmic gel formulations with various terpinen-4-ol concentrations and a fixed concentration of Carbopol-934 through the excised rabbit's cornea ($n = 3$). Reproduced from Reference [141] with permission from Elsevier, 2010.

Semifluorinated alkanes (SFAs) belong to the group of amphiphilic liquids that can dissolve lipophilic compounds forming clear solutions. Agarwal et al. [142] assessed the potential of two different SFAs for topical ocular drug delivery. Cyclosporin A (CsA) was dissolved in perfluorobutylpentane (F4H5) or perfluorohexyloctane (F6H8) and was compared with commercially available CsA ophthalmic emulsions, Restasis® and Ikervis®, in terms of corneal availability. The penetration of CsA through the cornea was evaluated by plotting the concentration of the corneal CsA per g of cornea (ng/g) against time and determining the mean area under curve of each formulation tested over 4 h (AUC (0–4 h)) (Figure 19). The permeability of the cornea was significantly enhanced for CsA after a single dose of 0.05% CsA in F4H5 and F6H8 was applied when compared to Restasis with the area under the curve over 4 h (AUC (0–4 h)) being at least eight-fold higher for both SFAs. Interestingly, the AUC (0–4 h) of 0.1% CsA in F4H5 was almost five-fold higher than with Ikervis. Thus, semifluorinated alkane-based CsA formulations may improve the therapeutic efficacy.

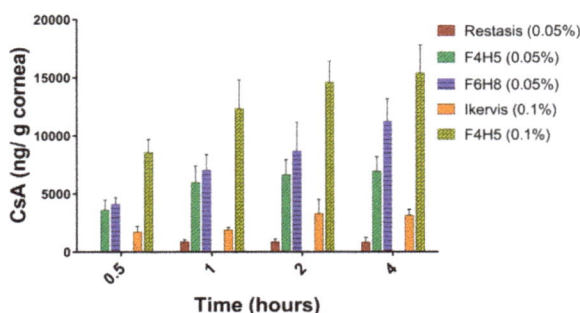

Figure 19. Corneal penetration of cyclosporin A (CsA) from the test formulations. The amount of CsA recovered (ng) per g of cornea after application of a single 50-μL dose was plotted against time (*n* = 5; mean ± standard error of the mean (SEM)). Reproduced from Reference [142] with permission from Elsevier, 2018.

6. Comparison of Different Penetration Enhancers

Different classes of penetration enhancers considered in this review are summarized in Table 2. Some of these compounds, such as EDTA and benzalkonium chloride, are already commonly used in ophthalmic formulations with different roles, e.g., as a buffering agent and antimicrobial preservative, respectively. However, these compounds may provide some permeability enhancement as an extra benefit. Cyclodextrins are used in some pharmaceutical formulations to facilitate the solubility of poorly soluble drugs; additionally, they could provide permeability-enhancing properties. Other amphiphilic molecules such as bile acids and Azone™ have established safety profiles but are not yet used in commercial ocular formulations. Crown ethers represent a relatively new class of permeability enhancers that will require more research into their efficiency and toxicological profile. Cell-penetrating peptides are highly promising permeability enhancers that received a lot of interest in the recent decade; more research is expected with these materials as they could potentially provide opportunities for formulating topical products for the delivery of biologicals.

Table 2. Different classes of penetration enhancers, their commercial applications, and possible mechanisms of action. EDTA—ethylenediamine-*N,N,N′,N′*-tetraacetic acid; TAT—trans-activating transcriptional activator; FDA—Food and Drug Administration.

Class of Enhancers	Examples of Compounds	Commercial Applications in Drug Delivery	Possible Mechanism of Penetration Enhancement
Cyclodextrins	α-, β-, γ-cyclodextrins	Some cyclodextrins are already used in commercial ocular formulations, e.g., Vitaseptol eye drops (Novartis). They are often used as enhancers of drug solubility.	Extraction of cholesterol and lipids from ocular membranes [68].
Chelating agents	EDTA	Disodium-EDTA is commonly used in ocular formulations as a buffering agent [143].	Extraction of Ca^{2+} from tight junctions [17].
Crown ethers	12-crown-4, 15-crown-5, 18-crown-6	None of these are currently used in commercial formulations for drug delivery.	Extraction of Ca^{2+} from tight junctions [100].
Surfactants	Benzalkonium chloride	Around 74% of ophthalmic preparations have benzalkonium chloride as a preservative [144].	Morphological changes in the epithelium [145].
Bile acids and salts	Deoxycholate, glycocholate, taurodeoxycholate	None of these are currently used in commercial formulations for drug delivery.	Different mechanisms leading to modification of the integrity of the corneal epithelium [121].
Cell-penetrating peptides	TAT, penetratin, poly(arginine), and poly(serine)	None of these are currently used in commercial formulations for drug delivery.	Direct translocation and endocytosis [133].
Other amphiphilic compounds	Azone™	Designed and widely researched mostly as a skin penetration enhancer. No FDA-approved products containing Azone™ on the market yet. It is recorded in Chinese Pharmacopoeia and widely used in China [146,147].	Changes in the structure and fluidity of biological membranes; facilitation of water influx leading to a more hydrated barrier [137].

7. Conclusions

Topical drug application is the most widely used treatment in ophthalmology due to its simplicity. However, some obstacles including low permeability of the cornea, tear reflex, blinking, and nasolacrimal drainage hamper drug delivery in this way. The analysis of physicochemical properties of various chemical compounds that cross ocular membranes, coupled with the histological structure of cornea, sclera, and conjunctiva, could be key in understanding the opportunities and obstacles in the ocular drug delivery. Penetration enhancers facilitate delivery of active pharmaceutical compounds through three main mechanisms or their combination: altering tear film stability and the mucous layer at the ocular surface, modifying membrane components such as lipid bilayers of associated epithelial cells, and loosening epithelial tight junctions. The variety of penetration enhancers (cyclodextrins, chelating agents, crown ethers, bile acids and bile salts, cell-penetrating peptides, and other amphiphilic compounds) enables an increase in the permeability of ocular membranes. However, ocular drug delivery remains one of the toughest problems in ophthalmology, and new formulations still need to be developed to allow better control of drug delivery and improved performance, whilst also minimizing undesired side effects.

Different penetration enhancers were identified and mechanisms of their action were researched in the past several decades. Many of these enhancers were also evaluated for their potential harmful effects on the eye. However, these toxicological studies were often done to evaluate short-term exposure of the ocular tissues to enhancers. Very little is known on the longer-term exposure and potential chronic applications.

Funding: This research received no external funding.

Acknowledgments: We thank Yurii A. Kriuchkov for providing images of the eye (Figures 1 and 2). The authors are also grateful to Nikolai Khutoryanskiy for proofreading the manuscript.

Conflicts of Interest: The authors declare no conflicts of interest. Fraser Steele is the employee of the MC2 therapeutics. The company had no role in the design of the study; in the collection, analyses, or interpretation of data; in the writing of the manuscript, and in the decision to publish the results.

References

1. World Health Organization. Available online: https://www.who.int/news-room/fact-sheets/detail/blindness-and-visual-impairment (accessed on 12 December 2018).
2. Haupt, C.; Huber, A.B. How axons see their way-axonal guidance in the visual system. *Front. Biosci.* **2008**, *13*, 3136–3149. [CrossRef] [PubMed]
3. Morrison, P.W.J.; Khutoryanskiy, V.V. Anatomy of the Eye and the Role of Ocular Mucosa in Drug Delivery. In *Mucoadhesive Materials and Drug Delivery Systems*, 1st ed.; Khutoryanskiy, V.V., Ed.; John Wiley & Sons, Ltd.: Chichester, UK, 2014; pp. 39–60, ISBN 9781119941439.
4. Kaur, I.P.; Smitha, R. Penetration enhancers and ocular bioadhesives: Two new avenues for ophthalmic drug delivery. *Drug Dev. Ind. Pharm.* **2002**, *28*, 353–369. [CrossRef] [PubMed]
5. Morrison, P.W.; Khutoryanskiy, V.V. Advances in ophthalmic drug delivery. *Ther. Deliv.* **2014**, *5*, 1297–1315. [CrossRef] [PubMed]
6. Lopath, P.; TecLens, C.L. Available online: https://player.vimeo.com/video/198253544 (accessed on 2 September 2018).
7. Del Amo, E.M.; Urtti, A. Current and future ophthalmic drug delivery systems. A shift to the posterior segment. *Drug Discov. Today* **2008**, *13*, 135–143. [CrossRef]
8. Zderic, V.; Clark, J.I.; Martin, R.W.; Vaezy, S. Ultrasound-enhanced transcorneal drug delivery. *Cornea* **2004**, *23*, 804–811. [CrossRef]
9. Vaka, S.R.; Sammeta, S.M.; Day, L.B.; Murthy, S.N. Transcorneal iontophoresis for delivery of ciprofloxacin hydrochloride. *Curr. Eye Res.* **2008**, *33*, 661–667. [CrossRef]
10. Jiang, J.; Gill, H.S.; Ghate, D.; McCarey, B.E.; Patel, S.R.; Edelhauser, H.F.; Prausnitz, M.R. Coated Microneedles for Drug Delivery to the Eye. *Investig. Ophthalmol. Vis. Sci.* **2007**, *48*, 4038–4043. [CrossRef]

11. Jiang, J.; Moore, J.S.; Edelhauser, H.F.; Prausnitz, M.R. Intrascleral drug delivery to the eye using hollow microneedles. *Pharm. Res.* **2009**, *26*, 395–403. [CrossRef]
12. Chen, H.; Jin, Y.; Sun, L.; Li, X.; Nan, K.; Liu, H.; Zheng, Q.; Wang, B. Recent Developments in Ophthalmic Drug Delivery Systems for Therapy of Both Anterior and Posterior Segment Diseases. *Colloid Interface Sci. Commun.* **2018**, *24*, 54–61. [CrossRef]
13. Williams, A.C.; Barry, B.W. Penetration enhancers. *Adv. Drug Deliv. Rev.* **2012**, *64*, 128–137. [CrossRef]
14. Lane, M.E. Skin penetration enhancers. *Int. J. Pharm.* **2013**, *447*, 12–21. [CrossRef] [PubMed]
15. Junginger, H.E.; Verhoef, J.C. Macromolecules as safe penetration enhancers for hydrophilic drugs-a fiction? *Pharm. Sci. Technol. Today* **1998**, *1*, 370–376. [CrossRef]
16. Sultana, Y.; Jain, R.; Aqil, M.; Ali, A. Review of ocular drug delivery. *Curr. Drug Deliv.* **2006**, *3*, 207–217. [CrossRef] [PubMed]
17. Morrison, P.W.J.; Khutoryanskiy, V.V. Enhancement in corneal permeability of riboflavin using calcium sequestering compounds. *Int. J. Pharm.* **2014**, *472*, 56–64. [CrossRef] [PubMed]
18. Chung, S.H.; Lee, S.K.; Cristol, S.M.; Lee, E.S.; Lee, D.W.; Seo, K.Y.; Kim, E.K. Impact of short-term exposure of commercial eyedrops preserved with benzalkonium chloride on precorneal mucin. *Mol. Vis.* **2006**, *12*, 415–421. [PubMed]
19. Burgalassi, S.; Chetoni, P.; Monti, D.; Saettone, M.F. Cytotoxicity of potential ocular permeation enhancers evaluated on rabbit and human corneal epithelial cell lines. *Toxicol. Lett.* **2001**, *122*, 1–8. [CrossRef]
20. Liu, R.; Liu, Z.; Zhang, C.; Zhang, B. Gelucire44/14 as a novel absorption enhancer for drugs with different hydrophilicities: In vitro and in vivo improvement on transcorneal permeation. *J. Pharm. Sci.* **2011**, *100*, 3186–3195. [CrossRef]
21. Loch, C.; Zakelj, S.; Kristl, A.; Nagel, S.; Guthoff, R.; Weitschies, W.; Seidlitz, A. Determination of permeability coefficients of ophthalmic drugs through different layers of porcine, rabbit and bovine eyes. *Eur. J. Pharm. Sci.* **2012**, *47*, 131–138. [CrossRef]
22. Bowling, B. *Kanski's Clinical Ophthalmology: A Systematic Approach*, 8th ed.; Saunders Ltd.: Philadelphia, PA, USA, 2015; p. 928, ISBN 978-0-7020-5572-0.
23. Järvinen, T.; Järvinen, K. Prodrugs for improved ocular drug delivery. *Adv. Drug Deliv. Rev.* **1996**, *19*, 203–224. [CrossRef]
24. Geerling, G.; Brewitt, H. *Surgery for the Dry Eye: Scientific Evidence and Guidelines for the Clinical Management of Dry Eye Associated Ocular Surface Disease*, 1st ed.; Karger: Basel, Switzerland, 2008; p. 325, ISBN 978-3-8055-8376-3.
25. Hodges, R.R.; Dartt, D.A. Conjunctival goblet cells. In *Encyclopedia of the Eye*, 1st ed.; Dartt, D.A., Besharse, J.C., Dana, R., Eds.; Academic Press: Oxford, UK, 2010; pp. 369–376, ISBN 978-0-12-374203-2.
26. Wang, L.; Li, T.; Lu, L. UV-induced corneal epithelial cell death by activation of potassium channels. *Investig. Ophthalmol. Vis. Sci.* **2003**, *44*, 5095–5101. [CrossRef]
27. Dua, H.S.; Faraj, L.A.; Said, D.G.; Gray, T.; Lowe, J. Human corneal anatomy redefined: A novel pre-Descemet's layer (Dua's layer). *Ophthalmology* **2013**, *120*, 1778–1785. [CrossRef] [PubMed]
28. Smith, G.T.; Dart, J.K.G. Cornea. In *Moorfields Manual of Ophthalmology*, 1st ed.; Jackson, T.L., Ed.; Mosby: Edinburgh, UK, 2008; pp. 144–221, ISBN 9781416025726.
29. Schlote, T.; Rohrbach, J.; Grueb, M.; Mielke, J. *Pocket Atlas of Ophthalmology*, 1st ed.; Thieme: Wemding, Germany, 2006; pp. 2–8, ISBN 3-13-139821-3.
30. Washington, N.; Washington, C.; Wilson, C.G. *Physiological Pharmaceutics: Barriers to Drug Absorption*, 2nd ed.; Taylor and Francis: New York, NY, USA, 2001; pp. 249–270, ISBN 9780748406104.
31. Shaikh, R.; Raj Singh, T.R.; Garland, M.J.; Woolfson, A.D.; Donnelly, R.F. Mucoadhesive drug delivery systems. *J. Pharm. Bioallied Sci.* **2011**, *3*, 89–100. [CrossRef] [PubMed]
32. Tsai, J.C.; Denniston, A.K.O.; Murray, P.I.; Huang, J.J.; Aldad, T.S. *Oxford American Handbook of Ophthalmology*, 1st ed.; Oxford University Press Inc.: New York, NY, USA, 2011; p. 768, ISBN 978-0-19-539344-6.
33. Goel, M.; Picciani, R.G.; Lee, R.K.; Bhattacharya, S.K. Aqueous humor dynamics: A review. *Open Ophthalmol. J.* **2010**, *4*, 52–59. [CrossRef] [PubMed]
34. Lang, G.K. *Ophthalmology: A Short Textbook*, 1st ed.; Thieme: Wemding, Germany, 2000; p. 586, ISBN 0-86577-936-8.
35. Caretti, L.; Buratto, L. *Glaucoma Surgery: Treatment and Techniques*, 1st ed.; Springer International Publishing: Cham, Switzerland, 2017; p. 133, ISBN 978-3-319-64854-5.

36. Sundaram, V.; Barsam, A.; Barker, L.; Khaw, P.T. *Training in Ophthalmology*, 2nd ed.; Oxford University Press: Gosport, UK, 2016; p. 568, ISBN 978-0-19-967251-6.

37. American Academy of Ophthalmology. Available online: https://www.aao.org/disease-review/anatomy-of-angle (accessed on 10 January 2019).

38. Albert, D.M.; Miller, J.W.; Azar, D.T.; Blodi, B.A. *Principles and Practice of Ophthalmology*, 3rd ed.; Saunders: Philadelphia, PA, USA, 2008; Volume 3, p. 5502, ISBN 978-1-4160-0016-7.

39. Andley, U.P. Crystallins in the eye: Function and pathology. *Prog. Retin. Eye Res.* **2007**, *26*, 78–98. [CrossRef] [PubMed]

40. Petrash, J.M. Aging and age-related diseases of the ocular lens and vitreous body. *Investig. Ophthalmol. Vis. Sci.* **2013**, *54*, ORSF54–ORSF59. [CrossRef]

41. Murphy, W.; Black, J.; Hastings, G. *Handbook of Biomaterial Properties*, 2nd ed.; Springer: New York, NY, USA, 2016; p. 676, ISBN 978-1-4939-3303-7.

42. Sebag, J. *Vitreous: In Health and Disease*, 1st ed.; Springer: New York, NY, USA, 2014; p. 925, ISBN 978-1-4939-1085-4.

43. Straatsma, B.R.; Landers, M.B.; Kreiger, A.E. The ora serrata in the adult human eye. *Arch. Ophthalmol.* **1968**, *80*, 3–20. [CrossRef] [PubMed]

44. Nag, T.C.; Kumari, C. Electron microscopy of the human choroid. In *Choroidal Disorders*, 1st ed.; Chhablani, J., Ruiz-Medrano, J., Eds.; Academic Press: Cambridge, MA, USA, 2017; pp. 7–20, ISBN 978-0-12-805313-3.

45. Schachat, A.P.; Wilkinson, C.P.; Hinton, D.R.; Sadda, S.V.R.; Wiedemann, P. *Ryan's Retina*, 6th ed.; Elsevier Health Sciences: Amsterdam, The Netherlands, 2017; Volume 1, p. 2976, ISBN 978-0-323-40197-5.

46. Agarwal, A. *Gass' Atlas of Macular Diseases*, 5th ed.; Saunders: Philadelphia, PA, USA, 2012; Volume 1, p. 1378, ISBN 978-1-4377-1580-4.

47. Kefalov, V.J. Phototransduction: Phototransduction in cones. In *Encyclopedia of the Eye*, 1st ed.; Dartt, D.A., Besharse, J.C., Dana, R., Eds.; Academic Press: Oxford, UK, 2010; pp. 389–396, ISBN 978-0-12-374203-2.

48. Denniston, A.K.O.; Murray, P.I. *Oxford Handbook of Ophthalmology*, 4th ed.; Oxford University Press: Oxford, Oxfordshire, UK, 2018; p. 1204, ISBN 978-0-19-881675-1.

49. Yanoff, M.; Duker, J.S. *Ophthalmology*, 5th ed.; Elsevier: Amsterdam, The Netherlands, 2018; p. 1440, ISBN 9780323528191.

50. Petroutsos, G.; Guimaraes, R.; Giraud, J.P.; Pouliquen, Y. Corticosteroids and corneal epithelial wound healing. *Br. J. Ophthalmol.* **1982**, *66*, 705–708. [CrossRef] [PubMed]

51. Dworkin, R.H.; Johnson, R.W.; Breuer, J.; Gnann, J.W.; Levin, M.J.; Backonja, M.; Betts, R.F.; Gershon, A.A.; Haanpaa, M.L.; McKendrick, M.W.; et al. Recommendations for the management of herpes zoster. *Clin. Infect. Dis. Off. Publ. Infect. Dis. Soc. Am.* **2007**, *44* (Suppl. 1), S1–S26. [CrossRef] [PubMed]

52. World Health Organization. Available online: http://origin.who.int/blindness/causes/priority/en/index1.html (accessed on 18 December 2018).

53. Chandra, P.; Hegde, K.R.; Varma, S.D. Possibility of topical antioxidant treatment of cataracts: Corneal penetration of pyruvate in humans. *Ophthalmologica* **2009**, *223*, 136–138. [CrossRef] [PubMed]

54. Zhao, L.; Chen, X.-J.; Zhu, J.; Xi, Y.-B.; Yang, X.; Hu, L.-D.; Ouyang, H.; Patel, S.H.; Jin, X.; Lin, D.; et al. Lanosterol reverses protein aggregation in cataracts. *Nature* **2015**, *523*, 607–611. [CrossRef] [PubMed]

55. Quigley, H.A. Use of animal models and techniques in glaucoma research: Introduction. In *Glaucoma: Methods and Protocols*, 1st ed.; Jakobs, T.C., Ed.; Humana Press: New York, NY, USA, 2018; pp. 1–10, ISBN 978-1-4939-7407-8.

56. Tham, Y.-C.; Li, X.; Wong, T.Y.; Quigley, H.A.; Aung, T.; Cheng, C.-Y. Global prevalence of glaucoma and projections of glaucoma burden through 2040: A systematic review and meta-analysis. *Ophthalmology* **2014**, *121*, 2081–2090. [CrossRef] [PubMed]

57. Jackson, T.L.; Egan, C.; Bird, A.C. Medical retina. In *Moorfields Manual of Ophthalmology*, 1st ed.; Jackson, T.L., Ed.; Mosby: Edinburgh, UK, 2008; pp. 412–518, ISBN 9781416025726.

58. Joseph, M.; Trinh, H.M.; Cholkar, K.; Pal, D.; Mitra, A.K. Recent perspectives on the delivery of biologics to back of the eye. *Expert Opin. Drug Deliv.* **2017**, *14*, 631–645. [CrossRef] [PubMed]

59. Burgalassi, S.; Monti, D.; Nicosia, N.; Tampucci, S.; Terreni, E.; Vento, A.; Chetoni, P. Freeze-dried matrices for ocular administration of bevacizumab: A comparison between subconjunctival and intravitreal administration in rabbits. *Drug Deliv. Transl. Res.* **2018**, *8*, 461–472. [CrossRef] [PubMed]

60. Davis, B.M.; Normando, E.M.; Guo, L.; Turner, L.A.; Nizari, S.; O'Shea, P.; Moss, S.E.; Somavarapu, S.; Cordeiro, M.F. Topical delivery of Avastin to the posterior segment of the eye in vivo using annexin A5-associated liposomes. *Small* **2014**, *10*, 1575–1584. [CrossRef]

61. Nayak, K.; Misra, M. A review on recent drug delivery systems for posterior segment of eye. *Biomed. Pharmacother.* **2018**, *107*, 1564–1582. [CrossRef] [PubMed]

62. Inokuchi, Y.; Hironaka, K.; Fujisawa, T.; Tozuka, Y.; Tsuruma, K.; Shimazawa, M.; Takeuchi, H.; Hara, H. Physicochemical Properties Affecting Retinal Drug/Coumarin-6 Delivery from Nanocarrier Systems via Eyedrop Administration. *Investig. Ophthalmol. Vis. Sci.* **2010**, *51*, 3162–3170. [CrossRef]

63. Duh, E.J.; Sun, J.K.; Stitt, A.W. Diabetic retinopathy: Current understanding, mechanisms, and treatment strategies. *JCI Insight* **2017**, *2*, 1–13. [CrossRef]

64. Prausnitz, M.R.; Noonan, J.S. Permeability of cornea, sclera, and conjunctiva: A literature analysis for drug delivery to the eye. *J. Pharm. Sci.* **1998**, *87*, 1479–1488. [CrossRef]

65. Edward, A.; Prausnitz, M.R. Predicted permeability of the cornea to topical drugs. *Pharm. Res.* **2001**, *18*, 1497–1508. [CrossRef]

66. Agarwal, P.; Rupenthal, I.D. In vitro and ex vivo corneal penetration and absorption models. *Drug Deliv. Transl. Res.* **2016**, *6*, 634–647. [CrossRef]

67. Kaluzhny, Y.; Kinuthia, M.W.; Truong, T.; Lapointe, A.M.; Hayden, P.; Klausner, M. New Human Organotypic Corneal Tissue Model for Ophthalmic Drug Delivery Studies. *Investig. Ophthalmol. Vis. Sci.* **2018**, *59*, 2880–2898. [CrossRef] [PubMed]

68. Morrison, P.W.; Connon, C.J.; Khutoryanskiy, V.V. Cyclodextrin-mediated enhancement of riboflavin solubility and corneal permeability. *Mol. Pharm.* **2013**, *10*, 756–762. [CrossRef] [PubMed]

69. Stefánsson, E.; Loftsson, T. Microspheres and nanotechnology for drug delivery. In *Retinal Pharmacotherapeutics*, 1st ed.; Nguyen, Q.D., Rodrigues, E.B., Farah, M.E., Mieler, W.F., Eds.; W.B. Saunders: Edinburgh, UK, 2010; pp. 86–90, ISBN 978-3318055641.

70. Cal, K.; Centkowska, K. Use of cyclodextrins in topical formulations: Practical aspects. *Eur. J. Pharm. Biopharm.* **2008**, *68*, 467–478. [CrossRef] [PubMed]

71. Loftsson, T.; Stefansson, E. Cyclodextrins in eye drop formulations: Enhanced topical delivery of corticosteroids to the eye. *Acta Ophthalmol. Scand.* **2002**, *80*, 144–150. [CrossRef]

72. Jarho, P.; Urtti, A.; Pate, D.W.; Suhonen, P.; Järvinen, T. Increase in aqueous solubility, stability and in vitro corneal permeability of anandamide by hydroxypropyl-β-cyclodextrin. *Int. J. Pharm.* **1996**, *137*, 209–216. [CrossRef]

73. Chordiya, M.A.; Senthilkumaran, K. Cyclodextrin in drug delivery: A review. *Res. Rev. Pharm. Pharm. Sci.* **2012**, *1*, 19–29.

74. Stella, V.J.; Rajewski, R.A. Cyclodextrins: Their future in drug formulation and delivery. *Pharm. Res.* **1997**, *14*, 556–567. [CrossRef]

75. Loftsson, T.; Brewster, M.E.; Másson, M. Role of cyclodextrins in improving oral drug delivery. *Am. J. Drug Deliv.* **2004**, *2*, 261–275. [CrossRef]

76. Loftssona, T.; Jarvinen, T. Cyclodextrins in ophthalmic drug delivery. *Adv. Drug Deliv. Rev.* **1999**, *36*, 59–79. [CrossRef]

77. Skowron, S. Cyclodextrin. Available online: https://commons.wikimedia.org/wiki/File:Cyclodextrin.svg (accessed on 9 May 2019).

78. Lisch, W.; Seitz, B. *Corneal Dystrophies*, 1st ed.; Karger: Basel, Switzerland, 2011; Volume 48, p. 159, ISBN 978-3-8055-9720-3.

79. Pescina, S.; Carra, F.; Padula, C.; Santi, P.; Nicoli, S. Effect of pH and penetration enhancers on cysteamine stability and trans-corneal transport. *Eur. J. Pharm. Biopharm.* **2016**, *107*, 171–179. [CrossRef]

80. Aktas, Y.; Unlu, N.; Orhan, M.; Irkec, M.; Hincal, A.A. Influence of hydroxypropyl beta-cyclodextrin on the corneal permeation of pilocarpine. *Drug Dev. Ind. Pharm.* **2003**, *29*, 223–230. [CrossRef] [PubMed]

81. Loftsson, T.; Stefansson, E. Cyclodextrins and topical drug delivery to the anterior and posterior segments of the eye. *Int. J. Pharm.* **2017**, *531*, 413–423. [CrossRef] [PubMed]

82. Abdulrazik, M.; Beher-Cohen, F.; Benita, S. Drug Delivery Systems for Enhanced Ocular Absorption. In *Enhancement in Drug Delivery*, 1st ed.; Touitou, E., Barry, B.W., Eds.; CRC Press: Boca Raton, FL, USA, 2006; pp. 489–526, ISBN 978-0-8493-3203-6.

83. Grass, G.M.; Wood, R.W.; Robinson, J.R. Effects of calcium chelating agents on corneal permeability. *Investig. Ophthalmol. Vis. Sci.* **1985**, *26*, 110–113.
84. Deli, M.A. Potential use of tight junction modulators to reversibly open membranous barriers and improve drug delivery. *Biochim. Biophys. Acta* **2009**, *1788*, 892–910. [CrossRef] [PubMed]
85. Kikuchi, T.; Suzuki, M.; Kusai, A.; Iseki, K.; Sasaki, H. Synergistic effect of EDTA and boric acid on corneal penetration of CS-088. *Int. J. Pharm.* **2005**, *290*, 83–89. [CrossRef] [PubMed]
86. Rodriguez, I.; Vazquez, J.A.; Pastrana, L.; Khutoryanskiy, V.V. Enhancement and inhibition effects on the corneal permeability of timolol maleate: Polymers, cyclodextrins and chelating agents. *Int. J. Pharm.* **2017**, *529*, 168–177. [CrossRef] [PubMed]
87. Andrés-Guerrero, V.; Vicario-de-la-Torre, M.; Molina-Martínez, I.T.; Benítez-del-Castillo, J.M.; García-Feijoo, J.; Herrero-Vanrell, R. Comparison of the In Vitro Tolerance and In Vivo Efficacy of Traditional Timolol Maleate Eye Drops versus New Formulations with Bioadhesive Polymers. *Investig. Ophthalmol. Vis. Sci.* **2011**, *52*, 3548–3556. [CrossRef]
88. Pedersen, C.J. Cyclic polyethers and their complexes with metal salts. *J. Am. Chem. Soc.* **1967**, *89*, 7017–7036. [CrossRef]
89. Pedersen, C.J. Macrocyclic Polyethers: Dibenzo-18-crown-6 Polyether and Dicyclohexyl-18-crown-6 Polyether. In *Organic Synthesis*; John Wiley & Sons: Hoboken, NJ, USA, 2003; Volume 52, ISBN 9780471264224.
90. Ouchi, M.; Inoue, Y.; Kanzaki, T.; Hakushi, T. Molecular design of crown ethers. 1. Effects of methylene chain length: 15- to 17-crown-5 and 18- to 22-crown-6. *J. Org. Chem.* **1984**, *49*, 1408–1412. [CrossRef]
91. Steed, J. First- and second-sphere coordination chemistry of alkali metal crown ether complexes. *Coord. Chem. Rev.* **2001**, *215*, 171–221. [CrossRef]
92. Boojar, M.M.; Goodarzi, F. Cytotoxicity and the levels of oxidative stress parameters in WI38 cells following 2 macrocyclic crown ethers treatment. *Clin. Chim. Acta* **2006**, *364*, 321–327. [CrossRef] [PubMed]
93. Capel-Cuevas, S.; de Orbe-Payá, I.; Santoyo-González, F.; Capitan-Vallvey, L.F. Double-armed crown ethers for calcium optical sensors. *Talanta* **2009**, *78*, 1484–1488. [CrossRef] [PubMed]
94. Song, M.Z.; Zhu, L.Y.; Gao, X.K.; Dou, J.M.; Sun, D.Z. Microcalorimetric study on host-guest complexation of naphtho-15-crown-5 with four ions of alkaline earth metal. *J. Zhejiang Univ. Sci. B* **2005**, *6*, 69–73. [CrossRef] [PubMed]
95. Marjanovic, M.; Kralj, M.; Supek, F.; Frkanec, L.; Piantanida, I.; Smuc, T.; Tusek-Bozic, L. Antitumor potential of crown ethers: Structure-activity relationships, cell cycle disturbances, and cell death studies of a series of ionophores. *J. Med. Chem.* **2007**, *50*, 1007–1018. [CrossRef] [PubMed]
96. Kralj, M.; Tušek-Božić, L.; Frkanec, L. Biomedical potentials of crown ethers: Prospective antitumor agents. *ChemMedChem* **2008**, *3*, 1478–1492. [CrossRef] [PubMed]
97. Muzzalupo, R.; Nicoletta, F.P.; Trombino, S.; Cassano, R.; Iemma, F.; Picci, N. A new crown ether as vesicular carrier for 5-fluoruracil: Synthesis, characterization and drug delivery evaluation. *Colloids Surf. B Biointerfaces* **2007**, *58*, 197–202. [CrossRef] [PubMed]
98. Darwish, I.; Uchegbu, I. The evaluation of crown ether based niosomes as cation containing and cation sensitive drug delivery systems. *Int. J. Pharm.* **1997**, *159*, 207–213. [CrossRef]
99. Chehardoli, G.; Bahmani, A. The role of crown ethers in drug delivery. *Supramol. Chem.* **2019**, *31*, 221–238. [CrossRef]
100. Morrison, P.W.J.; Porfiryeva, N.N.; Chahal, S.; Salakhov, I.A.; Lacourt, C.; Semina, I.I.; Moustafine, R.I.; Khutoryanskiy, V.V. Crown Ethers: Novel Permeability Enhancers for Ocular Drug Delivery? *Mol. Pharm.* **2017**, *14*, 3528–3538. [CrossRef]
101. Hartman. Surface-Active Compounds. BODE Science Centre. Available online: https://www.bode-science-center.com/center/glossary/surface-active-compounds.html (accessed on 21 September 2018).
102. Sekhon, B. Surfactants: Pharmaceutical and Medicinal Aspects. *J. Pharm. Technol. Res. Manag.* **2013**, *1*, 11–36. [CrossRef]
103. Jiao, J. Polyoxyethylated nonionic surfactants and their application in topical ocular drug delivery. *Adv. Drug Deliv. Rev.* **2008**, *60*, 1663–1673. [CrossRef] [PubMed]
104. Kumar, G.P.; Rajeshwarrao, P. Nonionic surfactant vesicular systems for effective drug delivery—An overview. *Acta Pharm. Sin. B* **2011**, *1*, 208–219. [CrossRef]
105. Marsh, R.J.; Maurice, D.M. The influence of non-ionic detergents and other surfactants on human corneal permeability. *Exp. Eye Res.* **1971**, *11*, 43–48. [CrossRef]

106. Saettone, M.F.; Chetoni, P.; Cerbai, R.; Mazzanti, G.; Braghiroli, L. Evaluation of ocular permeation enhancers: In vitro effects on corneal transport of four β-blockers, and in vitro/in vivo toxic activity. *Int. J. Pharm.* **1996**, *142*, 103–113. [CrossRef]

107. Ostacolo, C.; Caruso, C.; Tronino, D.; Troisi, S.; Laneri, S.; Pacente, L.; Del Prete, A.; Sacchi, A. Enhancement of corneal permeation of riboflavin-5'-phosphate through vitamin E TPGS: A promising approach in corneal trans-epithelial cross linking treatment. *Int. J. Pharm.* **2013**, *440*, 148–153. [CrossRef]

108. Li, X.; Pan, W.; Ju, C.; Liu, Z.; Pan, H.; Zhang, H.; Nie, S. Evaluation of Pharmasolve corneal permeability enhancement and its irritation on rabbit eyes. *Drug Deliv.* **2009**, *16*, 224–229. [CrossRef]

109. Montenegro, L.; Bucolo, C.; Puglisi, G. Enhancer effects on in vitro corneal permeation of timolol and acyclovir. *Pharmazie* **2003**, *58*, 497–501.

110. Kaur, I.P. Ocular Penetration Enhancers. In *Enhancement in Drug Delivery*, 1st ed.; Touitou, E., Barry, B.W., Eds.; CRC Press: Boca Raton, FL, USA, 2006; pp. 527–548, ISBN 978-0-8493-3203-6.

111. Sahoo, S.K.; Dilnawaz, F.; Krishnakumar, S. Nanotechnology in ocular drug delivery. *Drug Discov. Today* **2008**, *13*, 144–151. [CrossRef]

112. Shih, R.L.; Lee, V.H. Rate Limiting Barrier to the Penetration of Ocular Hypotensive Beta Blockers Across the Corneal Epithelium in the Pigmented Rabbit. *J. Ocul. Pharmacol.* **1990**, *6*, 329–336. [CrossRef]

113. Wilson, W.S.; Duncan, A.J.; Jay, J.L. Effect of benzalconium chloride on the stability of the precorneal film in rabbit and man. *Br. J. Ophthalmol.* **1975**, *59*, 667–669. [CrossRef]

114. Johannsdottir, S.; Jansook, P.; Stefánsson, E.; Myrdal Kristinsdottir, I.; Marta Asgrimsdottir, G.; Loftsson, T. Topical drug delivery to the posterior segment of the eye: The effect of benzalkonium chloride on topical dexamethasone penetration into the eye in vivo. *J. Drug Deliv. Sci. Technol.* **2018**, *48*, 125–127. [CrossRef]

115. Sasaki, H.; Yamamura, K.; Mukai, T.; Nishida, K.; Nakamura, J.; Nakashima, M.; Ichikawa, M. Modification of ocular permeability of peptide drugs by absorption promoters. *Biol. Pharm. Bull.* **2000**, *23*, 1524–1527. [CrossRef] [PubMed]

116. Van Der Bijl, P.; Engelbrecht, A.H.; Van Eyk, A.D.; Meyer, D. Comparative permeability of human and rabbit corneas to cyclosporin and tritiated water. *J. Ocul. Pharmacol. Ther.* **2002**, *18*, 419–427. [CrossRef] [PubMed]

117. Liu, Z.; Li, J.; Nie, S.; Guo, H.; Pan, W. Effects of Transcutol P on the corneal permeability of drugs and evaluation of its ocular irritation of rabbit eyes. *J. Pharm. Pharmacol.* **2006**, *58*, 45–50. [CrossRef] [PubMed]

118. Liu, Z.; Zhang, X.; Li, J.; Liu, R.; Shu, L.; Jin, J. Effects of Labrasol on the corneal drug delivery of baicalin. *Drug Deliv.* **2009**, *16*, 399–404. [CrossRef] [PubMed]

119. Russell, D.W. The enzymes, regulation, and genetics of bile acid synthesis. *Annu. Rev. Biochem.* **2003**, *72*, 137–174. [CrossRef]

120. Chiang, J. Bile Acids: Bile acids: Regulation of synthesis. *J. Lipid Res.* **2009**, *50*, 1955–1966. [CrossRef]

121. Stojančević, M.; Pavlović, N.; Goločorbin-Kon, S.; Mikov, M. Application of bile acids in drug formulation and delivery. *Front. Life Sci.* **2013**, *7*, 112–122. [CrossRef]

122. Rajput, T.; Chauhan, M. Bilosome: A bile salt based novel carrier system gaining interest in pharmaceutical research. *J. Drug Deliv. Ther.* **2017**, *7*, 4–16. [CrossRef]

123. Sasaki, H.; Igarashi, Y.; Nagano, T.; Nishida, K.; Nakamura, J. Different Effects of Absorption Promoters on Corneal and Conjunctival Penetration of Ophthalmic Beta-Blockers. *Pharm. Res.* **1995**, *12*, 1146–1150. [CrossRef]

124. Morimoto, K.; Nakai, T.; Morisaka, K. Evaluation of permeability enhancement of hydrophilic compounds and macromolecular compounds by bile salts through rabbit corneas in-vitro. *J. Pharm. Pharmacol.* **1987**, *39*, 124–126. [CrossRef] [PubMed]

125. Dai, Y.; Zhou, R.; Liu, L.; Lu, Y.; Qi, J.; Wu, W. Liposomes containing bile salts as novel ocular delivery systems for tacrolimus (FK506): In vitro characterization and improved corneal permeation. *Int. J. Nanomed.* **2013**, *8*, 1921–1933. [CrossRef]

126. Mahaling, B.; Katti, D.S. Understanding the influence of surface properties of nanoparticles and penetration enhancers for improving bioavailability in eye tissues in vivo. *Int. J. Pharm.* **2016**, *501*, 1–9. [CrossRef] [PubMed]

127. González de Llano, D.; Polo Sánchez, C. Peptides. In *Encyclopedia of Food Sciences and Nutrition*, 2nd ed.; Caballero, B., Ed.; Academic Press: Oxford, UK, 2003; pp. 4468–4473, ISBN 978-0-12-227055-0.

128. Dupont, E.; Prochiantz, A.; Joliot, A. Penetratin story: An overview. *Methods Mol. Biol.* **2011**, *683*, 21–29. [CrossRef] [PubMed]

129. Liu, C.; Tai, L.; Zhang, W.; Wei, G.; Pan, W.; Lu, W. Penetratin, a potentially powerful absorption enhancer for noninvasive intraocular drug delivery. *Mol. Pharm.* **2014**, *11*, 1218–1227. [CrossRef]
130. Pescina, S.; Sala, M.; Padula, C.; Scala, M.C.; Spensiero, A.; Belletti, S.; Gatti, R.; Novellino, E.; Campiglia, P.; Santi, P.; et al. Design and Synthesis of New Cell Penetrating Peptides: Diffusion and Distribution Inside the Cornea. *Mol. Pharm.* **2016**, *13*, 3876–3883. [CrossRef]
131. De Cogan, F.; Hill, L.J.; Lynch, A.; Morgan-Warren, P.J.; Lechner, J.; Berwick, M.R.; Peacock, A.F.A.; Chen, M.; Scott, R.A.H.; Xu, H.; et al. Topical Delivery of Anti-VEGF Drugs to the Ocular Posterior Segment Using Cell-Penetrating Peptides. *Investig. Ophthalmol. Vis. Sci.* **2017**, *58*, 2578–2590. [CrossRef]
132. Nemoto, E.; Takahashi, H.; Kobayashi, D.; Ueda, H.; Morimoto, Y. Effects of poly-L-arginine on the permeation of hydrophilic compounds through surface ocular tissues. *Biol. Pharm. Bull.* **2006**, *29*, 155–160. [CrossRef]
133. Pescina, S.; Ostacolo, C.; Gomez-Monterrey, I.M.; Sala, M.; Bertamino, A.; Sonvico, F.; Padula, C.; Santi, P.; Bianchera, A.; Nicoli, S. Cell penetrating peptides in ocular drug delivery: State of the art. *J. Control. Release* **2018**, *284*, 84–102. [CrossRef]
134. Kato, A.; Iwata, S. In vitro study on corneal permeability to bunazosin. *J. Pharm.-Dyn.* **1988**, *11*, 115–120. [CrossRef]
135. Kato, A.; Iwata, S. Studies on improved corneal permeability to bunazosin. *J. Pharm.-Dyn.* **1988**, *11*, 330–334. [CrossRef]
136. Antunes, A.; De Geest, B.; Vervaet, C.; Remon, J. Gelucire 44/14 based immediate release formulations for poorly water-soluble drugs. *Drug Dev. Ind. Pharm.* **2012**, *39*, 791–798. [CrossRef] [PubMed]
137. Tang-Liu, D.D.; Richman, J.B.; Weinkam, R.J.; Takruri, H. Effects of four penetration enhancers on corneal permeability of drugs in vitro. *J. Pharm. Sci.* **1994**, *83*, 85–90. [CrossRef] [PubMed]
138. Afouna, M.; Hussein, A.; Ahmed, O. Influence of the Interplay between Azone™ as Permeation Enhancer a and Carbopol-974® as a Mucoadhesive upon the in vitro Transcorneal Release and the in vivo Antiglaucoma Effect of S-Timolol Maleate Ophthalmic Gel Formulations. *Int. J. PharmTech Res.* **2014**, *6*, 298–315.
139. Afouna, M.I. Maximization of the In Vitro transcorneal release and the In Vivo IOP-lowering effects of Latanoprost Ophthalmic gel formulations using Azone as a penetration enhancer and Carbopol-974 as a mucoadhesive. *J. Excip. Food Chem.* **2016**, *7*, 20–35.
140. Yang, H.; Xun, Y.; Li, Z.; Hang, T.; Zhang, X.; Cui, H. Influence of borneol on in vitro corneal permeability and on in vivo and in vitro corneal toxicity. *J. Int. Med. Res.* **2009**, *37*, 791–802. [CrossRef] [PubMed]
141. Afouna, M.I.; Khedr, A.; Abdel-Naim, A.B.; Al-Marzoqi, A. Influence of various concentrations of terpene-4-ol enhancer and carbopol-934 mucoadhesive upon the in vitro ocular transport and the in vivo intraocular pressure lowering effects of dorzolamide ophthalmic formulations using albino rabbits. *J. Pharm. Sci.* **2010**, *99*, 119–127. [CrossRef] [PubMed]
142. Agarwal, P.; Scherer, D.; Gunther, B.; Rupenthal, I.D. Semifluorinated alkane based systems for enhanced corneal penetration of poorly soluble drugs. *Int. J. Pharm.* **2018**, *538*, 119–129. [CrossRef] [PubMed]
143. Epstein, S.P.; Ahdoot, M.; Marcus, E.; Asbell, P.A. Comparative toxicity of preservatives on immortalized corneal and conjunctival epithelial cells. *J. Ocul. Pharmacol. Ther.* **2009**, *25*, 113–119. [CrossRef] [PubMed]
144. European Medicines Agency. Available online: https://www.ema.europa.eu/en/documents/report/benzalkonium-chloride-used-excipient-report-published-support-questions-answers-benzalkonium_en.pdf (accessed on 27 June 2019).
145. Green, K.; Tonjum, A.M. The effect of benzalkonium chloride on the electropotential of the rabbit cornea. *Acta Ophthalmol.* **1975**, *53*, 348–357. [CrossRef]
146. Chen, Y.; Quan, P.; Liu, X.; Wang, M.; Fang, L. Novel chemical permeation enhancers for transdermal drug delivery. *Asian J. Pharm. Sci.* **2014**, *9*, 51–64. [CrossRef]
147. Jampilek, J. Azone® and Its Analogues as Penetration Enhancers. In *Percutaneous Penetration Enhancers Chemical Methods in Penetration Enhancement*, 1st ed.; Dragicevic, N., Maibach, H.I., Eds.; Springer: Berlin/Heidelberg, Germany, 2015; pp. 69–105, ISBN 978-3-662-47038-1.

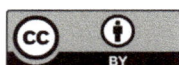

pharmaceutics

MDPI

Review

Strategies to Enhance Drug Absorption via Nasal and Pulmonary Routes

Maliheh Ghadiri *, Paul M. Young and Daniela Traini

Respiratory Technology, Woolcock Institute of Medical Research and Discipline of Pharmacology,
Faculty of Medicine and Health, The University of Sydney, Camperdown, NSW 2006, Australia;
paul.young@sydney.edu.au (P.M.Y.); daniela.traini@sydney.edu.au (D.T.)
* Correspondence: Maliheh.ghadiri@sydney.edu.au; Tel.: +61(2)911-40366

Received: 16 January 2019; Accepted: 5 March 2019; Published: 11 March 2019

Abstract: New therapeutic agents such as proteins, peptides, and nucleic acid-based agents are being developed every year, making it vital to find a non-invasive route such as nasal or pulmonary for their administration. However, a major concern for some of these newly developed therapeutic agents is their poor absorption. Therefore, absorption enhancers have been investigated to address this major administration problem. This paper describes the basic concepts of transmucosal administration of drugs, and in particular the use of the pulmonary or nasal routes for administration of drugs with poor absorption. Strategies for the exploitation of absorption enhancers for the improvement of pulmonary or nasal administration are discussed, including use of surfactants, cyclodextrins, protease inhibitors, and tight junction modulators, as well as application of carriers such as liposomes and nanoparticles.

Keywords: nasal; pulmonary; drug administration; absorption enhancers; nanoparticle; and liposome

1. Background

Absorption enhancers are functional excipients included in formulations to improve the absorption of drugs across biological barriers. They have been investigated for many years, particularly to enhance the efficacy of peptides, proteins, and other pharmacologically active compounds that have poor barrier permeability [1]. The ideal absorption enhancer should be one that protects biological agents against enzymatic degradation and causes a rapid opening of the relevant barrier while enhancing absorption transiently.

As a portal for non-invasive delivery, nasal and pulmonary administration has several advantages over traditional oral medication or injection. Nasal and pulmonary delivery are non-invasive routes of administration that target the delivered dose directly to the site of drug action [2,3]. Moreover, drug delivery to the respiratory area can also be used for systemic delivery of peptides and proteins due to the large surface area for drug absorption. Pulmonary and nasal administration bypasses first-pass metabolism that is observed in oral administration and the lung and nasal cavity have a low drug metabolizing environment [4]. Despite all these advantages, there is a significant challenge to enhance the absorption of the active agent via these routes. In nasal and pulmonary administration, absorption enhancers have been investigated over the last two decades, to increase the rate of absorption by targeting different mechanisms [5,6]. These mechanisms are either to improve the permeation of materials across the epithelial barrier via intracellular or paracellular mechanisms (Figure 1) or to enhance stability and mucus solubility of the drugs regionally. However, to date, no safe absorption enhancer for pulmonary administration of drugs has translated into commercial products. Their use has generated safety concerns due to potential irreversible alteration of the epithelial cell membrane, which could potentially make the lung susceptible to the entry of exogenous allergens. While there are no absorption enhancers for pulmonary drug administration on the market, quite a few appear to be at the threshold of becoming products for nasal administration.

This review critically assesses advances in the field of absorption enhancers for nasal and pulmonary drug administration. The various agents used to increase the absorption of poorly permeable drugs, their mechanisms of action, safety, and effectiveness are also presented.

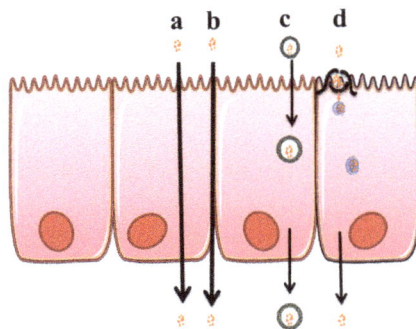

Figure 1. Mechanisms of absorption includes; (a) Transcellular diffusion, (b) Para cellular transport, (c) Vesicle mediated transport, and (d) Carrier mediated transport.

2. The Barriers

The first requirement for drug absorption is for the active pharmaceutical ingredient (API, or drug) to reach the absorbing barrier. For the respiratory system, the drug has to be deposited on the luminal surface of the epithelial membrane and be absorbed before being cleared or degraded. Furthermore, adequate absorption of the API may also require controlling its release profile as it passes through multiple biological barriers. These barriers include: (1) the surfactant layer, mucus layer, (2) epithelial layer, (3) interstitium and basement membrane, and (4) capillary endothelium (Figure 2).

The mucus layer is the first barrier. The deposited drug needs to be dissolved or transverse the mucus layer before degradation due to the enzymatic activity or clearance by mucociliary activity. Because the ciliary action is relatively fast in removing the drug from the absorption site, permeation enhancers must act rapidly to increase bioavailability. The understanding of mucus layer thickness and clearance rate is important to develop drug delivery strategies to overcome mucosal clearance mechanisms. In the lung, the thickness of the luminal mucus gel has been reported to be ~5–10 µm [7]. The underlying, less viscoelastic sol layer, also known as the periciliary liquid, covers the cilia and has an additional 5–10 µm thickness [7]. However, other studies based on confocal fluorescence microscopy suggest that airway mucus may range in thickness from 5 to 55 µm [8,9]. The nasal tract has a thin mucus layer which is readily accessible and considered highly permeable compared to other mucosal surfaces [10]. In the nasal tract, the ciliary motion transports mucus with the flow rate of about 5 mm per minute, and the mucus layer is renewed approximately every 20 min [11,12]. Similarly, the luminal gel layer of respiratory tract mucus is replaced every 10 to 20 min, [11]. While, the sol layer of respiratory mucus has a slower rate of clearance than the more solid-like luminal gel layer. Drug absorption via the nose is dependent on drug clearance from the nasal cavity, which is determined by nasal mucociliary clearance (MC). In a study by Inoue et al., the effect of nasal MC on in vivo absorption of norfloxacin after intranasal administration to rats was estimated quantitatively. This study resulted in a model to precisely estimate nasal drug absorption [13].

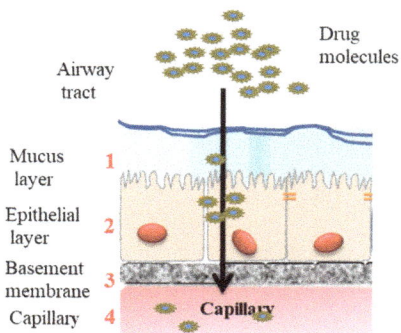

Figure 2. Barriers against drug absorption in pulmonary drug administration including; (1) mucus layer, (2) epithelial layer, (3) interstitium and basement membrane, and (4) capillary endothelium.

The second barrier is the epithelial cell membrane. It is comprised of a layer of pseudostratified columnar cells interconnected via tight junctions. Most drugs are primarily absorbed via transcellular diffusion, permeating through the epithelial cell membrane. Small hydrophobic molecules can partition across biological membranes via a concentration gradient. Hydrophilic molecules generally require some sort of selective transport system to cross the lipid bilayer. Large and polar drugs may be absorbed by a paracellular mechanism, and the tight junction structure represents the barrier to paracellular absorption.

Once a drug molecule has passed through to the basolateral side of the epithelium, the next barrier is the capillary endothelium for absorption into the blood. While this is not critical for locally acting drugs, it is important for systemically targeting APIs.

Strategies used to overcome these barriers to absorption include: A. Preventing degradation/metabolism; B. Enhancing barrier permeability via transient opening of tight junctions, C. Disruption of lipid bilayer packing/complexation/carrier/ion pairing; and D. Enhancing resident time/slowing down mucociliary clearance (Figure 3).

In the following sections, absorption enhancers utilized to overcome these barriers in nasal and pulmonary routes of administration are discussed.

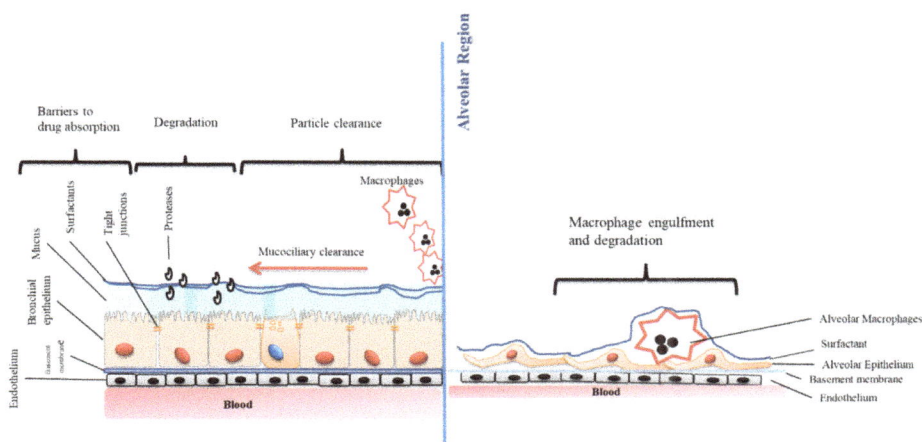

Figure 3. Hurdles for the absorption of drugs via inhalation.

3. Absorption Enhancers Investigated for Nasal and Pulmonary Drug Administration

The most common permeation enhancers investigated for nasal and pulmonary drug administration and their classification are listed in Table 1. Most of these agents have been divided into one of the following major classifications: (I) surfactants, (II) cyclodextrins, (III) protease inhibitors, (IV) cationic polymers, and (V) tight junction modulators. Each of these classifications are discussed in greater detail below.

Table 1. Common absorption permeation enhancers- application for nasal and pulmonary administration.

Class	Enhancers	Examples	References
Surfactants	Bile salts	Sodium taurocholate	[14,15]
		Sodium deoxycholate sodium	[16]
		Glycodeoxycholat	[17,18]
Surfactants	Fatty acids and derivatives	Palmitic acid	[19]
		Palmitoleic acid	
		Stearic acid	
		Oleyl alcohol	
		Oleic acid	
		Capric acid	[20,21]
		DHA, EPA	[20]
Surfactants	Phospholipids	Dipalmitoyl phophatidyl choline, soybean lecithin, phosphatidylcholine	[22,23]
Cationic polymers	Polymers	Chitosan and their derivatives	[24–26]
Enzyme inhibitors		Human neutrophil elastase inhibitor (ER143)	
Cyclodextrins		Beta-Cyclodextrin	[27]
Tight junction modulators	Claudine modulator	Clostridium perfringens enterotoxin	[28]
	ZO modulator	Zonula occludens toxin (ZOT)	[29]

3.1. Surfactants

Surface active agents, or surfactants, are amphiphilic molecules possessing both lipophilic and hydrophilic residues. Surfactants have various applications in pulmonary drug administration, due to their high interfacial activity; one of which is as an absorption enhancer [30]. Surfactants can enhance absorption with more than one mechanism; these include perturbing the cell membrane by leaching of membrane proteins, opening of tight junctions, or preventing enzymatic degradation of the drugs [31]. These surfactants are mainly used and studied in oral drug administration; however, there have been a few studies looking at their application in nasal and pulmonary drug delivery. Surfactants used as absorption enhancers can be classified as; (A) phospholipids [32], (B) bile salts, (such as sodium taurocholate etc.) [33], (C) non-ionic surfactants [31], (D) salt of fatty acids [20], and (E) alkyl glycosides (e.g., tetradecylmaltoside, *N*-lauryl-*b*-*d*-maltopyranoside etc.) [34].

(a) **Phospholipids**: Natural pulmonary surfactant is a complex mixture of phospholipids (90%) and proteins (10%). The main function of this surfactant is to reduce the surface tension at the alveolar air–liquid interface of the lungs to avoid alveolar collapse [35]. It has also been shown that phospholipids can enhance the absorption of active agents in the lung [36]. A review by Wauthoz extensively discussed their role in pulmonary drug administration [36]. For example, Dipalmitoylphosphatidylcholine (DPPC) is a main component of lung surfactant, representing 40% by weight [37]. DPPC has been used as a lung absorption enhancer in several studies [23,38,39]; for instance, it was used to optimize the absorption of parathyroid hormone 1-34 (PTH) from the lungs into the bloodstream [38]. Other lung surfactants, including phosphatidyl cholines (35%), phosphatidylglycerol (10%), phosphatidylinositol (2%), phosphatidylethanolamine (3%), sphingomyelin (2.5%), and neutral lipid (3%) have also been used as absorption enhancers. These natural pulmonary surfactants (PS) and their artificial substitute phospholipid hexadecanol tyloxapol (PHT) have been tested as absorption enhancers for promoting recombinant human insulin (Rh-ins) absorption in vivo from the lung in a diabetic rat model [40]. In another study, the same phospholipids were tested in vitro on Calu-3 ALI (air-liquid culture) model [41] to further investigate their absorption potential. This in vitro study demonstrated an enhanced permeation of Rh-ins and fluorescein isothiocyanate-labelled dextran (FD-4) (4000 Dalton molecular weight) through the cell layer. Hence, PS demonstrated a greater absorption enhancing effect than that of PHT. However, they could not identify the underlying mechanism of enhanced absorption. It was suggested that PS and PHT may interact directly with the tight junctions and increase the absorption via the paracellular pathway.

(b) **Bile salts**; one of the primary roles of bile salts and their derivatives in drug delivery is their ability to enhance absorption [42]. For pulmonary drug delivery applications, salts of cholate, deoxycholate, glycocholate, glycodeoxycholate, taurocholate, and taurodeoxycholate [43] have been tested as absorption enhancers. Sodium taurocholate is one of the most-used bile salts to increase bioavailability of proteins, especially insulin [33] via the pulmonary route. The ranking of enhancement by bile salts for insulin has been reported to be sodium deoxycholate > sodium cholate > sodium glycocholate > sodium glycodeoxycholate (GDCA) > sodium taurodeoxycholate [33]. Even though bile salts and derivatives have shown potential as absorption enhancers, their toxicity on the epithelial surface is a main challenge in clinical applications. In a recent study the effect of inhaled bile salts on lung surfactant function as absorption enhancers was investigated in two in vitro models and then correlated to in vivo lung effects [44]. This study demonstrated that bile salts in vitro disrupted surfactant function and in vivo induced pulmonary irritation. Therefore, even though the bile salts did not affect the barrier integrity or viability of human airway epithelial cells at the tested doses, they have shown toxicity to some extent.

(c) **Fatty acids**; Fatty acids, polyunsaturated fatty acids (PUFA), and their salts have also been investigated as absorption enhancers via the nasal and pulmonary route [21]. They have shown a tight junction modulatory effect to some extent, and enhanced permeation of drugs through the epithelial cell barrier. Although the exact mechanism is still unknown, previous studies have suggested that they may alter the membrane's permeability, increasing fluidity of the membrane or through Ca^{2+} dependent tight junction mechanisms [45]. Their potential as an absorption enhancer has been demonstrated in both in vitro [20] and in vivo studies [16]. For example, the effects of arachidonic acid as an absorption enhancer combined with amino acid Taurine enhanced absorption of fluorescein isothiocyanate 4000 (FD-4) via the pulmonary route [46]. Among the fatty acids, medium chain fatty acids such as capric acid and lauric acid have been studied extensively as absorption enhancers due to their safety and effectiveness [45,47]. The suggested mechanism for capric acid (sodium caprate) is most likely by activation of phospholipase-C and increase of intracellular calcium levels, resulting in contraction of actin microfilaments and dilation of the tight junctions [45].

(d) **Non-ionic surfactants**—Non-ionic surfactants, consisting of a hydrophilic head group and a hydrophobic tail, carry no charge and are relatively non-toxic [48]. Poloxamer 188, a non-ionic surfactant, has been widely studied as intranasal drug delivery system [49]. in vitro and in vivo studies demonstrated that poloxamer 188 played a key role in promoting intranasal absorption of both isosorbide dinitrate [49] and sumatriptan succinate [50] in rats. Incorporation of poloxamer 188 was reported to be able to influence the elasticity of nano-cubic vehicles for intranasal delivery [51]. Other non-ionic surfactants such as cremophor EL, laurate sucrose ester (SE), and sucrose cocoate have also shown absorption enhancement properties via nasal administration. SE has shown an efficient absorption-enhancing effect of poorly permeable drugs [31], furthermore, intranasal administration of an insulin formulation containing 0.5% sucrose cocoate showed a rapid and significant increase in plasma insulin level, with a concomitant decrease in blood glucose level [52]. Alkylglycosides (AGs) are a type of non-ionic surfactant class with groups such as maltose, sucrose or monosaccharides (e.g., glucose) attached to alkyl chains of variable length. Tetradecylmaltoside and *N*-lauryl-*b*-*d*-maltopyranoside are the most commonly used AGs. They have shown effective nasal absorption enhancement properties at extremely low concentrations. Pillion and his colleagues showed that AGs could be used effectively to enhance nasal absorption of insulin, calcitonin, and glucagon [53]. They synthesized a series of new glycosides with extended alkyl side-chains (C13–16) linked to maltose or sucrose and tested their efficacy as a penetration enhancer for delivery of nasal insulin in anesthetized rats [54]. Of the AGs tested, tetradecyl maltoside (TDM), a 14-carbon alkyl chain attached to a maltose ring, has been shown to be the most efficacious in enhancing nasal insulin absorption. The effects of TDM on the respiratory epithelium were shown to be reversible, with the epithelium reversing to its normal physiological barrier function 120 min after exposure to these agents. The molecular mechanism involved in these absorption-enhancing effects in vivo is unclear. It has been suggested that AGs have a direct effect on the epithelium layer, probably via the para cellular pathway [55]. Although AGs have shown absorption enhancing effect, they exhibit significant toxicity towards airway epithelial cells (Calu-3 cells), probably from a membrane-damaging effect [56].

(e) **Bio-surfactants**—Biosurfactants are surface-active substances synthesised by living cells such as bacteria, fungi, and yeast. Bio-surfactants are generally non-toxic, environmentally benign, and biodegradable. Biosurfactants have been investigated as drug absorption enhancers previously [57]. One of the most well characterized classes of biosurfactants are rhamnolipids. The effect of rhamnolipids on the epithelial permeability of FD-4 and FD-10 across Caco-2 and Calu-3 monolayers has been reported [58]. It was shown that rhamnolipids increased permeation of FD-4 and FD-10 across both cell lines at a safe concentration with a dose-dependent effect.

(f) **Animal derived surfactants**—The animal-derived surfactant poractant alfa (Curosurf®) was used to deliver polymyxin E and gentamicin to the lung in a neonatal rabbit model [59]. In this study, polymyxin E was mixed with poractant alfa and administered to a near-term rabbit. This mixture increased bactericidal effect of the antibiotics against Pseudomonas aeruginosa in vivo. This may be due to more efficient spreading mediated by interactions between drugs and surfactant.

3.2. Enzyme Inhibitors

Airway surface liquid and mucus contains a high number of enzymes including proteases, and nucleases that may degrade active agents before they are absorbed [60]. Among these enzymes, serine proteases and aminopeptidases constitute the majority of degrading enzymes present in the lung. Given the high number of enzymes in the lung, these may metabolize respiratory drugs before they reach the absorbing membrane. Peptide, proteins, and nucleic acid-based drugs are especially vulnerable to metabolism. Therefore, a strategy to protect drugs against enzymatic degradation within the lung and nasal cavity may be necessary in some cases. Some of the protease inhibitors studied over the last decade in pulmonary/nasal drug administration as absorption enhancers are: nafamostat mesilate [61], aprotinin [62], bacitracin [63], soybean trypsin inhibitor [63], phosphoramidon [15], leupeptin [64], and bestatin [65]. In one study, aprotinin, bacitracin, and soybean trypsin were used as protease inhibitors in combination with other absorption enhancers (sodium glycocholate, linoleic acid-surfactant mixed micelles, and *N*-lauryl-β-*d*-maltopyranoside) and tested on rat lung for the absorption of insulin and Asu (1,7)) eel-calcitonin (ECT) [62,63]. During the aforementioned study, rats received insulin with protease inhibitor via intra tracheal administration. The absorption of insulin from the lung was evaluated by their hypoglycemic and hypocalcemic response when used with these additives [62,63]. In the presence of protease inhibitors, the plasma concentration of glucose reached a minimum of 24.0–66.7% of baseline within 90 min of solution administration. It was also found that bacitracin (20 mM) was more effective at enhancing the pulmonary absorption of insulin than aprotinin and soybean trypsin inhibitor. In the same study, the effects of these protease inhibitors on the stability of insulin in rat lung homogenate were investigated, to elucidate the enhancing mechanisms of these protease inhibitors. All protease inhibitors were effective in reducing insulin degradation and these findings suggest that combination of absorption enhancers and protease inhibitors would be a useful approach for improving the pulmonary absorption of biologically active drugs. Studies have shown that when nafamostat mesilate, which strongly inhibits a variety of proteases, such as trypsin, plasmin, and kallikaren, was co-administered with insulin in the lung, the relative bioavailability of insulin was approximately twice that obtained when the peptide was administered alone [66].

During chronic lung inflammation and infection proteases such as neutrophil elastase (NE), a neutrophil-specific serine protease against P. aeruginosa, will be released into the lung lumen to fight pathogens involved in lung infections [67]. Excessive accumulation of NE in pulmonary fluids and tissues of patients with chronic lung infection is thought to reduce the absorption of inhaled drugs. Therefore, neutrophil elastase inhibitors (NEIs) have shown potential as absorption enhancers by protecting drug moieties from degradation by neutrophil elastase [68]. The potential use of NEIs, such as peptide chloromethyl ketones or reversible peptide aldehydes, tripeptide ketones, modified NE-specific β-lactams, or peptide boronic acids have been largely replaced by the development of EPI-HNE-4, a rapid acting and potent NE inhibitor [69] which can potentially be nebulized to CF patients [70]. However, clear clinical efficacy of this NE inhibitor remains to be demonstrated.

3.3. Cationic Polymers as Absorption Enhancers

Polymeric systems with positive charges or modified with cationic entities, incorporated on their backbone and/or side chains, are considered cationic polymers [71]. Cationic polymers have the potential to enhance absorption of macromolecules [72]. Cationated gelatins [72], cationated pullulans, poly-L-arginine, polyethylenamine (PEI), chitosan, and its derivatives are types of cationic polymers. Cationic polymers interact with the mucosal barriers and enhance the absorption of water-soluble macromolecules via tight junctions modification. For example, in the case of insulin with negative charges in neutral solutions, interaction between the cationic polymers and insulin is important to promote effective insulin absorption. An appropriate interaction can help insulin to access the cell surface; however, strong interaction can inhibit insulin absorption. PEI is a cationic and highly water-soluble polymer that has shown potential as a carrier for nasal drug administration. It was also demonstrated that the degree of positive charge was linearly correlated with absorption enhancing effect of PEI, suggesting that positive charge of PEI might be related to its absorption mechanisms for enhancing pulmonary absorption of insulin in rats [73]. Spermined dextran (SD), a cationic polymer, has been studied as absorption enhancer for pulmonary application of peptide drugs [74]. Its enhancing effects on the absorption of insulin and permeation of FD-4 through Calu-3 cells increased with an increase in the molecular weight of SD, over the range 10–70 kDa. The mechanism of action of SD is not fully understood yet, but it is hypothesized that the molecule may interact directly with the luminal surface of the mucus barriers via an ion-ion interaction, inducing the opening of tight junctions, resulting in intercellular permeation of water soluble drugs [74]. Chitosan and its derivatives are excellent examples of cationic polyelectrolytes. They have been extensively used to develop mucoadhesive polymers [25,75] and have favorable characteristics such as biocompatibility, biodegradation, and low toxicity. These aforementioned characteristics make them suitable as a pharmaceutical excipient [76]. Chitosan interacts electrostatically with the negatively charged mucin chains thereby demonstrating mucoadhesive properties. This mucoadhesion prolongs the residence time of the drug and thus enhances API absorption [77]. However, Chitosan derivatives are poorly soluble in water at physiological pH, limiting their application. Chitosan exhibits excellent mucoadhesive properties when dissolved in neutral or alkaline medium so to overcome solubility issues, different derivatives have been synthesized [78]. Chitosan oligomers [79], for example, have relatively high solubility in water compared to conventional chitosan and have been tested for their absorption enhancing potential via lung [25]. For example, the pulmonary absorption of interferon-α has been shown to be effective when using chitosan oligomers [25]. Of these chitosan oligomers, 0.5% w/v chitosan hexamer appeared to be more effective in enhancing the pulmonary absorption of IFN than other oligomers at the same concentration, and the AUC value of IFN with chitosan hexamer increased 2.6-fold when compared to control. In a recent study, O-palmitoyl chitosan, synthesized from chitosan and palmitoyl chloride, demonstrated improved mucoadhesive and absorption enhancing properties [80]. In addition, bioadhesive properties of chitosan may be useful in enhancing drug absorption following inhalation [81].

Sperminated pullulans (SP) have been shown to enhance pulmonary absorption of insulin in rats, with their enhancing effects correlated to the amino group content and their molecular weight [82]. SP acted as an enhancer for insulin absorption when a 0.1% w/v solution was applied with insulin simultaneously in vivo. Ikada et al. studied the use of negatively and positively charged gelatin microspheres for pulmonary administration of salmon calcitonin in rats [83]. The pharmacological effect after administration of salmon calcitonin in positively charged gelatin microspheres was significantly higher than that in negatively charged gelatin microspheres. Additionally, administration of salmon calcitonin in positively charged gelatin microspheres with smaller particle sizes led to a higher pharmacological effect. The pharmacological effect after pulmonary administration of salmon calcitonin in positively charged gelatin microspheres with particle sizes of 3.4 and 11.2 μm was approximately 50% [83].

Polyamines have also been tested for their absorption enhancing properties [84]. The polyamines spermidine and spermine are commonly found in all mammalian cells [84]. They are essential for the maintenance of cell growth in many tissues. Specifically, for the lungs, He et al. showed that polyamines, particularly spermine and spermidine, can effectively improve the pulmonary absorption of insulin and other water soluble macromolecules without any membrane damage of the lung tissues in rats [84]. It was suggested that the absorption-enhancing mechanism of spermine partly includes opening of the epithelial tight junctions. Sperminated dextrans have also been studied as absorption enhancers with different average molecular weights (MWs; 10, 40, and 70 kDa) and numbers of amino groups, prepared as cationized polymers [74]. Sperminated dextrans increased pulmonary absorption of insulin in rats and also permeation of FD-4 through Calu-3 cell monolayers in vitro [74].

3.4. Tight Junction Modulators

The intercellular spaces between adjacent epithelial cells are sealed by tight junctions (TJs). Modulation of TJs is an effective strategy for drug absorption via the paracellular pathway. The paracellular transport is not suitable for the transport of large macromolecules and is generally restricted to the compounds of molecular radii less than 11 Å. Hydrophilic drugs with low molecular weight, peptides, and proteins often have poor bioavailability. However, it has been shown that some peptide drugs, such as octreotide, desmopressin, and thyrotropin-releasing hormone are absorbed by this route in which tight junctions play a fundamental role [85]. Tight junction modulators effective on TJ proteins such as Claudin and ZO are extremely potent in opening these tight junctions, 400 fold stronger than other agents [86]. Until now they have mainly been tested on intestinal and dermal [87] tight junction barriers [88,89] and on the blood–brain barrier [90]. Of these modulators, two have been tested for pulmonary drug administration.

(A) Clostridium perfringens enterotoxin (CPE)—The C-terminal fragment of CPE (C-CPE) is known to modulate the barrier function of claudin [28]. Claudin is one of the key structural and functional components of the TJ-seal (70). Therefore, it has been suggested that claudin may be a potential target for paracellular API delivery. C-CPE is a potent absorption-enhancer and this enhancing activity is greater than clinically used enhancers. The main problem with tight junction modulators is their toxicity [91]; therefore, many variants of CPE have been synthesized to decrease toxicity [86]. In a study on nasal and pulmonary absorption of human parathyroid hormone hPTH in rats, C-CPE was used as an absorption enhancer. It was instilled into each nostril and after 4 h hPTH was delivered intranasally. A Micro-sprayer was used to spray C-CPE into rats' lungs, then after 4 h, hPTH was administered. This study showed C-CPE, and enhanced nasal but not pulmonary absorption of hPTH [89].

(B) Zonula occludens toxin (ZOT) are another tight junction modulator. Zot is a protein of Vibrio cholera, and zonulin is the Zot analogue that governs the permeability of intercellular TJs [92]. Zot and Zot derivatives are reversible TJ openers that enhance the delivery of drugs through the paracellular route. The active domain of zonula occludens toxin (ZOT) is called AT-1002 [93]. AT-1002, a hexamer peptide, induced tight junction disassembly in the epithelial layer in the trachea [29]. In this study, in vivo intratracheal administration of salmon calcitonin in rats with 1 mg of AT-1002 resulted in a 5.2-fold increase in absorption of calcitonin over the control group [29].

4. Other Strategies to Enhance Absorption

4.1. Nanoparticles (NPs)

Nanoparticles (NPs) have been used as drug carriers for overcoming mucociliary clearance and to avoid phagocytosis by alveolar macrophages, hence increasing the absorption of drugs in respiratory system [94]. It was shown that alveolar macrophages are less efficient to phagocytose ultrafine particles compared to larger particles [95] and NPs overcome the mucus barrier and achieve longer retention time at the cell surface, effectively penetrating the mucus layer and accumulating on the epithelial surface. In order to penetrate mucus, nanoparticles must avoid adhesion to mucin fibres and be small enough to avoid significant steric inhibition by the dense fibre mesh [96]. In a study by Schneider, variously sized, polystyrene-based muco-penetrating particles (MPP) were synthesized and their absorption in the lungs following inhalation investigated. They demonstrated that MPP as large as 300 nm exhibited uniform distribution and markedly enhanced retention in the lung [96]. NPs can also improve nose-to-brain drug delivery, since they are able to protect encapsulated drug from biological and/or chemical degradation, and from extracellular transport by P-gp efflux proteins [97]. Retention of bioadhesive NPs on the mucosal surface of the nasal cavity, as well as their ability of transiently opening of the tight junctions of the mucosal epithelium, should contribute to enhanced nasal absorption [98].

4.2. Liposomes

An approach to enhance mucosal penetration is to encapsulate drugs within liposomes. Liposomes consist of one or more phospholipid bilayers and can incorporate hydrophilic substances within their inner cavity and hydrophobic substances within the lipid bilayer. Liposomes and phospholipids have been investigated for the systemic absorption of proteins after intra tracheal administration [99]. It is suggested that the mechanism of absorption is driven by phospholipids in the liposomes being infused with the rapidly recycling lung surfactant that leads to enhanced uptake of the protein molecule into the systemic circulation [99]. Liposomes are also known to promote an increase in drug retention time and reduce the toxicity of drugs after administration [23]. Several factors influence drug release and absorption of drugs loaded into liposomes such as the composition of lipids and the size of the liposomes used [100]. The presence of cholesterol and phospholipids with saturated hydrocarbon chains have also been shown to increase drug residence time within the lung [23]. A number of nebulizable liposome formulations have reached clinical trial phase. For example, Arikace® (liposomal amikacin) and Pulmaquin® (liposomal ciprofloxacin) are antibacterial formulations currently in advanced stages of development.

Glycerosomes are vesicles composed of phospholipids, glycerol, and water, and have been used as novel vesicular carriers for trans-mucosal drug delivery. Glycerosomes are made from a diverse range of phospholipids and a high percent of glycerol (20–40%, *v/v*). They are flexible vesicular carriers, where the glycerol component alters the vesicle membrane fluidity, and are constituted by different substances such as cholesterol that enhance the lipidic bilayer stability. They also may contain basic or acidic lipid molecules which adjust the electrical charge of vesicular surfaces and decrease liposome aggregation. Glycerosomes can be prepared by the same common techniques that are used for the preparation of conventional liposomes.

As an example, curcumin was incorporated in glycerosomes for delivery into the lungs. In this study, curcumin was loaded into glycerosomes which were then combined with two polymers, sodium hyaluronate and trimethyl chitosan, to form polymer-glycerosomes [101]. The study showed that nebulized curcumin vesicles were able to protect in vitro A549 cells stressed with hydrogen peroxide, restoring healthy conditions, not only by directly scavenging free radicals but also by indirectly inhibiting the production of cytokine IL6 and IL8. Also, in vivo results in rats showed the high capacity of these glycerosomes to favor the curcumin accumulation in the lungs, confirming their potential use as a pulmonary drug delivery system. In another study, Rifampicin loaded glycerosomes, vesicles composed of phospholipids, glycerol, and water, were combined with trimethyl chitosan chloride (TMC) to prepare TMC-glycerosomes or with sodium hyaluronate (HY) to obtain HY-glycerosomes [102]. These new hybrid nanovesicles were tested as carriers for pulmonary delivery of rifampicin. Rifampicin nanoincorporation in vesicles reduced the in vitro drug toxicity on A549 cells, as well as increasing its efficacy against Staphylococcus aureus. Finally, the in vivo biodistribution and accumulation, evaluated after intra-tracheal administration to rats, confirmed the improvement of rifampicin accumulation in lung.

4.3. Dendrimers

Dendrimers possess high water solubility, and as highly efficient absorption promoters, they can easily penetrate through barriers. In addition, they can be used as carriers for different routes of drug administration [103,104]. Dendrimers have been studied intensively as a drug carrier in delivery systems [103,104]. As a novel class of artificial macromolecules, polyamidoamine (PAMAM) dendrimers have shown excellent performance in drug delivery systems due to their unique physical and chemical properties [105]. PAMAM dendrimers with generation 0 to generation 3 (G0–G3) and concentrations (0.1–1.0%) were tested in terms of their capacity to enhance pulmonary absorption of macromolecules [105]. The results showed that treatment with a 0.1% G3 PAMAM dendrimer could increase the secretion of organic cation transporters (OCTs), OCT1, OCT2, and OCT3, which might be related to the absorption-enhancing mechanisms of the pulmonary absorption of the macromolecule.

4.4. Exosomes

Exosomes are a subgroup of 30–100 nm size extracellular vesicles (EVs) secreted by cells into the extracellular environment. EVs have the distinct advantage that their membranes are structurally similar to the cell membrane. This means that EVs lipid composition, fluidity, protein membranes, and other fusogenic proteins are similar to what is found in cell membranes. Because of this unique property, cellular uptake of EVs surpasses that of more traditional carriers, such as liposomes or nanoparticles. Exosomes can be used as a biological nano-platform for enhanced drug delivery [106]. Their advantages include their small size for penetration into deep tissues, slightly negative zeta potential for long circulation, and deformable cytoskeleton, as well as their similarity to cell membranes [107]. In addition, some exosomes also exhibit an increased capacity to escape degradation or clearance by the immune system [108]. Exosomes have been developed as drug delivery vehicles for a variety of drugs [109,110]. Tumor-derived exosomes are of great significance for guiding the targeted therapy of lung cancer, and exosomes themselves can be a target for treatment. For example, GW4869, a neutral sphingomyelase inhibitor (regulates ceramide biosynthesis, promotes exosomes inward budding), tested in mice, demonstrated inhibition of exosomes production with reduced metastasis in lung cancer [111]. In another study, exosomes derived from curcumin-treated cells alleviated oxidative stress, tight junctions (ZO-1, claudin, occludin), adherent junction (VE-cadherin) proteins, and endothelial cell layer permeability [112]. A nano-formulation consisting of exosomes loaded with paclitaxel (PTX), a commonly used chemotherapeutic agent, developed by Batrakova et al. [113], showed efficacy in the treatment of multi-drug resistant cancer cells. Incorporation of PTX into exosomes increased cytotoxicity more than 50 times in drug resistant MDCKMDR1 (Pgp+) cells and showed a potent anticancer effect in the murine Lewis lung carcinoma pulmonary metastases model. It was shown that exosomes loaded with PTX may alter drug intracellular trafficking and bypass the drug efflux system. The potential of intranasally administered exosomes as delivery vehicles for the treatment of neuro inflammatory diseases has also been investigated. After intranasal administration of exosomes loaded with potent antioxidant, considerable amounts of catalase were detected in a Parkinson's disease (PD) mouse brain model. It provided significant neuroprotective effects in in vitro and in vivo models of PD [114]. Low molecular antioxidant [115], anticancer agents, doxorubicin (Dox) [116], and a model drug rhodamine [117], have also been loaded into exosomes or exosome-like vesicles for nasal drug delivery to enhance absorption and efficacy.

4.5. Cell Penetrating Peptides (CPPs)

Improving the translocation of drugs across the plasma membrane will significantly enhance their absorption. Therefore, using cell penetrating peptides (CPPs) to enhance drug penetration has the potential to significantly reduce the quantity of drug to be administered, thus reducing possible side effects. Cell-penetrating peptides are short peptides that enable cellular intake/uptake of various molecular moieties with poor permeability across epithelial and endothelial barriers [118]. Several types of cargoes, for example, proteins, nucleic acid based macromolecules such as siRNA, plasmid DNA, and small drug molecules, can be transported by CPPs to overcome the natural cellular biological barriers [119]. The mechanism of action of CPPs is still a matter of some debate. Some research suggests CPPs could pass through the plasma membrane via an energy-independent pathway, with others claiming the formation of micro-micelles at the membrane [120], or direct translocation through the lipid bilayer [121]. Multiple studies have consolidated the high efficiency of CPP-mediated drug delivery in vitro. For instance, CPPs have been used successfully to deliver macromolecules [122], oligonucleotides [119,123], and peptides [124] across different cellular barriers. Specifically, CPPs have been recently investigated in nasal and pulmonary drug administration [125–127], where they have been used as a conjugate to liposomes and nanoparticles to enhance absorption of model DNA [128]. Co-administration of CPPs could improve nose-to-brain drug transport. In Kamei's study, it was demonstrated that, insulin was transported into the brain when co-administered with amphipathic CPP, and eventually insulin reached the deeper regions of the brain such as the hippocampus in both mice and rat [126]. The immunohistological examination of the hippocampus demonstrated enhanced nose-to-brain delivery of insulin had a partial neuroprotective effect but unexpectedly increased amyloid β plaque deposition. Therefore, CPPs seem to hold great promise as delivery agents for biomacromolecules. However, CPP-mediated delivery is apparently not tissue- or cell-type specific, so for specific targeting purposes additional agents need to be included in the drug delivery system.

4.6. Surface Modification

To enhance the absorption of poorly permeable drugs, another strategy is to modify the inhaled particle surface with agents that enhance their absorption. For example, by coating particles with lipids, the disturbance of the particles on the cellular layer can be reduced [129]. Moreover, the lipid-coated particles can be readily enfolded by the surfactant layer to form vesicular structures that can fuse with the cell membrane. Polymer coating of nanoparticles and liposomes is another strategy to enhance the mucosal penetration of particles via nasal/pulmonary administration [130]. For example, spray dried polymer coated liposomes composed of soy phosphatidylcholine and phospholipid dimyristoyl phosphatidylglycerol coated with alginate, chitosan, or trimethyl chitosan, increased penetration of liposomes through the nasal mucosa over uncoated liposomes when delivered as a dry powder [130]. Surface-modified liposomes for pulmonary administration of peptides were also investigated. For example, chitosan oligosaccharide (oligoCS) and polyvinyl alcohol (PVA-R) with a hydrophobic anchor were used as surface modifiers [131]. The effect of surface modified liposomes on potential toxicity via inhalation was evaluated in vitro and in vivo. In vitro studies on alveolar epithelial cells (A549 cells) demonstrated that PVA-R modification reduced interaction with this cell line, whereas oligoCS modification electrostatically enhanced cellular interaction. The therapeutic efficacy of a peptide (elcatonin) after pulmonary administration to rats was significantly enhanced and prolonged for 48 h after separate administration with oligoCS- or PVA-R-modified liposomes. Furthermore, oligoCS-modified liposomes increased residency of liposomes in the lung and had a tight junction opening effect. On the other hand, PVA-R-modified liposomes induced long-term retention of elcatonin in the lung fluid, leading to sustained absorption. Lactoferrin, a natural iron binding protein whose receptor is highly expressed in both respiratory epithelial cells and neurons, was utilized to facilitate the nasal delivery of nucleic based therapeutic agents. For example, a Lactoferrin-modified PEG-*co*-PCL NPs was recently developed to enhance brain delivery of a neuroprotective peptide—NAPVSIPQ following intranasal administration [132]. In another study, rotigotine, dopamine agonist for the treatment of PD, was loaded in lactoferrin (Lf) modified poly(ethylene glycol)–poly(lactic-*co*-glycolic acid) (PEG-PLGA) nanoparticles. Following intranasal administration, brain delivery of rotigotine was more effective with Lf-NPs than with NPs alone. The brain distribution of rotigotine was heterogeneous, with a higher concentration in the striatum, the primary region affected in PD. This strongly suggested that Lf-NPs enable the targeted delivery of rotigotine for the treatment of PD.

4.7. Cyclodextrins (CDs)

Cyclodextrins (CDs) are a distinct family of chemical reagents that contain six, seven, or eight monosaccharide units in a cyclized ring with a central cavity that can accommodate other agents [133]. Hydrophobic drug molecules or hydrophobic parts of drugs are introduced into the CD apolar cavities, thereby presenting the potential to modify the properties of the inhaled drug. For example, Shimpi et al. showed that CDs have an effect on absorption of hydrophilic macromolecules through the pulmonary and nasal routes [27]. They have demonstrated many benefits in pulmonary drug administration, such as improvements in aqueous solubility, systemic absorption and bioavailability of drugs. It has also been shown that modified CDs, such as methylated β-cyclodextrin (M-β-CD), dimethyl-β-cyclodextrin (DM-β-CD), and hydroxypropyl-beta-cyclodextrin (HP-β-CD) as its derivatives notably enhance intranasal absorption of drugs [134]. β-cyclodextrins (β-CD) have been broadly studied as an intranasal absorption enhancer [49]. The effect of CDs on the respiratory cell layer permeability was investigated in vitro and shown to be concentration-dependent and variable according to the type of CDs, type of chemical modification, and degree of substitution [135]. It has been shown that CDs, in general, do not cause a decrease in cell viability at concentrations ≤1 mM, whereas differences between various CDs were observed at concentrations ≥2 mM [136,137]. HP-β-CD and natural-CDs are safest in terms of cytotoxicity, while M-β-CD were the least safe for pulmonary administration [138]. Particularly, it has been shown that CDs are more effective in animal studies compared to in vitro studies as absorption enhancers [134].

The mechanism of absorption enhancement with CDs is still unclear; however, there are reports that M-β-CD increase transcellular, as well as paracellular, movement of peptide drugs [135]. CDs may also have a direct disruptive effect on the alveolar epithelial membrane as evidenced by the extraction of membrane lipids and proteins [139]. CDs derivatives can also stimulate transmucosal absorption of peptide drugs. Importantly, M-β-CD, such as DM-β-CD, strongly enhance transmucosal insulin absorption, whereas unmodified-cyclodextrin has little effect on insulin absorption [139]. It is suggested that both DM-β-CD and tetradecyl-beta-maltoside cyclodextrin (TDM-CD) enhance absorption of insulin by different mechanisms. It has been demonstrated that CDs enhance transmucosal absorption of insulin by formation of an inclusion complex, with insulin or by direct action on the membrane [139]. The latter may involve removal of membrane proteins, complexation with different membrane components, or inhibition of proteolytic enzyme activity. However, it has been claimed that TDM-CD may act by opening cell–cell tight junctions. There is a commercial product of CDs available in the market called Kleptose® HPB (hydroxypropylβ-cyclodextrin) which has been suggested as an attractive excipient for nasal and pulmonary drug administration due to its potential in solubilizing drugs, enhancing absorption of drugs, and low toxicity profile.

5. Products in Development

Currently, there are few products in development that employ an absorption-enhancing technology for nasal and pulmonary formulations, as seen in Table 2.

Table 2. Nasal and Inhalation products in development that employ penetration enhancers.

Technology	Development Stage	Biological Products	Company	Absorption Enhancer Used in the Technology
Cyclopenta Decalactone	Marketed Phase 2	Testosterone (Testim) Nocturia	CPEX Pharmaceuticals Serenity	Surfactant
ChiSys™ PecSys™	Phase 2 Phase 2 Phase 3	Intranasal Apomorphine Intranasal Diazepam Intranasal fentanyl citrate (NasalFent)	Archimedes Pharma Ltd.	Chitosan based delivery
Intravail™	Phase 1 Phase 2 Phase 1	Proteins (IFN-β, EPO) and peptides (PTH, GLP-1), Sumatriptan Naltrexone, Nalmefene	Neurelis, Inc. (Aegis Therapeutics Inc.) Opiant Pharmaceuticals	Cationic polymers-Alkyl saccharide
GelSite® GelVac™ nasal dry powder	Phase 1	Vaccines	Carrington Labs (Delsite Biotech)	Cationic polymers-Poly saccharide
μco™	Phase II Phase 1	Granisetron-zolmitriptan Peptides: (insulin, PTH, FSH, GHRP) Nasal epinephrine formulation	SNBL, Ltd. G2B Pharma Inc.	Polymer-Micro crystalline cellulose (Powder)

6. Conclusions

Several technologies for enhancing the absorption of poorly permeable therapeutic biomolecules have progressed from early studies. They have demonstrated permeation enhancement in isolated barrier model, and a number of absorption-enhancing technologies, especially for nasal applications, are now in clinical trials. These absorption enhancers increase systemic absorption of biomolecules as indicated by improved bioavailability or bioactivity, and appear to represent possible alternatives to existing products, which have sub-optimal bioavailability. Still, one of the challenges towards clinical application of these agents is their lack of safety. Understanding the mechanism of absorption enhancement may be very useful toward reducing their side effects and improving their efficacy before these could be considered as future platforms for inhalation formulation of drugs with poor permeability.

Funding: This research received no external funding.

Conflicts of Interest: The authors declare no conflict of interest.

References

1. Helmstadter, A. Endermatic, epidermatic, enepidermatic-the early history of penetration enhancers. *Int. J. Pharm.* **2011**, *416*, 12–15. [CrossRef] [PubMed]
2. Thwala, L.N.; Preat, V.; Csaba, N.S. Emerging delivery platforms for mucosal administration of biopharmaceuticals: A critical update on nasal, pulmonary and oral routes. *Expert Opin. Drug Deliv.* **2017**, *14*, 23–36. [CrossRef] [PubMed]

3. Turker, S.; Onur, E.; Ozer, Y. Nasal route and drug delivery systems. *Pharm. World Sci.* **2004**, *26*, 137–142. [CrossRef] [PubMed]

4. Agu, R.U.; Ugwoke, M.I.; Armand, M.; Kinget, R.; Verbeke, N. The lung as a route for systemic delivery of therapeutic proteins and peptides. *Respir. Res.* **2001**, *2*, 198–209. [PubMed]

5. Fan, Y.; Chen, M.; Zhang, J.Q.; Maincent, P.; Xia, X.F.; Wu, W. Updated progress of nanocarrier-based intranasal drug delivery systems for treatment of brain diseases. *Crit. Rev. Ther. Drug* **2018**, *35*, 433–467. [CrossRef] [PubMed]

6. Zhu, Z.T.; Pan, J.H.; Wu, X.H.; Jiang, Z.T. [screen absorption enhancer for intranasal administration preparations of paeoniflorin based on nasal perfusion method in rats]. *Zhongguo Zhong yao za zhi = Zhongguo zhongyao zazhi = China J. Chin. Mater. Med.* **2017**, *42*, 493–497.

7. Sleigh, M.A.; Blake, J.R.; Liron, N. The propulsion of mucus by cilia. *Am. Rev. Respir. Dis.* **1988**, *137*, 726–741. [CrossRef] [PubMed]

8. Clunes, M.T.; Boucher, R.C. Cystic fibrosis: The mechanisms of pathogenesis of an inherited lung disorder. *Drug Discov. Today Dis. Mech.* **2007**, *4*, 63–72. [CrossRef] [PubMed]

9. Verkman, A.S.; Song, Y.; Thiagarajah, J.R. Role of airway surface liquid and submucosal glands in cystic fibrosis lung disease. *Am. J. Physiol. Cell Physiol.* **2003**, *284*, C2–C15. [CrossRef] [PubMed]

10. Rosen, H.; Abribat, T. The rise and rise of drug delivery. *Nat. Rev. Drug Discov.* **2005**, *4*, 381–385. [CrossRef] [PubMed]

11. Ali, M.S.; Pearson, J.P. Upper airway mucin gene expression: A review. *Laryngoscope* **2007**, *117*, 932–938. [CrossRef] [PubMed]

12. Mainardes, R.M.; Urban, M.C.; Cinto, P.O.; Chaud, M.V.; Evangelista, R.C.; Gremiao, M.P. Liposomes and micro/nanoparticles as colloidal carriers for nasal drug delivery. *Curr. Drug Deliv.* **2006**, *3*, 275–285. [CrossRef] [PubMed]

13. Inoue, D.; Tanaka, A.; Kimura, S.; Kiriyama, A.; Katsumi, H.; Yamamoto, A.; Ogawara, K.I.; Kimura, T.; Higaki, K.; Yutani, R.; et al. The relationship between in vivo nasal drug clearance and in vitro nasal mucociliary clearance: Application to the prediction of nasal drug absorption. *Eur. J. Pharm. Sci.* **2018**, *117*, 21–26. [CrossRef] [PubMed]

14. Karasulu, E.; Yavasoglu, A.; Evrensanal, Z.; Uvanikgil, Y.; Karasulu, H.Y. Permeation studies and histological examination of sheep nasal mucosa following administration of different nasal formulations with or without absorption enhancers. *Drug Deliv.* **2008**, *15*, 219–225. [CrossRef] [PubMed]

15. Kobayashi, S.; Kondo, S.; Juni, K. Study on pulmonary delivery of salmon-calcitonin in rats—Effects of protease inhibitors and absorption enhancers. *Pharm. Res.-Dordr.* **1994**, *11*, 1239–1243. [CrossRef]

16. Chavanpatil, M.D.; Vavia, P.R. The influence of absorption enhancers on nasal absorption of acyclovir. *Eur. J. Pharm. Biopharm.* **2004**, *57*, 483–487. [CrossRef] [PubMed]

17. Kim, I.W.; Yoo, H.; Song, I.S.; Chung, Y.B.; Moon, D.C.; Chung, S.J.; Shim, C.K. Effect of excipients on the stability and transport of recombinant human epidermal growth factor (rhegf) across caco-2 cell monolayers. *Arch. Pharm. Res.* **2003**, *26*, 330–337. [CrossRef] [PubMed]

18. Ikeda, K.; Murata, K.; Kobayashi, M.; Noda, K. Enhancement of bioavailability of dopamine via nasal route in beagle dogs. *Chem. Pharm. Bull.* **1992**, *40*, 2155–2158. [CrossRef] [PubMed]

19. Amancha, K.P.; Hussain, A. Effect of protease inhibitors on pulmonary bioavailability of therapeutic proteins and peptides in the rat. *Eur. J. Pharm. Sci.* **2015**, *68*, 1–10. [CrossRef] [PubMed]

20. Ghadiri, M.; Canney, F.; Pacciana, C.; Colombo, G.; Young, P.M.; Traini, D. The use of fatty acids as absorption enhancer for pulmonary drug delivery. *Int. J. Pharm.* **2018**, *541*, 93–100. [CrossRef]

21. Ghadiri, M.; Mamlouk, M.; Spicer, P.; Jarolimek, W.; Grau, G.E.R.; Young, P.M.; Traini, D. Effect of polyunsaturated fatty acids (pufas) on airway epithelial cells' tight junction. *Pulm. Pharmacol. Ther.* **2016**, *40*, 30–38. [CrossRef] [PubMed]

22. Li, F.; Yang, X.L.; Yang, Y.A.; Li, P.; Yang, Z.L.; Zhang, C.F. Phospholipid complex as an approach for bioavailability enhancement of echinacoside. *Drug Dev. Ind. Pharm.* **2015**, *41*, 1777–1784. [CrossRef] [PubMed]

23. Chono, S.; Fukuchi, R.; Seki, T.; Morimoto, K. Aerosolized liposomes with dipalmitoyl phosphatidylcholine enhance pulmonary insulin delivery. *J. Control. Release* **2009**, *137*, 104–109. [CrossRef] [PubMed]

24. Benediktsdottir, B.E.; Gudjonsson, T.; Baldursson, O.; Masson, M. N-alkylation of highly quaternized chitosan derivatives affects the paracellular permeation enhancement in bronchial epithelia in vitro. *Eur. J. Pharm. Biopharm.* **2014**, *86*, 55–63. [CrossRef] [PubMed]
25. Yamada, K.; Odomi, M.; Okada, N.; Fujita, T.; Yamamoto, A. Chitosan oligomers as potential and safe absorption enhancers for improving the pulmonary absorption of interferon-alpha in rats. *J. Pharm. Sci.-US* **2005**, *94*, 2432–2440. [CrossRef] [PubMed]
26. Yamamoto, A.; Yamada, K.; Muramatsu, H.; Nishinaka, A.; Okumura, S.; Okada, N.; Fujita, T.; Muranishi, S. Control of pulmonary absorption of water-soluble compounds by various viscous vehicles. *Int. J. Pharm.* **2004**, *282*, 141–149. [CrossRef] [PubMed]
27. Shimpi, S.; Chauhan, B.; Shimpi, P. Cyclodextrins: Application in Different Routes of Drug Administration. *Acta Pharm.* **2005**, *55*, 139–156. [PubMed]
28. Suzuki, H.; Kondoh, M.; Li, X.; Takahashi, A.; Matsuhisa, K.; Matsushita, K.; Kakamu, Y.; Yamane, S.; Kodaka, M.; Isoda, K.; et al. A toxicological evaluation of a claudin modulator, the c-terminal fragment of clostridium perfringens enterotoxin, in mice. *Pharmazie* **2011**, *66*, 543–546. [PubMed]
29. Gopalakrishnan, S.; Pandey, N.; Tamiz, A.P.; Vere, J.; Carrasco, R.; Somerville, R.; Tripathi, A.; Ginski, M.; Paterson, B.M.; Alkan, S.S. Mechanism of action of zot-derived peptide at-1002, a tight junction regulator and absorption enhancer. *Int. J. Pharm.* **2009**, *365*, 121–130. [CrossRef] [PubMed]
30. Shubber, S.; Vllasaliu, D.; Rauch, C.; Jordan, F.; Illum, L.; Stolnik, S. Mechanism of mucosal permeability enhancement of criticalsorb (r) (solutol (r) hs15) investigated in vitro in cell cultures. *Pharm. Res.-Dordr* **2015**, *32*, 516–527. [CrossRef] [PubMed]
31. Li, Y.; Li, J.; Zhang, X.; Ding, J.; Mao, S. Non-ionic surfactants as novel intranasal absorption enhancers: In vitro and in vivo characterization. *Drug Deliv.* **2016**, *23*, 2272–2279. [PubMed]
32. Brockman, J.M.; Wang, Z.D.; Notter, R.H.; Dluhy, R.A. Effect of hydrophobic surfactant proteins sp-b and sp-c on binary phospholipid monolayers ii. Infrared external reflectance-absorption spectroscopy. *Biophys. J.* **2003**, *84*, 326–340. [CrossRef]
33. Johansson, F.; Hjertberg, E.; Eirefelt, S.; Tronde, A.; Bengtsson, U.H. Mechanisms for absorption enhancement of inhaled insulin by sodium taurocholate. *Eur. J. Pharm. Sci.* **2002**, *17*, 63–71. [CrossRef]
34. Chen-Quay, S.C.; Eiting, K.T.; Li, A.W.A.; Lamharzi, N.; Quay, S.C. Identification of tight junction modulating lipids. *J. Pharm. Sci.-US* **2009**, *98*, 606–619. [CrossRef] [PubMed]
35. Griese, M. Pulmonary surfactant in health and human lung diseases: State of the art. *Eur. Respir. J.* **1999**, *13*, 1455–1476. [CrossRef] [PubMed]
36. Wauthoz, N.; Amighi, K. Phospholipids in pulmonary drug delivery. *Eur. J. Lipid Sci. Technol.* **2014**, *116*, 1114–1128. [CrossRef]
37. Veldhuizen, R.; Nag, K.; Orgeig, S.; Possmayer, F. The role of lipids in pulmonary surfactant. *BBA-Mol. Basis Dis.* **1998**, *1408*, 90–108. [CrossRef]
38. Hoyer, H.; Perera, G.; Bernkop-Schnurch, A. Noninvasive delivery systems for peptides and proteins in osteoporosis therapy: A retroperspective. *Drug Dev. Ind. Pharm.* **2010**, *36*, 31–44. [CrossRef] [PubMed]
39. Ventura, C.A.; Fresta, M.; Paolino, D.; Pedotti, S.; Corsaro, A.; Puglisi, G. Biomembrane model interaction and percutaneous absorption of papaverine through rat skin: Effects of cyclodextrins as penetration enhancers. *J. Drug Target* **2001**, *9*, 379–393. [CrossRef] [PubMed]
40. Zheng, J.H.; Zhang, G.; Lu, Y.; Fang, F.; He, J.K.; Li, N.; Talbi, A.; Zhang, Y.; Tang, Y.; Zhu, J.B.; et al. Effect of pulmonary surfactant and phospholipid hexadecanol tyloxapol on recombinant human-insulin absorption from intratracheally administered dry powders in diabetic rats. *Chem. Pharm. Bull.* **2010**, *58*, 1612–1616. [CrossRef] [PubMed]
41. Zheng, J.H.; Zheng, Y.; Chen, J.Y.; Fang, F.; He, J.K.; Li, N.; Tang, Y.; Zhu, J.B.; Chen, X.J. Enhanced pulmonary absorption of recombinant human insulin by pulmonary surfactant and phospholipid hexadecanol tyloxapol through calu-3 monolayers. *Pharmazie* **2012**, *67*, 448–451. [PubMed]
42. Stojancevic, M.; Pavlovic, N.; Golocorbin-Kon, S.; Mikov, M. Application of bile acids in drug formulation and delivery. *Front. Life Sci.* **2013**, *7*, 112–122. [CrossRef]
43. Moghimipour, E.; Ameri, A.; Handali, S. Absorption-enhancing effects of bile salts. *Molecules* **2015**, *20*, 14451–14473. [CrossRef] [PubMed]

44. Sørli, J.B.; Balogh Sivars, K.; Da Silva, E.; Hougaard, K.S.; Koponen, I.K.; Zuo, Y.Y.; Weydahl, I.E.K.; Åberg, P.M.; Fransson, R. Bile salt enhancers for inhalation: Correlation between in vitro and in vivo lung effects. *Int. J. Pharm.* **2018**, *550*, 114–122. [CrossRef] [PubMed]

45. Del Vecchio, G.; Tscheik, C.; Tenz, K.; Helms, H.C.; Winkler, L.; Blasig, R.; Blasig, I.E. Sodium caprate transiently opens claudin-5-containing barriers at tight junctions of epithelial and endothelial cells. *Mol. Pharm.* **2012**, *9*, 2523–2533. [CrossRef] [PubMed]

46. Miyake, M.; Minami, T.; Yamazaki, H.; Emoto, C.; Mukai, T.; Toguchi, H. Arachidonic acid with taurine enhances pulmonary absorption of macromolecules without any serious histopathological damages. *Eur. J. Pharm. Biopharm.* **2017**, *114*, 22–28. [CrossRef] [PubMed]

47. Coyne, C.B.; Ribeiro, C.M.P.; Boucher, R.C.; Johnson, L.G. Acute mechanism of medium chain fatty acid-induced enhancement of airway epithelial permeability. *J. Pharmacol. Exp. Ther.* **2003**, *305*, 440–450. [CrossRef] [PubMed]

48. Ujhelyi, Z.; Fenyvesi, F.; Varadi, J.; Feher, P.; Kiss, T.; Veszelka, S.; Deli, M.; Vecsernyes, M.; Bacskay, I. Evaluation of cytotoxicity of surfactants used in self-micro emulsifying drug delivery systems and their effects on paracellular transport in caco-2 cell monolayer. *Eur. J. Pharm. Sci.* **2012**, *47*, 564–573. [CrossRef] [PubMed]

49. Na, L.; Mao, S.; Wang, J.; Sun, W. Comparison of different absorption enhancers on the intranasal absorption of isosorbide dinitrate in rats. *Int. J. Pharm.* **2010**, *397*, 59–66. [CrossRef] [PubMed]

50. Kreuter, J. Mechanism of polymeric nanoparticle-based drug transport across the blood-brain barrier (bbb). *J. Microencapsul.* **2013**, *30*, 49–54. [CrossRef] [PubMed]

51. Salama, H.A.; Mahmoud, A.A.; Kamel, A.O.; Abdel Hady, M.; Awad, G.A.S. Phospholipid based colloidal poloxamer–nanocubic vesicles for brain targeting via the nasal route. *Colloids Surf. B Biointerfaces* **2012**, *100*, 146–154. [CrossRef] [PubMed]

52. Ahsan, F.; Arnold, J.J.; Meezan, E.; Pillion, D.J. Sucrose cocoate, a component of cosmetic preparations, enhances nasal and ocular peptide absorption. *Int. J. Pharm.* **2003**, *251*, 195–203. [CrossRef]

53. Maggio, E.T.; Pillion, D.J. High efficiency intranasal drug delivery using intravail (r) alkylsaccharide absorption enhancers. *Drug Deliv. Transl. Res.* **2013**, *3*, 16–25. [CrossRef] [PubMed]

54. Pillion, D.J.; Ahsan, F.; Arnold, J.J.; Balusubramanian, B.M.; Piraner, O.; Meezan, E. Synthetic long-chain alkyl maltosides and alkyl sucrose esters as enhancers of nasal insulin absorption. *J. Pharm. Sci.-US* **2002**, *91*, 1456–1462. [CrossRef] [PubMed]

55. Ahsan, F.; Arnold, J.; Meezan, E.; Pillion, D.J. Enhanced bioavailability of calcitonin formulated with alkylglycosides following nasal and ocular administration in rats. *Pharm. Res.-Dordr.* **2001**, *18*, 1742–1746. [CrossRef]

56. Vllasaliu, D.; Shubber, S.; Fowler, R.; Garnett, M.; Alexander, C.; Stolnik, S. Epithelial toxicity of alkylglycoside surfactants. *J. Pharm. Sci.-US* **2013**, *102*, 114–125. [CrossRef] [PubMed]

57. Wallace, C.J.; Medina, S.H.; ElSayed, M.E.H. Effect of rhamnolipids on permeability across caco-2 cell monolayers. *Pharm. Res.-Dordr.* **2014**, *31*, 887–894. [CrossRef] [PubMed]

58. Perinelli, D.R.; Vllasaliu, D.; Bonacucina, G.; Come, B.; Pucciarelli, S.; Ricciutelli, M.; Cespi, M.; Itri, R.; Spinozzi, F.; Palmieri, G.F.; et al. Rhamnolipids as epithelial permeability enhancers for macromolecular therapeutics. *Eur. J. Pharm. Biopharm.* **2017**, *119*, 419–425. [CrossRef] [PubMed]

59. Basabe-Burgos, O.; Zebialowicz, J.; Stichtenoth, G.; Curstedt, T.; Bergman, P.; Johansson, J.; Rising, A. Natural derived surfactant preparation as a carrier of polymyxin e for treatment of *pseudomonas aeruginosa* pneumonia in a near-term rabbit model. *J. Aerosol. Med. Pulm. Drug Deliv.* **2018**. [CrossRef] [PubMed]

60. Candiano, G.; Bruschi, M.; Pedemonte, N.; Musante, L.; Ravazzolo, R.; Liberatori, S.; Bini, L.; Galietta, L.J.; Zegarra-Moran, O. Proteomic analysis of the airway surface liquid: Modulation by proinflammatory cytokines. *Am. J. Physiol. Lung Cell. Mol. Physiol.* **2007**, *292*, L185–L198. [CrossRef] [PubMed]

61. Morita, T.; Yamamoto, A.; Takakura, Y.; Hashida, M.; Sezaki, H. Improvement of the pulmonary absorption of (asu(1,7))-eel calcitonin by various protease inhibitors in rats. *Pharm. Res.-Dordr.* **1994**, *11*, 909–913. [CrossRef]

62. Yamamoto, A.; Umemori, S.; Muranishi, S. Absorption enhancement of intrapulmonary administered insulin by various absorption enhancers and protease inhibitors in rats. *J. Pharm. Pharmacol.* **1994**, *46*, 14–18. [CrossRef] [PubMed]

63. Yamamoto, A.; Fujita, T.; Muranishi, S. Pulmonary absorption enhancement of peptides by absorption enhancers and protease inhibitors. *J. Control. Release* **1996**, *41*, 57–67. [CrossRef]

64. Yamahara, H.; Morimoto, K.; Lee, V.H.L.; Kim, K.J. Effects of protease inhibitors on vasopressin transport across rat alveolar epithelial-cell monolayers. *Pharm. Res.-Dordr.* **1994**, *11*, 1617–1622. [CrossRef]

65. Machida, M.; Hayashi, M.; Awazu, S. The effects of absorption enhancers on the pulmonary absorption of recombinant human granulocyte colony-stimulating factor (rhg-csf) in rats. *Biol. Pharm. Bull.* **2000**, *23*, 84–86. [CrossRef] [PubMed]

66. Okumura, K.; Iwakawa, S.; Yoshida, T.; Seki, T.; Komada, F. Intratracheal delivery of insulin absorption from solution and aerosol by rat lung. *Int. J. Pharm.* **1992**, *88*, 63–73. [CrossRef]

67. Hirche, T.O.; Benabid, R.; Deslee, G.; Gangloff, S.; Achilefu, S.; Guenounou, M.; Lebargy, F.; Hancock, R.E.; Belaaouaj, A. Neutrophil elastase mediates innate host protection against pseudomonas aeruginosa. *J. Immunol.* **2008**, *181*, 4945–4954. [CrossRef] [PubMed]

68. Gibbons, A.; McElvaney, N.G.; Cryan, S.A. A dry powder formulation of liposome-encapsulated recombinant secretory leukocyte protease inhibitor (rslpi) for inhalation: Preparation and characterisation. *AAPS PharmSciTech* **2010**, *11*, 1411–1421. [CrossRef] [PubMed]

69. Delacourt, C.; Herigault, S.; Delclaux, C.; Poncin, A.; Levame, M.; Harf, A.; Saudubray, F.; Lafuma, C. Protection against acute lung injury by intravenous or intratracheal pretreatment with epi-hne-4, a new potent neutrophil elastase inhibitor. *Am. J. Respir Cell Mol. Biol.* **2002**, *26*, 290–297. [CrossRef] [PubMed]

70. Grimbert, D.; Vecellio, L.; Delepine, P.; Attucci, S.; Boissinot, E.; Poncin, A.; Gauthier, F.; Valat, C.; Saudubray, F.; Antonioz, P.; et al. Characteristics of epi-hne4 aerosol: A new elastase inhibitor for treatment of cystic fibrosis. *J. Aerosol. Med.* **2003**, *16*, 121–129. [CrossRef] [PubMed]

71. Schulz, J.D.; Gauthier, M.A.; Leroux, J.C. Improving oral drug bioavailability with polycations? *Eur. J. Pharm. Biopharm.* **2015**, *97*, 427–437. [CrossRef] [PubMed]

72. Seki, T. Enhancement of insulin absorption through mucosal membranes using cationic polymers. *Yakugaku Zasshi* **2010**, *130*, 1115–1121. [CrossRef] [PubMed]

73. Zhang, H.; Huang, X.; Sun, Y.; Lu, G.; Wang, K.; Wang, Z.; Xing, J.; Gao, Y. Improvement of pulmonary absorption of poorly absorbable macromolecules by hydroxypropyl-β-cyclodextrin grafted polyethylenimine (hp-β-cd-pei) in rats. *Int. J. Pharm.* **2015**, *489*, 294–303. [CrossRef] [PubMed]

74. Morimoto, K.; Fukushi, N.; Chono, S.; Seki, T.; Tabata, Y. Spermined dextran, a cationized polymer, as absorption enhancer for pulmonary application of peptide drugs. *Pharmazie* **2008**, *63*, 180–184. [PubMed]

75. Zhang, J.; Zhu, X.; Jin, Y.; Shan, W.; Huang, Y. Mechanism study of cellular uptake and tight junction opening mediated by goblet cell-specific trimethyl chitosan nanoparticles. *Mol. Pharm.* **2014**, *11*, 1520–1532. [CrossRef] [PubMed]

76. Yamada, K. Control of pulmonary absorption of drugs by various pharmaceutical excipients. *Yakugaku Zasshi* **2007**, *127*, 631–641. [CrossRef] [PubMed]

77. Roy, S.; Pal, K.; Anis, A.; Pramanik, K.; Prabhakar, B. Polymers in mucoadhesive drug-delivery systems: A brief note. *Des. Monomers Polym.* **2009**, *12*, 483–495. [CrossRef]

78. Botelho da Silva, S.; Krolicka, M.; van den Broek, L.A.M.; Frissen, A.E.; Boeriu, C.G. Water-soluble chitosan derivatives and ph-responsive hydrogels by selective c-6 oxidation mediated by tempo-laccase redox system. *Carbohydr. Polym.* **2018**, *186*, 299–309. [CrossRef] [PubMed]

79. Jeon, Y.J.; Shahidi, F.; Kim, S.K. Preparation of chitin and chitosan oligomers amd their applications in physiological functional foods. *Food Rev. Int.* **2000**, *16*, 159–176. [CrossRef]

80. Zariwala, M.G.; Bendre, H.; Markiv, A.; Farnaud, S.; Renshaw, D.; Taylor, K.M.; Somavarapu, S. Hydrophobically modified chitosan nanoliposomes for intestinal drug delivery. *Int. J. Nanomed.* **2018**, *13*, 5837–5848. [CrossRef] [PubMed]

81. Sonia, T.A.; Rekha, M.R.; Sharma, C.P. Bioadhesive hydrophobic chitosan microparticles for oral delivery of insulin: In vitro characterization and in vivo uptake studies. *J. Appl. Polym. Sci.* **2011**, *119*, 2902–2910. [CrossRef]

82. Seki, T.; Fukushi, N.; Maru, H.; Kimura, S.; Chono, S.; Egawa, Y.; Morimoto, K.; Ueda, H.; Morimoto, Y. Effects of sperminated pullulans on the pulmonary absorption of insulin. *Yakugaku Zasshi* **2011**, *131*, 307–314. [CrossRef] [PubMed]

83. Morimoto, K.; Katsumata, H.; Yabuta, T.; Iwanaga, K.; Kakemi, M.; Tabata, Y.; Ikada, Y. Gelatin microspheres as a pulmonary delivery system: Evaluation of salmon calcitonin absorption. *J. Pharm. Pharmacol.* **2000**, *52*, 611–617. [CrossRef] [PubMed]

84. He, L.; Gao, Y.; Lin, Y.; Katsumi, H. Improvement of pulmonary absorption of insulin and other water-soluble compounds by polyamines in rats. *J. Control. Release* **2007**, *122*, 94–101. [CrossRef] [PubMed]

85. Pauletti, G.M.; Okumu, F.W.; Borchardt, R.T. Effect of size and charge on the passive diffusion of peptides across caco-2 cell monolayers via the paracellular pathway. *Pharm. Res.-Dordr.* **1997**, *14*, 164–168. [CrossRef]

86. Smedley, J.G.; Saputo, J.; Parker, J.C.; Fernandez-Miyakawa, M.E.; Robertson, S.L.; McClane, B.A.; Uzal, F.A. Noncytotoxic *clostridium perfringens* enterotoxin (cpe) variants localize cpe intestinal binding and demonstrate a relationship between cpe-induced cytotoxicity and enterotoxicity. *Infect. Immun.* **2008**, *76*, 3793–3800. [CrossRef] [PubMed]

87. Nakajima, M.; Nagase, S.; Iida, M.; Takeda, S.; Yamashita, M.; Watari, A.; Shirasago, Y.; Fukasawa, M.; Takeda, H.; Sawasaki, T.; et al. Claudin-1 binder enhances epidermal permeability in a human keratinocyte model. *J. Pharmacol. Exp. Ther.* **2015**, *354*, 440–447. [CrossRef] [PubMed]

88. Saaber, D.; Wollenhaupt, S.; Baumann, K.; Reichl, S. Recent progress in tight junction modulation for improving bioavailability. *Expert Opin. Drug Dis.* **2014**, *9*, 367–381. [CrossRef] [PubMed]

89. Uchida, H.; Kondoh, M.; Hanada, T.; Takahashi, A.; Hamakubo, T.; Yagi, K. A claudin-4 modulator enhances the mucosal absorption of a biologically active peptide. *Biochem. Pharmacol.* **2010**, *79*, 1437–1444. [CrossRef] [PubMed]

90. Helms, H.C.; Waagepetersen, H.S.; Nielsen, C.U.; Brodin, B. Paracellular tightness and claudin-5 expression is increased in the bcec/astrocyte blood-brain barrier model by increasing media buffer capacity during growth. *AAPS J.* **2010**, *12*, 759–770. [CrossRef] [PubMed]

91. Deli, M.A. Potential use of tight junction modulators to reversibly open membranous barriers and improve drug delivery. *BBA-Biomembranes* **2009**, *1788*, 892–910. [CrossRef] [PubMed]

92. Fasano, A.; Not, T.; Wang, W.L.; Uzzau, S.; Berti, I.; Tommasini, A.; Goldblum, S.E. Zonulin, a newly discovered modulator of intestinal permeability, and its expression in coeliac disease. *Lancet* **2000**, *355*, 1518–1519. [CrossRef]

93. Li, M.; Oliver, E.; Kitchens, K.M.; Vere, J.; Alkan, S.S.; Tamiz, A.P. Structure-activity relationship studies of permeability modulating peptide at-1002. *Bioorg. Med. Chem. Lett.* **2008**, *18*, 4584–4586. [CrossRef] [PubMed]

94. Porter, A.E.; Muller, K.; Skepper, J.; Midgley, P.; Welland, M. Uptake of c60 by human monocyte macrophages, its localization and implications for toxicity: Studied by high resolution electron microscopy and electron tomography. *Acta Biomater.* **2006**, *2*, 409–419. [CrossRef] [PubMed]

95. Kreyling, W.G.; Semmler-Behnke, M.; Moller, W. Ultrafine particle-lung interactions: Does size matter? *J. Aerosol. Med.* **2006**, *19*, 74–83. [CrossRef] [PubMed]

96. Schneider, C.S.; Xu, Q.; Boylan, N.J.; Chisholm, J.; Tang, B.C.; Schuster, B.S.; Henning, A.; Ensign, L.M.; Lee, E.; Adstamongkonkul, P.; et al. Nanoparticles that do not adhere to mucus provide uniform and long-lasting drug delivery to airways following inhalation. *Sci. Adv.* **2017**, *3*, e1601556. [CrossRef] [PubMed]

97. Mistry, A.; Stolnik, S.; Illum, L. Nanoparticles for direct nose-to-brain delivery of drugs. *Int. J. Pharm.* **2009**, *379*, 146–157. [CrossRef] [PubMed]

98. Kulkarni, A.D.; Vanjari, Y.H.; Sancheti, K.H.; Belgamwar, V.S.; Surana, S.J.; Pardeshi, C.V. Nanotechnology-mediated nose to brain drug delivery for parkinson's disease: A mini review. *J. Drug Target* **2015**, *23*, 775–788. [CrossRef] [PubMed]

99. Hussain, A.; Arnold, J.J.; Khan, M.A.; Ahsan, F. Absorption enhancers in pulmonary protein delivery. *J. Control. Release* **2004**, *94*, 15–24. [CrossRef] [PubMed]

100. Cupri, S.; Graziano, A.C.E.; Cardile, V.; Skwarczynski, M.; Toth, I.; Pignatello, R. A study on the encapsulation of an occludin lipophilic derivative in liposomal carriers. *J. Liposome Res.* **2015**, *25*, 287–293. [CrossRef] [PubMed]

101. Manca, M.L.; Peris, J.E.; Melis, V.; Valenti, D.; Cardia, M.C.; Lattuada, D.; Escribano-Ferrer, E.; Fadda, A.M.; Manconi, M. Nanoincorporation of curcumin in polymer-glycerosomes and evaluation of their in vitro–in vivo suitability as pulmonary delivery systems. *Rsc. Adv.* **2015**, *5*, 105149–105159. [CrossRef]

102. Melis, V.; Manca, M.L.; Bullita, E.; Tamburini, E.; Castangia, I.; Cardia, M.C.; Valenti, D.; Fadda, A.M.; Peris, J.E.; Manconi, M. Inhalable polymer-glycerosomes as safe and effective carriers for rifampicin delivery to the lungs. *Colloid Surf. B* **2016**, *143*, 301–308. [CrossRef] [PubMed]

103. Bai, S.; Thomas, C.; Ahsan, F. Dendrimers as a carrier for pulmonary delivery of enoxaparin, a low-molecular weight heparin. *J. Pharm. Sci.-US* **2007**, *96*, 2090–2106. [CrossRef] [PubMed]

104. Inapagolla, R.; Guru, B.R.; Kurtoglu, Y.E.; Gao, X.; Lieh-Lai, M.; Bassett, D.J.P.; Kannan, R.M. In vivo efficacy of dendrimer–methylprednisolone conjugate formulation for the treatment of lung inflammation. *Int. J. Pharm.* **2010**, *399*, 140–147. [CrossRef] [PubMed]

105. Lu, J.; Li, N.; Gao, Y.; Guo, Y.; Liu, H.; Chen, X.; Zhu, C.; Dong, Z.; Yamamoto, A. The Effect of Absorption-Enhancement and the Mechanism of the PAMAM Dendrimer on Poorly Absorbable Drugs. *Molecules* **2018**, *23*, 2001. [CrossRef] [PubMed]

106. Luan, X.; Sansanaphongpricha, K.; Myers, I.; Chen, H.; Yuan, H.; Sun, D. Engineering exosomes as refined biological nanoplatforms for drug delivery. *Acta Pharmacol. Sin.* **2017**, *38*, 754. [CrossRef] [PubMed]

107. Vader, P.; Mol, E.A.; Pasterkamp, G.; Schiffelers, R.M. Extracellular vesicles for drug delivery. *Adv. Drug Deliv. Rev.* **2016**, *106*, 148–156. [CrossRef] [PubMed]

108. Hood, J.L. Post isolation modification of exosomes for nanomedicine applications. *Nanomedicine (London, England)* **2016**, *11*, 1745–1756. [CrossRef] [PubMed]

109. Batrakova, E.V.; Kim, M.S. Using exosomes, naturally-equipped nanocarriers, for drug delivery. *J. Control. Release* **2015**, *219*, 396–405. [CrossRef] [PubMed]

110. Harding, C.V.; Heuser, J.E.; Stahl, P.D. Exosomes: Looking back three decades and into the future. *J. Cell Biol.* **2013**, *200*, 367–371. [CrossRef] [PubMed]

111. Fabbri, M.; Paone, A.; Calore, F.; Galli, R.; Gaudio, E.; Santhanam, R.; Lovat, F.; Fadda, P.; Mao, C.; Nuovo, G.J.; et al. Micrornas bind to toll-like receptors to induce prometastatic inflammatory response. *Proc. Natl. Acad. Sci. USA* **2012**, *109*, E2110–E2116. [CrossRef] [PubMed]

112. Kalani, A.; Kamat, P.K.; Chaturvedi, P.; Tyagi, S.C.; Tyagi, N. Curcumin-primed exosomes mitigate endothelial cell dysfunction during hyperhomocysteinemia. *Life Sci.* **2014**, *107*, 1–7. [CrossRef] [PubMed]

113. Batrakova, E.V.; Kim, M.S.; Haney, M.J.; Zhao, Y.; Deygen, I.; Klyachko, N.L.; Kabanov, A.V. Development of exosome-encapsulated paclitaxel to treat cancer metastases. *In Vitro Cell Dev.* **2017**, *53*, S9.

114. Haney, M.J.; Klyachko, N.L.; Zhao, Y.; Gupta, R.; Plotnikova, E.G.; He, Z.; Patel, T.; Piroyan, A.; Sokolsky, M.; Kabanov, A.V.; et al. Exosomes as drug delivery vehicles for parkinson's disease therapy. *J. Control. Release* **2015**, *207*, 18–30. [CrossRef] [PubMed]

115. Zhuang, X.; Xiang, X.; Grizzle, W.; Sun, D.; Zhang, S.; Axtell, R.C.; Ju, S.; Mu, J.; Zhang, L.; Steinman, L.; et al. Treatment of brain inflammatory diseases by delivering exosome encapsulated anti-inflammatory drugs from the nasal region to the brain. *Mol. Ther.* **2011**, *19*, 1769–1779. [CrossRef] [PubMed]

116. Tian, Y.; Li, S.; Song, J.; Ji, T.; Zhu, M.; Anderson, G.J.; Wei, J.; Nie, G. A doxorubicin delivery platform using engineered natural membrane vesicle exosomes for targeted tumor therapy. *Biomaterials* **2014**, *35*, 2383–2390. [CrossRef] [PubMed]

117. Yang, T.; Martin, P.; Fogarty, B.; Brown, A.; Schurman, K.; Phipps, R.; Yin, V.P.; Lockman, P.; Bai, S. Exosome delivered anticancer drugs across the blood-brain barrier for brain cancer therapy in danio rerio. *Pharm. Res.* **2015**, *32*, 2003–2014. [CrossRef] [PubMed]

118. Foged, C.; Nielsen, H.M. Cell-penetrating peptides for drug delivery across membrane barriers. *Expert Opin. Drug Deliv.* **2008**, *5*, 105–117. [CrossRef] [PubMed]

119. McClorey, G.; Banerjee, S. Cell-penetrating peptides to enhance delivery of oligonucleotide-based therapeutics. *Biomedicines* **2018**, *6*, 51. [CrossRef] [PubMed]

120. Derossi, D.; Calvet, S.; Trembleau, A.; Brunissen, A.; Chassaing, G.; Prochiantz, A. Cell internalization of the third helix of the antennapedia homeodomain is receptor-independent. *J. Biol. Chem.* **1996**, *271*, 18188–18193. [CrossRef] [PubMed]

121. Thorén, P.E.G.; Persson, D.; Esbjörner, E.K.; Goksör, M.; Lincoln, P.; Nordén, B. Membrane binding and translocation of cell-penetrating peptides. *Biochemistry-US* **2004**, *43*, 3471–3489. [CrossRef] [PubMed]

122. Tan, J.; Cheong, H.; Park, Y.S.; Kim, H.; Zhang, M.; Moon, C.; Huang, Y.Z. Cell-penetrating peptide-mediated topical delivery of biomacromolecular drugs. *Curr. Pharm. Biotechnol.* **2014**, *15*, 231–239. [CrossRef] [PubMed]

123. Kato, T.; Yamashita, H.; Misawa, T.; Nishida, K.; Kurihara, M.; Tanaka, M.; Demizu, Y.; Oba, M. Plasmid DNA delivery by arginine-rich cell-penetrating peptides containing unnatural amino acids. *Bioorg. Med. Chem.* **2016**, *24*, 2681–2687. [CrossRef] [PubMed]

124. Eudes, F.; Shim, Y.S. Cell-penetrating peptides trojan horse for DNA and protein delivery in plant. *In Vitro Cell Dev.* **2010**, *46*, S112–S113.

125. Dos Reis, L.G.; Svolos, M.; Hartwig, B.; Windhab, N.; Young, P.M.; Traini, D. Inhaled gene delivery: A formulation and delivery approach. *Expert Opin. Drug Deliv.* **2017**, *14*, 319–330. [CrossRef] [PubMed]

126. Kamei, N. Nose-to-brain delivery of peptide drugs enhanced by coadministration of cell-penetrating peptides: Therapeutic potential for dementia. *Yakugaku Zasshi* **2017**, *137*, 1247–1253. [CrossRef] [PubMed]

127. Kamei, N.; Tanaka, M.; Choi, H.; Okada, N.; Ikeda, T.; Itokazu, R.; Takeda-Morishita, M. Effect of an enhanced nose-to-brain delivery of insulin on mild and progressive memory loss in the senescence-accelerated mouse. *Mol. Pharm.* **2017**, *14*, 916–927. [CrossRef] [PubMed]

128. Zhang, X.; Lin, C.; Lu, A.; Lin, G.; Chen, H.; Liu, Q.; Yang, Z.; Zhang, H. Liposomes equipped with cell penetrating peptide br2 enhances chemotherapeutic effects of cantharidin against hepatocellular carcinoma. *Drug Deliv.* **2017**, *24*, 986–998. [CrossRef] [PubMed]

129. Xu, Y.; Li, S.; Luo, Z.; Ren, H.; Zhang, X.; Huang, F.; Zuo, Y.Y.; Yue, T. Role of lipid coating in the transport of nanodroplets across the pulmonary surfactant layer revealed by molecular dynamics simulations. *Langmuir* **2018**, *34*, 9054–9063. [CrossRef] [PubMed]

130. Chen, K.H.; Di Sabatino, M.; Albertini, B.; Passerini, N.; Kett, V.L. The effect of polymer coatings on physicochemical properties of spray-dried liposomes for nasal delivery of bsa. *Eur. J. Pharm. Sci.* **2013**, *50*, 312–322. [CrossRef] [PubMed]

131. Murata, M.; Nakano, K.; Tahara, K.; Tozuka, Y.; Takeuchi, H. Pulmonary delivery of elcatonin using surface-modified liposomes to improve systemic absorption: Polyvinyl alcohol with a hydrophobic anchor and chitosan oligosaccharide as effective surface modifiers. *Eur. J. Pharm. Biopharm.* **2012**, *80*, 340–346. [CrossRef] [PubMed]

132. Liu, Z.Y.; Jiang, M.Y.; Kang, T.; Miao, D.Y.; Gu, G.Z.; Song, Q.X.; Yao, L.; Hu, Q.Y.; Tu, Y.F.; Pang, Z.Q.; et al. Lactoferrin-modified peg-co-pcl nanoparticles for enhanced brain delivery of nap peptide following intranasal administration. *Biomaterials* **2013**, *34*, 3870–3881. [CrossRef] [PubMed]

133. Marttin, E.; Verhoef, J.C.; Merkus, F.W.H.M. Efficacy, safety and mechanism of cyclodextrins as absorption enhancers in nasal delivery of peptide and protein drugs. *J. Drug Target* **1998**, *6*, 17–36. [CrossRef] [PubMed]

134. Schipper, N.G.M.; Verhoef, J.; Romeijn, S.G.; Merkus, F.W.H.M. Absorption enhancers in nasal insulin delivery and their influence on nasal ciliary functioning. *J. Control. Release* **1992**, *21*, 173–185. [CrossRef]

135. Salem, L.B.; Bosquillon, C.; Dailey, L.A.; Delattre, L.; Martin, G.P.; Evrard, B.; Forbes, B. Sparing methylation of beta-cyclodextrin mitigates cytotoxicity and permeability induction in respiratory epithelial cell layers in vitro. *J. Control. Release* **2009**, *136*, 110–116. [CrossRef] [PubMed]

136. Kiss, T.; Fenyvesi, F.; Bacskay, I.; Varadi, J.; Fenyvesi, E.; Ivanyi, R.; Szente, L.; Tosaki, A.; Vecsernyes, M. Evaluation of the cytotoxicity of beta-cyclodextrin derivatives: Evidence for the role of cholesterol extraction. *Eur. J. Pharm. Sci.* **2010**, *40*, 376–380. [CrossRef] [PubMed]

137. Roka, E.; Ujhelyi, Z.; Deli, M.; Bocsik, A.; Fenyvesi, E.; Szente, L.; Fenyvesi, F.; Vecsernyes, M.; Varadi, J.; Feher, P.; et al. Evaluation of the cytotoxicity of alpha-cyclodextrin derivatives on the caco-2 cell line and human erythrocytes. *Molecules* **2015**, *20*, 20269–20285. [CrossRef] [PubMed]

138. Matilainen, L.; Toropainen, T.; Vihola, H.; Hirvonen, J.; Jarvinen, T.; Jarho, P.; Jarvinen, K. In vitro toxicity and permeation of cyclodextrins in calu-3 cells. *J. Control. Release* **2008**, *126*, 10–16. [CrossRef] [PubMed]

139. Hussain, A.; Yang, T.; Zaghloul, A.-A.; Ahsan, F. Pulmonary absorption of insulin mediated by tetradecyl-β-maltoside and dimethyl-β-cyclodextrin. *Pharm. Res.* **2003**, *20*, 1551–1557. [CrossRef] [PubMed]

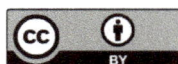

pharmaceutics

MDPI

Article

The Role of Combined Penetration Enhancers in Nasal Microspheres on In Vivo Drug Bioavailability

Giovanna Rassu [1], Luca Ferraro [2], Barbara Pavan [3], Paolo Giunchedi [1], Elisabetta Gavini [1,*] and Alessandro Dalpiaz [4]

[1] Department of Chemistry and Pharmacy, University of Sassari, via Muroni 23/a, 07100 Sassari, Italy; grassu@uniss.it (G.R.); pgiunc@uniss.it (P.G.)

[2] Department of Life Sciences and Biotechnology, University of Ferrara, via Borsari 46, 44121 Ferrara, Italy; frl@unife.it

[3] Department of Biomedical and Specialist Surgical Sciences, University of Ferrara, via Borsari 46, 44121 Ferrara, Italy; pvnbbr@unife.it

[4] Department of Chemical and Pharmaceutical Sciences, University of Ferrara, via Fossato di Mortara 19, 44121 Ferrara, Italy; dla@unife.it

* Correspondence: eligav@uniss.it; Tel.: +39-079-228-752; Fax: +39-079-228-733

Received: 21 September 2018; Accepted: 23 October 2018; Published: 26 October 2018

Abstract: Microspheres based on both methyl-β-cyclodextrins and chitosan were prepared by spray-drying as nasal formulations of a model polar drug to analyze, firstly, how the composition of the carrier affects drug permeation across synthetic membranes and, secondly, how it induces systemic or brain delivery of the drug. Microparticles with different weight ratios of the two penetration enhancers (10–90, 50–50, 90–10) were characterized with respect to morphology, size, structural composition, water uptake, and the in vitro drug permeation profile. The leader formulation (weight ratio of 50–50) was then nasally administered to rats; systemic and cerebrospinal fluid (CSF) drug concentrations were analyzed by high performance liquid chromatography (HPLC) over time. Microspheres obtained with a single enhancer, methyl-β-cyclodextrins or chitosan, were administered in vivo as a comparison. The in vitro properties of combined microspheres appeared modified with regard to the polymeric matrix ratio. In vivo results suggest that the optimal drug distribution between CSF and bloodstream can be easily obtained by varying the amount of these two penetration enhancers studied in the matrix of nasal microspheres.

Keywords: combined microsphere; chitosan; cyclodextrin; nasal delivery; nose to brain transport; penetration enhancer; nasal formulation; in vivo studies

1. Introduction

Absorption enhancers are agents included in formulations whose function is to increase absorption of a pharmacologically active drug by enhancing membrane permeation [1]. They are frequently employed in nasal formulations [2–5] in order to improve drug flux through nasal epithelia [6]. The main mechanisms involved in enhanced permeability of nasal membranes include (i) the transient opening of the tight junction between adjacent cells that favor paracellular diffusion through the intercellular space, and/or (ii) perturbation of lipid bilayer integrity and increased membrane fluidity promoting the transcellular permeation of drugs [1]. Permeation-enhancing excipients are investigated to develop formulations for hydrophilic drugs that have poor nasal membrane permeability [7]; among these, cyclodextrins (CDs) and chitosan are characterized by high biocompatibility, since they are able to induce their enhancing effects without causing damage to nasal mucosa [7].

Cyclodextrins, especially methylated-β-cyclodextrins, have proven to be excellent solubilizers and absorption enhancers in nasal drug delivery [2,8–10]. Owing to their ability to remove cholesterol and phospholipids from the outer half of the membrane bilayer, CDs can increase membrane fluidity [11]. Furthermore, methylated-β-cyclodextrins cause an increase in the paracellular permeability of epithelial cell layers because the cholesterol depletion influences the distribution of specific tight junction proteins (claudin 3, claudin 4, and occludin) [12]. Recently, Fenyvesi and co-workers [13] have shown that fluid-phase endocytosis of CDs can contribute to overcoming the mucosal barrier for poorly absorbed drugs.

Chitosan is one of the most-used penetration enhancers in nasal formulations [14–17]. A combination of mucoadhesion and transient opening of the tight junctions in the cell membrane allows polar drugs to pass by a paracellular pathway [2]. There are a number of chitosan salts that have better characteristics than chitosan itself; these include solubility, mucoadhesiveness, and penetration enhancement ability. The chitosan chloride salt form is the only kind of chitosan that has a specific monograph in the European Pharmacopoeia 8.0 [18].

In addition to high stability, powder formulations can also have an absorption promoting effect [2,17] by exerting a direct effect on the mucosa. Microspheres absorb water from mucus causing dehydration of the epithelial cells which leads to the opening of the tight junctions [19]. For these reasons, the formulation of solid microparticles in the presence of promotion enhancers appears advantageous for nose to brain delivery of drugs.

Traditionally cyclodextrin and chitosan have been used separately in nasal powder formulation [15,16,20] and no combination has been evaluated. Bshara and co-workers [21] formulated hydroxylpropyl-β-CD and chitosan aspartate in microemulsion and observed that the highest C_{max} and AUC values among all the formulations they tested (formulation without hydroxylpropyl-β-CD and chitosan aspartate and with chitosan aspartate alone) were most likely due to a synergistic effect of both materials on the intranasal permeation of drug.

Therefore, the aim of this work was to formulate methyl-β-cyclodextrins and chitosan in combination in spray-dried microspheres for nasal administration of a polar drug. In particular, the effects of the microparticles' composition on drug permeation across synthetic membranes were analyzed, and, then, related to systemic or brain delivery of the drug after intranasal administration.

Indeed, when administered nasally, a drug can be deposited on the respiratory or olfactory epithelia. In the first case, it may cross the respiratory mucosa by paracellular or transcellular transport, reaching the lamina propria and then blood vessel (systemic circulation) or peripheral trigeminal nerve (brainstem). If, on the other hand, the drug is deposited on the olfactory epithelium, transport to the central nervous system may be either paracellular through olfactory neurones, or transcellular through olfactory epithelial cells [7,22].

N^6-cyclopentyladenosine was selected as a model polar drug with low molecular weight.

2. Materials and Methods

2.1. Materials

Methyl-β-cyclodextrin, Cavasol® W7MPharma (Mw: 1300 g/mol; molecular substitution: 1.7) was purchased from Wacker-Chemie GmbH (München, Germany). Chitosan chloride, Protasan UP CL 113 (Mw: 160,000 g/mol; deacetylation degree, 86%) were purchased from NovaMatrix/FMC Biopolymer (Sandvika, Norway). Tegiloxan3™ silicon oil was kindly gift from Goldschmidth (Essen, Germany). N6-cyclopentyladenosine (CPA) (Mw: 335.36), N6-cyclohexyladenosine CHA, sodium acetate and acetic acid glacial were obtained from Sigma-Aldrich (Milan, Italy). Dimethylsulfoxide (DMSO) was obtained from Merck (Darmstadt, Germany). Methanol, acetonitrile, ethyl acetate, and water high performance liquid chromatography (HPLC) grade were purchased from Sigma-Aldrich (Milan, Italy). Male Wistar rats were purchased from Charles-River, Milan, Italy.

2.2. Preparation of Microspheres

Formulations of microspheres were prepared by spray drying technique with a Mini Büchi B-191 spray dryer (Büchi Laboratoriums-Technik AG, Flawil, Switzerland) using methyl-β-cyclodextrin and chitosan as excipients in different percentage ratios chosen on the basis of preliminary studies. Drug to polymer ratio 1/20 was chosen which guarantees an optimal dose for in vivo test and administration of powder amount suitable for rat nasal cavity [23]. The feed solution concentration was 0.5% (*w/v*). The microparticles containing both excipients in different weight ratio (10–90, 50–50, and 90–10) were prepared dissolving separately methyl-β-cyclodextrin and chitosan in water, under magnetic stirring, and solutions were mixed before the addition of CPA. The following operating conditions were utilized during spray drying: inlet and outlet temperature, 110 °C and 77 ± 2 °C, respectively; spray flow rate, 500 L/h; pump setting, 5% (1.74 ± 0.09 mL/min); and aspirator setting, 98% regardless solutions composition. The dry particles were put in a desiccator for at least 24 h. Unloaded microspheres based on methyl-β-cyclodextrin (MCb) and loaded microspheres based on chitosan (CH100) or methyl-β-cyclodextrin (MC100) were prepared as comparison.

The codes and composition of the microspheres are presented in Table 1.

Table 1. The polymer composition (% *w/w*), drug content (DC) and encapsulation efficiency (EE) of loaded microspheres.

Microsphere Codes	Methyl-β-Cyclodextrin	Chitosan	DC (%)	EE (%)	d_{vs} (μm)	SPAN
MC100	100	-	4.25 ± 0.05 [a]	88.78 ± 0.98 [a]	3.49 ± 0.10	2.20
MC90	90	10	4.25 ± 0.01 [a]	88.66 ± 0.22 [a]	2.74 ± 0.09	1.85
MC50	50	50	4.20 ± 0.07 [a]	87.87 ± 1.53 [a]	6.79 ± 1.84 [b,c]	2.24
MC10	10	90	3.81 ± 0.05	80.91 ± 1.13	6.55 ± 1.04 [b,c]	2.09
CH100 [#]	-	100	4.75 ± 0.06	95.0 ± 1.20	6.14 ± 0.84 [b,c]	1.66

[#] Prepared as reference for in vivo studies [23]. [a] $p < 0.05$ MC10 versus MC100; versus MC90; versus MC50. [b] $p < 0.05$ MC100 versus CH100; versus MC50; versus MC10. [c] $p < 0.05$ MC90 versus CH100; versus MC50; versus MC10.

The yields of production were calculated as the weight percentage of the final product after drying, with respect to initial total amounts of drug and excipients used for the preparation.

2.3. Microsphere Characterization

2.3.1. Determination of Drug Content and Encapsulation Efficiency

To determine the real amount of CPA loaded in microspheres, 0.5 mL of water was added to an exact amount of combined formulations (containing about 0.5 mg of drug); then, 45.5 mL of methanol were added and stirred until solution was obtained. Finally, spectrophotometric analysis (UV-160A UV–Visible Recording Spectrophotometer, Shimadzu, Tokyo, Japan) was performed at 270 nm and the drug in solutions was quantified by using the calibration curve obtained in concentrations range from 2.8 to 22.4 mg/L ($y = 0.067x + 0.027$, $R^2 = 0.9997$). Analyses were carried out in triplicate.

Furthermore, an exact amount of MC100 (corresponding to 0.5 mg of CPA) was dissolved in 50 mL of methanol and solution spectrophotometrically analyzed.

The drug loaded in microspheres (DC) was calculated as the experimentally detected amount of CPA in microspheres and expressed as percentage; encapsulation efficiency (EE), as percentage, was also calculated. The following equations were applied:

$$DC\ (\%) = \left(\frac{rCPA}{tCPA} \right) \times tDC$$

$$EE\ (\%) = \left(\frac{DC}{tDC} \right) \times 100$$

where rCPA is the detected amount of CPA in microspheres, tCPA is the drug amount solubilized in feed solution and tDC the percentage of the expected theoretical value.

2.3.2. Morphological Analysis

The morphology of the microspheres was determined by observation on a scanning electron microscope (VP-SEM; Zeiss EVO40XVP, Arese, Milan, Italy). The samples were placed on double-sided tape that had previously been secured to aluminum stubs and then analyzed under an argon atmosphere at an 18 kV acceleration voltage after gold sputtering.

2.3.3. Particle Size Analysis

The particle size and particle size distribution of the microspheres were determined by laser diffraction using a Coulter Laser Sizer LS100Q (Coulter LS 100Q Laser sizer, Beckman Coulter, Miami, FL, USA). All analyses were performed at room temperature. Two mg of microspheres were suspended in 1 mL of Tegiloxan by sonication (about 4–6 s) and then analyzed. The results reported are the averages of triplicate averages. The average particle size of the microspheres was reported as the mean volume-surface diameter, d_{vs} (μm). To quantify distribution width, SPAN was calculated as previously reported [24].

2.3.4. Powder X-ray Diffraction

Powder diffraction spectra were recorded, at room temperature, on a Bruker D-8 Advance diffractometer (Brucker, Karlsruhe, Germany) with graphite monochromatized Cu Kα radiation (λ = 1.5406 Å). The data were recorded at 2θ steps of 0.02° from 3° to 50° with 2 s/step.

2.3.5. Water Uptake

The investigation of water uptake capability was carried out by the modified Enslin apparatus as previously described [25]. Microspheres (10 mg) were uniformly dispersed on a cellulose filter disk saturated with MilliQ water, lying on the top of a fritted glass support, connected with a graduated capillary. The volume of water absorbed (μL) along the time (from 0.25 up to 60 min) was measured. The result obtained is the average of three determinations (n = 3; ±SD).

2.3.6. In Vitro Permeation Test of Microspheres

The in vitro drug permeation across synthetic membrane was performed using a modified Franz diffusion system incorporating three in-line flow-through diffusion cells [26]. Regenerated cellulose membranes (pore size 0.45 μm, 47 mm diameter, Sartorius, Goettingen, Germany) saturated with octanol were chosen as lipophilic layer [20]. An amount of microspheres containing about 1.0 mg of CPA was uniformly spread out above the membrane. Acceptor compartment was filled with 100 mL of pH 6.5 phosphate buffer at 37 ± 0.5 °C, to guarantee sink condition. The flux of the medium was 6 mL/min. Permeation system was automatically coupled to UV-spectrophotometer (UV-1800, UV–Visible Recording Spectrophotometer, Shimadzu, Tokyo, Japan) and the fluid was analyzed at 270 nm at predetermined times (from 30 up to 120 min). The permeated drug was quantified by using the calibration curve obtained in concentrations range from 2.8 to 22.4 mg/L (y = 0.0559x + 0.051 R^2 = 1). All experiments were performed in triplicate. As comparison, in vitro permeation test of raw CPA was carried out.

From the values obtained, the curves of accumulated amounts (mg/cm^2) versus permeation time (min) were drawn; then, the flux (J) was determined from the slope of the steady state portion as well as the lag time (T lag) values from the x-intercept of the slope at a steady state [27].

2.4. In Vivo Studies

2.4.1. In Vivo CPA Administration and Quantification

Male Wistar rats (200−250 g) anesthetized during the experimental period received a femoral intravenous infusion of 0.1 mg/mL CPA dissolved in a medium constituted by 20% (*v*/*v*) DMSO and 80% (*v*/*v*) physiologic solution, with a rate of 0.2 mL/min for 10 min. At the end of infusion and at fixed time points, blood samples (100 µL) were collected and cerebrospinal fluid (CSF) samples (50 µL) were withdrawn by the cysternal puncture method described by van den Berg and co-workers [28], which requires a single needle stick and allows the collection of serial (40–50 µL) CSF samples that are virtually blood-free [29]. Four rats were employed for femoral intravenous infusions. CSF samples (10 µL) were immediately injected into high performance liquid chromatography (HPLC) system for CPA detection.

The blood samples were hemolyzed immediately after their collection with 500 µL of ice-cold water, then 50 µL of 3N NaOH and 100 µL of internal standard (10 µM CHA) were added. The samples were extracted twice with 1 mL of water-saturated ethyl acetate, and, after centrifugation, the organic layer was reduced to dryness under a nitrogen stream. One hundred and fifty microliters of a mobile phase (see below) was added, and, after centrifugation, 10 µL was injected into the HPLC system for CPA detection.

The in vivo half-life of CPA in the blood was calculated by nonlinear regression (exponential decay) of concentration values in the time range within 90 min after infusion.

Nasal administration of CPA was performed to anaesthetized rats laid on their backs, following two procedures. The first way consisted on the introduction in each nostril of rats 20 µL of an aqueous suspension of CPA (5 mg/mL) using a semiautomatic pipette which was attached to a short polyethylene tubing [29]. After the administration, blood (100 µL) and CSF samples (50 µL) were collected at fixed time points, and they were analyzed with the same procedures described above. Four rats were employed for nasal administration of CPA suspension. The second way consisted on the insufflation of loaded CPA microparticles to each nostril of the anaesthetized rats by means of single dose Monopowder P1 insufflators [30]. The insufflators were loaded with about 2.4 mg of CH100, MC100 and MC50 and their content was administered to each nostril of rats. After the administration, blood (100 µL) and CSF samples (50 µL) were collected at fixed time points, then analyzed. Four rats were employed for nasal administration of each type of microparticulate powders.

All in vivo experiments were performed in accordance with the European Communities Council Directive of September 2010 (2010/63/EU) a revision of the Directive 86/609/EEC and were approved by the Italian Ministry of Health and by the Ethical Committee of the University of Ferrara. Any effort has been done to reduce the number of the animals and their suffering.

The area under concentration curves of CPA in the blood and CSF (AUC, $\mu g\ mL^{-1}$ min) were calculated by the trapezoidal method. All the calculations were performed by using the computer program Graph Pad Prism (GraphPad Software Incorporated, La Jolla, CA, USA).

2.4.2. HPLC Analysis

The quantification of CPA in all samples generated from the experimental procedures was performed by HPLC. The chromatographic apparatus consisted of a modular system (model LC-10 AD VD pump and model SPD-10A VP variable wavelength UV−vis detector; Shimadzu, Kyoto, Japan) and an injection valve with 20 µL sample loop (model 7725; Rheodyne, IDEX, Torrance, CA, USA). Separations were performed at room temperature on a 5 µm Hypersil BDS C-18 column (150 mm × 4.6 mm i.d.; Alltech Italia Srl, Milan, Italy), equipped with a guard column packed with the same Hypersil material. Data acquisition and processing were accomplished with a personal computer using CLASS-VP Software, version 6.12 SP5 (Shimadzu Italia, Milan, Italy). The detector was set at 269 nm. The mobile phase consisted of a ternary mixture of acetonitrile, methanol and 10 mM acetate buffer (pH 4) with a ratio of 4/40/56 (*v/v/v*). The flow rate was 0.8 mL/min and the retention time of CPA and CHA were 4.1 and 5.8 min, respectively.

The chromatographic precision, represented by relative standard deviations (RSD), was evaluated by repeated analysis (*n* = 6) of the same sample solution containing each of the examined compounds at a concentration of 10 μM. The solutes were diluted in water by 10^{-2} M stock solutions in DMSO. The RSD values ranged between 0.81% and 0.83% for the analyzed compounds. The calibration curve of peak areas versus concentration was generated in the range 0.1 to 20 μM of CPA and resulted linear (*n* = 9, *r* = 0.998, *p* < 0.0001). For CSF simulation, standard aliquots of balanced solution (PBS Dulbecco's without calcium and magnesium) in the presence of 0.45 mg/mL BSA were employed [31,32]. In this case, the chromatographic precision was evaluated by repeated analysis (*n* = 6) of the same sample solution containing 1.0 μM CPA whose RSD value was 0.92% and calibration curve of peak areas versus concentration was generated in the range 0.08 to 10 μM (corresponding to 26.8 to 3353 ng/mL), resulting linear (*n* = 8, *r* = 0.994, *p* < 0.0001). The LOD and LOQ values of CPA determination in the blood were 8.12 ng/mL (0.0002 nmoles/injection, signal-to-nose ratio of 3:1) and 26.8 ng/mL (0.0008 nmoles/injection, signal-to-noise ratio of 10:1), respectively. The accuracy of the analytical method for CPA extracted from rat whole blood was determined by comparing the peak areas of 10 μM CPA (corresponding to 3353 ng/mL) extracted at 4 °C (*n* = 3) with those obtained by injection of an equivalent concentration of the analyte dissolved in the mobile phase for HPLC analysis. The average recovery from rat whole blood ± S.E. was 86 ± 3%. The concentrations of CPA were therefore referred to as peak area ratio with respect to the internal standard CHA. The precision of this peak area ratio-based method is demonstrated by the RSD values of 1.03% for 10 μM CPA extracted from rat blood at 4 °C, whose calibration curve was linear over the range 0.15−30 μM (corresponding to 50.4 to 10,059 ng/mL; *n* = 9, *r* > 0.992, *p* < 0.0001). The LOD and LOQ values of CPA determination in the blood were 15.3 ng/mL (0.0005 nmoles/injection, signal-to-nose ratio of 3:1) and 50.4 ng/mL (0.0015 nmoles/injection, signal-to-noise ratio of 10:1), respectively.

2.5. Statistical Analysis

Data were analyzed using one-way ANOVA followed by Tukey or Bonferroni test (GraphPad Prism, version 6.02; GraphPad Software Incorporated). Difference was considered statistically significant at P values less than 0.05.

3. Results and Discussion

3.1. Preparation and Characterization of Microspheres

Spray drying appears to be a suitable method for the preparation of CPA-loaded microspheres containing methyl-β-cyclodextrin and chitosan chloride. The technique is simple and rapid as it only requires the preparation of a feed solution. Production yields were good (range from 63–72% (*w/w*)) with no significant differences between the formulations produced.

3.1.1. Determination of Drug Content and Encapsulation Efficiency

CPA content of the formulations and encapsulation efficiency are listed in Table 1. The drug contents of the formulations were relatively close to the theoretical values, and the encapsulation efficiency values ranged between 80% and 88%. The higher chitosan content of MC10 determined a significant decrease in drug encapsulation capacity compared to the other formulations (*p* < 0.05).

3.1.2. Morphological Analysis

Figure 1 illustrates that by increasing the percentage of methyl-β-cyclodextrin in the microspheres, the transition from a smooth to corrugated surface was gradual. In fact, CH100 and MC100 evidenced distinct morphologies. In particular, as reported in Figure 2, CH100 showed a spherical shape and smooth surface, whereas the surface of MC100 particles appeared corrugated in the presence of multiple invaginations.

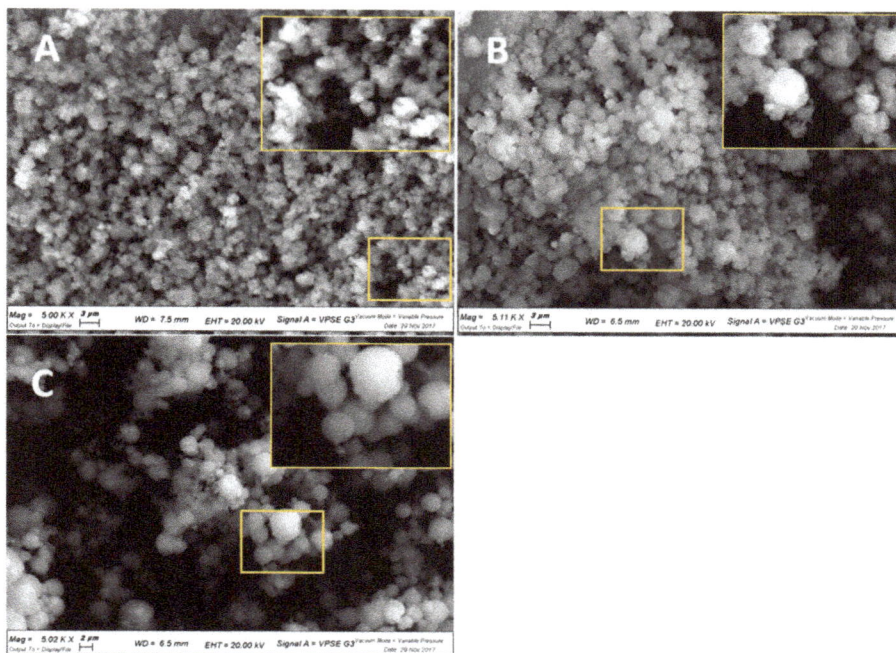

Figure 1. SEM micrographs with magnifications of 5000 times of: (**A**) MC90; (**B**) MC50; (**C**) MC10.

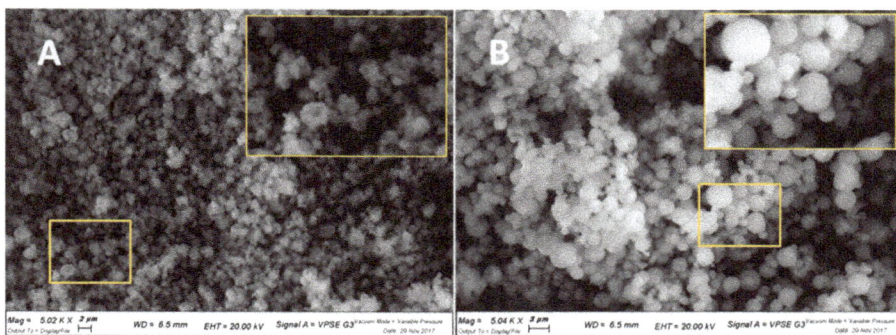

Figure 2. SEM micrographs with magnifications of 5000 times of: (**A**) MC100; (**B**) CH100.

3.1.3. Particle Size Analysis

The d_{vs} values of the formulations are reported in Table 1. The size of the microspheres, generated by spraying feed solutions with the same concentration, depends on the kind and ratio of excipients used. In fact, the weight ratio between two polymers affected the d_{vs}, which increased significantly from MC90 to MC50 and 10–90 ($p < 0.05$), but not particle size distribution ($p > 0.05$). In fact, SPAN index values were comparable, ranging between 1.85 and 2.24, indicating an almost narrow size distribution in all cases. Drug encapsulation did not significantly affect the particle size of methyl-β-cyclodextrin microspheres (MCb 4.52 ± 0.09). On the contrary, chitosan unloaded microparticles generally appeared bigger than the corresponding loaded particles. These last data would appear to be in accordance with those obtained in previous studies: indeed, size modification was observed for spray-dried chitosan microparticles as a consequence of the presence of metoclopramide [33] and CPA [23].

3.1.4. Powder X-ray Diffraction

Additional information on the solid state of the microparticles was obtained by powder X-ray diffraction. As illustrated in Figure 3A, pure CPA (black) exhibited distinct diffraction peaks. The diffractogram of the loaded microparticles did not exhibit any CPA diffraction peaks, indicating the absence of its crystalline state in the loaded form. In particular, the patterns of CH100 (red) and MC10 (blue) samples reported in Figure 3A are accordant with the pattern of chitosan, as shown in Figure 3B, showing a magnification of the comparison between pure chitosan (black) and the sample CH100 (red) diffractograms. Moreover, the patterns of MC100 (fuchsia) and MC90 (brown) samples reported in Figure 3A are accordant with the pattern of methyl-β-cyclodextrin, as may be seen in Figure 3C, showing a magnification of the comparison among pure methyl-β-cyclodextrin (red), MCb (black) and MC100 (blue) diffractograms. The pattern of MC50 sample (green) reported in Figure 3A evidenced the presence of both chitosan and methyl-β-cyclodextrin in the same sample.

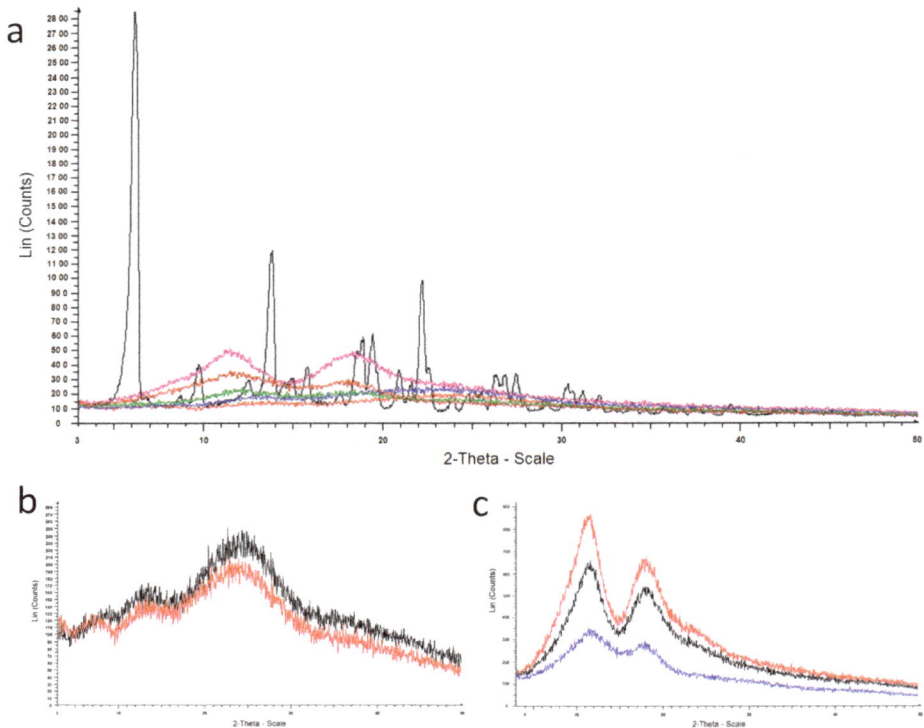

Figure 3. Powder X-ray diffraction patterns of: (**a**) CPA (black), MC90 (brown), MC50 (green) MC10 (blue), MC100 (fuchsia) and CH100 (red); (**b**) chitosan (black) and CH100 (red); (**c**) methyl-β-cyclodextrin (red), MCb (black) and MC100 (blue).

3.1.5. Water Uptake

The water uptake of formulations containing both excipients was affected by their weight ratio (Figure 4). It is well-known that methyl-β-cyclodextrin is a water soluble excipient that absorbs very little water and is then rapidly solubilized; on the contrary, chitosan salts are able to absorb water allowing them to swell and gel [20]. Consequently, the amount of water absorbed per milligram of microspheres markedly increased when the amount of chitosan was raised in the particle matrix.

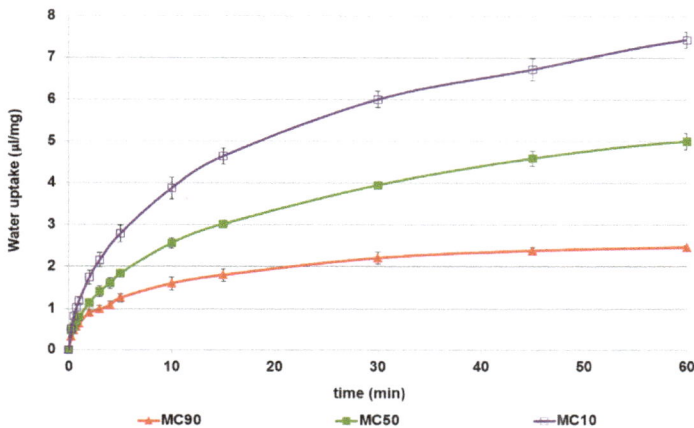

Figure 4. The water uptake capacity (μL/mg) of the microspheres. Data are reported as the mean value of three independent experiments. SD values were ≤0.17 of their corresponding means.

3.1.6. In Vitro Permeation Test of Microspheres

The in vitro permeation profiles of CPA released from microspheres, compared with those of the pure drug, are shown in Figure 5. CPA, as a hydrophilic drug, was able to permeate synthetic membrane with linear kinetic ($n = 11$, $r = 0.984$, $p < 0.0001$), reaching 80% of the amount tested in acceptor medium within 120 min. When encapsulated in microspheres the CPA permeation ability was modified in relation to the polymer and ratio employed as the polymeric matrix. In particular, cyclodextrin increased the flux and total amount of drug permeated when used alone (MC100), or at 90% (w/w) (MC90) (Table 2).

On the contrary, chitosan reduced the permeation of the loaded drug through lipophilic membranes (CH100: 30% of CPA permeated after 120 min). When the concentration of chitosan was 50% (MC50) and 90% (MC10) MC50, the CPA permeation flux and drug total amount significantly decreased (Table 2), reaching the zero values for MC10 sample at all time points tested (Figure 5). CPA's inability to permeate when encapsulated in MC10 could be due to the need of the elevated amount of water for its hydration (as demonstrated by the water uptake results), which was not available in the experimental conditions. Worthy of note is, firstly, chitosan's ability to reduce the permeation, and, secondly, methyl-β-cyclodextrin's ability to increase the passage of the loaded drug through lipophilic membranes regardless of the kind of drug encapsulated [20]. Among the combined formulations tested, of interest is the linear kinetic of CPA release from MC50 in the range from 20 min to 120 min ($R^2 = 0.9987$).

Lag time is the time required for the diffusion flow to become stable. During our experiments, it varied from 1.44 to 20.11 min (Table 2), and was affected by the hydration time of the matrix. These lag times could be considered appropriate for nasal formulations, taking into account that the half-life of clearance in nasal cavity is in the order of 15–20 min [7].

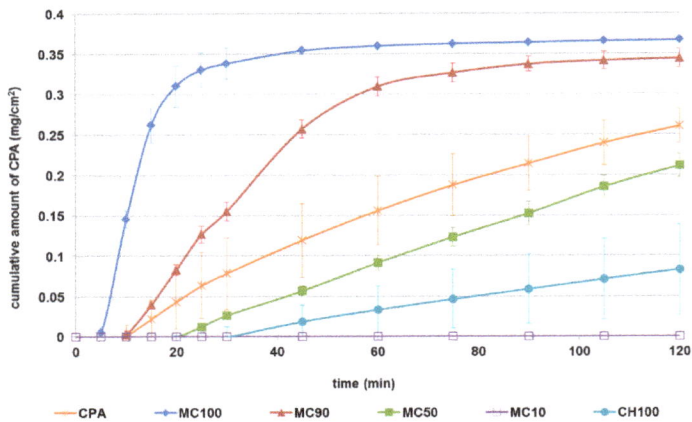

Figure 5. The permeation profiles of N6-cyclopentyladenosine (CPA) from formulations through lipophilic membranes. Profiles are compared with those of the raw drug. Data are reported as the mean ± standard deviation (SD) of three independent experiments.

Table 2. Values of flux (J), T lag and drug permeated for each formulation after 120 min.

Microsphere Codes	J (μg/cm^2 min)	T Lag (min)	Drug Permeated (%)
CPA	2.48 ± 0.65 [a,b,c]	1.44	83.55 ± 10.85 [d,e,g]
MC100	25.64 ± 2.14 [a]	4.64	112.56 ± 1.24 [d]
MC90	7.27 ± 0.18 [a,b]	8.96	105.87 ± 2.26 [e]
MC50	2.09 ± 0.14 [a,b]	17.62	65.46 ± 3.66 [d,e,f]
MC10	0.00 [a,b,c]	-	0.00
CH100	0.86 ± 0.53 [a,b]	20.11	22.26 ± 15.33 [d,e,f,g]

[a] $p < 0.01$ MC100 versus MC90; versus MC50; versus MC10; versus CH100 and CPA. [b] $p < 0.01$ MC90 versus MC50; versus MC10; versus CH100; versus CPA. [c] $p < 0.05$ MC10 versus CPA. [d] $p < 0.05$ MC100 versus MC50; versus CH100; versus CPA. [e] $p < 0.05$ MC90 versus MC50; versus CH100; CPA. [f] $p < 0.05$ MC50 versus CH100. [g] $p < 0.05$ CH100 versus CPA.

On the basis of the in vitro properties of microspheres made by combined penetration enhancers, MC50 was elected as the leader formulation to be in vivo tested. MC50 possessed good EE% as well as size and morphology, comparable to the other formulation containing a high amount of chitosan (MC10). Nevertheless, MC50 needed lower amounts of water to hydrate and showed a better drug release profile than MC10. On the other hand, MC90 had very similar in vitro properties to MC100, but as it is a formulation made by cyclodextrin alone, it would not be possible to evaluate the in vivo effect of the co-presence of the two penetration enhancers.

3.2. In Vivo CPA Administration and Quantification

The analysis of rat blood samples following the intravenous infusion of 0.2 mg of CPA indicated that the drug concentration in the blood stream was 6.11 ± 0.41 μg/mL at the end of infusion, and decreased with a terminal half-life of 6.8 ± 0.9 min. The AUC value of this profile was 37687 ± 1118 ng mL^{-1} min (Table 3). These data are in good agreement with those obtained in previous in vivo studies on CPA pharmacokinetics in rats [23,34]. On the other hand, no CPA was detected in the CSF of rats within 120 min after the end of the intravenous infusion. These results confirm that CPA is unable to reach the CNS from the bloodstream, as previously reported [23,35–37]. The microparticles (CH100, MC100 and MC50) were tested for nasal administration of CPA in order to verify its potential uptake into the CNS. Nasal administration of an aqueous suspension of CPA was also tested as control. Indeed, the nasal administration of pure CPA as powder was not performed, owing to the very low dose (200 µg in rats). Therefore, as control we employed a water suspension of the raw drug. No significant amounts of CPA were observed either in blood or in in the CSF of rats within 120 of the treatment (data not shown). A similar behavior was registered after the nasal administrations of rokitamicin [15], deferoxamine [20], and a zidovudine prodrug [16,29], as water suspensions, confirming that appropriate nasal formulations are needed in order to promote the drug uptake in the central nervous system.

Table 3. Area under concentration curves (AUC) obtained after CPA administration in rats for blood and CSF compartments.

Administration Way	Blood		CSF	
	AUC (ng mL^{-1} min)	Absolute Bioavailability	AUC (ng mL^{-1} min)	Relative Bioavailability
Intravenous	37,687 ± 1118	100	n.d.	0
Nasal (suspension)	n.d.	0	n.d.	0
Nasal (CH100)	699 ± 257	1.85%	32,910 ± 1199	100%
Nasal (MC50)	4830 ± 827 [a]	12.8%	39,900 ± 1520	121% [b]
Nasal (MC100)	13,590 ± 1451 [c]	36.0%	55,140 ± 1016	170% [c]

Data are reported as mean ± standard deviation, $n = 4$. Absolute bioavailability values are referred to AUC obtained by intravenous administration (100%); relative bioavailability values are referred to AUC obtained by nasal administration of CH100 microparticles (100%). n.d., not detectable. [a] $p > 0.05$ versus CH100; [b] $p < 0.05$ versus CH100; [c] $p < 0.001$ versus CH100.

On the contrary, nasal administration of the powder constituted by the loaded CH100, MC100 and MC50 microparticles (4.8 mg, about 200 µg of CPA) produced detectable levels of the drug in both blood and CSF, as reported in Figures 6 and 7, respectively. CH100 microparticles were previously described [23], but they were chosen as reference formulation in order to evaluate the effects induced by MC100 presence in the formulations. After nasal administration of CH100 particles, the peak concentration in the blood was detected at 60 min, with values just above the LOD of the analytical method (22 ± 12 ng/mL), indicating relatively poor CPA permeation from the nose to the bloodstream, as previously reported for this type of formulation [23]. Indeed, a comparison of the AUC values (Table 3) obtained after intravenous administration (37687 ± 1118 ng mL^{-1} min) and nasal administration (699 ± 257 ng mL^{-1} min) indicated an absolute bioavailability value of 1.85% for the microparticulate powders based on chitosan.

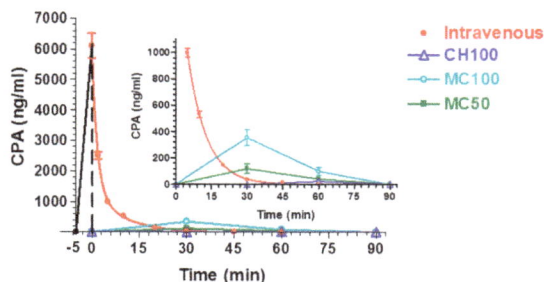

Figure 6. Blood CPA concentrations (ng/mL) after infusion or nasal administration of a 200-µg dose. The time ranging from −5 to 0 min refers to CPA IV infusion. In the inset: zoom of the same plot with expanded Y-scale (CPA blood concentration) from 0 to 1000 ng/mL. The inset highlights the concentration values obtained after administration of CH100, MC100 and MC50. Data are expressed as the mean ± standard deviation, $n = 4$.

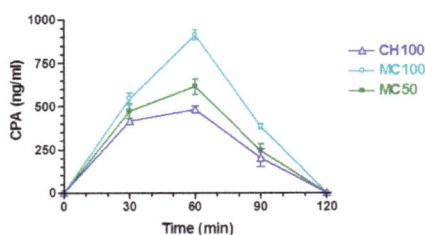

Figure 7. CPA concentrations (ng/mL) detected in the cerebrospinal fluid (CSF) after nasal administration of CH100, MC100 and MC50. Data are expressed as the mean ± standard deviation, $n = 4$.

The presence of cyclodextrins in the microparticulate nasal formulation induced an increase in CPA permeation in the bloodstream after nasal administration. Indeed, as evidenced in the inset of Figure 6, following the nasal administration of MC50 or MC100 particles, the peak plasma concentrations of CPA were detected at 30 min, with values of 118 ± 36 ng/mL or 354 ± 62 ng/mL, respectively. In this case the AUC values of MC50 or MC100 formulations were 4830 ± 827 or 13,590 ± 1451 ng mL^{-1} min, respectively, but only the MC100 value appeared significantly different from the AUC of CH100 (Table 3). The absolute bioavailability values were 12.8% and 36.0% for MC50 and MC100 samples, respectively. Table 3 summarizes the AUC and bioavailability values for the different administration routes of CPA. These data indicate that the progressive modifications of the morphology and structural composition of CH100 particles induced by the enhancement of the CDs in their composition reflects a progressive increase in systemic delivery of CPA, following their nasal administration.

Relevant amounts of CPA were detected in the CNS of rats after nasal administration of the solid microparticulate formulations. In particular, Figure 7 shows the CPA concentrations detected in the CSF: drug loaded chitosan microparticles (CH100 sample) may be seen to lead to an increase in CPA concentration values up to 481 ± 21 ng/mL within 60 min. Then, at 90 min the CPA concentration in CSF was significantly decreased (201 ± 50 ng/mL) and became undetectable at 120 min. The AUC value of this profile was found to be 32,910 ± 1199 ng mL^{-1} min. These data are in good agreement with those obtained in previous in vivo studies for this type of microparticles [23]. As registered in the bloodstream, the presence of cyclodextrins in the nasal formulations induced an increase in CPA amounts permeating in the CSF. Indeed, after nasal administration of the samples MC50 or MC100, the CPA concentrations in the CSF of rats increased up to 614 ± 44 and 911 ± 29 ng/mL, respectively, within 60 min after the nasal administration, then the values decreased to 243 ± 39 ng/mL for MC50 and 382 ± 16 ng/mL for MC100 at 90 min and became undetectable at 120 min. The AUC value of the MC50 and MC100 profiles were found to be 39,900 ± 1520 and 55,140 ± 1016 ng mL^{-1} min, respectively, with relative bioavailability values of 121% for MC50 and 170% for MC100, with respect to the CH100 formulation. These data seem to confirm that the presence of cyclodextrins in microparticulate nasal formulations can enhance drug permeation across nasal mucosa, with respect to formulations based on chitosan [20].

On the other hand, CH100 microparticles allowed us to obtain a CPA distribution between CSF and bloodstream resulting in a significantly higher ratio of concentrations than the ratios obtained by the nasal administration of the microparticles containing cyclodextrins. This aspect is evidenced in Figure 8, where the AUC ratios of CPA between CSF and bloodstream, obtained after nasal administration of the CH100, MC50 and MC100 microparticles, are reported. In particular, CH100 microparticles induced an AUC ratio of 47 ± 18, significantly higher ($p < 0.001$) than the AUC ratios obtained by nasal administration of MC50 (8.2 ± 1.6) and MC100 (3.9 ± 0.5) samples. A high AUC value can be very useful when a selective therapeutic activity of the drug is required in the central nervous system with respect to the bloodstream where the drug activity can induce severe side-effects. To the best of our knowledge, this is the first time that a modulation between the optimal uptake of a drug and its optimal distribution between CSF and bloodstream has been shown to be easily obtainable simply by varying the amount of cyclodextrins and chitosan in the microparticles.

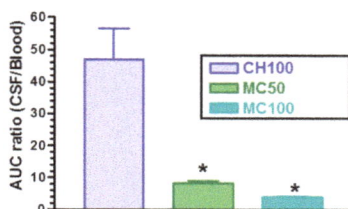

Figure 8. Ratios between CPA area under concentration curves (AUC) values between CSF and bloodstream obtained after nasal administration of the loaded microparticles CH100, MC50 and MC100. Data are expressed as the mean $\pm$ standard deviation, $n = 4$. * $p < 0.001$ versus CH100.

4. Conclusions

This study has demonstrated that the choice of penetration enhancer in nasal microspheres significantly affects the in vivo bioavailability of the encapsulated drug. In particular, methyl-β-cyclodextrin is more effective in enhancing drug permeation through respiratory and olfactory epithelia; this could be due to the changes in both paracellular and transcellular transports. On the contrary, chitosan has proven to be a selective excipient able to increase, above all, the paracellular transport of a drug through olfactory epithelia. This is, moreover, the first time that optimal drug distribution between CSF and bloodstream has been shown to be easily obtainable by varying the amount of these two penetration enhancers studied in the matrix of powder formulations.

Author Contributions: Conceptualization, E.G., P.G.; Investigation, G.R.; HPLC acquisition, analysis, validation and interpretation of data, A.D. and B.P.; Experiments on rats, L.F.; Project Administration, E.G.; Resources, P.G., A.D., L.F.; Writing—Original Draft Preparation, G.R., A.D., L.F.; Writing—Review & Editing, E.G., G.R., A.D.

Funding: This research received no external funding.

Acknowledgments: The authors thank Gabriele Bertocchi (Department of Chemical and Pharmaceutical Sciences, University of Ferrara, Italy) for powder X-ray diffraction measurements.

Conflicts of Interest: The authors declare no conflict of interest.

References

1. Aungst, B.J. Absorption Enhancers: Applications and Advances. *AAPS J.* **2012**, *14*, 10–18. [CrossRef] [PubMed]
2. Davis, S.S.; Illum, L. Absorption Enhancers for Nasal Drug Delivery. *Clin. Pharmacokinet.* **2003**, *42*, 1107–1128. [CrossRef] [PubMed]
3. Gavini, E.; Rassu, G.; Haukvik, T.; Lanni, C.; Racchi, M.; Giunchedi, P. Mucoadhesive microspheres for nasal administration of cyclodextrins. *J. Drug Target.* **2009**, *17*, 168–179. [CrossRef] [PubMed]
4. Gavini, E.; Rassu, G.; Ferraro, L.; Beggiato, S.; Alhalaweh, A.; Velaga, S.; Marchetti, N.; Bandiera, P.; Giunchedi, P.; Dalpiaz, A. Influence of polymeric microcarriers on the in vivo intranasal uptake of an anti-migraine drug for brain targeting. *Eur. J. Pharm. Biopharm.* **2013**, *83*, 174–183. [CrossRef] [PubMed]
5. Yalcin, A.; Soddu, E.; Turunc Bayrakdar, E.; Uyanikgil, Y.; Kanit, L.; Armagan, G.; Rassu, G.; Gavini, E.; Giunchedi, P. Neuroprotective Effects of Engineered Polymeric Nasal Microspheres Containing Hydroxypropyl-β-cyclodextrin on β-Amyloid (1-42)-Induced Toxicity. *J. Pharm. Sci.* **2016**, *105*, 2372–2380. [CrossRef] [PubMed]
6. Williams, A.C.; Barry, B.W. Penetration enhancers. *Adv. Drug Deliv. Rev.* **2012**, *64*, 128–137. [CrossRef]
7. Illum, L. Nasal drug delivery-possibilities, problems and solutions. *J. Control. Release* **2003**, *87*, 187–198. [CrossRef]
8. Merkus, F.W.H.M.; Verhoef, J.C.; Marttin, E.; Romeijn, S.G.; van der Kuy, P.H.M.; Hermens, W.A.J.; Schipper, N.G.M. Cyclodextrins in nasal drug delivery. *Adv. Drug Deliv. Rev.* **1999**, *36*, 41–57. [CrossRef]

9. Yang, T.; Hussain, A.; Paulson, J.; Abbruscato, T.J.; Ahsan, F. Cyclodextrins in nasal delivery of low-molecular-weight heparins: In vivo and in vitro studies. *Pharm. Res.* **2004**, *21*, 1127–1136. [CrossRef] [PubMed]

10. Zhang, X.; Zhang, X.; Wu, Z.; Gao, X.; Shua, S.; Wang, Z.; Li, C. β-Cyclodextrin grafting hyperbranched polyglycerols as carriers for nasal insulin delivery. *Carbohydr. Polym.* **2011**, *84*, 1419–1425. [CrossRef]

11. Challa, R.; Ahuja, A.; Ali, J.; Khar, R.K. Cyclodextrins in Drug Delivery: An Updated Review. *AAPS PharmSciTech* **2005**, *6*, E329–E357. [CrossRef] [PubMed]

12. Lambert, D.; O'Neill, C.A.; Padfield, P.J. Depletion of Caco-2 cell cholesterol disrupts barrier function by altering the detergent solubility and distribution of specific tight-junction proteins. *Biochem. J.* **2005**, *387*, 553–560. [CrossRef] [PubMed]

13. Fenyvesi, F.; Réti-Nagy, K.; Bacsó, Z.; Gutay-Tóth, Z.; Malanga, M.; Fenyvesi, É.; Szente, L.; Váradi, J.; Ujhelyi, Z.; Fehér, P.; et al. Fluorescently labeled methyl-beta-cyclodextrin enters intestinal epithelial Caco-2 cells by fluid-phase endocytosis. *PLoS ONE* **2014**, *9*, e84856. [CrossRef] [PubMed]

14. Casettari, L.; Illum, L. Chitosan in nasal delivery systems for therapeutic drugs. *J. Control. Release* **2014**, *190*, 189–200. [CrossRef] [PubMed]

15. Gavini, E.; Rassu, G.; Ferraro, L.; Generosi, A.; Rau, J.V.; Brunetti, A.; Giunchedi, P.; Dalpiaz, A. Influence of chitosan glutamate on the in vivo intranasal absorption of rokitamycin from microspheres. *J. Pharm. Sci.* **2011**, *100*, 1488–1502. [CrossRef] [PubMed]

16. Dalpiaz, A.; Fogagnolo, M.; Ferraro, L.; Capuzzo, A.; Pavan, B.; Rassu, G.; Salis, A.; Giunchedi, P.; Gavini, E. Nasal chitosan microparticles target a zidovudine prodrug to brain HIV sanctuaries. *Antiviral Res.* **2015**, *123*, 146–157. [CrossRef] [PubMed]

17. Rassu, G.; Soddu, E.; Cossu, M.; Gavini, E.; Giunchedi, P.; Dalpiaz, A. Particulate formulations based on chitosan for nose-to-brain delivery of drugs. A review. *J. Drug Deliv. Sci. Technol.* **2016**, *32*, 77–87. [CrossRef]

18. Council of Europe. *European Pharmacopoeia Chitosan Hydrochloride*, 8th ed.; Council of Europe: Strasbourg, France, 2014; p. 1841.

19. Türker, S.; Onur, E.; Ozer, Y. Nasal route and drug delivery systems. *Pharm. World Sci.* **2004**, *26*, 137–142. [CrossRef] [PubMed]

20. Rassu, G.; Soddu, E.; Cossu, M.; Brundu, A.; Cerri, G.; Marchetti, N.; Ferraro, L.; Regan, R.F.; Giunchedi, P.; Gavini, E.; et al. Solid microparticles based on chitosan or methyl-β-cyclodextrin: A first formulative approach to increase the nose-to-brain transport of deferoxamine mesylate. *J. Control. Release* **2015**, *201*, 68–77. [CrossRef] [PubMed]

21. Bshara, H.; Osman, R.; Mansour, S.; El-Shamy, A.E.A. Chitosan and cyclodextrin in intranasal microemulsion for improved brain buspirone hydrochloride pharmacokinetics in rats. *Carbohydr. Polym.* **2014**, *99*, 297–305. [CrossRef] [PubMed]

22. Lochhead, J.J.; Thorne, R.G. Intranasal delivery of biologics to the central nervous system. *Adv. Drug Deliv. Rev.* **2012**, *64*, 614–628. [CrossRef] [PubMed]

23. Dalpiaz, A.; Gavini, E.; Colombo, G.; Russo, P.; Bortolotti, F.; Ferraro, L.; Tanganelli, S.; Scatturin, A.; Menegatti, E.; Giunchedi, P. Brain uptake of an anti-ischemic agent by nasal administration of microparticles. *J. Pharm. Sci.* **2008**, *97*, 4889–4903. [CrossRef] [PubMed]

24. Gavini, E.; Rassu, G.; Ciarnelli, V.; Spada, G.; Cossu, M.; Giunchedi, P. Mucoadhesive drug delivery systems for nose-to-brain targeting of dopamine. *J. Nanoneurosci.* **2012**, *2*, 1–9. [CrossRef]

25. Rassu, G.; Gavini, E.; Jonassen, H.; Zambito, Y.; Fogli, S.; Breschi, M.C.; Giunchedi, P. New chitosan derivatives for the preparation of rokitamycin loaded microspheres designed for ocular or nasal administration. *J. Pharm. Sci.* **2009**, *98*, 4852–4865. [CrossRef] [PubMed]

26. Gavini, E.; Spada, G.; Rassu, G.; Cerri, G.; Brundu, A.; Cossu, M.; Sorrenti, M.; Giunchedi, P. Development of solid nanoparticles based on hydroxypropyl-β-cyclodextrin aimed for the colonic transmucosal delivery of diclofenac sodium. *J. Pharm. Pharmacol.* **2011**, *63*, 472–482. [CrossRef] [PubMed]

27. Kouchak, M.; Handali, S.; Boroujeni, B.N. Evaluation of the mechanical properties and drug permeability of chitosan/Eudragit RL composite film. *Osong Public Health Res. Perspect.* **2015**, *6*, 14–19. [CrossRef] [PubMed]

28. Van den Berg, M.P.; Romeijn, S.G.; Verhoef, J.C.; Merkus, F.W. Serial cerebrospinal fluid sampling in a rat model to study drug uptake from the nasal cavity. *J. Neurosci. Methods* **2002**, *116*, 99–107. [CrossRef]

29. Dalpiaz, A.; Ferraro, L.; Perrone, D.; Leo, E.; Iannuccelli, V.; Pavan, B.; Paganetto, G.; Beggiato, S.; Scalia, S. Brain uptake of a Zidovudine prodrug after nasal administration of solid lipid microparticles. *Mol. Pharm.* **2014**, *11*, 1550–1561. [CrossRef] [PubMed]

30. Sacchetti, C.; Artusi, M.; Santi, P.; Colombo, P. Caffeine microparticles for nasal administration obtained by spray drying. *Int. J. Pharm.* **2002**, *242*, 335–339. [CrossRef]

31. Felgenhauer, K. Protein Size and CSF Composition. *Klinische Wochensch.* **1974**, *52*, 1158–1164. [CrossRef]

32. Madu, A.; Cioffe, C.; Mian, U.; Burroughs, M.; Tuomanen, E.; Mayers, M.; Schwartz, E.; Miller, M. Pharmacokinetics of Fluconazole in Cerebrospinal Fluid and Serum of Rabbits: Validation of an Animal Model used to Measure Drug Concentrations in Cerebrospinal Fluid. *Antimicrob. Agents Chemother.* **1994**, *38*, 2111–2115. [CrossRef] [PubMed]

33. Gavini, E.; Rassu, G.; Sanna, V.; Cossu, M.; Giunchedi, P. Mucoadhesive microspheres for nasal administration of an antiemetic drug, metoclopramide: In-vitro/ex-vivo studies. *J. Pharm. Pharmacol.* **2005**, *57*, 287–294. [CrossRef] [PubMed]

34. Mathot, R.A.; Appel, S.; van Schaick, E.A.; Soudijn, W.; Ijzerman, A.P.; Danhof, M. High-performance liquid chromatography of the adenosine A1 agonist N6-cyclopentyladenosine and the A1 antagonist 8-cyclopentyltheophylline and its application in a pharmacokinetic study in rats. *J. Chromatogr.* **1993**, *620*, 113–120. [CrossRef]

35. Brodie, M.S.; Lee, K.; Fredholm, B.B.; Stahle, L.; Dunwiddie, T.V. Central versus peripheral mediation of responses to adenosine receptor agonists: Evidence against a central mode of action. *Brain Res.* **1987**, *415*, 323–330. [CrossRef]

36. Tamai, I.; Tsuji, A. Transporter-mediated permeation of drugs across the blood-brain barrier. *J. Pharm. Sci.* **2000**, *89*, 1371–1388. [CrossRef]

37. Schaddelee, M.P.; Read, K.D.; Cleypool, C.G.J.; Ijzerman, A.P.; Danhof, M.; de Boer, A.G. Brain penetration of synthetic A1 receptor agonists in situ: Role of the rENT1 nucleoside transporter and binding to blood constituents. *Eur. J. Pharm. Sci.* **2005**, *24*, 59–66. [CrossRef] [PubMed]

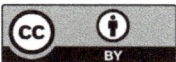

pharmaceutics

MDPI

Article

Chitosan-Coated Nanoparticles: Effect of Chitosan Molecular Weight on Nasal Transmucosal Delivery

Franciele Aline Bruinsmann [1,2], Stefania Pigana [2], Tanira Aguirre [3], Gabriele Dadalt Souto [1], Gabriela Garrastazu Pereira [1], Annalisa Bianchera [2], Laura Tiozzo Fasiolo [2,4], Gaia Colombo [4], Magno Marques [5], Adriana Raffin Pohlmann [1,6], Silvia Stanisçuaski Guterres [1] and Fabio Sonvico [2,*]

[1] Programa de Pós-Graduação em Ciências Farmacêuticas, Universidade Federal do Rio Grande do Sul, Porto Alegre 90610-000, Brazil; fbruinsmann@gmail.com (F.A.B.); gabrieledadalt@gmail.com (G.D.S.); garrastazugp@gmail.com (G.G.P.); adriana.pohlmann@ufrgs.br (A.R.P.); silvia.guterres@ufrgs.br (S.S.G.)
[2] Food and Drug Department, University of Parma, Parco Area delle Scienze 27/a, 43124 Parma, Italy; stefania.pigana@studenti.unipr.it (S.P.); annalisa.bianchera@unipr.it (A.B.); laura.tiozzofasiolo@studenti.unipr.it (L.T.F.)
[3] Programa de Pós-Graduação em Biociências, Universidade Federal de Ciências da Saúde de Porto Alegre, Porto Alegre RS 900500-170, Brazil; tanira@ufcspa.edu.br
[4] Department of Life Sciences and Biotechnology, University of Ferrara, Via Fossato di Mortara 17/19, 44121 Ferrara, Italy; clmgai@unife.it
[5] Programa de Pós-Graduação em Ciências Fisiológicas, Universidade Federal do Rio Grande, Rio Grande RS 96203-000, Brazil; magnomarques@aol.com
[6] Departamento de Química Orgânica, Instituto de Química, Universidade Federal do Rio Grande do Sul, Porto Alegre 91501-970, Brazil
*   Correspondence: fabio.sonvico@unipr.it; Tel.: +39-0521-906282

Received: 1 February 2019; Accepted: 15 February 2019; Published: 18 February 2019

Abstract: Drug delivery to the brain represents a challenge, especially in the therapy of central nervous system malignancies. Simvastatin (SVT), as with other statins, has shown potential anticancer properties that are difficult to exploit in the central nervous system (CNS). In the present work the physico–chemical, mucoadhesive, and permeability-enhancing properties of simvastatin-loaded poly-ε-caprolactone nanocapsules coated with chitosan for nose-to-brain administration were investigated. Lipid-core nanocapsules coated with chitosan (LNC_{chit}) of different molecular weight (MW) were prepared by a novel one-pot technique, and characterized for particle size, surface charge, particle number density, morphology, drug encapsulation efficiency, interaction between surface nanocapsules with mucin, drug release, and permeability across two nasal mucosa models. Results show that all formulations presented adequate particle sizes (below 220 nm), positive surface charge, narrow droplet size distribution (PDI < 0.2), and high encapsulation efficiency. Nanocapsules presented controlled drug release and mucoadhesive properties that are dependent on the MW of the coating chitosan. The results of permeation across the RPMI 2650 human nasal cell line evidenced that LNC_{chit} increased the permeation of SVT. In particular, the amount of SVT that permeated after 4 hr for nanocapsules coated with low-MW chitosan, high-MW chitosan, and control SVT was 13.9 ± 0.8 µg, 9.2 ± 1.2 µg, and 1.4 ± 0.2 µg, respectively. These results were confirmed by SVT ex vivo permeation across rabbit nasal mucosa. This study highlighted the suitability of LNC_{chit} as a promising strategy for the administration of simvastatin for a nose-to-brain approach for the therapy of brain tumors.

Keywords: nasal permeability; nose-to-brain; simvastatin; nanocapsules; mucoadhesion; CNS disorders; chitosan

1. Introduction

Statins are potent inhibitors of the hydroxymethyl glutaryl coenzyme A (HMG-CoA) reductase, and they are commonly administered for the treatment of cardiovascular disease [1]. However, in recent years, it has been suggested that the statin therapeutic indications might expand, due to their pleiotropic effects [2]. These non-cholesterol-related effects include their modulation of immune responses, the enhancement of endothelial function, the reduction of oxidative stress, and checking of inflammation processes [3,4]. The majority of pleiotropic effects are mediated by preventing the synthesis of isoprenoids, and the subsequent inhibition of small signaling proteins [5,6]. Among the diseases that could benefit from statin's pleiotropic effects are multiple sclerosis, rheumatoid arthritis, systemic lupus erythematosus, chronic obstructive pulmonary disease, neurodegenerative disorders, bacterial infections, and cancer [3].

In the field of cancer therapy, statins showed pro-apoptotic effects against various tumor cell lines [7,8], and numerous studies have examined their potential chemopreventive action [9]. Due to the inhibition of the enzyme HMG-CoA reductase, statins decrease the levels of mevalonate, the precursor of dolichol, geranylpyrophosphate (GPP), and farnesyl-pyrophosphate (FPP). Dolichol enhances DNA synthesis and is associated with several proteins found in tumor cells [10]. GPP and FPP are post-translational modifications of intracellular proteins as the G-proteins Ras and Rho, which regulate the signal transduction of several membrane receptors, and which are critical for the transcription of genes involved in cell proliferation, differentiation, and apoptosis. Ras and Rho gene mutations are found in a variety of tumor cells [7,11]. Furthermore, statins show apoptotic effects in human glioblastoma cell lines that induce the depletion of geranylgeranylated proteins, which is important for the transition to cell cycle phases [12]. Statins have also shown to play a role in the prevention of tumor metastases by the inhibition of epithelial growth factor–induced tumor cell invasion [13]. Moreover, statins, inducing the inactivation of nuclear factor kB, reduce urokinase and matrix metalloproteinase-9 expression, which are pivotal for tumor metastatic processes [7,14].

In the case of glioma cell lines, simvastatin (SVT) showed a suppression of cell proliferation and the induction of apoptosis [15,16]. However, when evaluated in an in vivo orthotopic model of the glioblastoma multiform model, simvastatin did not show tumor-inhibitory effects [17]. As in this experiment, the major factor for the failure of chemotherapies against central nervous system (CNS) tumors has been attributed to limited brain-blood barrier (BBB) permeability [18]. In addition, after oral administration statins are extensively metabolized in the liver, their hydrophilic metabolites are prevented from crossing the BBB [19].

Some new strategies have been proposed to deal with such limitations in order to increase the distribution of drugs in the CNS, such as the use of nose-to-brain route [20,21] and the development of nanocarriers [22–24]. In recent years, nose-to-brain delivery has attracted much attention as a means of delivering drugs more efficiently to the CNS bypassing the BBB. This is because the nasal cavity is anatomically connected to the CNS via the olfactory system [25]. Moreover, it offers advantages such as non-invasiveness, the avoidance of hepatic first-pass metabolism, practicality and the convenience of administration [26]. However, due to the presence of the rapid mucociliary clearance mechanism, nasal delivery applications for brain delivery are hindered by the short residence time of conventional formulations. Moreover, the barrier of the nasal epithelium, nasal metabolism, and the limited volume of administration are limiting aspects for the development of nose-to-brain drug delivery systems [25,27].

To increase bioavailability after nasal delivery, polymeric nanocapsules have been investigated [28–30]. These nanocarriers are considered a type of reservoir drug delivery system [31], and can be obtained by the interfacial deposition of pre-formed polymers [32]. Their structure is characterized by an oil core surrounded by a polymeric shell stabilized by a surfactant system [31,33]. The lipid-core nanocapsules (LNCs), developed by our research group, are composed of a dispersion of sorbitan monostearate (solid lipid) and medium-chain triacylglycerols (liquid lipids) in the core, surrounded by poly(ε-caprolactone), an aliphatic polyester as a polymeric wall, and polysorbate 80 as a stabilizing surfactant [34]. The lipid core dispersion, i.e., sorbitan monostearate dispersed in oil, confers different properties to this system, such as controlling the drug release and increasing the encapsulation efficiency when compared to the core of the conventional nanocapsules containing only liquid lipids [34–36]. These nanocarriers showed efficient brain delivery of drugs as resveratrol [37] and curcumin [38] when administered orally and intraperitoneally, as well as the reduction of the side effects of the antipsychotic drug olanzapine [39]. Furthermore, they demonstrated improved the vitro and in vivo antitumor effectiveness of resveratrol, methotrexate, and acetyleugenol when compared to the free drugs [40–42].

Bender and co-authors [43], developed a two-step process to obtain modified LNC stabilized simultaneously with polysorbate 80, and lecithin and coated with chitosan. Chitosan is a cationic biopolymer obtained by the partial deacetylation of chitin under alkaline conditions [44]. Chitosan demonstrated several interesting properties for pharmaceutical application, such as biodegradability, biocompatibility, antibacterial activity, and the controlled release of drugs [45,46]. Furthermore, chitosan showed mucoadhesive and penetration-enhancing properties, which are particularly desirable for its application in drug nasal delivery [47,48]. These actions are mediated by the structural reorganization of the tight junctions of the nasal epithelium, increasing the paracellular transport of drugs [49].

In the present study, LNC stabilized with lecithin and coated with chitosan was obtained by an innovative one-pot technique. Moreover, the pharmaceutical properties of formulations with chitosans of different molecular weights (MW), intended for the nose-to-brain delivery of simvastatin, were evaluated.

2. Materials and Methods

2.1. Materials

Poly (ε-caprolactone) (PCL) (MW = 14,000) and Span 60® (sorbitan monostearate) were purchased from Sigma-Aldrich (Strasbourg, France). Caprylic/capric triglyceride was obtained from Delaware (Porto Alegre, Brazil), and simvastatin (SVT) was purchased from Pharma Nostra (Rio de Janeiro, Brazil). Chitosan low MW (21 kDa—viscosity 9 cP) and high MW (152 kDa—viscosity 114 cP) was provided by Primex (Chitoclear FG, deacetylation degree 95%, Siglufjordur, Iceland). Soybean lecithin (Lipoid S75) was kindly donated by Lipoid AG (Ludwigshafen, Germany). Minimum essential medium (MEM), fetal bovine serum (FBS), phosphate-buffered saline (PBS), and Hank's Balanced Salt Solution (HBSS) were supplied by Gibco (Carlsbad, CA, USA). Transwell® cell culture inserts (1.12 cm^2 surface area, polyester, 0.4 µm pore size) were supplied by Corning Costar (Lowell, MA, USA). All of the other chemicals and solvents used were of analytical or pharmaceutical grade.

2.2. Preparation of the Lipid-Core Nanocapsules Coated using a One-Pot Technique

Chitosan-coated simvastatin-loaded lipid-core nanocapsules were prepared according to the method of interfacial deposition of pre-formed polymers already reported in literature [35]. An organic phase (25 mL of acetone) containing the polymer (PCL, 0.04 g), sorbitan monostearate (0.016 g), and caprylic/capric triglyceride (0.048 mL) was kept under magnetic stirring at 40 °C. After complete dissolution of the components, an ethanolic solution (4 mL) containing lecithin (0.025 g) was added into the organic phase, and finally, simvastatin (0.010 g) was added and completely dissolved. The aqueous phase (50 mL) contained 0.1% (w/v) chitosan, prepared as a dilution from a 0.5% (w/v) of chitosan solution in 1% (v/v) acetic acid. The organic phase was injected using a funnel into the aqueous phase under moderate magnetic stirring. The solvents were eliminated at 40 °C to a final volume of 10 mL, by the use of a rotary evaporator, Büchi® R-114 (Flawill, Switzerland). The formulations obtained were named LNC$_{SVT-LMWchit}$ when low-MW chitosan (viscosity 9 cP) was used, and LNC$_{SVT-HMWchit}$ when high-MW chitosan (viscosity 114cP) was used. Blank nanocapsules (LNC$_{LMWchit}$ and LNC$_{HMWchit}$) were also prepared, omitting the simvastatin from the organic phase preparation.

2.3. Drug Content and Encapsulation Efficiency

SVT quantification was carried out by high performance liquid chromatography with detection in the ultraviolet range (HPLC-UV), using a previously validated method [30]. The analysis was performed with a Shimadzu HPLC system (Kyoto, Japan) with detection at 238 nm and using a column Phenomenex Lichrosphere® C18 (4.6 × 250 mm, 5 μm). The composition of the mobile phase was 65% acetonitrile and 35% sodium dihydrogen phosphate buffer (25 mM, pH 4.5), the flow rate was 1.0 mL·min^{-1}, with an injection volume of 100 μL. Calibration curves ($n = 3$) were prepared to determine the linearity ($R > 0.99$) in the concentration range from 0.1 to 20 μg·mL^{-1}. The drug content in the formulations was determined by diluting a precise volume of nanoparticle suspension (100 μL) in 10 mL of the mobile phase. The samples were then sonicated for 30 min and filtered through a 0.45 μm membrane (Millipore®, Billerica, MA, USA) before being assayed by HPLC-UV. Free simvastatin was determined in the ultrafiltrate after ultrafiltration–centrifugation (Ultrafree-MC, cut-off of 30 kDa, Millipore) at 2688× g (Scilogex D3024, Rocky Hill, CT, USA) for 15 min and quantification by HPLC-UV. Encapsulation efficiency (EE) as a percentage was calculated by the difference between the total and free, i.e., non-encapsulated, drug amount, divided by the total drug amount multiplied by 100. All analyses were performed for triplicate batches ($n = 3$).

2.4. Physicochemical Characterization

The nanoparticle formulations were characterized with multiple techniques, as described below. All analyses, with the exception of transmission electron microscopy (TEM) ($n = 1$), were performed for triplicate batches ($n = 3$).

2.4.1. Laser Diffraction

Particle size and the size distribution were determined by laser diffraction (Mastersizer® 2000, Malvern Instruments, Malvern, UK), with the aim of detecting the eventual presence of micrometric particles or aggregates. The sample was directly added to water in the wet dispersion accessory (Hydro 2000SM-AWM2002, Malvern Instruments) until an obscuration level of 2% was reached. The particle size was then expressed by using the volume-weighted mean diameter (D[4,3]), and the diameters calculated at the 10th, 50th, and 90th percentiles ($d_{0.1}$, $d_{0.5}$, and $d_{0.9}$, respectively) of the cumulative size distribution curve, by volume (v) and by the number (n) of particles. The width of the distribution (*Span*) was determined according to Equation (1):

$$Span = \frac{d_{0.9} - d_{0.1}}{d_{0.5}}, \tag{1}$$

2.4.2. Dynamic Light Scattering

The mean particle size (Z-average diameter) and the polydispersity index (PDI) of the nanocapsules were evaluated by dynamic light scattering (DLS) at 25 °C, using a Zetasizer® Nano ZS (Malvern Instruments). After dilution of the samples (500×) in purified and filtered (0.45 μm) water, the correlogram was obtained by allowing the instrument software to determine the optimal time of acquisition, and the Z-average diameter and PDI were calculated by the method of Cumulants, with the same software.

2.4.3. Nanoparticle Tracking Analysis

The nanoparticles tracking analysis (NTA) method was used to determine the mean diameter and the concentration of nanocapsules per volume, expressed as the particle number density (PND) (NanoSight LM10, Malvern Pananalytical, UK). The analysis was carried out by diluting the samples in ultrapure water (1000×) and introducing them into the instrument sample chamber cell by a syringe. The chamber is located on an optical microscope, where a laser diode (635 nm) illuminates the particles in suspension. The NTA 3.2 software tracks single particles, which are in Brownian motion, and it can relate this particle movement to a sphere equivalent hydrodynamic radius, as calculated using the Stokes–Einstein equation (Equation (2)). The samples were evaluated at room temperature for 60 s, with automatic detection. The results correspond to the arithmetic average of the calculated sizes of all particles analyzed:

$$\overline{(x, y)^2} = \frac{4\,Tk_B}{3\pi\eta d_h}\,,\tag{2}$$

where k_B is the Boltzmann constant, and $\overline{(x, y)^2}$ is the mean-squared displacement of a particle during time t at temperature T, in a medium of viscosity η, with a hydrodynamic diameter of d_h.

2.4.4. pH and Zeta Potential

The pH values of the nanocapsules suspensions were determined using a calibrated potentiometer (DM-22 Digimed, São Paulo, Brazil) via direct measurements of the formulations at 25 °C. The zeta potential values were determined by electrophoretic mobility after the samples were diluted in 10 mM NaCl aqueous solution (500×), previously filtered (0.45 μm, Millipore®, Billerica, USA). The zeta potentials of the nanoparticles suspensions were also measured at different pH values, using the MPT-2 autotitrator for the Zetasizer® Nano ZS (Malvern Instruments, Malvern, UK). The samples (10 mL) were placed in the titration cell and titrated over acid (0.1 M HCl) towards a basic (0.05 M NaOH) pH range in 1.0 pH unit intervals. This combination allowed for automated titration over a wide pH range, and thus, made it possible to determine the isoelectric point (IEP) of the nanoparticles.

2.4.5. Morphology

TEM was used to evaluate the morphology of the formulations. TEM samples were diluted in ultrapure water (10×, *v/v*), and then deposited (10 μL) onto specimen grids (Formvar-Carbon support film, Electron Microscopy Sciences, Hatfield, PA, USA) and negatively stained with uranyl acetate solution (2% (*w/v*), Sigma-Aldrich, St.Louis, MO, USA). Analyses were performed using a transmission electron microscope (JEM 2200-FS, Jeol, Tokyo, Japan) operating at 80 kV. The images were processed with Digital Micrograph (Gatan Inc., Pleasanton, CA, USA) software.

2.5. *In Vitro Evaluation of the Interaction between Nanocapsules and Mucin*

The mucoadhesive properties of the formulations were assessed by using mucin from porcine stomach (Type II, Sigma-Aldrich, St. Louis, MO, USA), as previously described [29,50]. The mucin was dispersed in ultrapure water (0.5% (*w/v*)) by magnetic stirring for 3 h at room temperature. The suspension was centrifuged at 4000× *g* for 30 min. The supernatant was collected and lyophilized. Then, mucin solutions were prepared in a simulated nasal electrolytic solution (SNES) [51] at predetermined weight ratios f, determined as:

$$f = \frac{W_{mucin}}{W_{mucin} + WNC}\,,\tag{3}$$

where W_{mucin} is the mucin mass and WNC is the LNC$_{chit}$ nanocapsule mass.

The Z-average diameter and PDI before and after contact with mucin were measured by DLS as described above, after the dilution (500×) of the samples in mucin solutions. The mucoadhesive index values (MI) were determined as:

$$MI = \frac{d}{d_0}\,,\tag{4}$$

where d and d_0 are the diameters of the LNC$_{chit}$ nanocapsules before and after their interaction with mucin, respectively.

Furthermore, changes in the zeta potential were measured after the nanocapsules were diluted (500×) in mucin solutions containing 10 mM NaCl.

2.6. In Vitro Release Study

The in vitro release profiles of SVT from the formulations were determined by using the dialysis bag method. Briefly, 1 mL of each sample was placed in a dialysis bag (14 kDa molecular weight cut-off, Sigma-Aldrich, St. Louis, MO, USA) and suspended into 100 mL of SNES containing 0.5% of polysorbate 80, to improve SVT solubility and to reach the sink conditions. A free drug solution was placed in the dialysis bag in the control experiment (SVT$_{solution}$, simvastatin dissolved in 1% ethanol and 0.5% polysorbate 80). The dialysis bags were maintained in the medium under stirring, and maintained in a temperature-constant water bath (37 °C). One milliliter of release medium was collected at predetermined time intervals (from 0.16 to 8 h) and filtered (0.45 µm, Millipore®). The volume was replaced by adding one milliliter of fresh release medium pre-heated at 37 °C. The samples were analyzed by HPLC–UV, and the cumulative drug release was determined.

2.7. Transport Studies across an In Vitro Nasal Epithelial Cell Model

RPMI 2650 human nasal cells (human nasal septum tumor, ECACC, Salisbury, UK) were cultured in MEM media supplemented with 10% (v/v) fetal bovine serum (FBS). Cells were grown at 37 °C in an atmosphere of 95% air/5% CO$_2$. Transwell® cell culture inserts were used to establish an air–liquid interface (ALI) nasal model, as previously reported [52]. Briefly, 200 uL of cell suspensions (2.5×10^6 cell/mL) were seeded onto Transwell® and after 24 h, the media from apical compartment was removed, resulting in an ALI culture configuration. After 14 days from seeding, the Transwell® was removed and transferred to a 12-well plate containing 1.5 mL of pre-warmed HBSS. Then, 200 µL of LNC$_{SVT-LMWchit}$, LNC$_{SVT-HMWchit}$, and SVT$_{suspension}$ were added to the upper compartment, and samples of 200 µL were collected from the baso-lateral chamber at pre-determined time points (1, 2, 3 and 4 h) and replaced with the same volume of fresh HBSS buffer. The samples were quantified for simvastatin content using HPLC–UV ($n = 4$). TEER measurements were performed with a Millicell-ers® (Millipore) at the beginning and at the end of experiment, in order to confirm that the integrity of the cell layer was maintained.

2.8. Ex Vivo Transport Experiments across Rabbit Nasal Mucosa

The transport of simvastatin across rabbit nasal tissue was evaluated by using Franz-type vertical diffusion cells with a receptor volume of 4.5 mL and a diffusional area of 0.58 cm^2. On the day of the experiment, nasal mucosae were freshly excised from rabbits obtained from a local slaughterhouse (Pola, Finale Emilia, Italy), and cleaned to remove the adhering submucosal tissue [53]. The rabbit nasal mucosa were placed between the donor and the receptor compartments of the diffusion cells. Then, in order to check the mucosa integrity, the donor compartment was filled with medium to confirm that no liquid leaked into the cell receptor compartment. If the nasal mucosa passed this test, the donor compartment received 200 µL of one of the three tested preparations, i.e., LNC$_{SVT-LMWchit}$, LNC$_{SVT-HMWchit}$, or SVT$_{suspension}$, equivalent to 200 µg of SVT. The Franz cells were maintained at 37 °C under mild magnetic stirring. At predetermined time intervals, 500 µL of the receptor medium, SNES containing 0.5% w/v of polysorbate 80, was withdrawn, and the receptor compartment was refilled with an equivalent volume of fresh medium. All samples were analyzed by HPLC-UV. In order to evaluate the retention of SVT in the nasal tissue, mucosa samples were placed in a volumetric flask (10 mL) containing a solvent of extraction (acetonitrile), and subjected to vortexing (2 min) and sonication (15 min). The solvent of extraction was then filtered (0.45 µm, Millipore®) and simvastatin was quantified using HPLC–UV. The experiments were conducted in triplicate for each formulation.

2.9. Preliminary Nasal Toxicity Studies

Nasal toxicity studies were performed by using rabbit nasal mucosa in a similar way to the ex vivo permeation study mentioned above, in order to evaluate any damage to the mucosa. Each mucosa piece of uniform thickness was treated with LNC$_{SVT-LMWchit}$, LNC$_{SVT-HMWchit}$, SVT, or PBS pH 6.4 (negative control) by placing 200 μL in the donor compartments of the Franz diffusion cells. The acceptor contained 4.5 mL of SNES containing 0.5% (w/v) of polysorbate 80. After 4 h, for each condition, the nasal mucosa was washed with PBS, fixed in 10% (v/v) buffered formalin for 6 h, and embedded in histological paraffin. A rotatory microtome was used to perform transverse cuts to obtain sections (5 μm) that were stained with hematoxylin–eosin. Images of mucosa samples were observed by using an Olympus BX51 optical microscope with an attached DP72 camera (Olympus, Tokyo, Japan) [54].

2.10. Statistical Analysis

Data are presented as the mean ± standard deviation (SD) of the analysis of at least triplicate batches ($n = 3$). Statistical analysis was performed using the Student's t-test for two groups, or one-way analysis of variance (ANOVA) followed by Tukey's test for multiple groups, using GraphPad Prism Software 5.0 (GraphPad Software, Inc., San Diego, CA, USA). Differences were considered significant at $p < 0.05$.

3. Results

SVT-nanocapsules were prepared by using the interfacial deposition of pre-formed polymer method, and coated with chitosan with a one-pot technique. The surfaces of the NPs were coated with two different chitosan grades, characterized by different molecular weights, and hence different viscosities, in order to evaluate the effect of chitosan molecular weight on the mucoadhesive properties and permeability enhancement of the nanocapsules obtained.

3.1. Characterization of Nanocapsules

SVT nanocapsules appeared macroscopically as an opalescent white homogeneous dispersion. The total SVT content in the formulations was found to be 0.94 ± 0.04 mg·mL^{-1} for LNC$_{\text{SVT-LMWchit}}$ and 0.96 ± 0.02 mg·mL^{-1} for LNC$_{\text{SVT-HMWchit}}$. Regarding the encapsulation efficiency (EE), SVT was not detected in the ultrafiltrate for both formulations, indicating almost complete encapsulation. The high EE achieved is probably linked to the high SVT distribution coefficient (log D) of 4.72, which confirms its great affinity for the lipophilic phase, and its concentration in the core of the nanocapsules [55]. Laser diffraction (LD) analysis showed D[4,3] of 150 ± 7 nm (LNC$_{\text{LMWchit}}$), 157 ± 6 nm (LNC$_{\text{HMWchit}}$), 163 ± 2 nm (LNC$_{\text{SVT-LMWchit}}$), and 161 ± 3 nm (LNC$_{\text{SVT-HMWchit}}$), with Span values of 1.3 ± 0.1, 1.3 ± 0.1, 1.4 ± 0.03, and 1.2 ± 0.2, respectively. According to the results obtained with this technique, there were no significant differences in terms of the particle diameter and polydispersity, between the formulations with and without SVT ($p > 0.05$). The shapes of the curves in the radar chart presented in Figure 1 are fingerprints of the formulations, which demonstrate the narrow size distributions and confirm their low polydispersities [56]. All of the formulations showed similar behaviors and they had $d_{0.9}$ calculated both for the cumulative distribution by number, and by a volume lower than 300 nm (Figure 1).

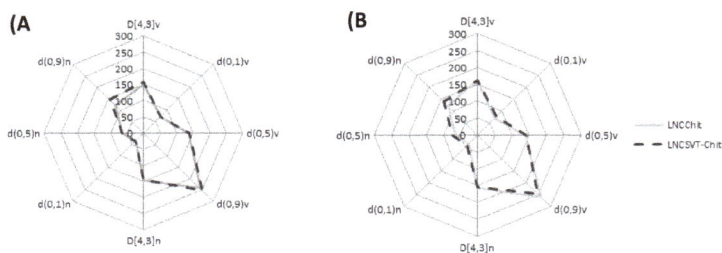

Figure 1. Radar chart presenting the volume-weighted mean diameters (D[4,3]) and the diameters at percentiles 10, 50, and 90 under the size distribution curves by volume and by the number of particles. Chitosan-coated simvastatin-loaded lipid-core nanocapsules developed with (**A**) low-MW chitosan and (**B**) high-MW chitosan.

The mean particle size was further confirmed by DLS and NTA analysis, as shown in Table 1. The DLS analysis showed a narrow particle size distribution for all of the formulations (PDI < 0.2). In particular, the encapsulation of SVT did not affect the particle size of the nanocapsules coated with low-MW chitosan. In fact, the diameters of $LNC_{LMWchit}$ and $LNC_{SVT-LMWchit}$ were not significantly different ($p > 0.05$).

Table 1. Physicochemical characterization of the nanocapsules ($n = 3$, Mean $\pm$ Standard Deviation).

Header	DLS		NTA		Zeta Potential (mV)	pH
	Z-Average (nm)	PDI	Mean (nm)	PND (Particles/mL)		
$LNC_{LMWchit}$	166 ± 5	0.13 ± 0.02	174 ± 5	$1.3 \pm 0.3 \times 10^{12}$	25.4 ± 4.1	4.1 ± 0.01
$LNC_{SVT-LMWchit}$	168 ± 5	0.12 ± 0.04	166 ± 7	$1.2 \pm 0.6 \times 10^{12}$	28.95 ± 2.1	4.1 ± 0.02
$LNC_{HMWchit}$	179 ± 14	0.13 ± 0.02	188 ± 7	$1.1 \pm 0.4 \times 10^{12}$	33.6 ± 3.9	4.1 ± 0.03
$LNC_{SVT-HMWchit}$	185 ± 7	0.16 ± 0.03	210 ± 10	$6.6 \pm 0.2 \times 10^{11}$	33.8 ± 5.5	4.4 ± 0.04

On the other hand, the presence of SVT led to a significant size increase ($p \leq 0.05$) in the case of $LNC_{SVT-HMWchit}$ (210 ± 10 nm) when compared with the blank nanocapsules ($LNC_{HMWchit}$, 188 ± 7 nm) according to the NTA analysis, but not according to the DLS data. This difference may be explained by the formation of a small number of particle agglomerates, compared to the formulation prepared without the drug. In addition, these agglomerates appeared to be detected more efficiently by the NTA technique compared to DLS. This is supported by the particle number density (PND) also measured by NTA, which evidenced, upon SVT encapsulation, almost a halving of the particle number density (PND), which was $1.1 \pm 0.4 \times 10^{12}$ particles/mL for $LNC_{HMWchit}$ and $6.6 \pm 0.2 \times 10^{11}$ particles/mL for $LNC_{SVT-HMWchit}$ (Table 1). Furthermore, in general, the nanocapsules coated with HMW chitosan showed a slightly higher mean diameter than those coated with LMW chitosan ($p > 0.05$), probably as a consequence of the higher molecular weight and higher viscosity of the chitosan in the water phase. In general, it has been reported that the higher the viscosity of the dispersion medium, the higher the mean diameter of the nanoparticles produced [57]. The zeta potentials of $LNC_{LMWchit}$ and $LNC_{HMWchit}$ were similar to those determined for the SVT-loaded nanocapsules. Therefore, the encapsulation of SVT did not significantly affect this parameter ($p > 0.05$). The pH value at which the nanoparticles do not exhibit any net charge is termed the isoelectric point (IEP). $LNC_{SVT-LMWchit}$ and $LNC_{SVT-HMWchit}$ showed an IEP at pH value 7.1 ± 0.2 and 7.2 ± 0.5, respectively. The positive zeta potential obtained for all the formulations prepared, and an IEP near the IEP of chitosan (IEP = 6.8) [58] is a good indicator that the chitosan was present at the external interface of the nanocapsules. $LNC_{SVT-LMWchit}$ and $LNC_{SVT-HMWchit}$ were further characterized in terms of their morphologies (Figure 2).

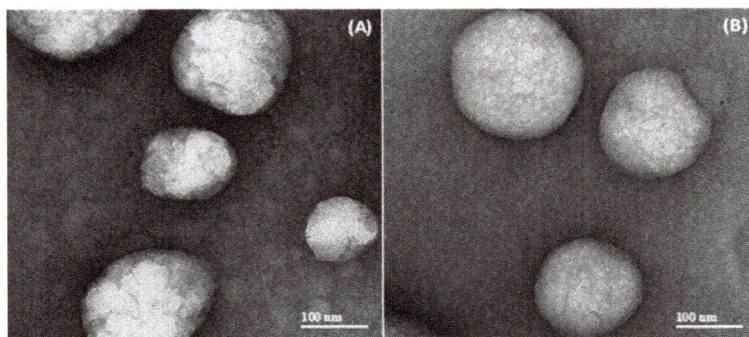

Figure 2. Transmission electron microscopy (TEM) micrographs (magnification 40,000×) of chitosan-coated lipid core nanocapsules: (**A**) $LNC_{SVT-LMWchit}$ and (**B**) $LNC_{SVT-HMWchit}$.

Concerning the nanocapsule morphology, TEM images clearly displayed spherical-shaped particles, with a core with low electron density, as expected for lipid nanocapsules. Also, from the results of the particle diameters, the images were in good agreement with the mean nanocapsule sizes determined with DLS, NTA, and LD.

3.2. Mucoadhesion Studies

To investigate the interaction between the formulations and mucin, a mucoadhesion index (MI), the PDI, and the zeta potentials of mixtures between the nanocapsules and mucin were determined for different mucin weight ratios f (Figure 3). For LNC$_{SVT-LMWchit}$ in the range of f values up to 0.3, particle sizes and MI values increased to a maximum of 474 ± 6 nm and 2.9 ± 0.1 ($f = 0.3$), respectively. Similarly, LNC$_{SVT-HMWchit}$ particle size and MI increased in the f range from 0 to 0.55, reaching a maximum of 557 ± 30 nm, 3.0 ± 0.3 ($f = 0.55$), respectively (Figure 3A). Despite the increase of the fraction by weight of mucin above f values of 0.3, for LNC$_{SVT-LMWchit}$, particle size and MI decreased to 318 ± 5 nm and 1.9 ± 0.1 for f values of 0.85. It has been hypothesized here that while at values of f of around 0.3, nanocapsules are able to form large agglomerates with mucin chains entangled and linked with more nanoparticles, above this value, the mucin is in such a large excess that almost all single particles are enrobed with mucins, leading to a decrease in the overall mean particle size. In fact, the MI values for f = 0.55 and 0.85 did not change significantly. On the other hand, for LNC$_{SVT-HMWchit}$ this decrease in the MI occurred only for f values above 0.55, with particle size and MI decreasing to 321 ± 7 nm, 1.7 ± 0.1 ($f = 0.85$). Therefore, the MI maximum was observed at lower f values (0.3) for LNC$_{SVT-LMWchit}$, and higher f values (0.55) for LNC$_{SVT-HMWchit}$, indicating a higher capacity to interact with larger quantities of mucin for nanoparticles coated with high MW chitosan, macroscopically translating to more efficient mucoadhesion.

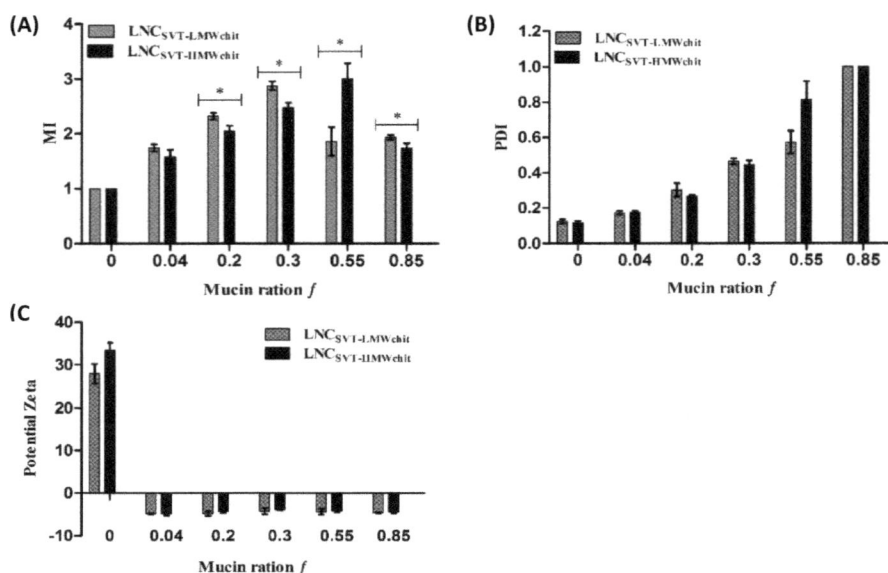

Figure 3. (A) Mucoadhesive index (MI) values, (B) PDI and (C) zeta potentials measured for various mixtures of mucin and nanocapsules. Values of the two formulations were obtained before ($f = 0$) and after incubation with different mucin weight ratios f.

The PDI before nanocapsule interaction with mucin was 0.12 ± 0.01 for LNC$_{SVT-LMWchit}$ and 0.11 ± 0.01 for LNC$_{SVT-HMWchit}$. After mixing the nanocapsules with mucin, PDI progressively increased for both formulations, up to 1 (*f* = 0.85), indicating the formation of agglomerates and the switch to highly polydispersed particle size distributions (Figure 3B). The zeta potentials of the formulations that were initially positive due to the chitosan coating immediately after interaction with even the smallest amount of mucin (*f* = 0.04), became negative for both formulations (-4.8 ± 0.1 mV for $LNC_{SVT\text{-}LMWchit}$ and -4.8 ± 0.7 mV for $LNC_{SVT\text{-}HMWchit}$) and remained roughly constant for both formulations, even with increasing f values (Figure 3C).

3.3. In Vitro Drug Release

The in vitro release profiles of the simvastatin-loaded chitosan coated lipid core nanocapsules were performed over 8 h (Figure 4). A solution of simvastatin was used as a control. It can be observed that $56.3 \pm 2.5\%$ of SVT diffused out from the dialysis bag when using the control simvastatin solution, within 8 h. On the other hand, the percentage of drug released from $LNC_{SVT\text{-}LMWchit}$ and $LNC_{SVT\text{-}HMWchit}$ after 8 h were $37.3 \pm 1.5\%$ and $31.0 \pm 1.1\%$, respectively. These results show that nanocapsules provided a controlled release of simvastatin, and that the different types of chitosan affected the drug release rate. Indeed, the release of SVT from $LNC_{SVT\text{-}HMWchit}$ was slower in comparison to the $LNC_{SVT\text{-}LMWchit}$.

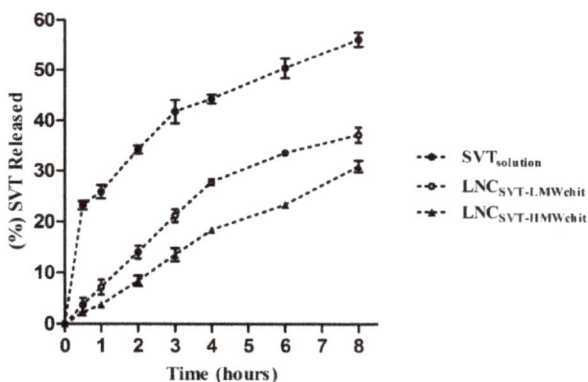

Figure 4. In vitro drug release profile from $LNC_{SVT\text{-}LMWchit}$, $LNC_{SVT\text{-}HMWchit}$ and from the control (SVT solution), using the dialysis bag method at 37 °C (*n* = 3, ± SD).

3.4. Transport Studies in a Nasal Cell Model

To confirm the potential permeability enhancement effects of the nanocapsules, the total amount of SVT transported across nasal mucosa model was determined by using RPMI2650 human nasal epithelial cells [52]. Figure 5 shows the amount of SVT transported when using the formulations, compared to a suspension of the raw material, over 4 h. After 1 h, the formulations already showed increased degrees of permeation compared to the control. However, no significant differences (*p* > 0.05) were observed at 1 h for the SVT permeation between $LNC_{SVT\text{-}LMWchit}$ and $LNC_{SVT\text{-}HMWchit}$. After the first hour however, each single time point showed an amount of SVT transported to be statistically different between the formulations (*p* < 0.05), confirming the greater permeation of $LNC_{SVT\text{-}LMWchit}$.

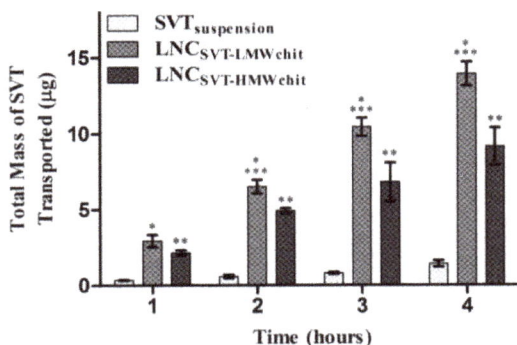

Figure 5. Amount (µg) of SVT transported across RPMI 2650 cells grown under air–liquid interface conditions ($n = 4$, $\pm$ SD). Significant difference ($p < 0.05$) is expressed considering the following comparisons: * SVT versus LNC$_{SVT-LMWchit}$, ** SVT versus LNC$_{SVT-HMWchit}$, *** LNC$_{SVT-LMWchit}$ versus LNC$_{SVT-HMWchit}$.

3.5. Ex Vivo Transport Experiments across Rabbit Nasal Mucosa

Figure 6A shows the SVT permeation across the excised rabbit nasal mucosa using Franz type vertical diffusion cells. The results of the ex vivo permeation studies on the rabbit nasal mucosa evidenced that the formulations significantly increased the permeation of SVT compared to the control. LNC$_{SVT-LMWchit}$ showed the highest percentage of SVT permeation after 4 h (19.2 $\pm$ 0.5%·cm^{-2}), followed by LNC$_{SVT-HMWchit}$ (11.0 $\pm$ 0.5%·cm^{-2}), while the control (SVT suspension) showed an extremely low degree of permeation (2.6 $\pm$ 0.2%·cm^{-2}). The results indicate that SVT permeation from LNC$_{SVT-LMWchit}$ was 1.74 and 7.4 times greater than LNC$_{SVT-HMWchit}$ and the SVT control, respectively.

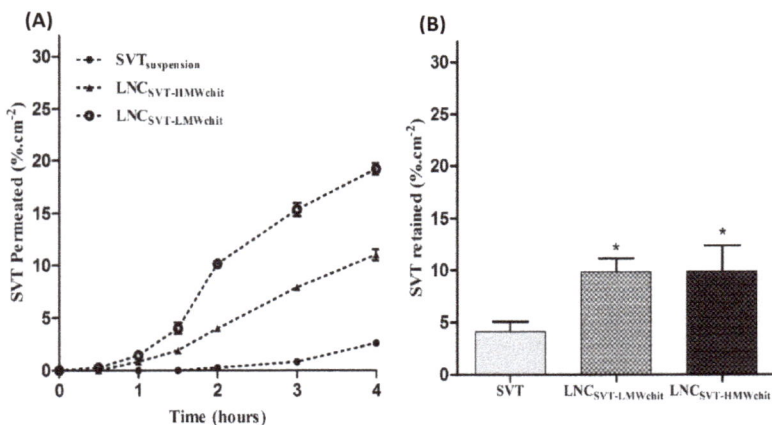

Figure 6. (**A**) Ex vivo SVT permeation across rabbit nasal mucosa up to 4 h in simulated nasal electrolytic solution (SNES) containing 0.5% of polysorbate 80 at 37 °C ($n = 3$, $\pm$ SD). (**B**) Percentage of SVT retained in nasal mucosa after 4 h of the permeation test in Franz-type diffusion cells ($n = 3$, $\pm$ SD). Asterisk (*) indicates significant differences between SVT versus LNC$_{SVT-LMWchit}$ and LNC$_{SVT-HMWchit}$.

The results of SVT retained in the mucosa tissue after 4 h experimental time are shown in Figure 6B. It can be seen that there was better retention of both formulations with respect to the control. The SVT fraction found in the tissue for the control was 4.2 $\pm$ 0.9%·cm^{-2}, while in the case of LNC$_{SVT-LMWchit}$ and LNC$_{SVT-HMWchit}$, the fraction of simvastatin found in the tissue was more than doubled, i.e., 9.8 ± 1.3 and $9.9 \pm 2.5\% \cdot cm^{-2}$, respectively. In this case, the difference between the amount of retained SVT from $LNC_{SVT-LMWchit}$ and $LNC_{SVT-HMWchit}$ was not statistically significant.

3.6. Preliminary Nasal Toxicity Studies

Nasal mucosa histopathology studies were performed to assess the integrity of the rabbit mucosa after 4 h of the permeation test. As shown in Figure 7, the mucosa treated with PBS pH 6.4 (negative control), SVT, $LNC_{SVT-LMWchit}$, and $LNC_{SVT-HMWchit}$ did not show any evident structural damage. The results from histological examinations indicated that the LNC nanocapsules did not cause any irritation or toxicity, and they can be considered to be biocompatible for nasal administration.

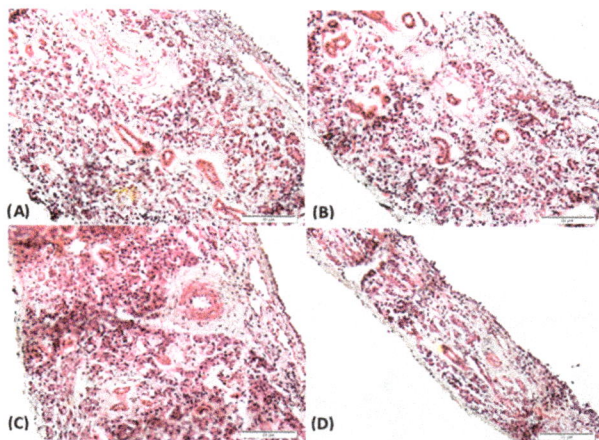

Figure 7. Histopathological sections of rabbit nasal mucosa after 4 h of permeation test in Franz-type diffusion cells treated with (**A**) PBS pH 6.4 (negative control), (**B**) SVT, (**C**) $LNC_{SVT-LMWchit}$, and (**D**) $LNC_{SVT-HMWchit}$. Sections are stained with hematoxylin and eosin.

4. Discussion

Over the past couple of decades, pharmaceutical nanotechnology has received considerable attention and demonstrated significant potential for the development of innovative medicinal products, both for the therapy and the diagnosis of severe diseases [59]. In this work, we report a new preparation method of lipid-core PCL nanocapsules, optimizing a two-step process (self-assembly step followed by a coating step) into a one-pot technique to develop chitosan-coated nanoparticles. Moreover, we compared the pharmaceutically relevant properties in terms of physicochemical characterization, mucoadhesive properties, drug release, and permeability studies of $LNC_{SVT-LMWchit}$ and $LNC_{SVT-HMWchit}$ coated by chitosan with low MW and high MW, in view of a nose-to-brain administration.

Polymeric nanocapsules containing poly(ε-caprolactone), capric/caprylic triglyceride, and sorbitan monostearate, and coated with chitosan, were developed. This formulation has the advantage of efficiently encapsulating lipophilic drugs such as simvastatin [34,35]. The production of positively-coated lipid-core nanocapsules in one step, avoiding the use of non-ionic surfactants in the aqueous phase, is the main novelty of this approach. Previously, we developed mucoadhesive amphiphilic nanocapsules based on a blend of PCL and poly(methyl methacrylate-b-2-(dimethylamino)ethyl methacrylate) for the nose-to-brain delivery of olanzapine. Nevertheless, the self-assembly of the nanocapsules by using this block copolymer (positive surface) avoids the use of sorbitan monostearate in the formulation. Indeed, the cores of those nanocapsules are composed exclusively of medium-chain triglycerides [29]. Sorbitan monostearate dispersed in core of the lipid-core nanocapsules has been demonstrated to provide an addition diffusional barrier to control the drug release, and an increase of the rigidity of the nanocapsules polymer wall [34,36]. Furthermore, a comparative study conducted with polymeric nanocapsules demonstrated that the presence of sorbitan monostearate instead of sorbitan monooleate in the core improved the anti-apoptotic and antioxidant effects of melatonin during bovine embryo development [60]. In the present development, it was possible to obtain in a one-step process, lipid-core nanocapsules incorporating sorbitan monostearate in the oily core, and decorated on the surface with chitosan, providing mucoadhesion and penetration-enhancing properties that appear to be fundamental for nose-to-brain delivery [21].

The combination between the composition and the interfacial deposition of the pre-formed polymer method produced nanocapsules with adequate particle sizes and narrow size distributions, as was confirmed by complementary techniques such as laser diffraction, DLS, and NTA. Besides that, coating the nanocapsules with chitosan with different molecular weights (21 kDa and 152 kDa) influenced their pharmaceutical properties. For example, chitosan molecular weight and viscosity in water affected the sizes of the nanoparticles. In fact, particle size could be reduced by using lower molecular weight chitosan [61,62]. Actually, for $LNC_{SVT\text{-}HMWchit}$, the higher mean particle hydrodynamic diameter could be attributed to the lengths of the chains of chitosan present on the particle surface, possibly expanding the water hydration shell of the nanoparticle. In addition, low-MW chitosan has been reported to have a higher aqueous solubility, and this, together with shorter polymer chains, contributes to forming smaller particles compared to high-MW chitosan [63]. The positive zeta potential obtained for all formulations is evidence of the polysaccharide coating. Furthermore, using different chitosan types did not cause significant changes in the zeta potentials of both formulations, probably due of a similar degree of deacetylation (95%) [64]. Mucoadhesive polymers such as chitosan represent a significant strategy for overcoming the nasal drug delivery limits of low membrane permeability, short residence time, and mucociliary clearance. The presence of polysaccharides on the nanocapsule surface is expected to prolong the permanence of the formulation in the nasal cavity, open the tight junctions between the nasal epithelial cells, and promote drug permeation through the biological barriers, granting access to the CNS [65–67]. For these reasons, the evaluation of the ability of nanocapsules to interact with mucin is of great interest for nasal administration. Mucous membranes internally delimit the body cavities (stomach, esophagus, cornea, oral cavity, reproductive and respiratory tracts), and are characterized by a superficial mucus layer with protective and lubricating functions [68]. The mucus is composed of water (approximately 95%), lipids, inorganic salts, and mucin, a glycoprotein composed of *N*-acetylgalactosamine, *N*-acetylglucosamine, fucose, galactose, and sialic acid, which is responsible for the adhesive properties and the viscosity of the mucus [66]. Lipophilic drugs show an affinity for mucus glycoproteins, reducing their adsorption and the bioavailability. This issue, together with the drugs' poor aqueous solubilities, are limiting factors for the nose-to-brain delivery of lipophilic drugs. To improve the transport of SVT through this barrier, we used nanoparticles as a drug delivery system [69].

Our results showed how, for both formulations, particle size and MI increased with the increase in the mucin weight ratio, to a critical point. A previous study [50] has led to the conclusion that the nanoparticles in mucin solution form agglomerates in which the nanoparticles are the points of contact between negatively charged mucin chains. Beyond the critical value of the mucin ratio, the repulsive forces among the mucin chains break these agglomerates. Our results support this theory; nevertheless it has to be stressed that the decrease of MI observed for high mucin weight ratio does not indicate a decrease in the mucoadhesive capacity of the formulations [50]. However, the results indicate how in mucin excess, smaller aggregates are formed in order to minimize the repulsive forces between the chains of mucin, and to maximize the points of contact between the positive charges of chitosan and the negative charges of the mucin chains. Moreover, it was noticed that the critical point of the formulations was different for the nanocapsules coated with chitosan with different characteristics ($LNC_{SVT\text{-}LMWchit}$ $f = 0.3$ and for $LNC_{SVT\text{-}HMWchit}$ $f = 0.55$). This difference could be attributed to the different chain lengths of the two chitosan batches [63]. Indeed, in a previous study conducted with a different method, Menchicchi and co-authors proposed that mucin interacts mostly with high molecular weight chitosan [70]. On the other hand, the results presented in this paper, compared to similarly uncoated LNC, demonstrate a large increase in the mucoadhesive capacity, due to the presence of chitosan. The uncoated LNC showed values of MI = 1.4, PDI = 0.51, and a zeta potential of −9.5 mV after contact with the maximum concentration of mucin (0.5% w/v) [71]. The PDI increase with the increase in the f mucin ratio corroborates the above-mentioned explanation. In fact, PDI results indicated that the heterogeneity of the distribution of the particle size in solution increased along with the mucin weight ratio, because of the formation of aggregates of different sizes. The oligosaccharide chains of mucin glycoproteins presenting terminal sialic acid residues confer a negative charge to the molecule; therefore, the variation of the particle zeta potential from positive to negative values demonstrates how the mucin enrobes the nanocapsules interacting with their surface layer of chitosan. This suggests that mucoadhesion mechanism is driven by the electrostatic interaction of the positively charged amine groups of D-glucosamine molecules of chitosan with the negatively charged sialic acid residues of mucin [72].

The SVT-loaded lipid core nanocapsules formulation was able to control drug release, due to the two diffusional barriers: the PCL polymer wall and the lipid dispersion present in the nanocapsule core. The nanoencapsulation reduced the diffusion rate of SVT across a dialysis membrane, confirming data that is frequently described in the literature as a property of polymeric nanoparticles [33]. Regarding the comparison between the two formulations, LNC$_{SVT-HMWchit}$ afforded better control of drug release. In order to explain the different release profiles, we evaluated the differences in terms of their physicochemical properties. Firstly, this can be explained by the higher viscosity of the chitosan used to develop the LNC$_{SVT-HMWchit}$. Previous studies demonstrated that the viscosity of the chitosan is an important factor for modulating the release control [73]. Moreover, nanoparticle size can influence in the release profile, which increases with decreasing particle size. Indeed, LNC$_{SVT-LMWchit}$ had a lower mean particle diameter than LNC$_{SVT-HMWchit}$, which could contribute to explaining their different release profiles, because of the greater available surface area [74,75].

The permeation across the RPMI 2650 human nasal cell line showed that the SVT transported across the nasal cell model by LNC$_{SVT-LMWchit}$ and LNC$_{SVT-HMWchit}$ can enhance drug transport across a cell pseudo-monolayer that also secretes mucin on its apical surface. The increase of SVT permeation across the human nasal cell layer can be explained by different mechanisms. In literature, chitosan is associated with an opening of tight junctions that increase cell layer permeability. However, this mechanism generally favors the permeation of water-soluble drugs, and it has been evidenced that it is slightly less efficient for chitosan bound to nanoparticles, compared to simple polysaccharide solutions [76]. More recently, it has been demonstrated that the biodegradation of nanocapsules by enzymes in the mucus barrier or intracellularly could be pivotal in enhancing the transcellular transport of lipophilic drugs [77]. The results of the ex vivo permeation studies on rabbit nasal mucosa confirmed and further added evidence for the fact that the nanoencapsulation of SVT significantly increased its permeation across excised nasal mucosa. In this case, the higher permeation evidenced for LNC$_{SVT-LMWchit}$ could be explained by a combination of factors. The smaller particle sizes of nanocapsules coated with low molecular weight chitosan could have facilitated its absorption into the mucosal tissue as reported before [78]. Moreover, an important factor is the bioadhesion of the nanostructures, as previously explained, given by the particles shell of chitosan, which interacts with electrostatic forces at the anionic sites of the nasal mucus [65]. However, from the mucoadhesion data, a better interaction with mucus could be expected from nanocapsules coated with the high molecular weight chitosan. However, the slower release kinetics evidenced for these particles have probably contributed to limiting the amount of drug permeated, especially considering that drug accumulation into the tissue is superimposable for the two nanocapsule formulations.

Previous findings [79,80], agree that chitosan-coated nanoparticles increase drug permeation across the nasal mucosa, compared to the free drug control. This controlled SVT permeation, together with the mucoadhesion effects, may be an important strategy for prolonging the effects of the drug when it is administered via the nasal route.

5. Conclusions

In the present investigation, the coating process of lipid-core nanocapsules, using a one-pot technique approach, was presented. Furthermore, two chitosan-coated simvastatin-loaded lipid core nanocapsules suitable for nasal administration were successfully developed. Both the nanoparticles produced with different types of chitosan were designed to have adequate physicochemical and mucoadhesive properties for a potential nose-to-brain application. The formulations prepared combine a controlled release of simvastatin, and mucoadhesion properties that are able to increase drug permeation across the nasal mucosa, as demonstrated by using two different models of nasal epithelium. In summary, simvastatin-loaded chitosan-coated lipid core nanocapsules seem to be a promising mucoadhesive system for the nose-to-brain delivery of poorly soluble anticancer drugs. Follow up studies will focus on the investigation of the potential of these nanoparticles for the treatment of brain tumors, involving studies with glioma cells, and an orthotopic intracranial tumor model in mice.

Author Contributions: Conceptualization, A.R.P., S.S.G., and F.S.; Methodology, F.A.B., S.P., T.A., G.D.S., G.G.P., M.M., L.T.F.; Investigation, F.A.B., S.P.; Resources, A.R.P., S.S.G.; Writing—Original Draft Preparation, F.A.B., S.P.; Writing—Review & Editing, F.A.B., F.S.; Supervision, A.B., G.C., F.S.

Funding: Franciele Aline Bruinsmann, Fabio Sonvico, Adriana Raffin Pohlmann, and Silvia Stanisçuaski Guterres would like to acknowledge the Brazilian government, as recipients of CNPq grants in the programs "Ciências sem Fronteiras" (BOLSA PESQUISADOR VISITANTE ESPECIAL—PVE 401196/2014-3) and "Produtividade em Pesquisa". This study was financed in part by the Coordenação de Aperfeiçoamento de Pessoal de Nível Superior—Brasil (CAPES)—Finance Code 001.

Conflicts of Interest: The authors declare no conflict of interest.

References

1. Chiang, K.H.; Cheng, W.L.; Shih, C.M.; Lin, Y.W.; Tsao, N.W.; Kao, Y.T.; Lin, C.T.; Wu, S.C.; Huang, C.Y.; Lin, F.Y. Statins, HMG-CoA Reductase Inhibitors, Improve Neovascularization by Increasing the Expression Density of CXCR4 in Endothelial Progenitor Cells. *PLoS ONE* **2015**, *10*, e0136405. [CrossRef] [PubMed]
2. Liao, J.K.; Ulrich, L. Pleiotropic effects of statins. *Annu. Rev. Pharmacol. Toxicol.* **2005**, *45*, 89–118. [CrossRef] [PubMed]
3. Davies, J.T.; Delfino, S.F.; Feinberg, C.E.; Johnson, M.F.; Nappi, V.L.; Olinger, J.T.; Schwab, A.P.; Swanson, H.I. Current and Emerging Uses of Statins in Clinical Therapeutics: A Review. *Lipid Insights* **2016**, *9*, 13–29. [CrossRef] [PubMed]
4. Jain, M.K.; Ridker, P.M. Anti-inflammatory effects of statins: Clinical evidence and basic mechanisms. *Nat. Rev. Drug Discov.* **2005**, *4*, 977–987. [CrossRef] [PubMed]
5. Liao, K.J. Isoprenoids as mediators of the biological effects of statins. *J. Clin. Investig.* **2002**, *110*, 285–288. [CrossRef] [PubMed]
6. Tanaka, S.; Fukumoto, Y.; Nochioka, K.; Minami, T.; Kudo, S.; Shiba, N.; Shimokawa, H. Statins exert the pleiotropic effects through small GTP-binding protein dissociation stimulator upregulation with a resultant Rac1 degradation. *Arter. Thromb. Vasc. Biol.* **2013**, *33*, 1591–1600. [CrossRef] [PubMed]
7. Hindler, K.; Cleeland, C.S.; Rivera, E.; Collard, C.D. The role of statins in cancer therapy. *Oncologist* **2006**, *11*, 306–315. [CrossRef] [PubMed]
8. Altwairgi, A.K. Statins are potential anticancerous agents (Review). *Oncol. Rep.* **2015**, *33*, 1019–1039. [CrossRef] [PubMed]
9. Gazzerro, P.; Proto, M.C.; Gangemi, G.; Malfitano, A.M.; Ciaglia, E.; Pisanti, S.; Santoro, A.; Laezza, C.; Bifulco, M. Pharmacological actions of statins: a critical appraisal in the management of cancer. *Pharmacol. Rev.* **2012**, *64*, 102–146. [CrossRef] [PubMed]
10. Wejde, J.; Hjertman, M.; Carlberg, M.; Egestad, B.; Griffiths, W.J.; Sjövall, J.; Larsson, O. Dolichol-like lipids with stimulatory effect on DNA synthesis: substrates for protein dolichylation. *J. Cell Biochem.* **1998**, *71*, 502–514. [CrossRef]

11. Bifulco, M. Therapeutic potential of statins in thyroid proliferative disease. *Nat. Clin. Pract. Endocrinol. Metab.* **2008**, *4*, 242–243. [CrossRef] [PubMed]

12. Chan, K.K.; Oza, A.M.; Siu, L.L. The statins as anticancer agents. *Clin. Cancer Res.* **2003**, *9*, 10–19. [PubMed]

13. Frick, M.; Dulak, J.; Cisowski, J.; Jozkowicz, A.; Zwick, R.; Alber, H.; Dichtl, W.; Schwarzacher, S.P.; Pachinger, O.; Weidinger, F. Statins differentially regulate vascular endothelial growth factor synthesis in endothelial and vascular smooth muscle cells. *Atherosclerosis* **2003**, *170*, 229–236. [CrossRef]

14. Denoyelle, C.; Vasse, M.; Körner, M.; Mishal, Z.; Ganné, F.; Vannier, J.P.; Soria, J.; Soria, C. Cerivastatin, an inhibitor of HMG-CoA reductase, inhibits the signaling pathways involved in the invasiveness and metastatic properties of highly invasive breast cancer cell lines: an in vitro study. *Carcinogenesis* **2001**, *22*, 1139–1148. [CrossRef] [PubMed]

15. Yanae, M.; Tsubaki, M.; Satou, T.; Itoh, T.; Imano, M.; Yamazoe, Y.; Nishida, S. Statin-induced apoptosis via the suppression of ERK1/2 and Akt activation by inhibition of the geranylgeranyl-pyrophosphate biosynthesis in glioblastoma. *J. Exp. Clin. Cancer Res.* **2011**, *30*, 74. [CrossRef] [PubMed]

16. Wu, H.; Jiang, H.; Lu, D.; Xiong, Y.; Qu, C.; Zhou, D.; Mahmood, A.; Chopp, M. Effect of simvastatin on glioma cell proliferation, migration, and apoptosis. *Neurosurgery* **2009**, *65*, 1087–1096. [CrossRef] [PubMed]

17. Bababeygy, S.R.; Polevaya, N.V.; Youssef, S.; Sun, A.; Xiong, A.; Prugpichailers, T.; Veeravagu, A.; Hou, L.C.; Steinman, L.; Tse, V. HMG-CoA Reductase Inhibition Causes Increased Necrosis and Apoptosis in an In Vivo Mouse Glioblastoma Multiforme Model. *Anticancer Res.* **2009**, *29*, 4901–4908. [PubMed]

18. Parrish, K.E.; Sarkaria, J.N.; Elmquist, W.F. Improving drug delivery to primary and metastatic brain tumors: strategies to overcome the blood-brain barrier. *Clin. Pharmacol. Ther.* **2015**, *97*, 336–346. [CrossRef] [PubMed]

19. Romana, B.; Batger, M.; Prestidge, C.A.; Colombo, G.; Sonvico, F. Expanding the therapeutic potential of statins by means of nanotechnology enabled drug delivery systems. *Curr. Top. Med. Chem.* **2014**, *14*, 1182–1193. [CrossRef] [PubMed]

20. Mittal, D.; Ali, A.; Md, S.; Baboota, S.; Sahni, J.K.; Ali, J. Insights into direct nose to brain delivery: current status and future perspective. *Drug Deliv.* **2014**, *21*, 75–86. [CrossRef] [PubMed]

21. Sonvico, F.; Clementino, A.; Buttini, F.; Colombo, G.; Pescina, S.; Guterres, S.S.; Pohlmann, A.R.; Nicoli, S. Surface-Modified Nanocarriers for Nose-to-Brain Delivery: From Bioadhesion to Targeting. *Pharmaceutics* **2018**, *10*, 34. [CrossRef] [PubMed]

22. Bernardi, A.; Braganhol, E.; Jäger, E.; Figueiró, F.; Edelweiss, M.I.; Pohlmann, A.R.; Guterres, S.S.; Battastini, A.M. Indomethacin-loaded nanocapsules treatment reduces in vivo glioblastoma growth in a rat glioma model. *Cancer Lett.* **2009**, *281*, 53–63. [CrossRef] [PubMed]

23. Patel, T.; Zhou, J.; Piepmeier, J.M.; Saltzman, W.M. Polymeric Nanoparticles for Drug Delivery to the Central Nervous System. *Adv. Drug Deliv. Rev.* **2012**, *64*, 701–705. [CrossRef] [PubMed]

24. Rodrigues, S.F.; Fiel, L.A.; Shimada, A.L.; Pereira, N.R.; Guterres, S.S.; Pohlmann, A.R.; Farsky, S.H. Lipid-Core Nanocapsules Act as a Drug Shuttle Through the Blood Brain Barrier and Reduce Glioblastoma After Intravenous or Oral Administration. *J. Biomed. Nanotechnol.* **2016**, *12*, 986–1000. [CrossRef] [PubMed]

25. Bahadur, S.; Pathak, K. Physicochemical and physiological considerations for efficient nose-to-brain targeting. *Expert Opin. Drug Deliv.* **2012**, *9*, 19–31. [CrossRef] [PubMed]

26. Comfort, C.; Garrastazu, G.; Pozzoli, M.; Sonvico, F. Opportunities and challenges for the nasal administration of nanoemulsions. *Curr. Top. Med. Chem.* **2015**, *15*, 356–368. [CrossRef] [PubMed]

27. Illum, L. Nasal drug delivery-possibilities, problems and solutions. *J. Control. Release* **2003**, *87*, 187–198. [CrossRef]

28. Prego, C.; Torres, D.; Alonso, M.J. Chitosan nanocapsules: a new carrier for nasal peptide delivery. *J. Nanosci. Nanotechnol.* **2006**, *6*, 2921–2928. [CrossRef] [PubMed]

29. Fonseca, F.N.; Betti, A.H.; Carvalho, F.C.; Gremião, M.P.; Dimer, F.A.; Guterres, S.S.; Tebaldi, M.L.; Rates, S.M.; Pohlmann, A.R. Mucoadhesive Amphiphilic Methacrylic Copolymer-Functionalized Poly(ε-caprolactone) Nanocapsules for Nose-to-Brain Delivery of Olanzapine. *Biomed. Nanotechnol.* **2015**, *11*, 1472–1481. [CrossRef]

30. Clementino, A.; Batger, M.; Garrastazu, G.; Pozzoli, M.; Del Favero, E.; Rondelli, V.; Gutfilen, B.; Barboza, T.; Sukkar, M.B.; Souza, S.A.; et al. The nasal delivery of nanoencapsulated statins—an approach for brain delivery. *Int. J. Nanomed.* **2016**, *11*, 6575–6590. [CrossRef] [PubMed]

31. Couvreur, P.; Barratt, G.; Fattal, E.; Vauthier, C. Nanocapsule Technology: A Review. *Crit. Rev. Ther. Drug Carrier Syst.* **2002**, *19*, 99–134. [CrossRef] [PubMed]

32. Mora-Huertas, C.E.; Fessi, H.; Elaissari, A. Polymer-based nanocapsules for drug delivery. *Int. J. Pharm.* **2010**, *385*, 113–142. [CrossRef] [PubMed]

33. Pohlmann, A.R.; Fonseca, F.N.; Paese, K.; Detoni, C.B.; Coradini, K.; Beck, R.C.; Guterres, S.S. Poly(e-caprolactone) microcapsules and nanocapsules in drug delivery. *Expert Opin. Drug Deliv.* **2013**, *10*, 623–638. [CrossRef] [PubMed]

34. Jäger, E.; Venturini, C.G.; Poletto, F.S.; Colomé, L.M.; Pohlmann, J.P.; Bernardi, A.; Battastini, A.M.; Guterres, S.S.; Pohlmann, A.R. Sustained release from lipid-core nanocapsules by varying the core viscosity and the particle surface area. *J. Biomed. Nanotechnol.* **2009**, *5*, 130–140. [CrossRef] [PubMed]

35. Venturini, C.G.; Jäger, E.; Oliveira, C.P.; Bernardi, A.; Battastini, A.M.O.; Guterres, S.S.; Pohlmann, A.R. Formulation of lipid core nanocapsules. *Colloids Surf. A Physicochem. Eng. Asp.* **2011**, *375*, 200–208. [CrossRef]

36. Fiel, L.A.; Rebêlo, L.M.; Santiago, T.M.; Adorne, M.D.; Guterres, S.S.; Sousa, J.S.; Pohlmann, A.R. Diverse Deformation Properties of Polymeric Nanocapsules and Lipid-Core Nanocapsules. *Soft Matter* **2011**, *7*, 7240–7247. [CrossRef]

37. Frozza, R.L.; Bernardi, A.; Paese, K.; Hoppe, J.B.; da Silva, T.; Battastini, A.M.; Pohlmann, A.R.; Guterres, S.S.; Salbego, C. Characterization of trans-resveratrol-loaded lipid-core nanocapsules and tissue distribution studies in rats. *J. Biomed. Nanotechnol.* **2010**, *6*, 694–703. [CrossRef] [PubMed]

38. Zanotto-Filho, A.; Coradini, K.; Braganhol, E.; Schröder, R.; de Oliveira, C.M.; Simões-Pires, A.; Battastini, A.M.; Pohlmann, A.R.; Guterres, S.S.; Forcelini, C.M.; et al. Curcumin-loaded lipid-core nanocapsules as a strategy to improve pharmacological efficacy of curcumin in glioma treatment. *Eur. J. Pharm. Biopharm.* **2013**, *83*, 156–167. [CrossRef] [PubMed]

39. Dimer, F.A.; Ortiz, M.; Pase, C.S.; Roversi, K.; Friedrich, R.B.; Pohlmann, A.R.; Burger, M.E.; Guterres, S.S. Nanoencapsulation of Olanzapine Increases Its Efficacy in Antipsychotic Treatment and Reduces Adverse Effects. *J. Biomed. Nanotechnol.* **2014**, *10*, 1137–1145. [CrossRef] [PubMed]

40. Figueiró, F.; Bernardi, A.; Frozza, R.L.; Terroso, T.; Zanotto-Filho, A.; Jandrey, E.H.; Moreira, J.C.; Salbego, C.G.; Edelweiss, M.I.; Pohlmann, A.R.; et al. Resveratrol-loaded lipid-core nanocapsules treatment reduces in vitro and in vivo glioma growth. *J. Biomed. Nanotechnol.* **2013**, *9*, 516–526.

41. Figueiró, F.; de Oliveira, C.P.; Rockenbach, L.; Mendes, F.B.; Bergamin, L.S.; Jandrey, E.H.; Edelweiss, M.I.; Guterres, S.S.; Pohlmann, A.R.; Battastini, A.M. Pharmacological Improvement and Preclinical Evaluation of Methotrexate-Loaded Lipid-Core Nanocapsules in a Glioblastoma Model. *J. Biomed. Nanotechnol.* **2015**, *11*, 1808–1818. [CrossRef] [PubMed]

42. Drewes, C.C.; Fiel, L.A.; Bexiga, C.G.; Asbahr, A.C.; Uchiyama, M.K.; Cogliati, B.; Araki, K.; Guterres, S.S.; Pohlmann, A.R.; Farsky, S.P. Novel therapeutic mechanisms determine the effectiveness of lipid-core nanocapsules on melanoma models. *Int. J. Nanomed.* **2016**, *11*, 1261–1279. [PubMed]

43. Bender, E.A.; Adorne, M.D.; Colomé, L.M.; Abdalla, D.S.P.; Guterres, S.S.; Pohlmann, A.R. Hemocompatibility of poly(epsilon-caprolactone) lipid-core nanocapsules stabilized with polysorbate 80-lecithin and uncoated or coated with chitosan. *Int. J. Pharm.* **2012**, *426*, 271–279. [CrossRef] [PubMed]

44. Muxika, A.; Etxabide, A.; Uranga, J.; Guerrero, P.; De la Caba, K. Chitosan as a bioactive polymer: Processing, properties and applications. *Int. J. Biol. Macromol.* **2017**, *105*, 1358–1368. [CrossRef] [PubMed]

45. Kim, I.Y.; Seo, S.J.; Moon, H.S.; Yoo, M.K.; Park, I.Y.; Kim, B.C.; Cho, C.S. Chitosan and its derivatives for tissue engineering applications. *Biotechnol. Adv.* **2008**, *26*, 1–21. [CrossRef] [PubMed]

46. Rodrigues, S.; Dionísio, M.; López, C.R.; Grenha, A. Biocompatibility of Chitosan Carriers with Application in Drug Delivery. *J. Funct. Biomater.* **2012**, *3*, 615–641. [CrossRef] [PubMed]

47. Ways, T.M.M; Lau, W.M.; Khutoryanskiy, V.V. Chitosan and Its Derivatives for Application in Mucoadhesive Drug Delivery Systems. *Polymers* **2018**, *10*, 267. [CrossRef]

48. Ali, A.; Ahmed, S. A review on chitosan and its nanocomposites in drug delivery. *Int. J. Biol. Macromol.* **2018**, *109*, 273–286. [CrossRef] [PubMed]

49. Bernkop-Schnürch, A.; Dünnhaupt, S. Chitosan-based drug delivery systems. *Eur. J. Pharm. Biopharm.* **2012**, *81*, 463–469. [CrossRef] [PubMed]

50. Eliyahu, S.; Aharon, A.; Bianco-Peled, H. Acrylated Chitosan Nanoparticles with Enhanced Mucoadhesion. *Polymers* **2018**, *10*, 106. [CrossRef]

51. Castile, J.; Cheng, Y.H.; Simmons, B.; Perelman, M.; Smith, A.; Watts, P. Development of in vitro models to demonstrate the ability of PecSys®, an in situ nasal gelling technology, to reduce nasal run-off and drip. *Drug Dev. Ind. Pharm.* **2013**, *39*, 816–824. [CrossRef] [PubMed]

52. Pozzoli, M.; Ong, H.X.; Morgan, L.; Sukkar, M.; Traini, D.; Young, P.M.; Sonvico, F. Application of RPMI 2650 nasal cell model to a 3D printed apparatus for the testing of drug deposition and permeation of nasal products. *Eur. J. Pharm. Biopharm.* **2016**, *107*, 223–233. [CrossRef] [PubMed]
53. Bortolotti, F.; Balducci, A.G.; Sonvico, F.; Russo, P.; Colombo, G. In vitro permeation of desmopressin across rabbit nasal mucosa from liquid nasal sprays: the enhancing effect of potassium sorbate. *Eur. J. Pharm. Sci.* **2009**, *37*, 36–42. [PubMed]
54. Vaz, G.R.; Hädrich, G.; Bidone, J.; Rodrigues, J.L.; Falkembach, M.C.; Putaux, J.L.; Hort, M.A.; Monserrat, J.M.; Varela Junior, A.S.; Teixeira, H.F.; et al. Development of Nasal Lipid Nanocarriers Containing Curcumin for Brain Targeting. *J. Alzheimers Dis.* **2017**, *59*, 961–974. [CrossRef] [PubMed]
55. Oliveira, P.; Venturini, C.G.; Donida, B.; Poletto, F.S.; Guterres, S.S.; Pohlmann, A.R. An algorithm to determine the mechanism of drug distribution in lipid-core nanocapsule formulations. *Soft Matter* **2013**, *9*, 1141–1150. [CrossRef]
56. Bianchin, M.D.; Külkamp-Guerreiro, I.C.; Oliveira, C.P.; Contri, R.V.; Guterres, S.S.; Pohlmann, A.R. Radar charts based on particle sizing as an approach to establish the fingerprints of polymeric nanoparticles in aqueous formulations. *J. Drug Deliv. Sci. Technol.* **2016**, *30*, 180–189. [CrossRef]
57. Frank, L.A.; Chaves, P.S.; D'Amore, C.M.; Contri, R.V.; Frank, A.G.; Beck, R.C.; Pohlmann, A.R.; Buffon, A.; Guterres, S.S. The use of chitosan as cationic coating or gel vehicle for polymeric nanocapsules: Increasing penetration and adhesion of imiquimod in vaginal tissue. *Eur. J. Pharm. Biopharm.* **2017**, *114*, 202–212. [CrossRef] [PubMed]
58. Gouda, M.; Elayaan, U.; Youssef, M.M. Synthesis and Biological Activity of Drug Delivery System Based on Chitosan Nanocapsules. *Adv. Nanopart.* **2014**, *3*, 148–158. [CrossRef]
59. Mir, M.; Ishtiaq, S.; Rabia, S.; Khatoon, M.; Zeb, A.; Khan, G.M.; Ur Rehman, A.; Ud Din, F. Nanotechnology: from In Vivo Imaging System to Controlled Drug Delivery. *Nanoscale Res. Lett.* **2017**, *12*, 500. [CrossRef] [PubMed]
60. Komninou, E.R.; Remião, M.H.; Lucas, C.G.; Domingues, W.B.; Basso, A.C.; Jornada, D.S.; Deschamps, J.C.; Beck, R.C.; Pohlmann, A.R.; Bordignon, V.; et al. Effects of Two Types of Melatonin-Loaded Nanocapsules with Distinct Supramolecular Structures: Polymeric (NC) and Lipid-Core Nanocapsules (LNC) on Bovine Embryo Culture Model. *PLoS ONE* **2016**, *11*, e0157561. [CrossRef] [PubMed]
61. Haliza, K.; Alpar, H.O. Development and characterization of chitosan nanoparticles for siRNA delivery. *J. Control. Release* **2006**, *115*, 216–225.
62. Sonvico, F.; Cagnani, A.; Rossi, A.; Motta, S.; Di Bari, M.T.; Cavatorta, F.; Alonso, M.J.; Deriu, A.; Colombo, P. Formation of self-organized nanoparticles by lecithin/chitosan ionic interaction. *Int. J. Pharm.* **2006**, *324*, 67–73. [CrossRef] [PubMed]
63. Zaki, S.S.O.; Ibrahim, M.N.; Katas, H. Particle Size Affects Concentration-Dependent Cytotoxicity of Chitosan Nanoparticles towards Mouse Hematopoietic Stem Cells. *J. Nanotechnol.* **2015**, *15*, 1–5.
64. Huang, M.; Khor, E.; Lim, L.Y. Uptake and cytotoxicity of chitosan molecules and nanoparticles: Effects of molecular weight and degree of deacetylation. *Pharm. Res.* **2004**, *21*, 344–353. [CrossRef] [PubMed]
65. Casettari, L.; Illum, L. Chitosan in nasal delivery systems for therapeutic drugs. *J. Control. Release* **2014**, *190*, 189–200. [CrossRef] [PubMed]
66. Mazzarino, L.; Coche-Guérente, L.; Labbé, P.; Lemos-Senna, E.; Borsali, R. On the mucoadhesive properties of chitosan-coated polycaprolactone nanoparticles loaded with curcumin using quartz crystal microbalance with dissipation monitoring. *J. Biomed. Nanotechnol.* **2014**, *10*, 787–794. [CrossRef] [PubMed]
67. Mistry, A.; Stolnik, S.; Illum, L. Nanoparticles for direct nose-to-brain delivery of drugs. *Int. J. Pharm.* **2009**, *379*, 146–157. [CrossRef] [PubMed]
68. Sosnik, A.J.; Neves, J.; Sarmento, B. Mucoadhesive polymers in the design of nano-drug delivery systems for administration by non-parenteral routes: A review. *Prog. Polym. Sci.* **2014**, *39*, 2030–2075. [CrossRef]
69. Sigurdsson, H.H.; Kirch, J.; Lehr, C.M. Mucus as a barrier to lipophilic drugs. *Int. J. Pharm.* **2013**, *453*, 56–64. [CrossRef] [PubMed]
70. Menchicchi, B.; Fuenzalida, J.P.; Bobbili, K.B.; Hensel, A.; Swamy, M.J.; Goycoolea, F.M. Structure of chitosan determines its interactions with mucin. *Biomacromolecules* **2014**, *15*, 3550–3558. [CrossRef] [PubMed]
71. Chaves, P.D.; Ourique, A.F.; Frank, L.A.; Pohlmann, A.R.; Guterres, S.S.; Beck, R.C. Carvedilol-loaded nanocapsules: Mucoadhesive properties and permeability across the sublingual mucosa. *Eur. J. Pharm. Biopharm.* **2017**, *114*, 88–95. [CrossRef] [PubMed]

72. Singh, I.; Rana, V. Enhancement of Mucoadhesive Property of Polymers for Drug Delivery Applications: A Critical Review. *Rev. Adhesion Adhesives* **2013**, *1*, 271–290. [CrossRef]
73. Chiou, S.H.; Wu, W.T.; Huang, Y.Y.; Chung, T.W. Effects of the characteristics of chitosan on controlling drug release of chitosan coated PLLA microspheres. *J. Microencapsul.* **2001**, *18*, 613–625. [PubMed]
74. Trotta, M.; Cavalli, R.; Chirio, D. Griseofulvin nanosuspension from triacetin-in-water emulsions. *S.T.P. Pharma Sci.* **2003**, *13*, 423–426.
75. Zili, Z.; Sfar, S.; Fessi, H. Preparation and characterization of poly-e-caprolactone nanoparticles containing griseofulvin. *Int. J. Pharm.* **2005**, *294*, 261–267. [CrossRef] [PubMed]
76. Vllasaliu, D.; Exposito-Harris, R.; Heras, A.; Casettari, L.; Garnett, M.; Illum, L.; Stolnik, S. Tight junction modulation by chitosan nanoparticles: comparison with chitosan solution. *Int. J. Pharm.* **2010**, *15*, 183–193. [CrossRef] [PubMed]
77. Barbieri, S.; Sonvico, F.; Como, C.; Colombo, G.; Zani, F.; Buttini, F.; Bettini, R.; Rossi, A.; Colombo, P. Lecithin/chitosan controlled release nanopreparations of tamoxifen citrate: loading, enzyme-trigger release and cell uptake. *J. Control. Release* **2013**, *167*, 276–283. [CrossRef] [PubMed]
78. Ahmad, J.; Singhal, M.; Amin, S.; Rizwanullah, M.; Akhter, S.; Kamal, M.A.; Haider, N.; Midoux, P.; Pichon, C. Bile salt stabilized vesicles (Bilosomes): a novel nano-pharmaceutical design for oral delivery of proteins and peptides. *Curr. Pharm. Des.* **2017**, *23*, 1575–1588. [CrossRef] [PubMed]
79. Colombo, M.; Figueiró, F.; de Fraga Dias, A.; Teixeira, H.F.; Battastini, A.M.O.; Koester, L.S. Kaempferol-loaded mucoadhesive nanoemulsion for intranasal administration reduces glioma growth in vitro. *Int. J. Pharm.* **2018**, *543*, 214–223. [CrossRef] [PubMed]
80. Khan, A.; Aqil, M.; Imam, S.S.; Ahad, A.; Sultana, Y.; Ali, A.; Khan, K. Temozolomide loaded nano lipid based chitosan hydrogel for nose to brain delivery: Characterization, nasal absorption, histopathology and cell line study. *Int. J. Biol. Macromol.* **2018**, *116*, 1260–1267. [CrossRef] [PubMed]

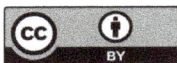

pharmaceutics

MDPI

Article

Chitosan Plus Compound 48/80: Formulation and Preliminary Evaluation as a Hepatitis B Vaccine Adjuvant

Dulce Bento [1,2], Sandra Jesus [1,2], Filipa Lebre [1,2], Teresa Gonçalves [1,3] and Olga Borges [1,2,*]

[1]   CNC-Center for Neuroscience and Cell Biology, University of Coimbra, 3004-0504 Coimbra, Portugal;
       dfbento@gmail.com (D.B.); sjesus.mg@gmail.com (S.J.); filipalebre@sapo.pt (F.L.);
       tgoncalves@fmed.uc.pt (T.G.)
[2]   Faculty of Pharmacy, University of Coimbra, Pólo das Ciências da Saúde, Azinhaga de Santa Comba,
       3000-548 Coimbra, Portugal
[3]   Faculty of Medicine, University of Coimbra, 3004-504 Coimbra, Portugal
*   Correspondence: olga@ci.uc.pt; Tel.: +(351)-239-488-428; Fax: +(351)-239-488-503

Received: 22 December 2018; Accepted: 4 February 2019; Published: 9 February 2019

Abstract: Current vaccine research is mostly based on subunit antigens. Despite the better toxicity profile of these antigens they are often poorly immunogenic, so adjuvant association has been explored as a strategy to obtain a potent vaccine formulation. Recently, mast cell activators were recognized as a new class of vaccine adjuvants capable of potentiating mucosal and systemic immune responses. In this study, a co-adjuvanted delivery system was developed and characterized, combining the mast cell activator C48/80 with chitosan nanoparticles (Chi-C48/80 NPs), and the results were compared with plain chitosan nanoparticles. The adsorption of model antigens onto the NP surface as well as the biocompatibility of the system was not affected by the incorporation of C48/80 in the formulation. The stability of the nanoparticles was demonstrated by studying the variation of size and zeta potential at different times, and the ability to be internalized by antigen presenting cells was confirmed by confocal microscopy. Vaccination studies with hepatitis B surface antigen loaded Chi-C48/80 NPs validated the adjuvanticity of the delivery system, demonstrating for the first time a successful association between a mast cell activator and chitosan nanoparticles as a vaccine adjuvant for hepatitis B virus, applied to a nasal vaccination strategy.

Keywords: compound 48/80; chitosan; nanoparticles; mast cell activator; vaccine adjuvant; nasal vaccination

---

1. Introduction

Traditional vaccines consisting of live attenuated or inactivated pathogens are highly immunogenic, but, due to safety concerns, development of new vaccines is being focused on the use of recombinant subunit antigens. Recombinant antigens are safer but they are often poorly immunogenic, requiring the use of adjuvants to enhance the resultant immune response. Therefore, different adjuvant approaches have been studied to enhance and/or modulate vaccine response to subunit antigens. Among them is the use of nanotechnology, a strategy that has been extensively explored and holds great promise [1,2]. Formulation of antigens in nanoparticles may offer several attractive features, namely an enhanced uptake by antigen presenting cells (APCs) [3], a depot effect with gradual release of the antigen [1,4], a cross-presentation of antigens [1,5], slower antigen processing than antigens in solution, which can result in a prolonged antigen presentation [6], and the co-delivery of antigens and adjuvants to the same cell population [2]. Besides, particulate antigens are generally more immunogenic than soluble antigens [7] and can be used to modulate the type of immune response [1]. Different nano-sized platforms such as virus-like particles, liposomes, immune stimulating complexes

(ISCOMs), nanoemulsions, and polymeric nanoparticles have been explored as potential vaccine delivery systems [8,9]. Chitosan and its derivatives are among the most studied compounds for development of polymeric vaccines [10,11] because of their attractive characteristics for biomedical applications. Chitosan is a biocompatible, biodegradable, and non-toxic polysaccharide [12], obtained by deacetylation of chitin, consisting of β-(1-4)-linked D-glucosamine and N-acetyl-D-glucosamine monomer units. Its cationic nature, mucoadhesivity and immunostimulating properties [10] make it an attractive polymer, particularly for the design of nanoparticulate vaccines for mucosal delivery.

Despite the potential of nanoparticles as vaccine adjuvants, it is possible to obtain a more potent adjuvant formulation by association with immunopotentiators. In fact, the concept of concomitant delivery of antigens and immunostimulatory molecules through delivery systems gained increased attention and has been appointed as a promising approach in vaccine development [2,13,14].

Mast cells (MCs), strategically located at the host surface contact with pathogens, have been recognized in recent years as important players in the development of protective immune responses [15–17], and the use of mast cell activators as a new class of vaccine adjuvants has begun to be explored [18]. Since then, additional studies confirmed the immunopotentiator properties of the mast cell activator compound 48/80 (C48/80) [19–21]. In this study, we explore the feasibility of combining the mast cell activator with chitosan nanoparticles to prepare a new adjuvant formulation for nasal vaccination. The strategy proposed here could be advantageous because, while chitosan could extend the residence time of the antigen on the nasal mucosa, MC activation could promote a local environment favorable to the development of an immune response. In particular, the application of this strategy to the hepatitis B recombinant antigen could allow the development of a nasal vaccine suitable for developing countries, where the possibility of self-administration could improve patient ease of access and compliance. Additionally, nasal vaccines are known to induce the generation of mucosal immune responses in the genital tract [22,23], which is highly attractive considering the sexual transmission of the virus. One of the biggest obstacles for vaccine development is the lack of knowledge on how to formulate complex adjuvant systems combining immunopotentiators and delivery systems [24]. Therefore, the publication of innovative methodologies for the preparation of these co-adjuvanted formulations is of utmost importance. These approaches would allow other researchers to have access to a broader range of adjuvants to test as vaccine candidates. Considering this, the present paper describes the design and characterization of a novel co-adjuvanted formulation consisting of chitosan nanoparticles associated with the mast cell activator C48/80. Stability, biocompatibility, and uptake by macrophages of the obtained nanoparticles were assessed in vitro. Finally, we tested the potential of C48/80 loaded chitosan NPs to modulate the adaptive immune response following nasal immunization using the recombinant hepatitis B surface antigen (HBsAg). To the authors' knowledge, this was the first time C48/80 was used as a co-adjuvant for hepatitis B vaccination.

2. Materials and Methods

2.1. Materials

A low molecular weight chitosan (deacetylation degree 95%) was purchased from Primex BioChemicals AS (Avaldsnes, Norway). Compound 48/80, bovine serum albumin (BSA), MTT (3-[4, 5-dimethylthiazol-2-yl]-2,5-diphenyl tetrazolium bromide), albumin-fluorescein isothiocyanate conjugate (FITC-BSA), trehalose, Dulbecco's modified Eagle medium (DMEM) and Roswell Park Memorial Institute (RPMI) 1640 were obtained from Sigma-Aldrich (Sintra, Portugal). Bicinchoninic acid (BCA) assay and micro BCA kits were obtained from Pierce Chemical Company (Rockford, IL, USA). FITC was purchased to Santa Cruz Biotechnology (Santa Cruz, CA, USA). Fetal bovine serum (FBS), wheat germ agglutinin Alexa Fluor® 350 Conjugate and Lysotracker® Red DND 99 were obtained from Life Technologies Corporation (Paisley, UK). HBsAg was purchased from Aldevron. All other reagents used were of analytical grade.

2.2. Chitosan Purification

Chitosan was purified by a method described elsewhere [25] with slight modifications. Briefly, 1 g of chitosan was suspended in 10 mL of a 1 M NaOH solution, and stirred for 3 h at 50 °C. The mixture was then filtered (0.45 μm membrane, MerckMillipore, Darmstadt, Germany), and the resultant pellet washed with 20 mL of deionized water. The recovered chitosan was dissolved in 200 mL of 1% (v/v) acetic acid solution and stirred for 1 h. The solution was filtered (0.45 μm membrane), and 1 M NaOH was used to adjust the filtrate to pH 8.0, resulting in purified chitosan in the form of precipitates. Purified chitosan was freeze-dried for 48 h with a Labconco freeze-dryer, model 77530 (Labconco, Kansas City, MO, USA) equipment.

2.3. Characterization of the Purified Chitosan by Fourier-Transform Infrared Spectroscopy (FTIR)

The FTIR spectra of purified and non-purified chitosan were recorded using an FTIR spectrometer (Spectrum 400, PerkinElmer, Villepinte, France) with an attenuated total reflection (ATR) top-plate accessory. The instrument operated with a resolution of 2 cm^{-1}, and 30 scans were collected for each sample. Spectra were recorded between 650 and 4000 cm^{-1}.

2.4. Nanoparticle Preparation

C48/80 loaded chitosan nanoparticles (Chi-C48/80 NPs) were prepared by adding dropwise 3 mL of an alkaline solution (5 mM NaOH) of C48/80 and Na$_2$SO$_4$ (0.3 mg/mL and 2.03 mg/mL, respectively) to 3 mL of a chitosan solution (1 mg/mL in acetic acid 0.1%) under high-speed vortexing. The nanoparticles were formed after further maturation for 60 min under magnetic stirring. Blank chitosan particles (Chi NPs) were obtained by preparing nanoparticles in exactly the same conditions but without C48/80.

To evaluate the stability after freeze-drying, nanoparticles were lyophilized with 1%, 2.5%, or 5% of trehalose as cryoprotectant. All samples were lyophilized for 48 h with a Labconco freeze-dryer, model 77530 (Labconco, Kansas City, USA), at −50 °C and 100 mbar.

Chitosan–aluminum nanoparticles (Chi-Al NPs) and chitosan–poly epsilon caprolactone (Chi-PCL) NPs used in the immunogenicity study were produced as previously described by our group [26,27]

2.5. Characterization of Nanoparticles

2.5.1. Size and Zeta Potential

Particle size was measured by dynamic light scattering (DLS) using a Delsa^{TM} Nano C (Beckman Coulter). Samples were diluted in milli-Q water and analyzed at a detection angle of 160° and a temperature of 25 °C. Zeta potential was measured by electrophoretic light scattering (ELS), after dispersion of the nanoparticles in a solution of 1 mM NaCl.

2.5.2. Morphology

Particle morphology was evaluated by scanning electron microscopy (SEM) in a field emission scanning electron microscope (FEI Quanta 400 FEG ESEM, ThermoFisher Scientific, Waltham, MA, USA). One drop of nanoparticle suspension was mounted on a microscope stub using a double-stick carbon tape and allowed to dry overnight. Prior to image acquisition, samples were coated with gold.

2.5.3. Quantification of C48/80 Loading Efficacy

In order to evaluate the loading efficacy (LE) of C48/80, nanoparticles were centrifuged for 20 min at 8000 g, and C48/80 was quantified in the supernatant using a method validated by our group [28]. Briefly, 25 μL of carbonate buffer pH 9.6 was added to 175 μL of sample in a 96-well plate. Subsequently,

50 µL of a 15% acetaldehyde solution containing 1.5% of sodium nitroprusside was added and the absorbance measured at 570 nm. The loading efficacy was calculated according to Equation (1).

$$\text{C48/80 LE (\%)} = \frac{\text{total C48/80 (µg/mL)} - \text{free C48/80 in supernatant (µg/mL)}}{\text{total C48/80 (µg/mL)}} \times 100 \quad (1)$$

2.5.4. FTIR Analysis

FTIR analysis of lyophilized chitosan, C48/80, Chi NPs, and Chi-C48/80 NPs was performed according to Section 2.3.

2.6. Stability Studies

The short term stability of freshly prepared nanoparticle suspensions stored either at 4 °C or at room temperature (RT) was studied for a period of 15 days. Size, polydispersity index (PI), and zeta potential of three independent batches of Chi-C48/80 NPs and Chi NPs were measured. Samples were withdrawn and characterized at Days 0, 3, 5 and 15.

The stability of lyophilized Chi-C48/80 NPs was also investigated after storage for a period of 4 months at RT. At the end of the test period, samples were resuspended in milli-Q water, NPs were characterized, and the parameters were compared to the values before lyophilization.

2.7. Evaluation of Loading Efficacy and Loading Capacity of Model Antigens

Loading of model antigens on a nanoparticle surface was performed by physical adsorption. Nanoparticles were centrifuged for 30 min at 4500 g and resuspended in acetate buffer, pH 5.7, 25 mM. Nanoparticles at a final concentration of 2.5 mg/mL were incubated with BSA, ovalbumin (OVA), or myoglobin in acetate buffer for 60 min at RT. Ratios from 7:1 to 1:1 (NP/protein) were tested for BSA, while OVA and myoglobin were incubated at a fixed weight ratio of 7:1. After incubation, particles were centrifuged at 12,000 g for 20 min, and the supernatant was collected. The amount of protein loaded on nanoparticles was determined indirectly by measuring the concentration of non-bound protein in the nanoparticle supernatant using the BCA or Micro-BCA protein assay (Pierce, ThermoFisher Scientific, Waltham, MA, USA) according to the manufacturer's instructions. Loading efficacy and loading capacity (LC) were determined by Equations (2) and (3), respectively.

$$\text{LE (\%)} = \frac{\text{total amount of BSA} - \text{non bound BSA}}{\text{total amount of BSA}} \times 100 \quad (2)$$

$$\text{LC (\%)} = \frac{\text{total amount of BSA} - \text{non bound BSA}}{\text{weight of nanoparticles}} \times 100. \quad (3)$$

2.8. In Vitro Cytotoxicity Studies

Single cell suspensions of spleens from 8-week old female C57BL/6 mice (Charles River) were prepared according to a method previously described [29]. Cells were seeded in a 96-well plate at a density of 1×10^6 cells/well in an RPMI 1640 medium (supplemented with 10% (v/v) fetal bovine serum, 2 mM glutamine, 1% (v/v) penicillin/streptomycin, and 20 mM HEPES) and incubated together with different concentrations of nanoparticles. After 24 h of incubation, cellular viability was assessed by MTT assay. Briefly, 20 µL of 5 mg/mL MTT in PBS, pH 7.4, was added to each well and incubated for more 4 h. The plate was centrifuged for 25 min, at 800 g, and the supernatants were removed. Finally, the formazan crystals produced by viable cells were solubilized with 200 µL of DMSO per well, and the optical density values were measured at 540 nm with 630 nm as a wavelength reference. The viability of non-treated cells (culture medium only) was defined as 100% and the relative cell viability calculated using Equation (4).

$$\text{Cell viability } (\%) = \frac{\text{OD sample } (540 \text{ nm}) - \text{OD sample } (630 \text{ nm})}{\text{OD control } (540 \text{ nm}) - \text{OD control } (630 \text{ nm})} \times 100. \tag{4}$$

A549 cells (American Type Culture Collection, ATCC) were seeded in a 96-well plate at a density of 10^5 cells/mL, at 37 °C and 5% CO_2, in a nutrient mixture F12-Ham with 10% (*v/v*) fetal bovine serum supplemented with 1% (*v/v*) penicillin/streptomycin, and incubated with different concentrations of nanoparticles. MTT assay was performed as described previously for spleen cells with minor modifications: incubation with MTT was performed over 1.5 h, and the cell supernatants were directly removed without centrifuging.

2.9. Particle Uptake by Macrophages

FITC-labeled NPs were prepared by the method described in Section 2.4 using FITC-labeled chitosan. The synthesis of FITC-labeled chitosan was based on the reaction between the isothiocyanate group of FITC (Ex/Em—490/525) and the primary amino group of chitosan established by our group [30]. Briefly, chitosan was labeled by mixing 35 mL of dehydrated methanol containing 25 mg of FITC to 25 mL of a 1% (*w/v*) chitosan in 0.1 M acetic acid. After 3 h of reaction in the dark at RT, the FITC-labeled chitosan was precipitated with 0.2 M NaOH until pH 10. FITC-labeled chitosan was obtained by centrifugation for 30 min at 4500 *g* and the resultant pellet was washed 3 times with a mixture of methanol/water (70:30, *v/v*). The labeled chitosan was resuspended in 15 mL of 0.1 M acetic acid and stirred overnight. A polymer solution was dialyzed in the dark against 2.5 L of deionized water for 3 days before freeze-drying using a freeze-dry system (FreezeZone 6, Labconco, Kansas City, MO, USA).

The ability of nanoparticles to be internalized by antigen presenting cells was assessed on the mouse macrophage cell line RAW 264.7 (ECACC, Salisbury, UK). Cells were maintained in Dulbecco's modified Eagle medium (DMEM, Sigma Aldrich, Sintra, Portugal) supplemented with 1 mM HEPES, 1 mM sodium pyruvate, and 10% of non-inactivated FBS. To evaluate the uptake of nanoparticles, RAW 264.7 cells were seeded on glass coverslips in 12-well plates at a density of 2.5×10^5 cells per well and cultured at 37 °C in 5% CO_2 overnight. On the next day, RAW 264.7 were pre-labeled with 300 nM Lysotracker® Red DND 99 (Ex/Em—577/590 nm) for 30 min at 37 °C, and the culture medium was replaced by a fresh one. The cells were then incubated for 4 h with FITC-Chi NPs and FITC-Chi-C48/80 NPs at 100 µg/mL or FITC-BSA loaded nanoparticles at 50 µg/mL in DMEM.

Following uptake, cells were washed three times with phosphate-buffered saline pH 7.4 (PBS) and fixed with 4% paraformaldehyde in PBS for 15 min at 37 °C. The plasma membrane of pre-fixed cells was then labeled with 5 µg/mL of wheat germ agglutinin Alexa Fluor 350 conjugate (Ex/Em—346/442 nm) in PBS for 10 min at RT. After labeling, cells were washed twice with PBS and the coverslips mounted in microscope slides with DAKO mounting medium and examined under an inverted laser scanning confocal microscope (Zeiss LSM 510 META, Carl Zeiss, Oberkochen, Germany) equipped with imaging software (LSM 5 software, version 3.2, Carl Zeiss, Oberkochen, Germany).

2.10. Immunogenicity Study

2.10.1. Nasal Vaccination

Female C57BL/6 mice of 6–8 weeks of age were purchased from Charles River (Écully, France) and housed in the Center for Neuroscience and Cell Biology (CNC) animal facility (Coimbra, Portugal) and provided food and water ad libitum. All experiments were carried out in accordance with institutional ethical guidelines and with national (Dec. No. 1005/92, 23 October 2018) and international (normative 2010/63 from EU) legislation. Groups of 5 mice were intranasally immunized on Days 0, 7, and 21 with 15 µL of vaccine formulation (7.5 µL per nostril), under slight isoflurane anesthesia. All mice, except for those in the naïve group (Group I), received 10 µg of HBsAg adsorbed onto Chi-C48/80 NPs (Group II), Chi-Al NPs (Group III), or Chi-PCL NPs (Group IV).

Samples were collected and processed as previously described [31]. Briefly, blood was collected by a submandibular lancet method on Days 21 and 42 and allowed to coagulate for 30 min prior to centrifugation at 1000 g for 10 min. Nasal and vaginal washes were collected on Day 42. Vaginal washes were collected by instilling 100 µL of PBS into the vaginal cavity, and the lavage fluid was flushed in and out a few times before collection. Samples were centrifuged at 11,500 g for 10 min, and supernatants were stored. Nasal lavage samples were collected from euthanized mice. The lower jaw of the mice was cut way and the nasal lavage collected by instilling 200 µL of sterile PBS posteriorly into the nasal cavity. Fluid exiting the nostrils was collected and spun at 11,500 g at 4 °C for 20 min. Collected and processed samples were stored until further analysis.

2.10.2. Determination of Serum IgG, IgG1, IgG2c, and Secretory IgA

Quantification of immunoglobulins was performed using a protocol optimized by our group [27,30]. The endpoint titers presented in the results represent the antilog of the last log2 dilution, for which the OD values were at least two-fold higher than that of the naive sample, equally diluted. The log 2 end-point titers were used for statistical analysis.

2.11. Statistical Analysis

Statistical analysis was performed with GraphPad Prism v 5.03 (GraphPad Software Inc., La Jolla, CA, USA). Student's t-test and ANOVA followed by Tukey's post-test were used for two samples or multiple comparisons, respectively. A p-value <0.05 was considered statistically significant (* $p < 0.05$; ** $p < 0.01$; *** $p < 0.001$).

3. Results and Discussion

3.1. Purification of Chitosan

Before use chitosan was submitted to a purification process to ensure the removal of any possible impurities. FTIR analysis was performed before and after the purification process to confirm the preservation of structure and integrity of the commercial polymer. The spectra obtained were in agreement with previously published data [32,33]. FTIR spectrum of chitosan showed a broad band between 3500 and 3200 cm^{-1} (Figure 1) corresponding to the stretching vibration of O–H. The peak of N–H stretching from primary amine groups was overlapped in the same region. The peak at 2869 cm^{-1} indicates C–H stretching vibrations. Peaks at 1650 and 1588 cm^{-1} correspond to C=O stretch and N–H bending, respectively. The peak at 1419 cm^{-1} belongs to the N–C stretching and the bands at 1150 and 1025 cm^{-1} are characteristic of the CO stretching vibration. No differences were observed between the spectra of non-purified and purified chitosan, which indicates that the purification process had no effect on the structure of the polymer.

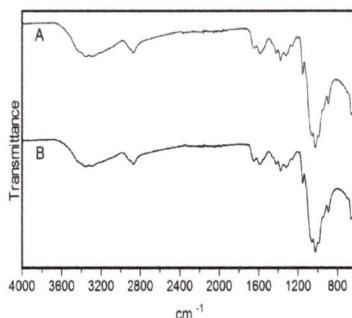

Figure 1. Fourier-transform infrared spectroscopy (FTIR) spectra of chitosan after and before the purification process. (A) Purified chitosan. (B) Non-purified chitosan.

3.2. Development and Physicochemical Characterization of C48/80-Chitosan Nanoparticles

C48/80 loaded chitosan nanoparticles were prepared by ionotropic gelation of cationic chitosan with sulfate anions from Na_2SO_4. C48/80 was added to a crosslink solution and entrapped during NP formation. This method of nanoparticle preparation is extremely simple and involves mixing two aqueous solutions at RT. Despite the simplicity of the method, different conditions were tested in the laboratory before getting the final nanoparticle formulation. Based on previous data collected from our group, different concentrations of the nanoparticles components, as well as different pH and incubation conditions, were tested in order to achieve nanoparticles with the desired characteristics: submicron size, a good polydispersity, and a reasonable encapsulation of the mast cell activator C48/80. The main challenge was to associate a cationic compound, the mast cell activator C48/80, with the also positively charged chitosan. Typically, interactions with chitosan amine group are electrostatic, which favors the interaction of the polymer with anionic compounds. Consequently, the association of cationic compounds with chitosan can be trickier due to partial repulsion, since both are positively charged [34]. At the end, the preparation of chitosan nanoparticles loaded with the mast cell activator C48/80 was possible by mixing the compound with an alkalinized sodium sulfate solution prior to the preparation of the nanoparticles.

Figure 2A summarizes Chi NP and Chi-C48/80 NP characteristics. The unloaded Chi NPs had an average size of 396.2 ± 35.0 nm, while the formulation loaded with the mast cell activator, Chi-C48/80 NPs, had an average size of 500.9 ± 65.15 nm. Images from scanning electron microscopy confirmed the size measured by DLS (Figure 2B1,B2). Both formulations had a narrow size distribution (PI < 0.170) and were positively charged. The incorporation of C48/80 in Chi NPs led to an increase of about 100 nm in the nanoparticle size (p < 0.001, Student's t-test), but the nanoparticle surface charge remained unaltered. The increased mean size was a good indicator of the association of C48/80 in the nanoparticles, but the incorporation was definitively confirmed after quantification of the amount of C48/80 in the nanoparticles by a validated method [28]. The results showed that the compound was successfully incorporated into Chi NPs with a loading efficacy of 18.6%. Even if the attempts to correlate particle size and the resultant immune responses lead to conflicting findings [4,35], previous studies showed that 500 nm is in the optimal size range for uptake by APCs [36]. Therefore, not only the Chi-C48/80 NPs and Chi NPs have a suitable size for uptake, but also their positive charge is an advantage since it favors mucoadhesion, through interaction with the negatively charged sites on cell surfaces, and should also facilitate the uptake by antigen-presenting cells.

A

Formulation	Size (nm)	PI[a]	ZP (mV)[b]	% LE (C48/80)[c]
Chi-C48/80 NP	500.9 ± 65.2	0.161 ± 0.051	+ 23.83 ± 3.76	18.6
Chi NP	396.2 ± 35.0	0.156 ± 0.037	+ 21.59 ± 2.81	·

[a]Polydispersity index; [b] Zeta Potential; [c] C48/80 loading efficacy

B

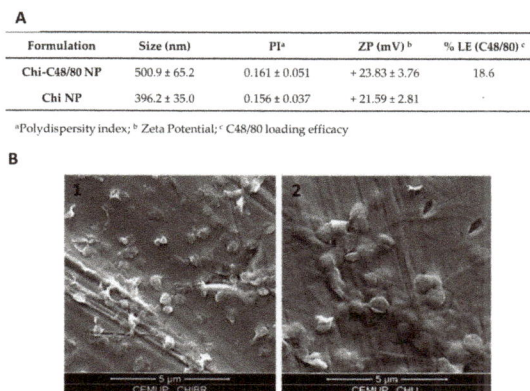

Figure 2. Characterization of C48/80 loaded and unloaded chitosan nanoparticles. (**A**) Size and zeta potential were measured by dynamic light scattering and electrophoretic light scattering, respectively, with a Delsa™ Nano C. C48/80 loading efficacy was measured by a colorimetric method. Mean ± SD, n ≥ 3. (**B**) SEM images of (**1**) Chi NP and (**2**) Chi-C48/80 NP. Magnification 15,000×, scale 5 μm.

3.3. FTIR Analysis of Nanoparticles

FTIR is an important tool to analyze the interactions between groups and useful for the study of nanomaterial surface [37]. Therefore, chitosan, Chi NPs, Chi-C48/80 NPs, and C48/80 were analyzed by FTIR to characterize any potential interactions in the nanoparticles. Comparison of chitosan polymer (Figure 3A) with Chi NPs (Figure 3B) showed a shift of peaks from 1650 and 1558 cm^{-1} to 1631 and 1532 cm^{-1}, respectively. This difference can be explained by the interaction between the amino groups of chitosan and sulfate ions, which resulted in the formation of the NPs by ionic crosslink [33]. The broad band between 3500 and 3200 cm^{-1} attributed to O–H and N–H bonds shifted to a lower wavelength in Chi NPs, indicating an enhancement of the hydrogen bonds interactions [38]. The same band appeared to be broader in Chi-C48/80 NPs (Figure 3C) than in Chi NPs, which also indicates enhanced hydrogen bonding in the loaded formulation [32]. No peak exclusively characteristic from C48/80 (Figure 3D) was observed on the FTIR spectrum of Chi-C48/80 NPs. This may be due to the small amount of C48/80 and therefore its chemical groups, present in the nanoparticles, which may be masked by the much higher amount of chitosan.

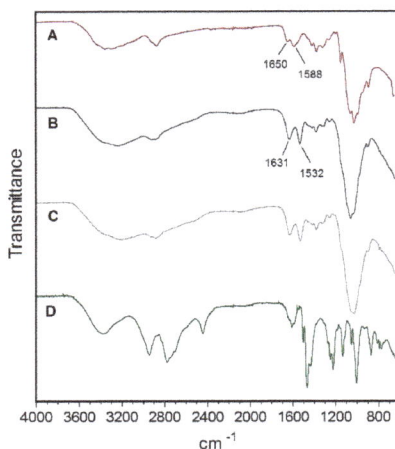

Figure 3. FTIR spectra of (A) Chitosan, (B) Chi NPs, (C) Chi-C48/80 NPs, and (D) C48/80.

3.4. Stability Studies of the Nanoparticles

A particle-based vaccine should be stable in relation to size throughout the process of preparation, storage, and administration. Considering this, the short-term stability of aqueous suspensions of Chi-C48/80 NPs was assessed by measuring the size, PI, and zeta potential during storage at 25 °C or at 4 °C for 15 days. Chi-C48/80 NPs showed a consistent particle size with a uniform size distribution during the test period (Figure 4A,B). Additionally, no changes in zeta potential of nanoparticles were observed (Figure 4C,D).

The results showed that Chi-C48/80 NPs were stable up to 15 days at the tested conditions. However, it should be noted that the target function of these formulation is to act as an adjuvant for nasal vaccination after association with an antigen of interest. It is known that instability during the storage of vaccines can lead to physicochemical changes of the formulation and antigen degradation, often requiring additional steps to improve its long-term stability [4]. One effective way to guarantee this stability and to prevent antigen degradation is to lyophilize the vaccine formulation [39]. It is important that this procedure does not affect the original particle size and size distribution of the formulation since it would also influence the immune responses. Thus, the potential impact of these processes should be investigated at early stages of formulation design [4]. Considering this, we explored the feasibility of lyophilizing the developed formulations by evaluating the impact of this technique on the physicochemical properties of Chi-C48/80 NPs and Chi NPs. The preliminary data obtained revealed that freeze-drying of the developed formulations without any cryoprotectant resulted in great particle aggregation (data not shown). This destabilization of nanoparticle suspensions is very common and most likely is a result of the stress of freezing and dehydration inherent to the technique [40]. Therefore, to avoid that, in this study a fixed concentration of nanoparticles (2 mg/mL) was lyophilized with different concentrations of trehalose (1%, 2.5%, and 5% (w/v)). The physicochemical characteristics of the delivery systems were then measured after reconstitution in water and compared to the initial ones (pre-lyophilization) to see if the concentrations of cryoprotectant used were sufficient to stabilize the formulations (Figure 5).

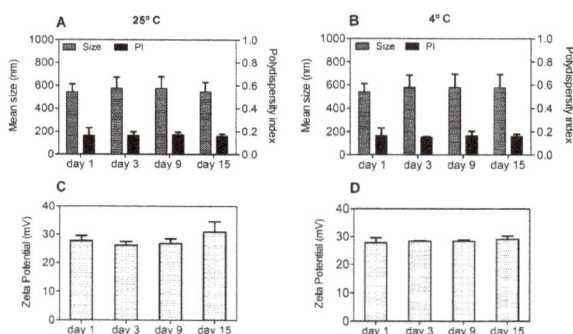

Figure 4. Short-term stability of Chi-C48/80 NPs at 25 °C (**A,C**) and 4 °C (**B,D**). Size, polydispersity index (PI), and zeta potential of the C48/80 loaded formulation were measured during storage up to 15 days at 25 °C or at 4 °C. Data are expressed as mean ± standard deviation (SD), n = 3.

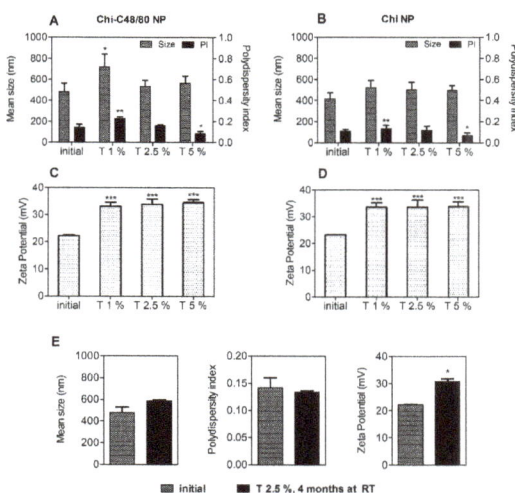

Figure 5. Effect of lyophilization with different concentrations of trehalose on the characteristics of nanoparticles. Size, polydispersion index, and zeta potential of Chi-C48/80 NPs (**A,C**) and Chi NPs (**B,D**) were measured before and after liophilization with 1%, 2.5%, and 5% of trehalose. (**E**) To evaluate the long-term stability of the lyophilized nanoparticles, Chi-C48/80 NPs plus 2.5% of trehalose were characterized after 4 months at room temperature (RT). Data are expressed as mean ± SD, n = 3.

Trehalose was selected as a cryoprotectant because it has been successfully used to preserve not only the characteristics of chitosan nanoparticles [38] but also the bioactivity of both C48/80 and an antigen [21]. The size of Chi NPs remains the same after lyophilization with all trehalose concentrations tested (Figure 5A,B). On the other hand, differences in size and PI for Chi-C48/80 NPs indicate that an adequate reconstitution was only achieved when using 2.5% or 5% of the cryoprotectant. Zeta potential of nanoparticles increased after the lyophilization with trehalose (Figure 5C,D). This can result from either a change in charge distribution on the NP surface or from the presence of trehalose on the on the NP suspension. The results suggest that 2.5% of trehalose was sufficient to achieve a successful cryopreservation of both delivery systems.

To assess if the lyophilized nanoparticles would be feasible to avoid the cold chain, Chi-C48/80 NPs lyophilized with 2.5% of trehalose were characterized after storage at RT for 4 months. Results showed that nanoparticles preserved the initial size and polydispersity for at least 4 months of storage (Figure 5E).

Overall, the results suggest that the stability of Chi NPs was not impaired by the association with C48/80. However, it is noteworthy that, even if these studies on the stability of the nanoparticles provided us with an indication about the potential of the formulations for long-term storage, they do not exclude the requirement of a more complete stability study, including antigen potency evaluation over time, for guarantee that the immunogenicity of the vaccine candidate is not affected. That would be particularly important during the development of vaccines designed to avoid the cold chain.

3.5. Loading of Model Antigens

In this study, BSA, OVA, and myoglobin were used as model antigens to confirm the adsorption of proteins onto the surface of nanoparticles. The use of three different proteins with different isoelectric points (IPs) allowed us to assess the suitability of the developed delivery systems for loading different antigens of interest. The loading of proteins on nanoparticles was made by physical adsorption, a mild technique that involves simply the incubation of nanoparticles with an aqueous solution of the antigen. This approach not only helps to preserve the structure of antigen but also allows a repetitive antigen display to the APC, which mimics pathogens [1].

Initially different NP/BSA ratios were tested to evaluate the more efficient weight ratio of NP/protein for loading. BSA loading efficacies were very similar for both Chi-C48/80 NPs and Chi NPs (Figure 6A,B). The LE was dependent on the ratio NP/BSA: the higher the ratio, the higher the amount of protein adsorbed on NP surface, ranging from 50.8% to 94.1% and from 52.2% and 95.5%, for Chi-C48/80 NPs and Chi NPs, respectively. The LC of nanoparticles was also calculated; it represents the amount of protein that the nanoparticles are able to carry. Unlike LE, the LC of the nanoparticles decreased with the increase in the NP/BSA ratio. Loading capacity was maximum at the lower ratio tested (1:1) for both Chi NPs and Chi-C48/80 NPs. However, even if the incubation with higher amounts of protein allows the nanoparticles to carry a higher amount of the protein of interest, generally it is preferable to use the NP/protein ratio that allows the highest LE because the antigen is usually the most expensive component of the vaccine. The LE near 95%, achieved for NP/BSA = 7:1, is very favorable in formulation development since almost the entire amount of antigen used would be associated with the nanoparticles. Therefore, this ratio was selected to test the loading of OVA and myoglobin on the NP surface.

LE of OVA and myoglobin on nanoparticles was around 70% and 10%, respectively, for both Chi-C48/80 NPs and Chi NPs (Figure 6C). These values were significantly lower than those observed for BSA. The isoelectric points of BSA, OVA, and myoglobin (4.7, 4.9, and 7.2, respectively) can help one to understand the observed results. BSA and OVA displayed high adsorption efficacies to the surface of the NPs that can be associated with the electrostatic interactions between the positively charged amino groups of chitosan and the negatively charged carboxyl groups of the proteins. On the other hand, at pH 5.7, both nanoparticles and myoglobin are positively charged, which explains the very low LE % observed for this protein. However, despite the similarity in the isoelectric points of BSA and

OVA, the adsorption of these proteins was different within the same delivery system. That is because, even if the IP is helpful for predicting the loading of proteins on the NP surface, the adsorption is a complex process depending on several other factors [41]. Overall, the results suggested that the developed formulations are suitable for loading negatively charged antigens and that the adsorption of protein onto the Chi NP surface was not affected by the presence of C48/80.

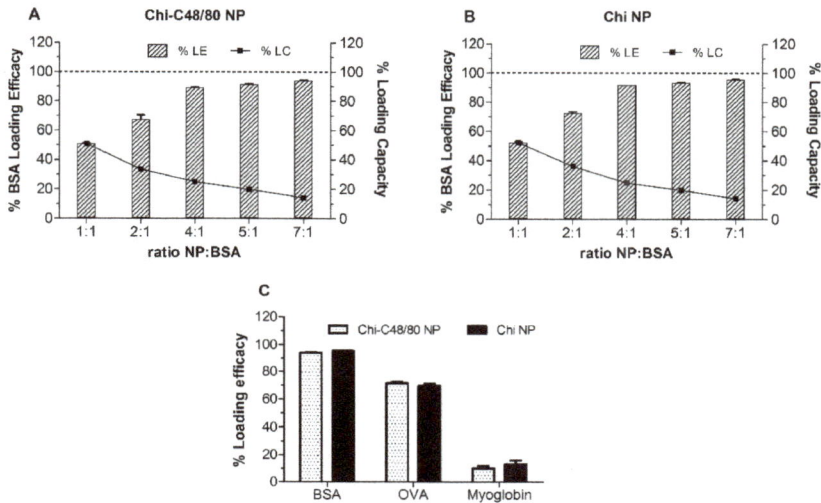

Figure 6. Loading of model antigens. Effect of NP/protein ratio on the protein adsorption to (**A**) Chi-C48/80 NPs and (**B**) Chi NPs. (**C**) Loading efficacy for bovine serum albumin (BSA), ovalbumin (OVA) and myoglobin at the NP/protein ratio of 7:1. Nanoparticles were incubated with different proteins for 60 min in acetate buffer, pH = 5.7 at RT. Loading efficacy (% LE) and loading capacity (% LC) were determined after quantification of unbound protein in the supernatant using the Bicinchoninic acid (BCA) assay. Bars represent mean $\pm$ SD, n = 3.

3.6. Cytotoxicity

The cytotoxicity of Chi-C48/80 NPs and Chi NPs was evaluated in spleen cells and in the A549 cell line using the MTT assay. Spleen cells were chosen because they are a good representation of the different cells of the immune system and have been already used to test the toxicity of vaccine delivery systems [29,42]. Since the aim of this study was to evaluate the incorporation of a mast cell activator in a delivery system, the A549 cell line, a model of alveolar basal epithelium, was used to evaluate the potential harmful effect of the nanoparticles at the administration site. As expected, the results show that cytotoxicity was concentration-dependent. Higher concentrations of nanoparticles resulted in a decreased cell viability (Figure 7).

In spleen cells, the incorporation of C48/80 in Chi NPs did not affect the toxicity of formulations, with both formulations showing no cytotoxicity for concentrations up to 2000 µg/mL (Figure 7A). With the A549 cell line, cell viability was above 70% for concentrations up to 750 µg/mL, for both formulations (Figure 7B). However, in these cells, the presence of C48/80 in the nanoparticles reduced the cell viability more rapidly than did Chi NPs. Note that 1500 µg/mL is a very high concentration and out of the range normally used in in vitro studies. These results are in agreement with others that have demonstrated that chitosan nanoparticles are nontoxic [29,43,44].

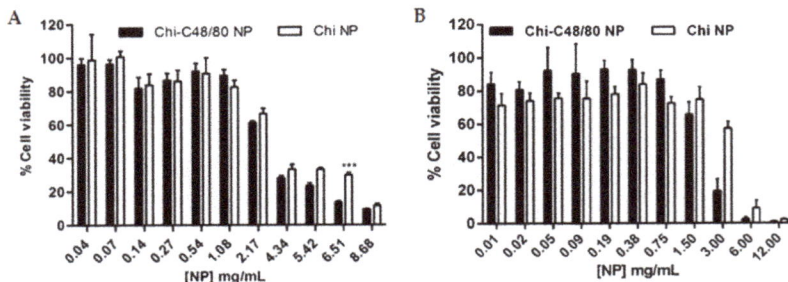

Figure 7. Effect of Chi-C48/80 NPs and Chi NPs on viability of spleen cells (**A**) and epithelial A549 cells (**B**). Different concentrations of nanoparticles were incubated with cells for 24 h. The cell viability was measured by MTT assay. Each result is representative of two independent experiments performed in quadruplicate for spleen cells and three independent experiments performed in quadruplicate for A549 cells (mean ± SD).

3.7. Uptake Studies

The uptake of nanoparticles by antigen presenting cells is favorable to an adaptive immune response [45]. Therefore, we investigated the ability of both developed formulations to be internalized by RAW 264.7 cells, a macrophage cell line widely used to explore the uptake and immune effect of vaccine delivery systems [3,7]. To visualize particle uptake by the macrophage cell line RAW 264.7, cells were incubated with FITC-labeled Chi NPs or Chi-C48/80 NPs. The intracellular location of nanoparticles was analyzed by labeling the cells with Lysotracker Red, which accumulates in the acidic endolysosomes. The results showed that the NPs were efficiently taken up by macrophages (Figure 8A). After 4 h of incubation, the FITC-NPs (green) were mostly detected on the cell cytoplasm. However, some of the compartments enclosing NPs showed acidification, as observed in the merged images between green fluorescent NPs and red fluorescent vesicles, appearing in yellow, indicating maturation of the phagolysosome (Figure 8A). To confirm that not only the nanoparticles but also the associated antigens would be internalized by antigen presenting cells, uptake studies were repeated with nanoparticles loaded with a fluorescently labeled protein. The confocal images showed an extensive internalization of FITC-BSA loaded on both Chi-C48/80 NPs and Chi NPs (Figure 8B). Similarly to what was observed with FITC-labeled NPs, the fluorescence signal of BSA was detected mostly on cell cytoplasm with only a few yellow co-localization signals observed.

These results suggest that NPs and protein-loaded NPs might escape from the endosomes to cytoplasm which can facilitate cross-presentation and potentially mediate the MHC I antigen presentation pathway, associated with an induction of CD8+ T cell response [3]. In fact, it was demonstrated by others that chitosan-based nanoparticles could escape from endosomes [46] and that antigens delivered by Chi NPs mediate antigen presentation through both MHC I and MHC II pathways [7]. This escape mechanism and consequent cross-presentation of antigens is particularly important for the development of vaccines that require cellular immune response.

Overall, the results showed that there were no significant differences regarding the uptake and distribution of Chi-C48/80 NPs and Chi NPs. This means that the association of the mast cell activator with the NPs not only did not impair the characteristics of nanoparticle and antigen uptake by antigen-presenting cells but also proved to be an effective antigen delivery system.

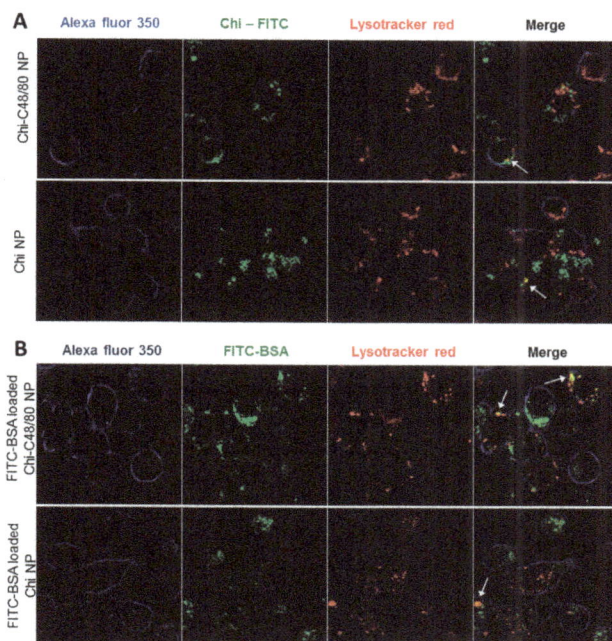

Figure 8. Evaluation of uptake by macrophages. (**A**) Uptake of nanoparticles was assessed by incubating 4 h, 100 µg/mL RAW 264.7 cells with Chi-C48/80 NPs or Chi NPs prepared with fluorescein isothiocyanate (FITC)-labeled chitosan (green). (**B**) Uptake of the antigen loaded on nanoparticles was evaluated by incubating the cells with FITC-BSA loaded Chi-C48/80 NPs or Chi NPs. Cells were labeled with Alexa Fluor© 350 WGA (blue) to identify the membrane, and Lysotracker© Red identifies the acidic endosomes and lysosomes. Arrows in the merge image show co-localization.

3.8. Immunogenicity Study

Chi-C48/80 NPs' ability to act as a nasal vaccine adjuvant for hepatitis B surface antigen was tested and compared with other particulate adjuvants by performing an immunogenicity study using C57BL/6 mice. The immunization schedule comprised a primary nasal immunization followed by two nasal boosts at Days 7 and 21. Therefore, in this study, we included two other established chitosan-based nano-delivery systems developed by our group, Chi-Al NPs [26] and Chi-PCL NPs [27], in order to compare adjuvanticity elicited by the new system.

As depicted in Figure 9A, although all formulations were able to induce detectable IgG titers at Day 21, at Day 42 Chi-C48/80 NPs and Chi-Al NPs induced significantly higher titers than Chi-PCL NPs. All delivery systems tested induced a Th2-type immune response, since the predominant IgG subclass elicited was the IgG1 (Figure 9B). Therefore, Chi-PCL NPs despite being an excellent adjuvant when administered by a subcutaneous route, was shown in this work to have a lower value when used in the intranasal route.

The main reason to develop new and effective mucosal vaccine delivery systems, besides its ease of access and administration, is the possibility to induce mucosal antibodies at the site of entry of pathogens, actively preventing the infection. Our results showed that Chi-C48/80 NPs were able to induce mucosal anti-HBsAg IgA in the vaccinated mice (Figure 9C). Indeed, the nasal washes revealed mucosal IgA titers in 80% of the Chi-C48/80 NP-vaccinated mice, similar to Chi-Al NPs, but vaginal washes revealed 60% of responder mice in comparison to the 40% of Chi-Al NPs. All nanoparticles used in this experiment presented a positive zeta potential, characteristic of a chitosan presence (Figure 9D). Nevertheless, sizes presented a higher variation between formulations, with a Chi-C48/80 NP size about two times larger than the other nanoparticles.

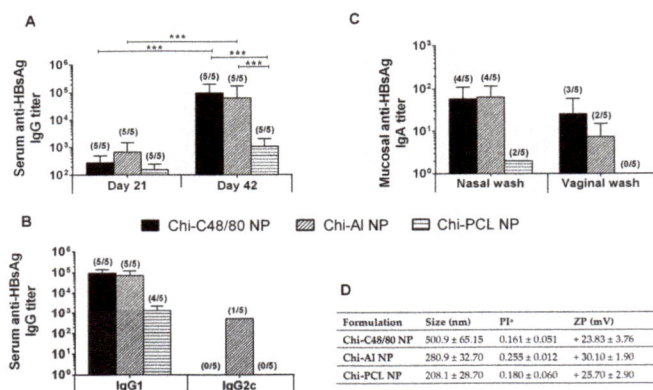

Figure 9. Immune profile of C57BL/6 mice after intranasal immunization. Serum anti-HBsAg IgG (**A**), IgG1 and IgG2c (**B**) and mucosal IgA (**C**) titers obtained with 10 µg HBsAg loaded into Chi-C48/80 NPs, Chi-Al NPs, or Chi-PCL NPs. Blood was collected by submandibular lancet method on Days 21 and 42, and nasal and vaginal washes were collected on Day 42. Numbers above bars represent the number of mice in which antibody levels were detected. Data (mean ± SD) correspond to responder mice of each group. Table with summary of nanoparticle size, polydispersity index, and zeta potential of the formulations used during the immunization studies (**D**).

These results suggest that the adjuvant Chi-C48/80 NPs is a valuable strategy to improve the efficacy of nasal recombinant vaccines. Immunoglobulin results were slightly higher than the ones obtained with Chi-Al NPs, which adjuvanticity was already established by our group [26,30,47] and particularly for the nasal route. In fact, Lebre et al. [30] observed Chi-Al NPs complexed with pDNA from HBsAg, were able to induce humoral and mucosal antibodies against HBV. Moreover, in opposition to free HBsAg, Lebre et al. [47] also reported that HBsAg loaded Chi-Al NPs elicited HBsAg-specific IgG in nasal and vaginal washes when the vaccine was subcutaneously administered. On the other hand, when compared to Chi-PCL NPs, Chi-C48/80 NPs demonstrated a superior adjuvant activity. Chi-PCL NP adjuvanticity through subcutaneous and nasal routes was also validated by our group in a direct comparison with free HBsAg [27,48,49]. In detail, through the nasal route, free HBsAg did not induce specific IgG titers, while Chi-PLC NPs elicited a detectable immune response with an HBsAg dose 10 times lower than the control [27]. Moreover, the conclusion that Chi-C48/80 NPs are able to increase the immune response to HBsAg is reinforced when the results are compared to Chi-Al NPs and Chi-PCL NPs, since those delivery systems were already compared in vaccination studies with the commercially available HBV vaccine (Engerix®) [47,49]. In those studies, both delivery systems were able to induce better IgG titers than Engerix® at same dose.

Interestingly, a recent article, published by Schubert et al. [50] observed that the adjuvant activity of C48/80 for the specific immune response against ovalbumin upon intranasal immunization is independent of the MC presence. Therefore, further work aimed to elucidate the mechanistic of action of Chi-C48/80 NPs as a mucosal vaccine adjuvant would be insightful to clarify if its adjuvant activity is related with a C48/80 ability to activate MC, or if it is a mechanism similar to chitosan, that largely stems from the fact that it is a cationic polymer. In fact, chitosan nanoparticles alone are able to activate mast cells, a finding recently made by our group [51].

Overall, the association of C48/80 with chitosan NPs was found to produce a good adjuvant and thus to be a suitable approach to improving the activity of the HBsAg, through mucosal routes of administration.

4. Conclusions

Chitosan is a biomaterial with appealing properties for vaccine delivery. Considering this, we designed and developed a new chitosan-based vaccine delivery system by efficiently incorporating the mast cell activator C48/80 into chitosan nanoparticles. Overall, the data obtained showed that the versatility of chitosan was associated with additional adjuvants without significantly affecting the physicochemical and biocompatible properties of the polymer. This is a characteristic of chitosan that deserves to be further explored in order to support the design of improved delivery systems or immunopotentiators to better modulate the immune response of the antigens. The delivery system was shown to have interesting features for vaccine delivery, namely, the ability to adsorb high amounts of antigen, internalization by antigen-presenting cells, and stability after lyophilization, which can be a useful future development of a cold chain-free vaccine formulation. Chi-C48/80 NPs also demonstrated adjuvant activity for the hepatitis B antigen similar to Chi-Al NPs and superior to Chi-PCL NPs, confirming its feasibility as a vaccine adjuvant through demanding but promising routes, such as the nasal route. To better design nanoparticulate immunopotentiators, it is desirable that the mechanism of the adjuvants be better studied, with the certainty that for each adjuvant we are not talking about a single mechanism, but most likely more than one that, the other way, may be competitive. This knowledge is absolutely essential, so that in the near future it will be possible to design adjuvants with more predictable immunomodulatory action.

Author Contributions: Conceptualization, D.B. and O.B.; investigation, D.B., S.J., and F.L.; writing—original draft preparation, D.B.; writing—review and editing, D.B., T.G., and O.B.; funding acquisition, O.B.

Funding: This work was financed by the European Regional Development Fund (ERDF), through the Centro 2020 Regional Operational Programme, under project CENTRO-01-0145-FEDER-000008:BrainHealth 2020, and through the COMPETE 2020—Operational Programme for Competitiveness and Internationalisation. This work was also financed by Portuguese national funds via FCT (Foundation for Science and Technology), I.P., under strategic project POCI-01-0145-FEDER-007440 as well as projects POCI-01-0145-FEDER-030331 and ProSafe/0001/2016 and via FCT doctoral fellowship SFRH/BD/65141/2009. SEM analysis was performed in CEMUP (under REEQ/1062/CTM/2005 and REDE/1512/RME/2005 funding contracts from FCT).

Acknowledgments: We thank Luisa Cortes for expert technical assistance with confocal microscopy.

Conflicts of Interest: The authors declare no conflict of interest.

References

1. Smith, D.M.; Simon, J.K.; Baker, J.R., Jr. Applications of nanotechnology for immunology. *Nat. Rev. Immunol.* **2013**, *13*, 592–605. [CrossRef] [PubMed]
2. De Temmerman, M.L.; Rejman, J.; Demeester, J.; Irvine, D.J.; Gander, B.; De Smedt, S.C. Particulate vaccines: on the quest for optimal delivery and immune response. *Drug Discov. Today* **2011**, *16*, 569–582. [CrossRef] [PubMed]
3. Akagi, T.; Shima, F.; Akashi, M. Intracellular degradation and distribution of protein-encapsulated amphiphilic poly(amino acid) nanoparticles. *Biomaterials* **2011**, *32*, 4959–4967. [CrossRef] [PubMed]
4. Oyewumi, M.O.; Kumar, A.; Cui, Z. Nano-microparticles as immune adjuvants: correlating particle sizes and the resultant immune responses. *Expert Rev. Vaccines* **2010**, *9*, 1095–1107. [CrossRef] [PubMed]
5. Shen, H.; Ackerman, A.L.; Cody, V.; Giodini, A.; Hinson, E.R.; Cresswell, P.; Edelson, R.L.; Saltzman, W.M.; Hanlon, D.J. Enhanced and prolonged cross-presentation following endosomal escape of exogenous antigens encapsulated in biodegradable nanoparticles. *Immunology* **2006**, *117*, 78–88. [CrossRef] [PubMed]
6. Thomann-Harwood, L.J.; Kaeuper, P.; Rossi, N.; Milona, P.; Herrmann, B.; McCullough, K.C. Nanogel vaccines targeting dendritic cells: contributions of the surface decoration and vaccine cargo on cell targeting and activation. *J. Control. Release* **2013**, *166*, 95–105. [CrossRef] [PubMed]
7. Koppolu, B.; Zaharoff, D.A. The effect of antigen encapsulation in chitosan particles on uptake, activation and presentation by antigen presenting cells. *Biomaterials* **2013**, *34*, 2359–2369. [CrossRef]
8. Gao, Y.; Wijewardhana, C.; Mann, J.F.S. Virus-Like Particle, Liposome, and Polymeric Particle-Based Vaccines against HIV-1. *Front. Immunol.* **2018**, *9*. [CrossRef]

9. Barclay, T.; Petrovsky, N. Vaccine Adjuvant Nanotechnologies. In *Micro and Nanotechnology in Vaccine Development*; Elsevier Science: Oxford, UK, 2017; pp. 127–147. [CrossRef]
10. Arca, H.C.; Gunbeyaz, M.; Senel, S. Chitosan-based systems for the delivery of vaccine antigens. *Expert Rev. Vaccines* **2009**, *8*, 937–953. [CrossRef]
11. Amidi, M.; Mastrobattista, E.; Jiskoot, W.; Hennink, W.E. Chitosan-based delivery systems for protein therapeutics and antigens. *Adv. Drug Deliv. Rev.* **2010**, *62*, 59–82. [CrossRef]
12. Baldrick, P. The safety of chitosan as a pharmaceutical excipient. *Regul. Toxicol. Pharmacol. RTP* **2010**, *56*, 290–299. [CrossRef] [PubMed]
13. Mutwiri, G.; Gerdts, V.; van Drunen Littel-van den Hurk, S.; Auray, G.; Eng, N.; Garlapati, S.; Babiuk, L.A.; Potter, A. Combination adjuvants: the next generation of adjuvants? *Expert Rev. Vaccines* **2011**, *10*, 95–107. [CrossRef] [PubMed]
14. Schijns, V.E.; Lavelle, E.C. Trends in vaccine adjuvants. *Expert Rev. Vaccines* **2011**, *10*, 539–550. [CrossRef] [PubMed]
15. Abraham, S.N.; St John, A.L. Mast cell-orchestrated immunity to pathogens. *Nat. Rev. Immunol.* **2010**, *10*, 440–452. [CrossRef] [PubMed]
16. Metz, M.; Maurer, M. Mast cells–key effector cells in immune responses. *Trends Immunol.* **2007**, *28*, 234–241. [CrossRef] [PubMed]
17. Marshall, J.S. Mast-cell responses to pathogens. *Nat. Rev. Immunol.* **2004**, *4*, 787–799. [CrossRef] [PubMed]
18. McLachlan, J.B.; Shelburne, C.P.; Hart, J.P.; Pizzo, S.V.; Goyal, R.; Brooking-Dixon, R.; Staats, H.F.; Abraham, S.N. Mast cell activators: A new class of highly effective vaccine adjuvants. *Nat. Med.* **2008**, *14*, 536–541. [CrossRef] [PubMed]
19. Staats, H.F.; Fielhauer, J.R.; Thompson, A.L.; Tripp, A.A.; Sobel, A.E.; Maddaloni, M.; Abraham, S.N.; Pascual, D.W. Mucosal targeting of a BoNT/A subunit vaccine adjuvanted with a mast cell activator enhances induction of BoNT/A neutralizing antibodies in rabbits. *PLoS ONE* **2011**, *6*, e16532. [CrossRef]
20. McGowen, A.L.; Hale, L.P.; Shelburne, C.P.; Abraham, S.N.; Staats, H.F. The mast cell activator compound 48/80 is safe and effective when used as an adjuvant for intradermal immunization with Bacillus anthracis protective antigen. *Vaccine* **2009**, *27*, 3544–3552. [CrossRef]
21. Wang, S.H.; Kirwan, S.M.; Abraham, S.N.; Staats, H.F.; Hickey, A.J. Stable dry powder formulation for nasal delivery of anthrax vaccine. *J. Pharm. Sci.* **2012**, *101*, 31–47. [CrossRef]
22. Kiyono, H.; Fukuyama, S. NALT- versus Peyer's-patch-mediated mucosal immunity. *Nat. Rev. Immunol.* **2004**, *4*, 699–710. [CrossRef] [PubMed]
23. Neutra, M.R.; Kozlowski, P.A. Mucosal vaccines: The promise and the challenge. *Nat. Rev. Immunol.* **2006**, *6*, 148–158. [CrossRef]
24. Reed, S.G.; Bertholet, S.; Coler, R.N.; Friede, M. New horizons in adjuvants for vaccine development. *Trends Immunol.* **2009**, *30*, 23–32. [CrossRef] [PubMed]
25. Gan, Q.; Wang, T. Chitosan nanoparticle as protein delivery carrier—Systematic examination of fabrication conditions for efficient loading and release. *Colloids Surf. B Biointerface* **2007**, *59*, 24–34. [CrossRef]
26. Lebre, F.; Bento, D.; Ribeiro, J.; Colaco, M.; Borchard, G.; de Lima, M.C.P.; Borges, O. Association of chitosan and aluminium as a new adjuvant strategy for improved vaccination. *Int. J. Pharm.* **2017**, *527*, 103–114. [CrossRef]
27. Jesus, S.; Soares, E.; Costa, J.; Borchard, G.; Borges, O. Immune response elicited by an intranasally delivered HBsAg low-dose adsorbed to poly-epsilon-caprolactone based nanoparticles. *Int. J. Pharm.* **2016**, *504*, 59–69. [CrossRef]
28. Bento, D.; Borchard, G.; Goncalves, T.; Borges, O. Validation of a new 96-well plate spectrophotometric method for the quantification of compound 48/80 associated with particles. *AAPS PharmSciTech* **2013**, *14*, 649–655. [CrossRef] [PubMed]
29. Borges, O.; Cordeiro-da-Silva, A.; Romeijn, S.G.; Amidi, M.; de Sousa, A.; Borchard, G.; Junginger, H.E. Uptake studies in rat Peyer's patches, cytotoxicity and release studies of alginate coated chitosan nanoparticles for mucosal vaccination. *J. Control. Release* **2006**, *114*, 348–358. [CrossRef]
30. Lebre, F.; Borchard, G.; Faneca, H.; Pedroso de Lima, M.C.; Borges, O. Intranasal Administration of Novel Chitosan Nanoparticle/DNA Complexes Induces Antibody Response to Hepatitis B Surface Antigen in Mice. *Mol. Pharm.* **2016**, *13*, 472–482. [CrossRef]

31. Jesus, S.; Soares, E.; Borges, O. Poly-epsilon-caprolactone/Chitosan and Chitosan Particles: Two Recombinant Antigen Delivery Systems for Intranasal Vaccination. *Method Mol. Biol.* **2016**, *1404*, 697–713. [CrossRef]
32. Dudhani, A.R.; Kosaraju, S.L. Bioadhesive chitosan nanoparticles: Preparation and characterization. *Carbohydr. Polym.* **2010**, *81*, 243–251. [CrossRef]
33. Borges, O.; Borchard, G.; Verhoef, J.C.; de Sousa, A.; Junginger, H.E. Preparation of coated nanoparticles for a new mucosal vaccine delivery system. *Int. J. Pharm.* **2005**, *299*, 155–166. [CrossRef]
34. Lim, S.T.; Martin, G.P.; Berry, D.J.; Brown, M.B. Preparation and evaluation of the in vitro drug release properties and mucoadhesion of novel microspheres of hyaluronic acid and chitosan. *J. Control. Release* **2000**, *66*, 281–292. [CrossRef]
35. Zhao, L.; Seth, A.; Wibowo, N.; Zhao, C.X.; Mitter, N.; Yu, C.; Middelberg, A.P. Nanoparticle vaccines. *Vaccine* **2014**, *32*, 327–337. [CrossRef]
36. Foged, C.; Brodin, B.; Frokjaer, S.; Sundblad, A. Particle size and surface charge affect particle uptake by human dendritic cells in an in vitro model. *Int. J. Pharm.* **2005**, *298*, 315–322. [CrossRef]
37. Mudunkotuwa, I.A.; Minshid, A.A.; Grassian, V.H. ATR-FTIR spectroscopy as a tool to probe surface adsorption on nanoparticles at the liquid-solid interface in environmentally and biologically relevant media. *Analyst* **2014**, *139*, 870–881. [CrossRef]
38. Rampino, A.; Borgogna, M.; Blasi, P.; Bellich, B.; Cesaro, A. Chitosan nanoparticles: preparation, size evolution and stability. *Int. J. Pharm.* **2013**, *455*, 219–228. [CrossRef]
39. Sloat, B.R.; Sandoval, M.A.; Cui, Z. Towards preserving the immunogenicity of protein antigens carried by nanoparticles while avoiding the cold chain. *Int. J. Pharm.* **2010**, *393*, 197–202. [CrossRef]
40. Abdelwahed, W.; Degobert, G.; Stainmesse, S.; Fessi, H. Freeze-drying of nanoparticles: formulation, process and storage considerations. *Adv. Drug Deliv. Rev.* **2006**, *58*, 1688–1713. [CrossRef]
41. Dee, K.C.; Puleo, D.A.; Bizios, R. Protein-Surface Interactions. In *An Introduction To Tissue-Biomaterial Interactions*; John Wiley & Sons, Inc.: Hoboken, NJ, USA, 2003; pp. 37–52. [CrossRef]
42. Eyles, J.E.; Bramwell, V.W.; Singh, J.; Williamson, E.D.; Alpar, H.O. Stimulation of spleen cells in vitro by nanospheric particles containing antigen. *J. Control. Release* **2003**, *86*, 25–32. [CrossRef]
43. Grenha, A.; Grainger, C.I.; Dailey, L.A.; Seijo, B.; Martin, G.P.; Remunan-Lopez, C.; Forbes, B. Chitosan nanoparticles are compatible with respiratory epithelial cells in vitro. *Eur. J. Pharm. Sci.* **2007**, *31*, 73–84. [CrossRef]
44. Kean, T.; Thanou, M. Biodegradation, biodistribution and toxicity of chitosan. *Adv. Drug Deliv. Rev.* **2010**, *62*, 3–11. [CrossRef]
45. O'Hagan, D.T.; Valiante, N.M. Recent advances in the discovery and delivery of vaccine adjuvants. *Nat. Rev. Drug Discov.* **2003**, *2*, 727–735. [CrossRef]
46. Yue, Z.G.; Wei, W.; Lv, P.P.; Yue, H.; Wang, L.Y.; Su, Z.G.; Ma, G.H. Surface charge affects cellular uptake and intracellular trafficking of chitosan-based nanoparticles. *Biomacromolecules* **2011**, *12*, 2440–2446. [CrossRef]
47. Lebre, F.; Pedroso de Lima, M.C.; Lavelle, E.C.; Borges, O. Mechanistic study of the adjuvant effect of chitosan-aluminum nanoparticles. *Int. J. Pharm.* **2018**, *552*, 7–15. [CrossRef]
48. Jesus, S.; Soares, E.; Borchard, G.; Borges, O. Poly–caprolactone/chitosan nanoparticles provide strong adjuvant effect for hepatitis B antigen. *Nanomedicine* **2017**, *12*, 2335–2348. [CrossRef]
49. Jesus, S.; Soares, E.; Borchard, G.; Borges, O. Adjuvant Activity of Poly-epsilon-caprolactone/Chitosan Nanoparticles Characterized by Mast Cell Activation and IFN-gamma and IL-17 Production. *Mol. Pharm.* **2018**, *15*, 72–82. [CrossRef]
50. Schubert, N.; Lisenko, K.; Auerbach, C.; Weitzmann, A.; Ghouse, S.M.; Muhandes, L.; Haase, C.; Häring, T.; Schulze, L.; Voehringer, D.; et al. Unimpaired Responses to Vaccination With Protein Antigen Plus Adjuvant in Mice With Kit-Independent Mast Cell Deficiency. *Front. Immunol.* **2018**, *9*. [CrossRef]
51. Bento, D.; Staats, H.F.; Gonçalves, T.; Borges, O. Development of a novel adjuvanted nasal vaccine: C48/80 associated with chitosan nanoparticles as a path to enhance mucosal immunity. *Eur. J. Pharm. Biopharm.* **2015**, *93*, 149–164. [CrossRef]

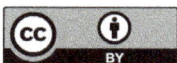

pharmaceutics

Article

Nasal Administration and Plasma Pharmacokinetics of Parathyroid Hormone Peptide PTH 1-34 for the Treatment of Osteoporosis

Richard G. Pearson [1,*], Tahir Masud [2], Elaine Blackshaw [3], Andrew Naylor [4], Michael Hinchcliffe [5], Kirk Jeffery [4], Faron Jordan [4], Anjumn Shabir-Ahmed [4], Gareth King [4], Andrew L. Lewis [4], Lisbeth Illum [6] and Alan C. Perkins [3]

[1] Division of Rheumatology, Orthopaedics and Dermatology, School of Medicine, Queen's Medical Centre, University of Nottingham, Nottingham NG7 2UH, UK
[2] Nottingham University Hospitals NHS Trust, Queen's Med Centre, University of Nottingham, Nottingham NG7 2UH, UK; tahir.masud@nuh.nhs.uk
[3] Radiological Sciences, School of Medicine, Queen's Medical Centre, University of Nottingham, Nottingham NG7 2UH, UK; elaine.blackshaw@nottingham.ac.uk (E.B.); alan.perkins@nottingham.ac.uk (A.C.P.)
[4] Critical Pharmaceuticals Ltd., Bio City, Pennyfoot Street, Nottingham NG1 1GF, UK; anaylor@upperton.com (A.N.); kjeffery@upperton.com (K.J.); faron.jordan@hotmail.co.uk (F.J.); anjumnshabir@yahoo.com (A.S.-A.); gareth.king@catapult-ventures.com (G.K.); andrew.lewis@quotientsciences.com (A.L.L.)
[5] Paracelsis Ltd., BioCity Nottingham, Pennyfoot Street, Nottingham NG1 1GF, UK; mh@paracelsis.com
[6] Identity, 19 Cavendish Crescent North, The Park, Nottingham NG71BA, UK; lisbeth.illum@illumdavis.com
*   Correspondence: richard.pearson@nottingham.ac.uk; Tel.: +44-(0)-115-8231-119

Received: 30 April 2019; Accepted: 24 May 2019; Published: 7 June 2019

Abstract: Nasal delivery of large peptides such as parathyroid 1-34 (PTH 1-34) can benefit from a permeation enhancer to promote absorption across the nasal mucosa into the bloodstream. Previously, we have published an encouraging bioavailability (78%), relative to subcutaneous injection in a small animal preclinical model, for a liquid nasal spray formulation containing the permeation enhancer polyethylene glycol (15)-hydroxystearate (Solutol® HS15). We report here the plasma pharmacokinetics of PTH 1-34 in healthy human volunteers receiving the liquid nasal spray formulation containing Solutol® HS15. For comparison, data for a commercially manufactured teriparatide formulation delivered via subcutaneous injection pen are also presented. Tc-99m-DTPA gamma scintigraphy monitored the deposition of the nasal spray in the nasal cavity and clearance via the inferior meatus and nasopharynx. The 50% clearance time was 17.8 min (minimum 10.9, maximum 74.3 min). For PTH 1-34, mean plasma C_{max} of 5 pg/mL and 253 pg/mL were obtained for the nasal spray and subcutaneous injection respectively; relative bioavailability of the nasal spray was ≤1%. Subsequently, we investigated the pharmacokinetics of the liquid nasal spray formulation as well as a dry powder nasal formulation also containing Solutol® HS15 in a crossover study in an established ovine model. In this preclinical model, the relative bioavailability of liquid and powder nasal formulations was 1.4% and 1.0% respectively. The absolute bioavailability of subcutaneously administered PTH 1-34 (mean 77%, range 55–108%) in sheep was in agreement with published human data for teriparatide (up to 95%). These findings have important implications in the search for alternative routes of administration of peptides for the treatment of osteoporosis, and in terms of improving translation from animal models to humans.

Keywords: PTH 1-34; teriparatide; nasal delivery; pharmacokinetics; osteoporosis; man; sheep; clinical trial; preclinical

1. Introduction

Fragility fractures are associated with osteoporosis, a skeletal disease that occurs mainly in the older population, and are associated with a reduced bone mineral density (BMD), with alterations in bone microarchitecture such that the bone exhibits a reduced capacity to resist fracture [1,2]. Osteoporosis is a significant contributor to non-traumatic hip fractures and vertebral fractures worldwide. In 2017, there were 66,668 hip fractures in those aged 60 years or over in the UK alone. The human cost in this patient group is high, with a mortality rate of 6.7%. A 30 day survival for patients with hip fracture can be accurately estimated using the Nottingham Hip Fracture Score [3,4]. This is mirrored by a huge health economic burden, and costs for the NHS and social care of £1 billion per year in the UK [5].

PTH 1-34 injections (teriparatide) are currently the only anabolic therapy specifically designed for the treatment of osteoporosis by promoting the deposition of bone to increase bone density as opposed to preventing bone loss. Poor compliance of between 25–30% at 12 months is widely reported in patient populations prescribed teriparatide treatment [6,7]. When this patient group is questioned, there is a reluctance to be prescribed teriparatide due to the need for repeated injection [8]. Therefore, we are researching nasal spray formulations as an alternative to daily injection, as a strategy for improving patient compliance which could afford improved patient outcomes and reduced economic healthcare/social care burden. In addition, there could be economic benefits due to reduced manufacturing costs.

Nasal spray delivery systems can facilitate easy, painless administration of a drug, and are convenient for patients to self-administer. However, large hydrophilic molecules such as peptides and proteins are poorly transported across the nasal membrane, and hence require the use of a permeation enhancer to achieve a therapeutically relevant bioavailability. Furthermore, it can be a challenge to develop a suitable nasal formulation since many permeation enhancers are poorly tolerated by the nasal membrane [9–11]. Enabling technologies in the form of both nasal delivery devices and nasal mucosal permeation enhancers are presently being developed for effective nasal delivery of peptides/proteins. Such technologies are being pursued in clinical trials [12,13]. The nasal delivery system investigated here contains a permeation enhancer aimed at promoting absorption of the PTH 1-34 (4.1 kDa 34 N-terminal amino acid peptide) across the nasal mucosa in a safe manner [9]. The selected permeation enhancer is a pharmaceutical excipient, polyethylene glycol (15)-hydroxystearate, also known as Macrogol (15)-hydroxystearate, polyoxyethylated 12-hydroxystearic acid, Solutol® HS 15, Kolliphor® HS 15 or CriticalSorb™ [10].

The therapeutic efficacy of the intranasal spray formulation of PTH 1-34 is dependent upon pharmacokinetics. To investigate this, the rat preclinical model was previously utilised, and showed that serum levels of PTH 1-34 were significantly greater when delivered in nasal formulations containing Solutol® HS15, compared to a simple PTH 1-34 formulation [14]. We have also previously demonstrated that Solutol® HS15 is an essential excipient for the enhancement of human growth hormone delivery via the intranasal route [10]. Solutol® HS15, a mixture of mono- and diesters of 12-hydroxystearate (macrogol 15-hydroxystearate), is a non-ionic surfactant with a hydrophilic–lipophilic balance value of 14–16. Due to its amphiphilic nature, Solutol® HS15 in solution forms micelles approximately 13 nm in diameter. Importantly, when peptides or proteins are dissolved in an aqueous solution comprising Solutol® HS15, they retain their tertiary structure [15]. The mechanism of action of Solutol® HS15 is considered to arise primarily from a combination of effects on the cell membrane (transcellular enhancement mechanism), and from an impact on the organization of the actin in the cell cytoskeleton resulting in tight junction opening (paracellular enhancement mechanism). Solutol® HS15 enhances the transport of drugs across the mucosal membrane without demonstrating toxicity to mucosal tissue [9]. The formulation is compliant with the European Medicines Agency guidelines on pharmaceutical quality of inhalation and nasal products (EMEA/CHMP/QWP/49313/2005).

Our previously published preclinical data in rats for a liquid nasal spray formation were encouraging, showing that the nasal systemic absorption of PTH 1-34 was increased considerably when administered in a formulation containing Solutol® HS15. The mean C_{max} obtained for the nasal spray (13.7 ng/mL after administering 100 µg/kg PTH 1-34) was comparable to that after subcutaneous injection (14.8 ng/mL after a 80 µg/kg dose), and the relative bioavailability was 78% [14]. These data led to the initiation of the clinical study assessing the liquid nasal spray formulation. This was carried out to assess nasal deposition, clearance and pharmacokinetics in human subjects [16]. In addition, on review of the clinical data obtained, we followed up this research using a large animal (ovine) model reported to be reliable and predictive of human intranasal drug delivery [17]. This replicated the evaluation of the liquid nasal spray formulation that was given to healthy human volunteers, in addition to piloting an intranasal dry powder formulation containing the same absorption enhancer excipient [18].

2. Materials

The PTH 1-34 acetate used for the nasal formulation was chemically synthesised (Polypeptide Inc., Torrance, CA, USA), and recombinant PTH 1-34 known as teriparatide was the active formulation ingredient (API) in the commercially available subcutaneous injection pen, Forsteo®, obtained from Lilly France S.A.S, Fegersheim, France. HyPure WFI Quality Water (Ph.Eur.) (Thermo Fisher Scientific, Loughborough, UK), Solutol® HS15 (BASF, Ludwigshafen, Germany). All other materials were supplied by Sigma Aldrich, Gillingham, UK: glacial acetic acid USP, sodium acetate USP, D-mannitol (Ph.Eur.) and L-methionine (Ph.Eur.). Gellan gum, Gelzan™ CM (CP Kelco), and trehalose USP Tc-99m-DTPA (Diethylenetriamine pentaacetate) supplied by the radiopharmacy unit of Queen's Medical Centre, University of Nottingham.

3. Methods

3.1. Preparation of Nasal Formulations for Clinical Study

The nasal formulation comprised 0.1% *w/v* PTH 1-34 (Polypeptide Inc., Torrance, CA, USA), 7.5% *w/v* polyethylene glycol (15)-hydroxystearate (Ph.Eur.), 5% *w/v* D-mannitol (Ph.Eur.), 3% *w/v* L-methionine (Ph.Eur.), 0.15% sodium acetate (Ph.Eur.), and 0.8% *w/v* acetic acid (Ph.Eur.) in water for injection (Ph.Eur.) containing the radiolabel (Tc-99m-DTPA). To achieve a 90 µg dose of PTH 1-34, 90 µL of the formulation was atomised in each actuation using a Standard Rexam 3959 winged spray actuator, SP270-90 pump (Rexam Healthcare, London, UK). In brief, for manufacture of the radiolabel (Tc-99m-DTPA) containing formulation, Solutol® HS15 was rendered molten by raising the temperature to 60 ± 10 °C. Molten Solutol® HS15 was then dissolved in 0.2 M acetate buffer (pH 4.0) containing the D-mannitol and L-Methionine at 50 ± 5 °C. The resulting 11% *w/v* Solutol HS15 was allowed to cool and was used to prepare the 1 mg/mL PTH 1–34, Tc-99m-DTPA (3–5 MBq activity), 7.5% Solutol® HS15 formulation in 0.1 M acetate buffer pH4 using water for injection (Ph.Eur.) as the diluent. Preparation of the formulations was performed at the GMP facility at the Queen's Medical Centre, Nottingham, UK.

The droplet size from the nasal spray was assayed for a 45 µL dose volume by Rexam (Suresnes, France) using a Spraytec (Malvern Panalytical, Malvern, UK) instrument, activation speed: 60 mm/s, acceleration: 2500 mm/s^2, with a symmetric profile. All parameters were analysed during the stabilization phase of the spray, with actuator positioned 6 cm from the laser. D10: Droplet diameter such that 10% of the total liquid volume consist of droplets of smaller diameter (in µm), similarly for D50 and D90. SPAN is a measure of the droplet size distribution and is defined by SPAN = (D90 − D10)/D50. D10 = 29.2 (26.8–33.5) µm, D50 = 59.7 (51.4–75.3) µm, D90 = 127.3 (102.7–155.6) µm, SPAN 1.64 (1.48–1.76).

A HPLC based analytical method was used to determine stability of the nasal formulation and was defined as 97.0–103.0 percent (*n* = 4) of the initial drug concentration in the formulation following storage (2–8 °C) over a period of 48 h, the maximum time elapsed between manufacture and dosing of the patients. Column: Discovery Bio wide pore C18 (25 mm × 4.6 mm i.d., 5 µm); Mobile Phase: Phase A: 0.1 M Sodium Perchlorate, pH 2.7, Phase B: Acetonitrile; Flow Rate: 1.0 mL/min; Run Time 50 min;

Injection Volume: 15 µL; Column Temperature: 60 °C; Auto Sampler Temperature: 2–8 °C; Detection: 210 nm.

3.2. Preparation of Nasal Formulations for Ovine Study

The liquid nasal formulation used in the sheep was prepared identically to that for the human study, with the exception that it was manufactured in the Critical Pharmaceutical Laboratories (CPL) and did not contain the Tc-99m-DTPA label. The dry powder formulation was also prepared at CPL as 1% *w/w* PTH (1-34) with 39% Gellan gum, 40% Solutol® HS15, 20% Trehalose. In brief, 97.5 mg Gellan gum was dissolved in 50 mL ultra-pure water overnight. Solutol® HS15 was rendered molten (60 ± 10 °C), and 100 mg was added to the Gellan gum solution and mixed for 30–45 min at 60 °C. 50 mg of trehalose was added and mixed for a further 10 min. A total 5 mg of PTH 1-34 was dissolved in 5 mL of ultra-pure water, and 2.5 mL was added to the formulation. Particles were prepared using a spray dryer Mini Spray Dryer B-290 (Buchi UK Ltd., Oldham, UK) with the inlet set at 85 °C (outlet modified by inlet temperature), the aspirator 100%, the pump set at 006 equivalent to 2 mL/ min, the spray pressure at 4 bar. Particle size of the dry powder formulation manufactured for use in the sheep was not measured, due to limited availability of material due to batch size. However, the particle size of similar formulations when prepared for loading into the delivery devices was monitored using Helos/BF (Sympatec GmbH, Clausthal-Zellerfeld, Germany) during formulation development, where the VMD was 73.7–91.8 µm (×10 = 10.6–23.7 µm, ×50 = 51.5–98.1 µm, ×90 = 142–153 µm). A total 2.4–2.8% of particles were below 10 µm. As the vast majority of particles were >10 µm, the formulations would be expected to be nasally deposited. The integrity of the spray dried PTH 1-34 was monitored during formulation development by HPLC analysis, which consistently revealed a purity of >82.5% PTH 1-34.

3.3. Healthy Human Volunteer Pharmacokinetic/Gamma Scintigraphy Study

The study was conducted in accordance with the Declaration of Helsinki, and the protocol for the clinical study was given a favourable opinion (12 September 2013) by the NRES committee London Westminster (ref 13/LO/1037, IRAS ID 126447). All participants gave their informed consent before they participated in the study. This included regulatory approvals from the Medicines and Healthcare products Regulatory Agency (MHRA), Nottingham University Hospitals NHS Trust Research & Innovation (NUH NHS Trust R&I) and certification from the Administration of Radioactive Substances Advisory Committee (ARSAC). The study was registered at https://clinicaltrials.gov/ website and with the Trent Comprehensive Local Research Network (Trent CLRN). A dose escalation component was included within the approved study using a developmental delivery device, however, the data are not reported here due to commercial sensitivities.

The focus of the study was to investigate the plasma pharmacokinetics of parathyroid hormone PTH 1-34 delivered in a liquid nasal spray formulation containing the excipient polyethylene glycol (15)-hydroxystearate (Solutol® HS15). Furthermore, the nasal deposition and clearance of the formulation was investigated using gamma scintigraphy. The pharmacokinetics and the deposition and clearance of the nasal spray by gamma scintigraphy were investigated in the same clinical study.

3.3.1. Pharmacokinetics

An open cross-over clinical IMP (investigative medicinal product) study was conducted in seven healthy female subjects aged over 55 years (mean age 67.7, range 58 to 81 years). Each participant provided informed consent in accordance with ethical committee requirements and good clinical practice. Pre-study screening assessments were carried out within 21 days of the participants receiving their first dose (Supplementary Materials: Section S1). Inclusion and exclusion criteria were applied (Supplementary Materials: Section S2). Participants were admitted to the study centre on the morning of dosing, having abstained from alcohol and smoking for at least 24 h previously and fasted from midnight. Participants were given a light meal on arrival. A cannula was then positioned in the participant's arm or hand to facilitate the collection of blood samples. The pre-dose sample was taken.

Participants received a single subcutaneous injection of 20 µg teriparatide into the abdomen at their first trial visit. Following a seven day wash out period, each participant self-administered 90 µg PTH 1-34 from the nasal spray formulation using the Rexam SP270 nasal spray device; the patients had previously been trained in operation of the Rexam device. Any episodes of sneezing after administration of the nasal formulation were recorded. The nasal spray formulation contained Tc-99m-DTPA, 3–5 MBq per Rexam SP270 nasal spray dose, resulting in an effective radiation dose of less than 0.14 mSv to each participant.

Following either subcutaneous or intranasal dosing, 10 mL blood samples (Becton Dickinson sodium heparin) were taken at 5, 15, 30, 60 120, 180, 240, 300 and 360 min. After each sample was taken, the cannula was flushed with 10 mL 0.9% saline. Blood was stored on ice and centrifuged within 30 min to prepare plasma (4 °C, 1100–1300 g, 10 min). These samples were stored at −20 °C before dispatching to Simbec Research Ltd. (Merthyr Tydfil, UK) for quantification by validated ELISA, in compliance with The UK Good Laboratory Practice Regulations 1999 (Statutory Instrument No. 310 6) and subsequent amendment, OECD Principles of Good Laboratory Practice (Paris 1998) and EC Commission Directive 2004/10/EC of February 2004.

Pharmacokinetic data were analysed using Phoenix® WinNonlin® 5.1 (Certara USA, Inc., Princeton, NJ, USA) from quantified PTH 1-34 in the plasma, using recorded sampling times. Summary statistics (mean, median, SD, coefficient of variation [CV%], minimum, maximum, *n*) and the following plasma pharmacokinetic parameters were calculated:

- C_{max}
- T_{max}
- Terminal half-life ($t_{1/2}$)
- AUC to 2 h (AUC_{0-2h})
- AUC to last measured time point (AUC_{last}) and corresponding F_{rel} for nasal formulation

3.3.2. Gamma Scintigraphy

For the gamma scintigraphy part of the study, a custom designed, rigid frame was attached to a single head X ring gamma camera (Mediso Ltd., Budapest, Hungary) and used to support the chin of the participant. This maintained a fixed position of the nose in a sagittal view relative to the camera, and negated the need to register the longitudinal image series. From immediately post-dose, a 20 min continuous (dynamic) image acquisition was recorded comprising 40 × 30 s frames. In addition, 30 min post administration, a 30 s frame was acquired which was repeated every 30 min thereafter, terminating at 2 h post-dose. Participants returned for a safety follow-up between 1 and 14 days after their final study procedure.

All seven participants attended the University of Nottingham MRI clinical facility (Sir Peter Mansfield Imaging Centre, School of Medicine) prior to the clinical study to generate a sagittal view of the head and neck to provide an anatomical image of the nasal cavity. The acquisition sequence protocol was: 3 plane localiser, Asset Calibration, Coronal STIR, Sagittal T_2 and Sagittal T_1 using a GE 750 3T MRI fitted with a 32 channel head coil.

Using a HERMES image workstation (Hermes Medical Solutions, Gravesend, UK) the scintigraphic images were superimposed upon the DICOM MRI images to enable reference of the nasal spray deposition site and to define formulation clearance relative to anatomical position within the nasal cavity. Using the sagittal MRI anatomical view, four regions of interest (ROI) were defined: one around the anterior site of deposition in the nasal cavity, the second covering the nasal cavity and nasopharynx to the level of the oropharynx, a third covering the entire region and a fourth distal region to obtain the background counts. The counts obtained from the ROIs were subject to various corrections to account for image time, background activity and radioactive decay. The time for 50% clearance of the total amount of radioactivity deposited in the nasal region ($T_{50\%}$) was calculated for each subject. $T_{50\%}$ was calculated from corresponding activity–time profiles by fitting 4 parameter logistic regression

(GraphPad Prism 6). For data where this program was unable to make a satisfactory curve fit, the $T_{50\%}$ was obtained by straight line interpolation.

3.3.3. Ovine Study

Research was conducted in accordance with the requirements of the Animals (Scientific Procedures) Act 1986 (ASPA) under Procedural Project Licence (PPL) number 40/3552 (Protocol 19b/1), between 26 April 2016 and 24 May 2016, at the University of Nottingham, Nottingham, UK (Procedural Establishment Licence (PEL) number PCD 40/2406). The overarching protocol (as detailed in the PPL) was subject to full review by the Animal Welfare and Ethical Review Board (AWERB), and the study-specific protocol received a more localised review by the Named Animal Care and Welfare Officer (NACWO) and Named Veterinary Surgeon (NVS). This research governance is compliant with recommended ethical review processes. In view of the clinical data obtained in the present study, the pharmacokinetics of the Solutol® HS15-based formulation of PTH 1-34 were further investigated in sheep. The sheep study replicated the clinical trial in that it tested the nasal solution formulation of PTH 1-34 as well as a subcutaneous injection, but also evaluated pharmacokinetics of PTH 1-34 following intravenous injection and an intranasal PTH1-34 dry powder formulation.

The study was conducted according to a four-way randomised cross-over study in four (Mule crossbred) female sheep (obtained from a reputable commercial supplier). The sheep were group housed in a heat and ventilation air conditioned (HVAC) facility for the duration of the study, and were uniquely identified by a combination of ear tag and electronic transponder. On arrival, the animals were also randomly assigned a unique identifier by the facilities Research Animal Facility Management system (LabTracks, Locus Technology Inc., Manchester, MD, USA) and an abbreviated study number (1, 2, 3 and 4). To aid identification during the study, the fleece of each animal was marked with the abbreviated study number by spraying with a commercial stockmarker (dye). The animals were acclimatised for 17 days prior to initiation of treatments. The animals were subject to a health inspection by the NVS prior to and after use in the study, and were monitored during the study by the PPL holder and facility personnel supported by the NACWO, NVS and University of Nottingham personnel. Animals were weighed weekly during the study (Supplementary Materials: Section S3).

The sheep were housed in a temperature and humidity controlled facility (14.2–22.2 °C and humidity from 42–70%) for the duration of the study. On the four study legs, temperature and humidity during the experimental period ranged from 17.6–19.8 °C and 51–61%, respectively. Sheep were routinely fed twice daily with hay and standard grower diet (pellets), with water ad libitum. The sheep were provided with food (approximately double rations of hay) to last overnight on the day prior to each study leg; remaining food was removed approximately 60 min before the start of dosing on each leg. Water was available throughout. Sheep were fed as normal following collection of the last blood sample on each study leg. At the end of the study, the animals were euthanised by overdose of anaesthetic.

Administration of the PTH 1-34 was either as an intranasal liquid, intranasal dry powder, subcutaneous injection or intravenous injection. The treatments were randomised according to a Latin Square design using an online randomisation programme (Experimental Design Generator and Randomiser (Edgar) accessed from: http://www.edgarweb.org.uk/) with a minimum of a two day washout period between study legs. Immediately prior to dosing, the four sheep were sedated by an intravenous injection of ketamine hydrochloride (100 mg/mL solution administered at 2.25 mg/kg). This provided approximately 3 min sedation, during which period the sheep were dosed.

The formulations were prepared at Critical Pharmaceuticals' Laboratories and transported, refrigerated, to the study facility. The intranasal liquid was administered via the right nostril using a LMA™ MAD110 Nasal™ Intranasal mucosal atomization device (MAD110) (Wolfe-Tory Medical, Inc., Salt Lake City, UT, USA) customised for use in sheep (to allow circumvention of the nostril and delivery of the dose to the respiratory mucosa of the nasal cavity). The intranasal powder formulation was also administered via the right nostril using a 5 mm oral/nasal tracheal tube Portex® Blueline 100/111/050,

(Smiths Medical, Ashford, UK) and one-way bellows. The amount of powder administered to each animal, and thus the nominal dose of PTH 1-34, was determined by weighing the devices before and after the nasal administrations. The subcutaneous and intravenous bolus injections of PTH 1-34 were administered into the flank and a jugular vein, respectively. Further details relating to dose administration are provided in Table 1. It has been reported in the literature that injections into the thigh as opposed to the abdomen have been estimated to result in a 21% slower rate of absorption, resulting in an 18% reduction in maximum plasma teriparatide concentrations (C_{max}) and 1.5 min prolongation in the time to reach peak concentration (T_{max}) [19]. Therefore, care was taken to mirror the subcutaneous injection site (flank) in the sheep model.

Table 1. Dosing of four female sheep (Mule crossbred) with PTH 1-34.

Formulation	Route	Nominal PTH Concentration (µg/mL)	Dose Volume (mL)	Dose Weight (mg)	Nominal PTH Dose (µg)
Solution [#]	intranasal	1000	0.2 †	not applicable	200
Powder	intranasal	10 **	not applicable	20 † (13 ± 1.5) §	200 (130 ± 15) §
Solution *	subcutaneous	40	0.5	not applicable	20
Solution *	Intravenous	40	0.5 ‡	not applicable	20

[#] nasal spray formulation as described for clinical study; * injection formulations did not contain 7.5% *w/v* polyethylene glycol (15)-hydroxystearate (Ph.Eur.); ** µg/mg; † nasal doses administered via single (right) nostril; ‡ intravenous doses given as a bolus injection; § Mean (± SE) powder and PTH 1-34 dose weights in parentheses calculated by weighing devices before and after dosing.

A qualitative assessment of local tolerability to the administered intranasal formulations (animals dosed by injection served as controls) was made by recording the incidences of sneezing/snorting in the first 60 min following dosing and any evidence of nasal discharge prior to dosing, at 15 min intervals in the first 60 min, and then at subsequent blood sampling time points thereafter. As part of the monitoring procedure, any other 'remarkable' observation was noted.

For pharmacokinetic evaluation, blood samples (3 mL) were collected by direct venepuncture of a cephalic vein (both veins used interchangeably) under local anaesthesia (topical application of EMLA™ Cream 5%, Astra Zeneca). For intranasal and subcutaneous treatments, blood samples were collected at time 0 (prior to dosing), 5, 10, 15, 30, 45, 60, 120, 180 and 240 min post-dose administrations. For the intravenous treatment, blood samples were collected at time 0 (prior to dosing), and at 2, 5, 15, 30, 45, 60, 120, 180 and 240 min post-dose administration. Each blood sample was dispensed into a BD Vacutainer and stored on crushed ice prior to centrifugation at 2000× *g* (3135 rpm) for 10 min at 4 °C (Sorvall™ legend RV refrigerated centrifuge). The samples were stored at −20 °C prior to PTH 1-34 quantification by ELISA kit (Immunotopic, San Clemente, CA USA) as directed by the manufacturer; optical densities were measured using an LT-4000 Microplate Reader (Labtech International Ltd, Heathfield, UK).

Pharmacokinetic analysis of the plasma PTH 1-34 concentration–time data was performed using Phoenix® WinNonlin® 6.4 (Certara USA, Inc., Princeton, NJ, USA) and Excel 2016 (Microsoft, Redmond, WA, USA). The following were used as the principal measures to evaluate intranasal and subcutaneous absorption of PTH 1-34 in the sheep compared to intravenous injection: C_{max}; T_{max}; $t_{1/2}$; AUC_{last}; and AUC_{INF} (definitions as before); C_0 (initial plasma concentration estimated by back-extrapolating from the first two concentration values) was also estimated after intravenous administration only. F_{rel} (bioavailability of intranasal (IN) or intravenous (IV) PTH 1-34, relative to subcutaneous (SC) injection) and F_{ab} (absolute bioavailability of IN or SC PTH 1-34, relative to IV) were estimated as follows:

$$F_{rel} (\%) = (AUC_{INF(IN \text{ or } IV)} \times Dose_{(SC)}) \div (AUC_{INF(SC)} \times Dose_{(IN \text{ or } IV)}) \times 100$$

$$F_{ab} (\%) = (AUC_{INF(IN\ or\ SC)} \times Dose_{(IV)}) \div (AUC_{INF(IV)} \times Dose_{(IN\ or\ SC)}) \times 100$$

4. Results

4.1. Clinical Study

All seven healthy volunteers completed the clinical study and all pre- and post-clinical assessments were acceptable. There were no serious adverse events during this study and no participant sneezed after nasal dosing.

4.1.1. Pharmacokinetics

The mean pharmacokinetic profiles of PTH 1-34 when delivered as a liquid nasal spray formulation or as a subcutaneous injection to healthy volunteers and corresponding summary pharmacokinetic data are presented in Figure 1 and Table 2, respectively. The mean profile obtained following subcutaneous administration (20 µg dose) of teriparatide was consistent with those obtained in individual subjects (not shown) and showed rapid absorption (mean C_{max} 253 pg/mL with range in C_{max} values of 141.8 to 406.5 pg/mL and mean T_{max} of 21 min) and elimination (mean $t_{1/2}$ approximately 1 h). Teriparatide concentrations returned to zero by 6 h. This was in contrast to PTH 1-34 delivered by liquid nasal spray (90 µg dose) with plasma concentrations only being measured above baseline in two of the seven subjects at 15 and 30 min (14.0–18.9 pg/mL) or 30 and 60 min (17.7–15.4 pg/mL) post-dose administration (for all seven subjects mean C_{max} 5 pg/mL with T_{max} 9 min; $t_{1/2}$ could not be calculated as PTH 1-34 was only measured in the plasma at two time points in these participants, where the concentration was observed to increase with time). The bioavailability of PTH 1-34 after intranasal dosing was approximately 1% (for the subjects with measurable plasma concentrations, but 0.26% if all seven subjects were included in the calculations) compared to the subcutaneous injection of Forsteo®. The pharmacokinetic parameters—C_{max}, T_{max}, AUC_{0-2h} and AUC_{0-last}—for the two delivery routes differed markedly (Table 2).

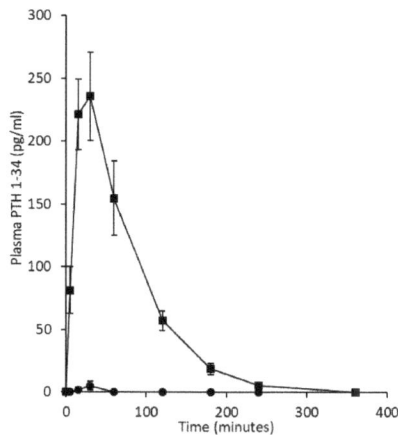

Figure 1. Pharmacokinetics of a single dose of either a liquid intranasal spray formulation containing the excipient Solutol® HS15 or a subcutaneous injection of teriparatide by a pen to healthy female subjects aged over 55 years (mean age 67.7, range 58 to 81 years). Circles represent the mean ± SE of the PTH 1-34 plasma concentration delivered from a Rexam SP270 nasal spray device (*n* = 7). Squares depict the PTH 1-34 plasma concentration in participants following subcutaneous injection using a commercially available formulation and injection pen (Eli Lilly).

Table 2. Pharmacokinetics of a single dose of an intranasal liquid spray formulation containing the excipient Solutol® HS15 or of a commercially available subcutaneous teriparatide injection formulation.

	Subcutaneous Injection (20 µg Teriparatide) *	Intranasal Spray (90 µg PTH 1-34) ‡
C_{max} (pg/mL)	252.5	5.2
t_{max} (min)	21.4	8.6
$t_{1/2}$ (min)	64.8	NC
AUC_{0-2h} (pg·min/mL)	17,381.9	242.3
AUC_{0-last} (pg·min/mL)	20,725.6	242.3

* $n = 7$ volunteers, each dose was given within a cross-over study with a one week washout between doses. ‡ $n = 7$, values were not detectable in 5 of the 7 volunteers. NC: not calculable.

4.1.2. Gamma Scintigraphy

An overview of the deposition and clearance of the nasal spray formulation delivered using a Rexam SP270 device is presented as a time series of scintigraphy images (Figure 2 and Supplementary Materials: Section S4). This represents the anatomical location of the Tc-99m-DTPA containing formulation, plotted as a density plot superimposed upon the sagittal view MRI of the participant. These data are a typical example and depicts Subject 2 in this study. The time series of images, 3, 15, 30, 60, 90 and 120 min, illustrates that the formulation was deposited in the anterior of the nasal cavity, extending to the mid-part of the nasal cavity in the region corresponding to the inferior meatus/turbinate, and was subsequently cleared from the inferior turbinates to the nasopharynx. The mean clearance curve obtained for the nasal spray formulation is shown in Figure 3. This depicts the amount of radioactivity (Tc^{99m}) that was present in the nasal cavity at each image timepoint. To adjust for variation between subjects in terms of the precise dose of Tc-99m-DTPA deposited, the counts obtained after analysis of the first frame (i.e., after 30 s) were taken as the total counts (100%) for each subject. The scintigraphy clearance data identified that the administered formulation underwent a rapid initial clearance phase (0–20 min) from the nasal cavity. The second phase demonstrated clearance at a slower rate (30–120 min). There was some variability in the clearance data between participants, graphically represented using 95% CI (Figure 3). These data can be summarised as having a median value for $T_{50\%}$ of 17.8 min (minimum 10.9, maximum 74.3 min).

4.1.3. Ovine Study

The mean pharmacokinetic profiles of PTH 1-34 in sheep when delivered nasally, as a liquid nasal spray formulation or dry powder, or by subcutaneous injection is shown in Figure 4. Corresponding summary pharmacokinetic data are presented in Table 3. The ovine study data replicate the clinical study regarding the liquid nasal spray formulation containing Solutol® HS15 making comparison to the subcutaneous injection. As in humans, the subcutaneous profile obtained in sheep showed rapid absorption and elimination of PTH 1-34; C_{max} for the 20 µg subcutaneous injection was 121 ± 47 pg/mL (mean, SE), with a median T_{max} of 10 min (range 5–15 min) and an elimination half-life of 54 ± 8 min (range 43–71 min, $n = 3$). A 200 µg intranasal dose of the PTH 1-34 liquid formulation produced a C_{max} of 47 ± 21 pg/mL and T_{max} of 10 min (range 10–15 min), and concentrations had returned to near baseline values by 30 min post-dose. The dry powder formulation was introduced to the experimental design in an attempt to improve upon the pharmacokinetic profile obtained for the liquid nasal spray. However, this formulation resulted in poor absorption of PTH 1-34 across the nasal mucosa following administration of a nominal 200 µg dose (actual dose based on weighing devices before and after administration ranged from 100–170 µg): C_{max} 8 ± 3 pg/mL. The intravenous injection provided reference pharmacokinetic data and facilitated calculation of absolute bioavailability (Figure 5). The intravenous pharmacokinetic profile of the PTH 1-34 plasma concentration demonstrated rapid elimination of PTH 1-34. The observed C_{max} for a 20 µg dose was 1142 ± 198 pg/mL at 2 min post-injection, returning to near baseline at 30–45 min. The bioavailabilities (F_{rel}) of PTH 1-34 from the liquid nasal formulation containing Solutol® HS15 and dry powder formulation, relative to subcutaneous injection, were 1.4 ± 0.3% and 1.0 ± 0.1%, respectively. The absolute bioavailability of subcutaneous injection of PTH 1-34 was 77.0 ± 13.7%.

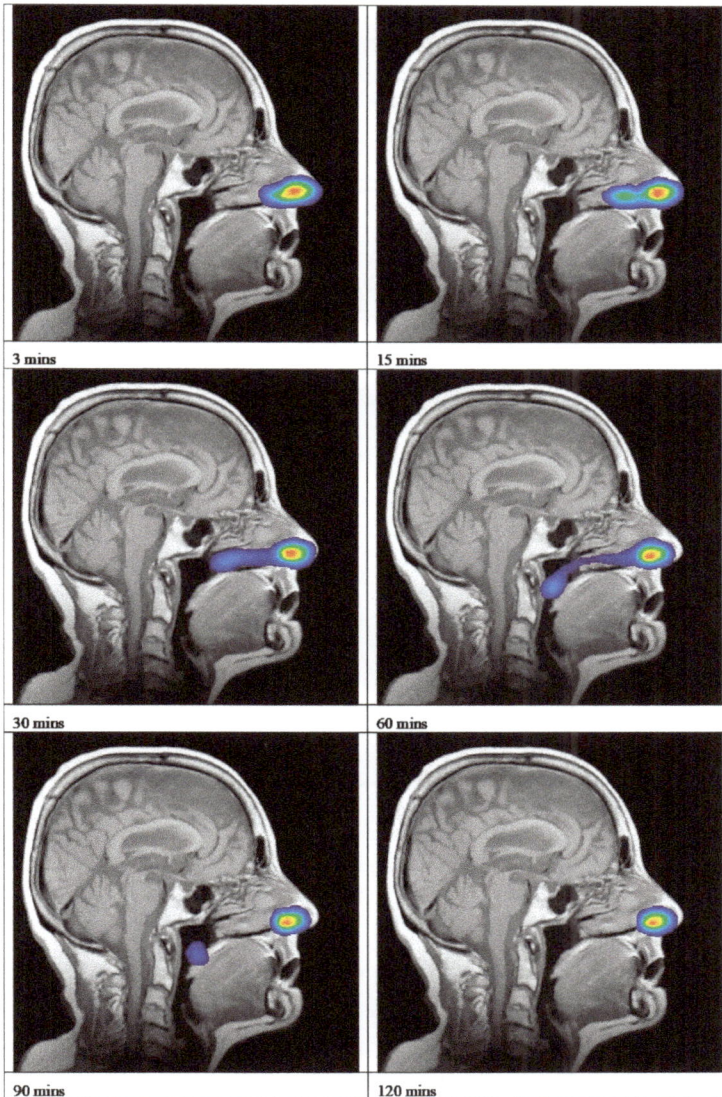

Figure 2. Deposition and clearance of nasal spray formulations delivered using a Rexam SP270 device. Scintigraphic images superimposed upon the MRI sagittal image of Subject 2, showing the clearance of the Tc^{99m}-DTPA nasal spray formulation. (The highest levels of activity are shown in red and yellow.).

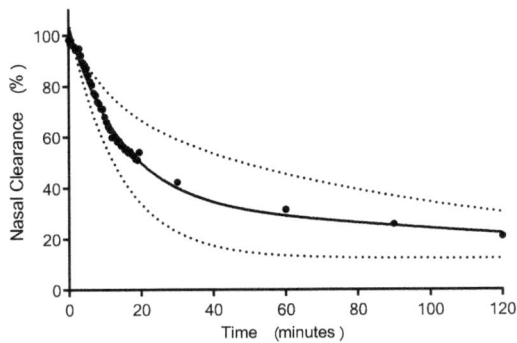

Figure 3. The clearance of Tc-99m-DTPA PTH 1-34 liquid formulation, delivered from a Rexam SP270 nasal spray device fitted with a Rexam 3959 standard winged applicator to healthy female subjects aged over 55 years (two phase decay clearance curve (Prism 7.03) fitted to mean values = solid line, ±95% CI = dotted line, *n* = 7).

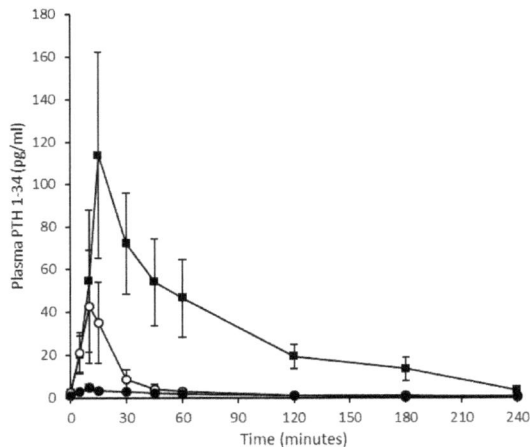

Figure 4. Pharmacokinetic profile of change of plasma PTH (1-34) concentration with time when delivered to an ovine model. Quantification of PTH (1-34) in plasma prepared from blood sampled at 5, 10, 15, 30, 45, 60, 120, 180, 240 min. Squares represent subcutaneous injection (20 µg), open circles represent intranasal liquid formulation (200 µg) and solid circles represent Gellan gum dry powder formulation (130 µg). (Mean values ± SE, *n* = 4 with the exception of the subcutaneous injection where *n* = 3.).

Monitoring of body weight (Supplementary Materials: Section S3) and adverse effects was conducted during the sheep study. One animal, Sheep 1, was withdrawn from the study prior to dosing on study leg 4 due to the animal suffering what appeared to be a seizure, further details are provided in Supplementary Materials, Section S3. All other general observations with regards to adverse effects monitoring were considered unremarkable.

In terms of monitoring for local tolerability, one incidence of sneezing/snorting was recorded across the four sheep that received the intravenous injection of PTH 1-34, and one incidence across the three sheep that received the subcutaneous injection. After administration of the PTH 1-34 liquid nasal spray formulation, there were six incidences of sneezing/snorting across three of four study animals, compared to ten incidences across three of four study animals after administration of the dry powder formulation. However, 9 of these 16 incidences were in Sheep 1, which, as stated above, was subsequently withdrawn due to ill health. Slight nasal discharge was noted on a single occasion in each of the two sheep that received subcutaneous and intravenous injections. Slight nasal discharge was observed in three of four study animals after intranasal administration of solution (one, two or four incidences observed) and powder (one, two or three incidences) formulations. Similarly, 7 of the 13 incidences of sneezing/snorting in nasally dosed animals were observed in Sheep 1. (Further details relating to incidences of sneezing/snorting and nasal discharge in sheep are summarised in Supplementary Materials, Section S5.)

Table 3. Summary of ovine pharmacokinetic parameters obtained for PTH 1-34 following intranasal (200 μg dose), subcutaneous (20 μg dose) and intravenous (20 μg dose) administration of PTH 1-34.

	Intranasal Liquid (200 μg)	Intranasal Powder (200 μg [1])	Subcutaneous Injection (20 μg)	Intravenous Injection (20 μg)
C_{max} (pg/mL)	47 ± 21	8 ± 3	121 ± 47	1142 ± 198 [2]
T_{max} (min)	10 ± 2.0 (10)	11 ± 6.6 (8)	12 ± 1.5 (10)	2 ± 0 (2)
$t_{1/2}$ (min)	109 ± 43.7 (77)	96 ± 29.8 (71)	54 ± 8.7 (47)	75 ± 18.1 (78)
AUC_{0-last} (pg·min/mL)	1094 ± 410	317 ± 49	7197 ± 2204	10,660 ± 1888
AUC_{INF} (pg·min/mL)	1222 ± 370	442 ± 41	7460 ± 2220	10,799 ± 1900 [3]
F_{rel} (%) [4]	1.4 ± 0.31	1.0 ± 0.12	100	155.8 ± 24.0
F_{ab} (%) [5]	1.1 ± 0.26	0.7 ± 0.03	77.0 ± 13.71	100

Data presented as mean ± SE (median values presented in parentheses where applicable); $n = 4$ except in the subcutaneous injection group, where $n = 3$. Except in the case of F_{rel}/F_{ab} values, no correction has been made to the data to account for the dose of PTH 1-34 administered. [1] For the powder formulation, this represents the nominal dose; the estimated dose, based on emitted dose weight of powder, was 100 μg Sheep 1, 170 μg Sheep 2, 130 μg Sheep 3 and 120 μg Sheep 4 (mean ± SE 130 ± 15μg); [2] C_0 was 2182 ± 696 pg/mL following extrapolation to $t = 0$; [3] Since the subcutaneous injection group only comprised data from three animals (Sheep 2, 3, and 4) the corresponding mean AUC_{INF} ± SE value from these three animals was 9361 ± 1758 pg/mL·min; [4] relative to subcutaneous injection for each individual animal, where subcutaneous data were missing (Sheep 1), the average AUC_{INF} ($n = 3$) was used in the calculation (in the case of the intravenous injection, the calculated F_{rel} for $n = 4$ was approximately 156% compared to 140% for $n = 3$, the nominal PTH 1-34 used throughout except for the powder formulation, where the estimated dose, as given above, was used; [5] relative to intravenous injection, the nominal PTH 1-34 dose was used throughout except for the powder formulation, where the estimated dose, as given above, was used.

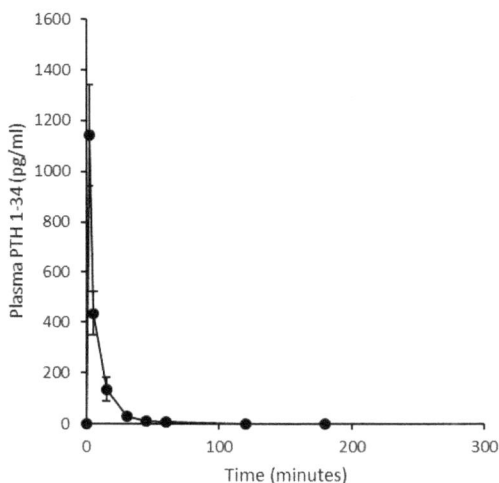

Figure 5. Plasma pharmacokinetic profile of an intravenous injection (20 μg) of PTH (1-34) in an ovine model. Quantification of PTH (1-34) in plasma prepared from blood sampled at 2, 5, 15, 30, 45, 60, 120, 180, 240 min. (Mean ± SE, $n = 4$.).

5. Discussion

Currently, in the UK and also globally, bisphosphonates are the first line of drug treatment for osteoporosis in the majority of patients. Subcutaneous injection of teriparatide has received regulatory approval for the treatment of post-menopausal women with osteoporosis, men with hypogonadal or idiopathic osteoporosis, and men and women with glucocorticoid-induced osteoporosis at high risk for fracture. In the UK, this is a second-line treatment in the National Health Service (NHS). At present, the course of treatment is up to 24 months [20]. Teriparatide has an imminent patent expiry date, which is of commercial interest [21]. Greater costs are incurred in the manufacture of injectable formulations compared to those for nasal delivery. An economic consideration regarding teriparatide prescription exists, as it is considerably more expensive than a course of bisphosphonate treatment [22]. Research indicates that patients poorly adhere to the long course of injections prescribed, and therefore a therapeutically efficient simple nasal spray, while cheaper to produce, would also be welcomed by patients being treated with PTH 1-34 [6–8].

An absolute bioavailability of 95% (i.e., intravenous injection 100%) has previously been reported for PTH 1-34 in human subjects when administered by subcutaneous injection into the abdominal wall [23]. Our clinical study did not attempt to replicate an assessment of absolute bioavailability, but instead focused on the current clinical route of administration of PTH 1-34 as a comparator for the nasal formulation under investigation, and therefore relative bioavailability to this delivery route. Our study data showed a plasma PTH 1-34 $t_{1/2}$ of 65 min post subcutaneous injection, which is similar to previously published values [19]. C_{max} for this delivery route was 253 pg/mL which is also comparable to those reported [24]. The pharmacokinetics we report for subcutaneous injection represent the consensus option in the literature [25–27]. As detailed above, the relative bioavailability of the intranasally dosed liquid nasal spray was approximately 0.26–1% of the subcutaneous injection of Forsteo® (Lilly France S.A.S, France) [28]. Published literature regarding nasal spray formulations are sparse, and those that are available tend to lack formulation and or pharmacokinetic data, making comparison difficult [28,29].

We consider the scintigraphy data to be an important aspect of our study, which demonstrated that the liquid nasal spray was deposited predominantly anteriorly in the nasal cavity. There is sparse literature regarding how the anatomical site of the deposition of the nasal spray formulation within the nasal regions influences transmucosal entry of peptides into the blood [30]. Deposition of the formulation is reported to be required posterior to the nasal valve, possibly within a larger and supra region of the turbinates than we achieved in order to attain optimal absorption of teriparatide [31–34]. The liquid formulation delivered to the nasal cavity in humans was rapidly cleared, and, hence, the time available for absorption was limited. It is not possible from the scintigraphic images obtained in the study to determine the percentage of formulation that did not reach (and deposit) past the nasal valve. Hence, suboptimal deposition could have contributed to the low bioavailability obtained. Similarly, we do not have data regarding how the excipient polyethylene glycol (15)-hydroxystearate, included in the formulation to promote absorption of PTH 1-34 into the plasma, interacted with the nasal mucosal surface. Perhaps a longer residency could improve drug plasma concentration, and this warrants further research. However, the $T_{50\%}$ median clearance time of 17.8 min (minimum 10.9, maximum 74.3 min) is comparable to published data on nasal clearance of liquid formulation [35].

The present clinical study showed disappointing relative bioavailability following delivery in a liquid formulation via the nasal route. This was not consistent with the previous data from our small animal preclinical studies [14]. In the preceding preclinical conscious rat model, we reported the pharmacokinetic performance of an intranasally administered PTH 1-34 subcutaneous formulation, an intranasal liquid formulation with no enhancer and an intranasal solution containing Solutol® HS15. PTH 1-34 doses of 80 µg/kg by subcutaneous injection and 100 µg/kg intranasally were given to rats. The C_{max} and T_{max} were approximately 14 ng/mL at 10 min, with 78% relative bioavailability for intranasally administered PTH 1-34 for the Solutol® HS15-based formulation, compared to 2 ng/mL,

13 min and 8% for the intranasal delivery without enhancer. We therefore expected that a relative bioavailability of at least 10% in humans should have been achievable.

Our sheep pharmacokinetic data for the SC and IV injections of PTH 1-34 are comparable with published values in human subjects. A 20 µg PTH 1-34 subcutaneous dose delivered to post-menopausal women with osteoporosis has been reported in a peer reviewed manuscript by the manufacturers of the commercial formulation to have a C_{max} in the region of 150 pg/mL and an elimination half-life of approximately 1 h. As previously stated, the absolute bioavailability of PTH SC injection in human subjects is approximately 95%. F_{ab} obtained in sheep herein was 77 ± 14% (range 55–108%). The relative bioavailability (F_{rel}) of the liquid intranasal formulation in the sheep was 1.4% ± 0.43%, close to that calculated for humans in the clinical study of approximately 1%. The mean C_{max} value in sheep of 47 ± 21 pg/mL can be put in context against reported values for the typical basal endogenous PTH concentration for post-menopausal women (28 pg/mL) and the 65 pg/mL upper limit in premenopausal women for endogenous PTH, yet at the dose given, were below the therapeutic concentrations currently used in treatment of osteoporosis [19,23].

With the aim of improving upon the pharmacokinetics of the liquid nasal spray in humans, our continued research evaluated a bioadhesive powder formulation within a large animal (ovine) model. This is a model known to be highly representative of intranasal drug delivery that closely replicates the clinical findings [17,36]. When using the ovine model to assess the dry powder formulation containing the same absorption enhancer, excipient delivered via the intranasal dry powder formulation did not improve upon the pharmacokinetics of the liquid nasal formulation. Likewise, we have published on the nasal administration in conscious rats of human growth hormone (hGH) (MW 22kDa), a molecular mass approximately five times that of PTH 1-34, with the permeation enhancer Solutol® HS15 (10%) added to the liquid formulation. For the first 2 h after administration, there was a relative bioavailability of 49% [11]. Powder formulations of the hGH with Solutol® HS15 were subsequently administered to human volunteers and compared to a subcutaneous injection of hGH. The relative bioavailability was found to be about 3%, although clinically relevant plasma concentrations could be reached with a twice daily hGF intranasal dose [18].

Observations made during the clinical study with healthy human subjects did not concur with the indicated mild irritation caused to the nasal cavities of the sheep (Supplementary Materials: Section S5) after administration of the nasal formulations [37]. However, the dose of PTH 1-34 in sheep was increased to 200 µg from the 90 µg delivered in the clinical study. A previously published clinical study reported in the literature, where 250, 500 and 1000 µg doses were delivered, reported some symptoms indicative of nasal irritation [28].

6. Conclusions

In conclusion, our study shows that PTH 1-34 was poorly absorbed from a liquid nasal spray containing the permeation enhancer Solutol® HS15 in healthy individuals with a 1% relative bioavailability. The scintigraphy imaging confirmed the anatomical site of deposition and rapid clearance of the administered dose in humans. The $T_{50\%}$ median was 17.8 min (minimum 10.9, maximum 74.3 min). When increasing the dose in the liquid nasal spray to 200 µg of PTH 1-34, this dose then resulted in a mean C_{max} value of 47 pg/mL in sheep. This value is between one third and one fifth of the C_{max} values for the drug administered at the prescribed dose of 20 µg as a subcutaneous injection for the treatment of osteoporosis in men and women.

The results discussed here for PTH 1-34 in two animal models, rats and sheep, and in humans, together with the results previously reported for hGH in rat and humans, highlights the issue of translation from animal models to humans, not only for the therapeutic effects of drugs but also for the effect of specific drug delivery systems, such as the Solutol® HS15 permeation enhancer. Many nasal delivery systems that include permeation enhancers for peptide drugs have been tested in various animal models, such as rats, rabbits and dogs, where they have been shown to effectively promote the uptake of peptide drugs, only to fail in clinical trials. The translation of effects seen in animal models

Pharmaceutics **2019**, *11*, 265

to humans may depend on many factors, such as the type of intervention, study protocol, animal model and case specific factors. There are opposing opinions in the research community about the relevance of animal models [38]. However from our data, we consider that for peptide nasal delivery, the sheep model provides a better indication of the potential of translation to humans than the rat. Translational research has recently been made a priority both in the US by NIH (budget $500 million per year), in the EU (budget €6 billion) and in the UK (budget £500 million over five years) in order to assess the likelihood of successful cross-species translation [39].

Supplementary Materials: The following are available online at http://www.mdpi.com/1999-4923/11/6/265/s1, Section S1: Clinical Trial: Screening Visit Assessment and Familiarisation with Device; Section S2: Clinical Trial: Inclusion and Exclusion Criteria; Section S3: Body Weight of Study Animals and Adverse Event; S4: Formulation Nasal Clearance in Health Volunteers—Clinical Study: Section S5: Nasal Tolerability in Sheep.

Author Contributions: Conceptualization, A.L.L., L.I., T.M., A.C.P. and R.G.P.; methodology, R.G.P., A.N., M.H., K.J., F.J., A.S.-A., A.C.P.; formal analysis, R.G.P, M.H., F.J., G.K., A.C.P.; investigation, R.G.P., E.B., A.N., M.H., K.J., F.J., G.K., A.C.P.; resources, R.G.P., T.M., M.H., G.K., A.C.P.; data curation, R.G.P., F.J., G.K., M.H., A.C.P.; writing—original draft preparation, R.G.P.; writing—review and editing, R.G.P., T.M., A.N, M.H., G.K., A.L.L., L.I., A.C.P.; visualization, R.G.P., M.H., A.C.P.; supervision, R.G.P., T.M., G.K., A.C.P.; project administration, R.G.P., T.M., G.K., A.C.P.; funding acquisition, R.G.P., T.M., A.L.L., L.I., A.C.P.

Funding: This research was funded by a Technology Strategy Board (17223-124195)/Engineering and Physical Sciences Research Council (Grant ref: EP/K502364/1). In addition funds were also made available from the EPSRC Impact Acceleration Account Knowledge Transfer Secondments (Grant ref: EP/K503800/1).

Acknowledgments: The authors would like to acknowledge the support of Robin Spiller for holding the ARSAC licence for the human administration of the radiolabelled formulation.

Conflicts of Interest: The authors declare no conflict of interest. The sponsors had no role in the design, execution, interpretation, or writing of the study.

References

1. Baron, R.; Hesse, E. Update on Bone Anabolics in Osteoporosis Treatment: Rationale, Current Status, and Perspectives. *J. Clin. Endocrinol. Metab.* **2012**, *97*, 311–325. [CrossRef] [PubMed]
2. Dhiman, P.; Andersen, S.; Vestergaard, P.; Masud, T.; Qureshi, N. Does bone mineral density improve the predictive accuracy of fracture risk assessment? A prospective cohort study in Northern Denmark. *BMJ Open* **2018**, *8*, 018898. [CrossRef] [PubMed]
3. Moppett, I.K.; Wiles, M.D.; Moran, C.G.; Sahota, O. The Nottingham Hip Fracture Score as a predictor of early discharge following fractured neck of femur. *Age Ageing* **2012**, *41*, 322–326. [CrossRef] [PubMed]
4. Maxwell, M.J.; Moran, C.G.; Moppett, I.K. Development and validation of a preoperative scoring system to predict 30 day mortality in patients undergoing hip fracture surgery. *Br. J. Anaesth.* **2008**, *101*, 511–517. [CrossRef] [PubMed]
5. Bunning, T.; Dickinson, R.; Fagan, E.; Inman, D.; Johansen, A.; Judge, A.; Hannaford, J.; Liddicoat, M.; Wakeman, R. *National Hip Fracture Database (NHFD) Annual Report 2018*; Royal College of Physicians: London, UK, 2017.
6. Modi, A.; Sajjan, S.; Insinga, R.; Weaver, J.; Lewiecki, E.M.; Harris, S.T. Frequency of discontinuation of injectable osteoporosis therapies in US patients over 2 years. *Osteoporos. Int.* **2017**, *28*, 1355–1363. [CrossRef] [PubMed]
7. Chan, D.C.; Chang, C.H.C.; Lim, L.C.; Brnabic, A.J.M.; Tsauo, J.Y.; Burge, R.; Hsiao, F.Y.; Jin, L.; Gurbuz, S.; Yang, R.S. Association between teriparatide treatment persistence and adherence, and fracture incidence in Taiwan: Analysis using the National Health Insurance Research Database. *Osteoporos. Int.* **2016**, *27*, 2855–2865. [CrossRef] [PubMed]
8. Fraenkel, L.; Gulanski, B.; Wittink, D. Patient treatment preferences for osteoporosis. *Arthritis Care Res. Off. J. Am. Coll. Rheumatol.* **2006**, *55*, 729–735. [CrossRef] [PubMed]
9. Brayden, D.J.; Bzik, V.A.; Lewis, A.L.; Illum, L. CriticalSorb promotes permeation of flux markers across isolated rat intestinal mucosae and Caco-2 monolayers. *Pharm. Res.* **2012**, *29*, 2543–2554. [CrossRef] [PubMed]
10. Illum, L. Nasal drug delivery—Recent developments and future prospects. *J. Control. Release* **2012**, *161*, 254–263. [CrossRef] [PubMed]

11. Illum, L.; Jordan, F.; Lewis, A.L. CriticalSorb (TM): A novel efficient nasal delivery system for human growth hormone based on Solutol HS15. *J. Control. Release* **2012**, *162*, 194–200. [CrossRef] [PubMed]

12. Rohrer, J.; Lupo, N.; Bernkop-Schnurch, A. Advanced formulations for intranasal delivery of biologics. *Int. J. Pharm.* **2018**, *553*, 8–20. [CrossRef] [PubMed]

13. Maggio, E.T. Intravail™: Highly effective intranasal delivery of peptide and protein drugs AU-Maggio. *Expert Opin. Drug Deliv.* **2006**, *3*, 529–539. [CrossRef] [PubMed]

14. Williams, A.J.; Jordan, F.; King, G.; Lewis, A.L.; Illum, L.; Masud, T.; Perkins, A.C.; Pearson, R.G. In vitro and preclinical assessment of an intranasal spray formulation of parathyroid hormone PTH 1-34 for the treatment of osteoporosis. *Int. J. Pharm.* **2018**, *535*, 113–119. [CrossRef] [PubMed]

15. Shubber, S.; Vllasaliu, D.; Rauch, C.; Jordan, F.; Illum, L.; Stolnik, S. Mechanism of Mucosal Permeability Enhancement of CriticalSorb (R) (Solutol (R) HS15) Investigated In Vitro in Cell Cultures. *Pharm. Res.* **2015**, *32*, 516–527. [CrossRef] [PubMed]

16. Soane, R.J.; Frier, M.; Perkins, A.C.; Jones, N.S.; Davis, S.S.; Illum, L. Evaluation of the clearance characteristics of bioadhesive systems in humans. *Int. J. Pharm.* **1999**, *178*, 55–65. [CrossRef]

17. Illum, L. Nasal delivery. The use of animal models to predict performance in man. *J. Drug Target.* **1996**, *3*, 427–442. [CrossRef]

18. Lewis, A.L.; Jordan, F.; Patel, T.; Jeffery, K.; King, G.; Savage, M.; Shalet, S.; Illum, L. Intranasal Human Growth Hormone (hGH) Induces IGF-1 Levels Comparable With Subcutaneous Injection With Lower Systemic Exposure to hGH in Healthy Volunteers. *J. Clin. Endocrinol. Metab.* **2015**, *100*, 4364–4371. [CrossRef]

19. Satterwhite, J.; Heathman, M.; Miller, P.D.; Marin, F.; Glass, E.V.; Dobnig, H. Pharmacokinetics of Teriparatide (rhPTH 1–34) and Calcium Pharmacodynamics in Postmenopausal Women with Osteoporosis. *Calcif. Tissue Int.* **2010**, *87*, 485–492. [CrossRef]

20. Joint Formulary Committee. *British National Formulary*, 72th ed.; BMJ Group and Pharmaceutical Press: London, UK, 2018.

21. Takacs, I.; Jokai, E.; Kovats, D.E.; Aradi, I. The first biosimilar approved for the treatment of osteoporosis: Results of a comparative pharmacokinetic/pharmacodynamic study. *Osteoporos. Int.* **2019**, *30*, 675–683. [CrossRef]

22. Basu, P.; Joglekar, G.; Rai, S.; Suresh, P.; Vernon, J. Analysis of Manufacturing Costs in Pharmaceutical Companies. *J. Pharm. Innov.* **2008**, *3*, 30–40. [CrossRef]

23. Eli_Lilly. *Highlights of Prescribing Information*; AbbVie Inc.: North Chicago, IL, USA, 2014; Available online: https://pi.lilly.com/us/forteo-pi.pf (accessed on 20 November 2018).

24. Haemmerle, S.P.; Mindeholm, L.; Launonen, A.; Kiese, B.; Loeffler, R.; Harfst, E.; Azria, M.; Arnold, M.; John, M.R. The single dose pharmacokinetic profile of a novel oral human parathyroid hormone formulation in healthy postmenopausal women. *Bone* **2012**, *50*, 965–973. [CrossRef] [PubMed]

25. Forssmann, W.-G.; Tillmann, H.-C.; Hock, D.; Forssmann, K.; Bernasconi, C.; Forssmann, U.; Richter, R.; Hocher, B.; Pfuetzner, A. Pharmacokinetic and Pharmacodynamic Characteristics of Subcutaneously Applied PTH-1-37. *Kidney Blood Press. Res.* **2016**, *41*, 507–518. [CrossRef]

26. Henriksen, K.; Andersen, J.R.; Riis, B.J.; Mehta, N.; Tavakkol, R.; Alexandersen, P.; Byrjalsen, I.; Valter, I.; Nedergaard, B.S.; Teglbjaerg, C.S.; et al. Evaluation of the efficacy, safety and pharmacokinetic profile of oral recombinant human parathyroid hormone rhPTH(1-31)NH$_2$ in postmenopausal women with osteoporosis. *Bone* **2013**, *53*, 160–166. [CrossRef] [PubMed]

27. Liu, Y.; Shi, S.; Wu, J.; Li, Z.; Zhou, X.; Zeng, F. Safety, Tolerability, Pharmacokinetics and Pharmacodynamics of Recombinant Human Parathyroid Hormone after Single- and Multiple-Dose Subcutaneous Administration in Healthy Chinese Volunteers. *Basic Clin. Pharmacol. Toxicol.* **2012**, *110*, 154–161. [CrossRef] [PubMed]

28. Matsumoto, T.; Shiraki, M.; Hagino, H.; Iinuma, H.; Nakamura, T. Daily nasal spray of hPTH(1–34) for 3 months increases bone mass in osteoporotic subjects: A pilot study. *Osteoporos. Int.* **2006**, *17*, 1532–1538. [CrossRef] [PubMed]

29. Brandt, G.C.; Spann, B.M.; Sileno, A.P.; Costantino, H.R.; Li, C.; Quay, S.C. Teriparatide nasal spray: Pharmacokinetics and safety versus subcutaneous teriparatide in healthy volunteers. *Calcif. Tissue Int.* **2006**, *78*, S45.

30. Djupesland, P.G. Nasal drug delivery devices: Characteristics and performance in a clinical perspective—A review. *Drug Deliv. Transl. Res.* **2013**, *3*, 42–62. [CrossRef] [PubMed]

31. McInnes, F.J.; O'Mahony, B.; Lindsay, B.; Band, J.; Wilson, C.G.; Hodges, L.A.; Stevens, H.N.E. Nasal residence of insulin containing lyophilised nasal insert formulations, using gamma scintigraphy. *Eur. J. Pharm. Sci.* **2007**, *31*, 25–31. [CrossRef]

32. Takala, A.; Kaasalainen, V.; Seppala, T.; Kalso, E.; Olkkola, K.T. Pharmacokinetic comparison of intravenous and intranasal administration of oxycodone. *Acta Anaesthesiol. Scand.* **1997**, *41*, 309–312. [CrossRef]

33. Djupesland, P.G.; Skretting, A. Nasal Deposition and Clearance in Man: Comparison of a Bidirectional Powder Device and a Traditional Liquid Spray Pump. *J. Aerosol Med. Pulm. Drug Deliv.* **2012**, *25*, 280–289. [CrossRef]

34. Charlton, S.; Jones, N.S.; Davis, S.S.; Illum, L. Distribution and clearance of bioadhesive formulations from the olfactory region in man: Effect of polymer type and nasal delivery device. *Eur. J. Pharm. Sci.* **2007**, *30*, 295–302. [CrossRef] [PubMed]

35. Al-Ghananeem, A.; Sandefer, E.; Doll, W.; C Page, R.; Chang, Y.; A Digenis, G. Gamma scintigraphy for testing bioequivalence: A case study on two cromolyn sodium nasal spray preparations. *Int. J. Pharm.* **2008**, *357*, 70–76. [CrossRef] [PubMed]

36. Soane, R.J.; Hinchcliffe, M.; Davis, S.S.; Illum, L. Clearance characteristics of chitosan based formulations in the sheep nasal cavity. *Int. J. Pharm.* **2001**, *217*, 183–191. [CrossRef]

37. Masud, T.; Pearson, R.G. Nasally and sc Administered Teriparatide in Healthy Volunteers (NINTTO). Available online: https://clinicaltrials.gov/ct2/show/NCT01913834 (accessed on 5 June 2019).

38. Ioannidis, J.P.A. Extrapolating from Animals to Humans. *Sci. Transl. Med.* **2012**, *4*, 15. [CrossRef] [PubMed]

39. Woolf, S.H. The meaning of translational research and why it matters. *JAMA J. Am. Med. Assoc.* **2008**, *299*, 211–213. [CrossRef]

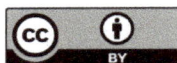

pharmaceutics

MDPI

Article

A Tailored Thermosensitive PLGA-PEG-PLGA/Emulsomes Composite for Enhanced Oxcarbazepine Brain Delivery via the Nasal Route

Ghada M. El-Zaafarany [1], Mahmoud E. Soliman [1], Samar Mansour [1,2], Marco Cespi [3], Giovanni Filippo Palmieri [3], Lisbeth Illum [4], Luca Casettari [5,*] and Gehanne A. S. Awad [1]

[1] Department of Pharmaceutics and Industrial Pharmacy, Faculty of Pharmacy, Ain Shams University, Monazzamet Elwehda Elafrikeya Street, Abbaseyya, Cairo 11566, Egypt; ghada@pharma.asu.edu.eg (G.M.E.-Z.); mahmoud.e.soliman@pharma.asu.edu.eg (M.E.S.); samar.mansour@guc.edu.eg (S.M.); gawad@pharma.asu.edu.eg (G.A.S.A.)
[2] Department of Pharmaceutical Technology, Faculty of Pharmacy and Biotechnology, German University in Cairo, Al-Tagmoaa Alkhames, Cairo 11835, Egypt
[3] School of Pharmacy, University of Camerino, Via S. Agostino 1, 62032 Camerino (MC), Italy; marco.cespi@unicam.it (M.C.); gianfilippo.palmieri@unicam.it (G.F.P.)
[4] IDentity, 19 Cavendish Crescent North, The Park, Nottingham NG7 1BA, UK; lisbeth.illum@illumdavis.com
[5] Department of Biomolecular Sciences, School of Pharmacy, University of Urbino, Piazza del Rinascimento 6, 61029 Urbino (PU), Italy
* Correspondence: luca.casettari@uniurb.it; Tel.: +39-0722303332

Received: 10 October 2018; Accepted: 1 November 2018; Published: 5 November 2018

Abstract: The use of nanocarrier delivery systems for direct nose to brain drug delivery shows promise for achieving increased brain drug levels as compared to simple solution systems. An example of such nanocarriers is emulsomes formed from lipid cores surrounded and stabilised by a corona of phospholipids (PC) and a coating of Tween 80, which combines the properties of both liposomes and emulsions. Oxcarbazepine (OX), an antiepileptic drug, was entrapped in emulsomes and then localized in a poly(lactic acid-*co*-glycolic acid)-poly(ethylene glycol)-poly(lactic acid-*co*-glycolic acid) (PLGA-PEG-PLGA) triblock copolymer thermogel. The incorporation of OX emulsomes in thermogels retarded drug release and increased its residence time (MRT) in rats. The OX-emulsome and the OX-emulsome-thermogel formulations showed in vitro sustained drug release of 81.1 and 53.5%, respectively, over a period of 24 h. The pharmacokinetic studies in rats showed transport of OX to the systemic circulation after nasal administration with a higher uptake in the brain tissue in case of OX-emulsomes and highest MRT for OX-emulsomal-thermogels as compared to the IN OX-emulsomes, OX-solution and Trileptal® suspension. Histopathological examination of nasal tissues showed a mild vascular congestion and moderate inflammatory changes around congested vessels compared to saline control, but lower toxic effect than that reported in case of the drug solution.

Keywords: nose to brain delivery; antiepileptic drug; drug delivery; block copolymers; thermogel system

---

1. Introduction

Hydrogels that are prepared from "intelligent" or "smart" polymers and capable of exhibiting a physicochemical response in a nonlinear manner to an external stimuli, such as temperature [1,2], pH [3], light [4], counter-ion changes [5] and biological molecules [6] have been extensively investigated in the literature. These polymers have great potential in drug delivery and tissue engineering [7–9], in addition to sensors and valves [10].

Thermosensitive polymers are a subcategory of smart polymers that undergo temperature-induced reversible sol-gel transition upon heating/cooling of the aqueous polymer solution. Drugs/formulations sequestered within these copolymers by simple mixing are administered as a solution that gels at body temperature at the desired site of application [11], and are used particularly in the field of controlled drug release.

Thermosensitive di-block copolymers that are composed of hydrophilic polyethylene glycol (PEG) as block A and hydrophobic biodegradable polyesters as block B e.g., poly(lactic acid) (PLA); poly(glycolic acid) (PGA); polyethylene terephthalate (PET); and polycaprolactone (PCL), have been studied as controlled release drug carriers [12–14]. Particularly, the di-block copolymer PEG/PLGA hydrogels are attractive polymers for the delivery of drugs since they are biodegradable with a good safety profile and their compositions can be tailored to provide sustained drug delivery [15–17].

Tri-block thermosensitive copolymers are used in either ABA or BAB configuration, with the poloxamers (ABA) (PEG-PPO-PEG) being of interest due to their commercial availability in a wide range of molecular weights and block ratios [18]. However, they show slow biodegradation kinetics and the inability to provide sustained drug delivery over more than just a few days [19,20]. Therefore, triblock copolymers consisting of PEG and PLGA copolymer moieties are regarded as good alternatives, being non-toxic, water-soluble biocompatible, biodegradable according to copolymer ratio used, and thus, can have tailor-made properties [21].

The gelation mechanisms of thermosensitive hydrogels based on PLGA-PEG-PLGA are illustrated in Figure 1. The cited copolymer self-assembles in micellar formations in aqueous media. A rise in temperature results in the dehydration of the PEG chains, causing the micelle formations to shrink, thus enhancing the interaction between the PEG and PLGA blocks [22]. At temperatures below the critical gelation temperature (CGT), the bridging between micelles are usually unstable due to the low hydrophobicity of PLGA [23]. With increasing temperatures that approach CGT and exceed it, a firm bridged micellar network forms because of the increase in hydrophobic interaction between the chains, thus enhancing inter micellar interaction and aggregation, leading to subsequent gelation [24,25].

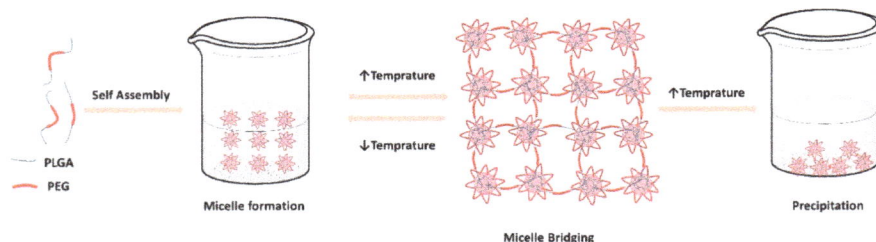

Figure 1. Schematic diagram of the sol-gel transition of BAB type poly(lactic acid-*co*-glycolic acid)-poly(ethylene glycol)-poly(lactic acid-*co*-glycolic acid) (PLGA-PEG-PLGA) tri-block copolymer aqueous solution in response to temperature.

In the present study we adopted a PLGA-PEG-PLGA tri-block copolymer (PLGA (3:1) M_W 1.88 kDa and PEG M_W 1.5 kDa) that was first synthesized by Zentner et al., 2001. Gelling of an aqueous solution of a PLGA-PEG-PLGA copolymer is initiated at around 32 °C, while at 37 °C, the flow of the copolymer solution decreases dramatically as the gel state is established, maintaining the gel in situ for prolonged periods of time. Hence, it is an excellent candidate for prolonging residence time of the sequestered drug/formulation on the nasal mucosa after IN application [26].

Oxcarbazepine (OX), which is used as a model drug in this study, is employed for the treatment of partial and generalized seizures that are associated with epilepsy. OX is usually administered via the oral route exhibiting distribution to non-targeted tissues, a high first pass metabolism, with potential drug-drug interactions as well as undesirable side effects [27]. OX is a microsomal enzyme inducer that necessitates the use of high therapeutic doses which support the interest in a direct transport of the drug to the brain such as what may be achieved by nose to brain delivery [28].

Emulsomes are nanocarriers prepared with lipid cores either in the solid or liquid crystalline state at 25 °C, coated with a phospholipid bilayer. These nanocarriers combine the characteristics of lipid spheres (apolar core) and liposomes (hydrophilic surface) [29]. Due to the apolar solid core, emulsomes can entrap higher amounts of lipophilic drugs [30]. Being composed of triglycerides that are surrounded by phospholipids, emulsomes form particles similar to micelles, hence, vastly increasing the solubility, as well as the bioavailability of poorly soluble drugs [31]. Previous studies from our laboratories optimised the emulsomes in terms of physicochemical characteristics, especially in terms of a prolonged release profile and nose to brain delivery of OX. It was found that the emulsomes delivery system showed a significantly higher brain C_{max} and a higher brain $AUC_{0-1440min}$ than an IV injection of OX and the oral administration of the marketed OX product.

The aim of this study was to investigate whether a combination of the thermo-responsive hydrogel and lipid-based nanoparticles (emulsomes) would enhance the promising results obtained previously for the OX emulsomes alone in delivery of the drug from nose to brain.

In the first instance the thermogelling PLGA-PEG-PLGA copolymer was synthesized and characterized using NMR, GPC, DSC, DLS, and its rheological behaviour investigated. Oxcarbazepine (OX)-loaded emulsomes was than mixed with PLGA-PEG-PLGA tri-block copolymer to develop a 2-phase drug depot system and the formed thermogel was characterized in terms of sol-gel transition temperature, viscosity, drug release and mucoadhesion.

Finally, the delivery system was evaluated in rats for the transport of OX from the nasal cavity to the systemic circulation and the brain tissue, and the histopathology of the OX-emulsome-thermogel delivery system in the nasal cavity investigated.

2. Materials and Methods

2.1. Materials

Oxcarbazepine (OX) was a gift from Novartis Pharmaceutical Co. (Cairo, Egypt). Triolein (TO) (Captex GTO) was generously supplied by Abitec Corp. (Janesville, WI, USA). Soya phosphatidylcholine (PC) and Tween 80 (Tw) were purchased from Sigma Chemical Co. (St. Louis, MO, USA). Chloroform and methanol were purchased from ADWIC, El Nasr Pharmaceutical Co. (Cairo, Egypt). The dialysis membrane made from standard grade regenerated cellulose (molecular weight cut off 12–14 Da) was purchased from Spectrum Laboratories Inc. (Rancho Dominguez, CA, USA). Di-hydroxyl-terminated polyethylene glycol (M_w 1.5 kDa) (PEG 1.5 kDa) and stannous-2-ethyl-hexanoate were purchased from Sigma-Aldrich (Steinheim, Germany). 3,6-dimethyl-1,4-dioxane-2,5-dione (D,L-lactide) and 1,4-dioxane-2,5-dione (glycolide) were kindly supplied by PURAC Biochem (Gorinchem, Netherlands). All other chemical used were of analytical grade.

2.2. Synthesis of PLGA-PEG-PLGA Tri-Block Copolymers

The composition and choice of molecular weights of the PEG and the PLGA components of the PLGA-PEG-PLGA copolymer was designed to have similar sol-gel forming properties as those that were previously synthesized by Chen et al. [32]. They found that the gel-to-sol and sol-to-gel transition only occurred with appropriate molecular weight and molar mass dispersity of the copolymer.

The PLGA-PEG-PLGA copolymer was produced by the method described by Zentner et al. [7]. Briefly, PEG 1.5 kDa was initially dried by azeotropic distillation in toluene under an atmosphere of nitrogen, followed by drying at 130 °C under vacuum, then allowed to melt by placing 6 g in a three-neck flask under vacuum with continuous agitation at150 °C for 3 h, thus generating a viscous liquid mass [33]. D,L-lactide and glycolide were then added with respective amounts of 6 and 1.5 g to maintain a fixed molar ratio of 3:1.

The reaction mixture was maintained at 150 °C under vacuum for another 30 min with constant mixing to allow the fusion of D,L-lactide and glycolide. Stannous-2-ethyl-hexanoate was subsequently added and the reaction mixture was further heated for 1 h [7].

In order to remove the unreacted monomers at the end of the reaction, the raw copolymer was dissolved in dichloromethane and poured dropwise into ethyl ether kept in an ice bath. The pure copolymer was precipitated, then separated by filtration, dried under vacuum and kept refrigerated [34].

2.3. Characterization of PLGA-PEG-PLGA Copolymers

In order to verify polymer formation and determine its chemical structure and molecular weight, the following characterisation methods were utilized on PLGA-PEG-PLGA copolymer solutions:

2.3.1. Nuclear Magnetic Resonance (^{1}H-NMR)

Structural analysis of the PLGA-PEG-PLGA copolymer, initial determination of its molecular weight and estimation of the lactide:glycolide ratio, was carried out via NMR spectroscopy. The copolymer was dissolved in deuterated acetone and analysis was done using NMR spectroscopy (Varian Mercury 400 MHz spectrometer, Varian Inc., Palo-Alto, CA, USA) operating at 400 MHz [35]. Subsequently, the molecular weight was calculated by comparing the integral of the signal for PEG protons chemical shift at 3.6 ppm with the integrals of glycolide at 4.8 ppm and those of lactide at 1.6 and 5.2 ppm.

2.3.2. Gel Permeation Chromatography (GPC)

7.5 mg of the PLGA-PEG-PLGA copolymer was dissolved in tetrahydrofuran and acetonitrile and then placed in a water bath at 40 °C for one hour. Vial contents were filtered through a regenerated cellulose syringe filter (diameter 13 mm and 0.45 μm pore size) then analyzed by a high performance liquid chromatography system (HPLC, Agilent Series 1100 LCsystem (Agilent Technologies, Waldbronn, Germany), equipped with a Gel permeation column (TSKGel 2500HHR from Tosoh Bioscience LLC, Montgomeryville, PA, USA) maintained at 37 °C, with tetrahydrofuran as the eluent at a flow rate of 1 mL/min [36].

The molecular weight was quantified by use of a calibration curve resulting from a series of PEG standards with low polydispersity and known molecular weights ranging from 106 Da to 21.3 kDa (PEG Calibration Kit PL 2070-0100, Varian Inc., Palo-Alto, CA, USA). Data were analyzed using the software DATAAPEX (DataApex Ltd., Prague, Czech Republic). Accordingly, the molecular weights of the copolymer were computed, expressed as number average molecular weight, M_n, and weight average molecular weight, M_w.

2.3.3. Differential Scanning Calorimetry (DSC)

Thermal analysis of the PLGA-PEG-PLGA copolymer was carried out in a DSC apparatus (PerkinElmer 8500, Perkin Elmer, Waltham, MA, USA) equipped with an intracooler in inert nitrogen atmosphere. A sample of the copolymer was placed in a closed aluminium pan and heated with a two-stage program at a rate of 10 °C/min. The 1st heating run was conducted from ambient temperature to 150 °C to remove the thermal history of the polymer (i.e., remaining solvent and humidity) and the 2nd run from −40 to 210 °C to determine the sample specific data. Both heating cycles were separated by a cooling run that was conducted at a rate of 10 °C/min [37].

2.3.4. Size Measurement of Copolymer Solution by Dynamic Light Scattering (DLS)

The DLS equipment (Zetasizer Nano ZS, Malvern Instrument, Malvern, UK) was adopted to measure the hydrodynamic diameter and size distribution of the PLGA-PEG-PLGA copolymer micelles, using a detector laser beam fixed at an angle of 90° [38]. To investigate the formation of micelles and the variation in micellar size in relation to temperature, a copolymer solution of 20% *w/w* in deionized water was prepared. 1 mL of the sample was analyzed at increasing temperatures from 10 to 40 °C. The experiment was performed in triplicate.

2.4. Preparation and Characterization of PLGA-PEG-PLGA Thermogel Solutions Loaded with Emulsomes

2.4.1. Sample Preparation

An optimised emulsome formulation (TO17-TW) was chosen from previous studies comprising a 3:1 ratio of PC:TG (TG ~Triolein), a total lipid content of 30 mg and coated with Tween 80 [36,37]. The emulsomes were prepared and characterized as a lipid mixture of PC and TO, as previously described [39,40]. Briefly, 10 mgs OX were introduced into a clean, dry round bottom flask, dissolved in chloroform, and then mixed with 30 mg lipid mixture composed of PC:TG (3:1). The organic solvent was removed using a rotary evaporator (Model RVO5, Janke and Kunkel, IKA Laboratories, Staufen, Germany). The formed thin film was hydrated by agitation for 1 h at room temperature with phosphate buffer (pH 6.8) containing 5% tween 80. The formed dispersion was sonicated for 1 min (Bath sonicator model 275T, Crest Ultrasonics Carp, Trenton, NJ, USA), then extruded through 450 nm cellulose nitrate membranes, and stored at 4 °C. The size of the emulsomes has previously been found to be in the order of 101.5 ± 2.9 nm [40].

For characterization of the final thermogel, different formulation concentrations (5, 10, 20, and 30% *w/w*) of aqueous PLGA-PEG-PLGA copolymer solutions were investigated. The solutions were prepared by dissolving pre-cooled PLGA-PEG-PLGA copolymer in deionized water via continuous magnetic stirring of the mixture in an ice bath until complete dissolution. This was followed by the addition of emulsomes in different loading concentrations (0, 10, 25, and 50% *v/v*) by physical mixing. Table 1 shows the coding, compositions and gelation temperature of all prepared thermogel formulations with G1-G16 indicating the individual compositions.

Table 1. Coding, compositions and gelation temperatures of prepared thermogels.

Emulsome Concentration % *v/v*	Gelation Temperature (°C ± SD)			
	PLGA-PEG-PLGA Copolymer (% *w/w*)			
	5%	10%	20%	30%
0%	G1 No gelation	G2 Opaque solution	G3 30.2 ± 0.05 °C	G4 28.5 ± 0.1 °C
10%	G5 No gelation	G6 Opaque solution	G7 31.5 ± 0.1 °C *	G8 29.0 ± 0.06 °C *
25%	G9 No gelation	G10 Opaque solution	G11 32.0 ± 0.06 °C *	G12 30.1 ± 0.05 °C *
50%	G13 No gelation	G14 Opaque solution	G15 33.4 ± 0.05 °C *	G16 31.0 ± 0.0 °C *

* Significantly different ($p < 0.05$) from emulsome free gel.

2.4.2. Macroscopic Phase Behaviour of Aqueous Copolymer Solutions and Determination of Gelation Temperature

The sol-gel transition temperatures of the aqueous copolymer solutions with the addition of 0–50% emulsomes were investigated by a tube inversion method [38]. Briefly, 0.5 mL of each solution (G1-G16) was placed in a thermoset circulating water bath where the temperature increased stepwise (0.5 °C) from 20 to 52 °C, with an equilibrium time of 3 min. At each temperature setting, tubes were inverted to check the flow properties. Solutions were considered to be in the gel state if the appearance changed from transparent to opaque with no observed flow for 30 s following the tube inversion [41].

2.4.3. Viscosity Measurement

The viscosities of the copolymer solutions that completely gelled at a temperature ranging between room (25 °C) and body temperatures (37 °C) were measured using a programmable Brookfield viscometer (Brookfield engineering laboratories Inc. model HADV-II, Middleboro, MA, USA) connected to a digital thermostatically controlled water bath (Polyscience Inc. model 9101, Niles, IL, USA). A sample of 0.5 g thermogel was applied onto the lower plate of the viscometer, adjusted at 37 °C. Rheological measurements were conducted at rpm range of 1–100 (shear rate 2–200 s^{-1}), using CPE-52 spindle.

2.5. In Vitro Drug Release

Franz type diffusion cells (Variomag Telesystem, H+P Labortechnik, Oberschleißheim, Germany) were used to compare the release and transport of OX from OX-emulsomes [40] to that from OX-emulsomal gel (G16) through a dialysis membrane in. An amount of the OX-emulsomes or the OX-emulsomal gel equivalent to 3 mg OX was introduced to the donor compartment of the diffusion cell. The detailed methodology was as described elsewhere [40].

2.6. Mucoadhesion Studies

The mucoadhesive strengths of the G16 emulsomal thermogel in comparison to its corresponding plain thermogel G4 and 0.5% Carbopol 980 gel as a positive control were determined by measuring the force that is required to detach the formulation from freshly excised sheep nasal mucosa, using a texture analyser CT3 (Brookfield Engineering Laboratories, Inc., Middleboro, MA, USA) in tension mode. The sheep nasal mucosa was obtained from the local slaughter house. The mucosal membrane was separated from underlying fat and loose tissues, then washed with distilled water followed by phosphate buffer (pH 6.8) at 37 °C and cut into pieces that fit the stainless-steel cylindrical probe of the device of 10 mm in diameter (3.14 cm^2).

A cut sample of the nasal mucosa was glued to the upper probe using a cyanoacrylate adhesive, keeping the mucosal side exposed. Fixed amounts of the appropriate thermogel were attached to the lower probe of the instrument with double-sided adhesive tape. The upper probe with the nasal tissue was lowered until the tissue contacted the surface of the gelled sample with a downward trigger force of 4 N for a contact time of 5 min to ensure intimate contact between the tissues and the samples [42]. The probe was then moved vertically upwards at a constant speed of 3 mm/s [43]. Work of adhesion, mJ, peak detachment force, N, deformation peak, mm, and final load, N, were all calculated from force-distance plots using the built-in Texture Exponent software.

2.7. In Vivo Studies

2.7.1. Pharmacokinetic Study

- Administration of OX containing formulations to rats

Male Wister albino rats weighing 200–250 g were divided into two groups, each containing forty eight rats. Group 1 received OX IN in phosphate buffer solution (pH 6.8) intranasally (IN), Group 2 received IN OX-emulsomes dispersion, Group 3 received IN G16 emulsomal thermogel and Group 4 received Oral Trileptal suspension. The drug dose was adjusted to be 0.32 mg/kg.

Results obtained from Group 2 and Group 4 were taken from identical experiments reported in El-Zaafarany et al. [40] for comparative reasons.

Conscious, non-anaesthetised rats were fixed in a prostrate position and 80 µL/kg of the formulations were administered into each of the two nostrils using a microinjector [44]. Blood samples were collected from the retro-orbital vein of four rats at predetermined time intervals and introduced into heparinized tubes. Plasma was separated from blood samples by centrifugation at 4000 rpm for 10 min and OX was analysed using a LC-MS/MS technique [40]. At each time interval, the animals were sacrificed and the brain tissues (not including the olfactory bulb) were separated, homogenized with saline and stored at −80°C until further assay. Ethical approval of this protocol was given by the "Experiments and Advanced Pharmaceutical Research Unit" of the Faculty of Pharmacy, Ain Shams University, Cairo, Egypt and National Institutes of Health guidelines for the use and care of Laboratory animals were followed in the course of this study (Project No.: 6 10 2016 approved on December 2016).

- Assay of OX content in plasma and brain samples

Chromatographic conditions (LC–MS/MS analysis parameters) and pharmacokinetic analysis of OX in plasma and brain (Peak plasma and brain concentrations (C_{max}), the time to reach these peaks (t_{max}) were determined, area under OX concentration-time curve ($AUC_{0-2880min}$), time to reach half the maximum plasma concentration ($t_{1/2}$), and the mean residence time (MRT)), as reported in our previous publication [40].

2.7.2. Histopathological Study

20 μL of the Ox loaded G16 emulsomal thermogel was applied daily to one nostril of male Wister rats (group size *n* = 3) weighing 180–220 g for 14 consecutive days, while the other nostril was used as control and treated with normal saline. Rats were then sacrificed and the nasal septa with their covering membranes were separated, formalin-fixed for one day, decalcified, washed with tap water, and then dehydrated by sequential exposure to methyl, ethyl and absolute alcohol).

Specimens were cleared by xylene, embedded in paraffin blocks, sectioned by slide microtome. Sections were deparaffinized and stained with hematoxylin and eosin and examined with a light microscope (Olympus optical microscope, Tokyo, Japan).

2.8. Statistical Analysis

Experiments were done in triplicates and all data that are shown in this study are expressed as a mean ± standard deviation (SD). Comparison of means was undertaken using Student *t*-test for dual comparisons and ANOVA test followed by Tukey-Kramer post-Hoc test for multiple comparisons using a statistical software program (GraphPad Instat, La Jolla, CA, USA). $p < 0.05$ were considered to be statistically significant.

3. Results

3.1. Preparation and Characterization of PLGA-PEG-PLGA Triblock Copolymers

PLGA-PEG-PLGA triblock copolymers were synthesized via ring-opening polymerization of D,L-lactide and glycolide initiated with PEG. The copolymer formed appeared as a sticky yellowish-brown semisolid. PLGA-PEG-PLGA is a non-ionic triblock copolymer consisting of hydrophilic PEG segments and hydrophobic PLGA segments. The process of polymer synthesis is shown in the supplementary part Figure S1.

3.1.1. NMR Spectroscopy

A typical NMR spectrum of PLGA-PEG-PLGA triblock copolymer is shown in the supplementary part Figure S2, showing the same characteristic signals as those reported in the literature [37]. Respective methyl (–CH₃) and methine (–CH–) proton peaks pertaining to lactide monomer were observed at 1.6 and 5.2 ppm. A peak at 4.8 ppm, corresponding to methene protons (–CH₂–) of glycolide monomer was obtained, as well as a peak at 3.6 ppm relative to methene in PEG monomer which was used for the calculation of the PEG:PLGA ratio.

By comparing the peak areas of specific types of prominent protons at corresponding chemical shifts or by the total number of these protons, the molecular weight of the polymer was calculated [36,37,45]. By analyzing the value of the integrals of peaks that are related to lactide and glycolide, the chain number molecular weight (M_n) of the tri-block copolymer was determined to be 5.2 kDa

3.1.2. GPC

Figure S3 in the supplementary part shows the GPC chromatograms of PEG and the prepared PLGA-PEG-PLGA block copolymer. It is obvious that the copolymer was eluted at a shorter time (at 6.76 min) than PEG, indicating that polymerization was successful and products of lower retention time have been formed. In addition, the unimodal GPC curve reflects that the purity of the prepared copolymer is sufficiently high. The number average molecular weight (M_n) was found to be 4.4 kDa, which corresponds to that obtained by NMR. Also, the weight average molecular weight (M_w) was determined to be 7.6 kDa, with a calculated PDI of 1.69.

3.1.3. DSC

DSC thermograms shown in Figure S4 of the supplementary part illustrate that PEG had a melting point at 49.2 °C with a melting enthalpy of 160.5 J/g. On the other hand, PLGA-PEG-PLGA exhibited glass transition at a temperature of −13.3 °C, which is comparable to what has been reported in the literature of PEG containing copolymers that show crystallization in the range of −25 to 0 °C [46].

3.1.4. DLS

Copolymers composed of hydrophilic and hydrophobic portions can when in solution be present both as individual hydrated molecules or as spherical aggregates (micelles) [37]. When these copolymers are exposed to aqueous conditions, the hydrophilic PEG and glycol portions will be oriented on the outside of the micelle in contact with water, and the hydrophobic PLGA parts will be located in the inner part of the micelle due to their hydrophobic intermolecular interactions. Thus, self-assembled micelles are formed [47]. Hence, DLS can be used as a method to highlight the transition of non-hydrated molecules to micelles i.e., copolymer association.

Figure S5 of the supplementary part shows the average micellar sizes of PLGA-PEG-PLGA copolymer samples that were prepared at 20% *w/v* and measured by DLS at temperatures ranging from 10–40 °C. No significant differences were encountered in the micellar sizes of the copolymer samples measured in the tested temperature range, as indicated by nearly overlapping peaks, always achieving results comparable to those relating to micellar systems (in the range of 4–20 nm). The observed larger size of samples measured at temperatures between 35–40 °C may be regarded as indication of system aggregation due to thermogelation [48,49].

3.2. Preparation and Characterization of Plain and Emulsome-Loaded PLGA-PEG-PLGA Thermogel Solutions

In order to study the physicochemical characteristics of PLGA-PEG-PLGA triblock copolymer solutions, either plain or emulsome-loaded, the solutions were prepared in different concentrations of the copolymer (5, 10, 20, and 30% *w/w*). Likewise, emulsomes were loaded into the copolymer solutions in concentrations of 0, 10, 25, and 50% *v/v*. For all of the prepared thermogel solutions, sol-gel transition temperature and viscosity were measured. Rheological properties of plain thermogels were studied as shown in the supplementary part (Figure S6).

3.2.1. Thermogelation of the Copolymer Solutions

The phase transition temperatures of thermogel solutions G1 to G16 were evaluated using the inverted tube method by increasing temperatures from 20 to 52 °C while checking phase changes.

Before insertion of the copolymer solution in the water bath, and below its transition temperature, the copolymer solution was clear (Figure 2A). Upon heating, the copolymer solutions became opaque without gelation (Figure 2B) or they formed a gel with an absence of flowability upon inversion (Figure 2C). Subsequent temperature decrease transforms the gel into its initial liquid state.

(A)   (B)   (C)

(D)

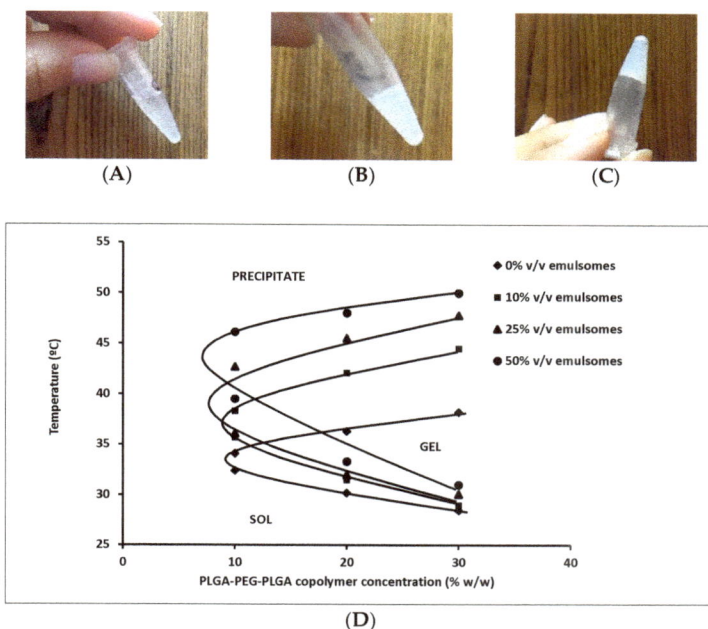

Figure 2. (**A**,**B**) are the photographs of a PLGA-PEG-PLGA copolymer solution prior to sol-gel transition (**A**) and formation of opaque solution (**B**), thermogels produced after sol-gel transition retain their position (**C**). (**D**) is the phase diagrams of polymers prepared from different PLGA-PEG-PLGA copolymer concentrations with different emulsomes loading, showing sol-gel and gel-precipitate transitions).

The sol-gel transition temperatures of all the prepared polymer solutions (G1-G16) are given in Table 1. Plain or drug loaded polymer solutions that were prepared from 5 and 10% *w/w* PLGA-PEG-PLGA copolymer (formulations G1, G5, G9, and G13) and (formulations G2, G6, G10, and G14), respectively, remained either clear or they formed turbid solutions showing no gelation till 52°C. Non-gelling opaque solutions were formed. However, formulations with higher concentrations of PLGA-PEG-PLGA (20 and 30% *w/w*) gelled, completely, at temperatures ranging between 28.50 and 33.37 °C. With temperature rise, up to 52 °C, copolymers prepared from 10, 20, and 30% *w/w* PLGA-PEG-PLGA underwent gel-precipitate transition in which the polymers reverted to a sol state (resol) but as a turbid suspension in which the polymer eventually precipitated. This thermo-reversible behavior of PLGA-PEG-PLGA copolymers has been reported in the literature [23,24,50,51]. Similar to our results, Duvvuri et al., (2005) reported the sol-gel transition temperature of 20–25% *w/v* aqueous polymer solution to be 32 °C [34]. The phase diagram of the copolymer with different emulsome loads is shown in Figure 2D.

The effect of varying PLGA-PEG-PLGA and emulsomes concentrations on the thermogelation temperatures of the copolymer solutions is shown in Table 1. At the same polymer concentration, increasing the emulsomes concentration resulted in a statistically significant increase in the transition temperatures from 30.2 ± 0.05 to 33.4 ± 0.05 °C at 20% *w/w* polymer and from 28.5 ± 0.1 to 31 ± 0.0 °C at 30% *w/w* polymer ($p > 0.05$). The increase in emulsomes concentration hinders PLGA interaction leading to retardation in gelation. The hydrophilic Tween 80 coated emulsomes with their polyoxyethylene chains are expected to render the interaction of hydrophobic blocks of PLGA-PEG-PLGA more difficult and they increase transition temperature of the composite. Similar behaviour was recorded upon increasing the concentration of hydrophilic nanoparticles incorporated in PDEGMMA block copolymer based hydrogels [51]. On the other hand, it was also found that increasing the copolymer concentration resulted in a reduction in the phase transition temperatures. On a similar basis, Qiao et al. [45] reported a decrease in gelation temperature that was associated with increasing the same copolymer concentrations from 15 to 25% *w/w*.

Hydrogelation demands two contradictory forces: strong inter-chain interaction in order to form junction points in the hydrogel network, yet the chain should not exclude the solvent (water) to prevent polymer precipitation. The polymer dissolution of the block copolymer at lower temperatures is due to the hydrogen bond between the hydrophilic PEG and water. The rise in temperature weakens the hydrogen bonding prevailing the hydrophobic forces of PLGA blocks, leading to the gel transition state. Accordingly, higher copolymer concentrations enhances the hydrophobic interactions and with the insufficiency of polymer hydration with the available amount of water causes a decrease in the sol-gel transition temperature [52].

In terms of properties of associated copolymer, PLGA-PEG-PLGA triblock copolymers form micellar structures, with a PLGA core and a PEG corona. At a temperature lower than CGT, individual and grouped micelles coexist in the sol state. With temperature rise, the fraction of individual micelles decreases and the size of grouped micelle grows rapidly causing initial sol-gel transition. The aggregation and packing interaction between micelles increase forming an opaque gel (Figure 2). If the temperature is further raised, then the hydrophobic PLGA chains of the micellar core shrink tightly and the hydrophilic PEG blocks undergo dehydration. Highly shrunk micellar groups will eventually precipitate in water, and the system becomes separated into two phases, water and polymer (Figure 1) [24].

3.2.2. Viscosity Measurement

The viscosities of all polymer solutions, post gelation at 37 °C, prepared using 20 and 30% *w/w* PLGA-PEG-PLGA copolymer and 0, 10, 25, and 50% *v/v* emulsomes, and measured at rpms ranging from 1 to 100 are shown in Figure 3. The figure shows that the rheological behavior of both plain and emulsome-loaded thermogels was concentration-dependent. Generally, an increase in viscosity accompanied the increase in copolymer and emulsome concentrations, especially when measured at the lowest rpm due to the preservation of the gel network structure.

Figure 3A shows that at 20% *w/w* copolymer concentration the viscosities were in the order: G15 > G11 > G7 > G3, at lower rpms ($p < 0.05$), directly correlated to with increasing emulsome concentration. However, G15 showed the absolute highest viscosity at all rpm values due to its 50% emulsomal content ($p < 0.01$). A similar trend was observed for G16 containing 30% *w/w* copolymer Figure 3B.

The incorporation of emulsomes will contribute to the formation of a stronger gel matrix. The presence of emulsomes caused a delay in PLGA interaction and micellar formation. Better polymer hydration occurred with the formation of highly viscous gel. A suggestion confirmed by the increase in gelation temperature by the incorporation of emulsomes. Likewise, Guo et al. [53] reported a concentration dependent rheological behavior of methoxyestradiol solid lipid nanoparticles loaded into a PLGA-PEG-PLGA thermosensitive hydrogel accompanied with viscosity increase.

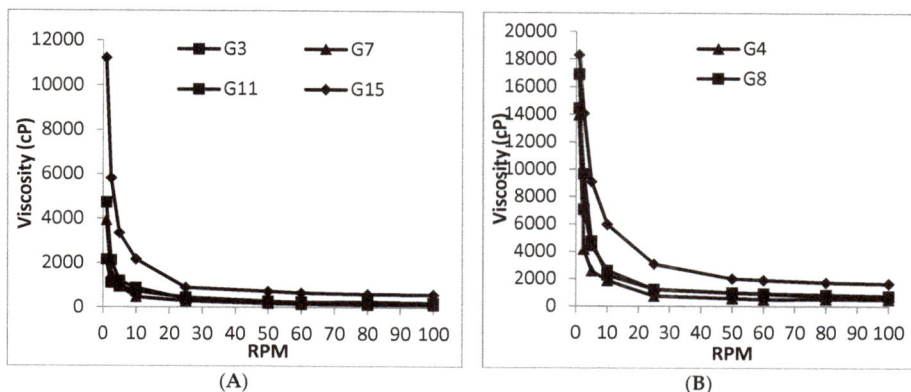

Figure 3. Rheograms of thermogels G3, G7, G11 and G15 prepared from 20% *w/w* PLGA-PEG-PLGA copolymer solution (**A**) and thermogels G4, G8, G12 and G16 prepared from 30% *w/w* PLGA-PEG-PLGA copolymer solution (**B**) in combination with 0, 10, 25, and 50% *v/v* emulsomes measured at 37 °C.

The study also revealed that significantly higher viscosities were encountered ($p < 0.01$) for 30% *w/w* copolymer (formulations: G4, G8, G12, and G16), at all emulsomal concentrations, than for 20% (formulations: G3, G7, G11, and G15). This was an expected behavior because higher copolymer concentration is translated into a denser thermogel matrix, and hence, higher viscosity [38,54]. Due to its high viscosity, G16 emulsomal thermogel was selected for further studies. The G16 emulsomal thermogel showed viscosity values of 3090 cp and 1656 cp at shear rate of 50 and 200 s^{-1} (sneezing produce a maximum shear rate of only >180 s^{-1} [55]). Knowing that IN formulations may leave the nasal cavity by gravity when their viscosity is less than about 2500 centipoise [56], G16 emulsomal thermogel represents a good candidate for IN delivery of OX.

3.3. In Vitro Release Study

Three mechanisms for controlling drug release from PLGA based matrices have previously been described, namely (i) Fickian diffusion through the polymer matrix, (ii) diffusion through water-filled pores (aqueous channels) formed by water penetration into the matrix, and (iii) liberation by erosion of the polymer matrix [57]. The actual drug release from these polymer matrices may be controlled by a combination of these three mechanisms [58].

Figure 4 shows the cumulative average amounts of OX released from emulsomes in comparison with G16 emulsomal thermogel for up to 24 h. Both formulations showed similar release profiles with no significant difference ($p < 0.05$) during the first 8 h. However, after 24 h, the OX release was reduced significantly from 81.1 to 53.5% ($p < 0.01$) in the G16 emulsomal thermogel as compared to the OX-emulsomes. The lack of initial difference in release profile between emulsomes and emulsomal thermogel may be due to the low solubility of OX, which would enhance its retention in both emulsomes and emulsomal thermogel up to 8 h of release. However, after 24 h more OX dissolved from the emulsomal core, and was released directly to the medium in case of emulsomes in comparison with emulsomes dispersed in hydrogel which showed a retarded OX release. Similar behaviour has been shown in situ with emulsomal thermosensitive gel, which was loaded with sparfloxacin for ocular delivery. A release profile that depended on drug solubility for up to 8–10 h was shown, however, when drug release was assessed at longer times it increased dramatically [59].

Moreover, drug release from hydrogel depots can be influenced by many factors, including pore size, rate of degradability of the hydrogel, size and morphology of the matrix, concentration of drug, interactions between the hydrogel and the loaded drug delivery system, polymer molecular weight, lactide/glycolide copolymer ratio, as well as matrix fabrication method [60].

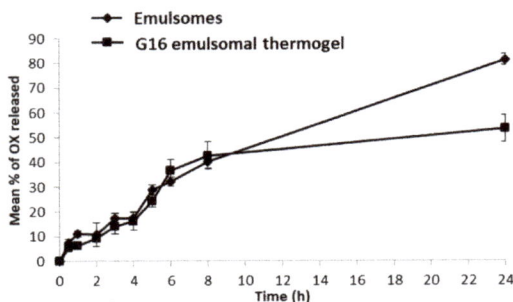

Figure 4. Release profiles of Oxcarbazepine (OX) from emulsomes and G16 emulsomal thermogel.

3.4. Mucoadhesion Study

One important design feature of formulations designed for IN administration is the ability to exhibit retention within the nasal cavity with the constant exposure to mucocilliary clearance and enzymatic degradation. Table 2 shows the mucoadhesion parameters (peak detachment, deformation peak, work of adhesion, final load) measured for plain (thermogel G4) and emulsome-loaded PLGA-PEG-PLGA copolymer (G16 emulsomal thermogel), as compared with a 0.5% carbopol gel as a positive standard.

Table 2. Mucoadhesion parameters measured for plain (G4) and G16 emulsome-loaded PLGA-PEG-PLGA thermogel compared with a standard Carbopol 980 gel.

Parameter	Plain G4 Thermogel (Mean ± SD)	G16 Emulsomal Thermogel (Mean ± SD)	Carbopol 980 Gel (Mean ± SD)
Peak detachment force (N)	21.9 ± 1.7 *	18.7 ± 2.3 *	10.52 ± 0.1
Deformation peak (mm)	10.5 ± 2 *	8.2 ± 1.3	5.4 ± 0.8
Work of adhesion (mJ)	788.3 ± 23.7 *	746.6 ± 52.2 *	304.8 ± 35
Final load (N)	20.2 ± 1.7	17.84 ± 2.9	15.41 ± 1.9

* Significantly different from Carbopol 980 gel ($p < 0.05$).

The "work of adhesion", also termed "adhesiveness", describes the work that is required to overcome the attractive forces between the surface of the sample and the surface of the probe [61]. This infers that probe removal occurs due to cleavage of both internal bonds within the sample (cohesive bonds), as well as, bonds occurring between the sample and the surface of the probe (adhesive bonds) [62].

The G4 and G16 gels both showed statistically significant higher adhesive properties for all mucoadhesive parameters, when compared to the Carbopol980 gel standard ($p < 0.05$). During optimal contact time between formulation and mucosa that ensures maximal adhesion, gel hydration occurs, which allows for exposure of its adhesive sites. This facilitates interpenetration of the gel adhesive moieties and entanglement with mucus glycoproteins of the nasal mucosa, to a sufficient depth that enables the creation of adhesive bonds [63], thus creating mucoadhesion. On a similar basis, Yu and co-workers proved that PLGA-PEG nanoparticles can penetrate human mucus secretions due to strong interactions with mucin [64]. Besides the results show that the increase in viscosity might help, but it is not crucial for mucoadhesion [65]. Thus, G16 emulsomal thermogel would be expected to show prolonged retention in the nasal cavity through the formation of adhesive bonds with the tissues lining the nasal mucosa. Since the half-life of clearance from the nasal cavity in humans, even for bioadhesive materials is in the order of 1–2 h [66], the differences in OX release after 8 h between the OX-emulsomes and the G16 emulsomal thermogel will likely not affect the nasal absorption of the OX in humans.

It is worthy to note that emulsomes had no influence on the mucoadhesive characters of PLGA-PEG-PLGA copolymer, probably because the binding with mucin occurs via hydrophilic interaction with the PEG chains of the polymer while emulsomes only interact with hydrophobic PLGA domains.

3.5. Pharmacokinetic Study

3.5.1. Plasma Pharmacokinetic Parameters

Nose-to-brain drug delivery represents a potential route for targeting drugs to the CNS and avoiding large systemic losses after drug administration. Figure 5A shows plasma concentration-time profiles of OX after the administration of Trileptal® suspension, IN solution, IN emulsomes, and IN G16 emulsomal thermogel loaded with the drug, with the corresponding PK parameters given in Table 3. Data of OX-emulsomes and Trileptal® suspension were incorporated into the paper for comparative purposes.

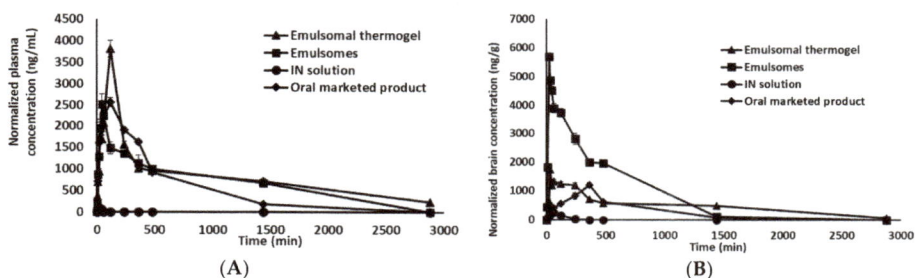

Figure 5. Mean OX concentrations in plasma (**A**) in brain (**B**) of rat groups receiving IN administration of emulsomes, G16 emulsomal thermogel, OX solution and Oral Trileptal® suspension. Data of IN administration of emulsomes, and Oral Trileptal® suspension reproduced with permission from El-Zaafarany et al. [40], Elsevier, 2016.

Table 3. Pharmacokinetic parameters for OX in rat plasma/brain following the IN administration of emulsomes, G16 emulsomal thermogel, OX solution and Oral Trileptal® suspension.

Parameter	Plasma				Brain			
	IN Emulsomes *	IN Emulsomal Thermogel	IN OX Solutions	Trileptal® Suspension *	IN Emulsomes *	IN Emulsomal Thermogel	IN OX Solutions	Trileptal® Suspension *
C_{max} (ng/mL)/(ng/g)	2514.4	3818.8	80.9	2567.6	5699.9	1733.2	249.1	1198.9
T_{max} (min)	45	120	20	120	20	30	60	360
$AUC_{0-2880min}$ (μg/mL·min)/(μg/g·min)	1943.4	2757.7	111.2	1524.6	2445.1	1440.5	57.7	742.8
$T_{1/2}$ (min)	1581.8	1919.6	302.1	364	250.9	734	197.4	285.6
MRT (min)	2024.3	2638.1	34.5	465.4	378	1007.8	95.4	504.5

* Data reproduced with permission from El-Zaafarany et al. [40], Elsevier, 2016.

In terms of plasma concentrations, the results revealed that the highest C_{max} of 3818.8 ng/mL ($p < 0.01$) was encountered after the instillation of IN G16 emulsomal thermogel at a T_{max} of 120 min, followed by Trileptal® suspension and IN emulsomes, which reached C_{max} value of 2567.6 and 2514.4 ng/mL at T_{max} value of 45 and 120 min, respectively, and finally the IN OX solution had the lowest C_{max} of 80.9 ng/mL after 20 min. The largest AUC $_{0-2880min}$ was obtained after administration of the IN G16 thermogel, followed by the IN OX emulsomes, Trileptal® suspension then IN OX solution ($p < 0.05$).

Furthermore, emulsomes and G16 thermogel formulations showed an MRT in plasma 58.7 and 76.5 times that of the IN OX solution respectively. Significantly larger residual amounts of OX after

2880 min were found in the plasma for G16 thermogel than for the OX emulsomes and IN OX solution ($p < 0.01$) (Figure 6). On the other hand, the OX administered IN in emulsomes and G16 thermogel resided in the plasma for up to 34 and 44 h, respectively. The plasma half-life of the G16 thermogel was found to be 1.2 times that of the IN OX emulsomes and significantly higher i.e., 6.4 and 5.3 times that of the IN OX solution and Trileptal® suspension, respectively ($p < 0.05$).

The long residence in plasma of OX when administered in combination with emulsomes (as opposed to the OX solution) might be explained by the lipophilic nature of the emulsomes that may allow for the partitioning of the OX in the emulsome particles (and/or the free OX) into the nasal epithelial cell membranes and further into the systemic circulation. The high absorption of OX, as shown by the AUC $_{0-2880min}$ and long mean residence time from the IN G16 emulsomal thermogel compared to IN OX-solution could be partly attributed to the high viscosity of the gel formulation which prolonged the contact time with nasal mucosa, thus enhancing the penetration of OX-emulsomes and/or free OX through the nasal mucosa into the systemic circulation [67]. The pharmacokinetic results suggest that the encapsulation of OX in emulsomes slowed its elimination, retained a high concentration in the bloodstream for a longer time period, and increased the circulation time of OX in rats, when compared to the free drug [68].

3.5.2. Brain Pharmacokinetic Parameters

OX concentrations in the brains of rats after the administration of IN OX-emulsomes, IN G16 OX-emulsomal thermogel, IN OX solution, and Trileptal® suspension of OX at predetermined time intervals are depicted in Figure 5B, with the corresponding pharmacokinetic parameters given in Table 3.

The OX concentration in the brain after administration in an IN OX solution was detected after 10 min of administration, showed a low C_{max} and reached baseline in 6 h. This observation and the low C_{max} in the plasma support the reported low ability of OX to cross mucosal membranes [69–71].

OX released from emulsomes and G16 thermogel was detected in the brain only 5 min after administration, but with significantly ($p < 0.01$) higher brain concentration (5 times) for the OX- emulsome formulation, as compared with that of the G16 OX-emulsomal thermogel formulation. Furthermore, the nasal administration of OX-emulsomes resulted in the highest OX brain C_{max} which was nearly 3.3, 22.9, and 4.8 times that of G16 OX-emulsomal thermogel, IN solution and Trileptal® suspension, respectively, with earlier T_{max} for emulsomes than all tested formulations. In contrast to the plasma data, the OX-emulsomes showed higher brain AUC $_{0-2880min}$ than G16 OX-emulsomal thermogel, IN OX solution and Trileptal® suspension. This could be attributed to the structure of emulsomes that comprises its lipidic phospholipid sheath, the Tween 80 coat and the small size (100–200 nm), all which are contributing factors to enable transcellular diffusion of OX (free or encapsulated) through the blood brain barrier [72]. Detection of OX in the brain within a time frame of 10–20 min after IN administration of emulsomes indicates that direct nose-to-brain transport was a main route for brain uptake from the nasal mucosa [73], in addition to its systemic absorption.

On the other hand, G16 OX-emulsomal thermogel had longer mean residence times in the brain, which exceeded that of the OX-emulsomes, IN OX solution and Trileptal® suspension. Also, the G16 emulsomal thermogel was the only tested formulation in which OX was detected in the brain after 48 h of its IN instillation (data not shown) which could result in a better control of seizures in patients for a longer time period. These results are in accordance with previously reported studies in animals that proved that formulations with a prolonged residence in the nasal cavity using either mucoadhesive systems or gels with very high viscosity can enhance the nose to brain delivery of drugs due to reduced mucociliary clearance and increased residence which ensure higher absorption. Furthermore, it has also been reported that some mucoadhesive polymer-containing systems may directly change epithelial tight junctions and thus, increase drug absorption [74,75].

Although the IN adminstration of emulsomal thermogel showed a lower C_{max} in the brain, it showed higher MRT values. It was previously reported that it is more advisable to use extended-action formulations for antiepileptic drugs with short half-lives (OX $t_{1/2}$ = 1–5 h) for a more efficient way of treating epilepsy [76].

When compared with formulations that rapidly release antiepileptic drugs, products with extended residence in the brain not only allow for a long dosing interval, which improve patient compliance but also decrease the risk of seizure breakthrough after missing a dose. Furthermore it was found that the use of sustained OX formulations for the treatment of focal epilepsy showed better tolerability and higher maintenance dosages to be reached than immediate action formulations [77].

3.6. Histopathological Examination

Nasal histopathology studies on rats were done to check the probable changes in the nasal mucosa caused by G16 emulsomal thermogel, in comparison to normal saline treated nasal epithelium. The control group showed normal, well defined histological structures without any signs of vascular or inflammatory changes (Figure 6A). The histopathology of the treated group revealed some signs of very low toxicity after administration of the G16 OX-emulsome thermogel (Figure 6B). This toxicity was lower than that reported for the drug alone and it is seen here as mild vascular congestion and moderate inflammatory changes around congested vessels.

The safety of PLGA-PEG-PLGA thermogels for a variety of biological applications has been previously reported [32,78–80]. Hence, this mild inflammation probably pertains to the effect of the drug on the nasal mucosa due to its controlled release throughout the study, since OX has been reported to have an irritant effect on cells by NADPH dependant DNA intercalation [81].

This observation of mild cell toxicity induced by OX is in agreement with previous finding [40,82] that showed OX as an agent that can cause anatomic and organizational disruption in cell layers, nuclear shrinkage, and cell atrophy. Conclusively, these findings would add to our previous finding that emulsomes can shield OX cell damaging effects [40] the ability of G16 emulsomal thermogel composite to further protect nasal cells from the severe effect of OX. Thus, adopted PLGA-PEG-PLGA thermogel matrices could be used to enhance safety and reduce the nasal damage of many other cell membrane damaging drugs.

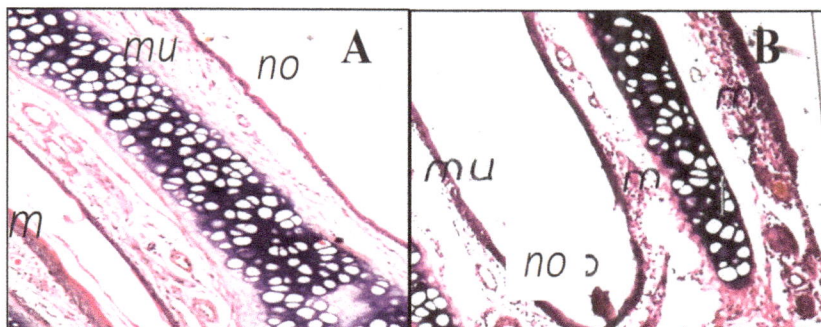

Figure 6. Light micrograph of (**A**) untreated nasal rat epithelium (with saline only) showing normal structure of the nose (no) with intact mucosal epithelium (mu). (**B**) nasal rat epithelium treated with OX-loaded G16 emulsomal thermogel showing intact mucosal epithelium (mu) with minimal focal inflammatory cells infiltration (m). (Maginifcation 16×).

4. Conclusions

A successful PEG-initiated ring opening polymerization of lactide and glycolide to prepare PLGA-PEG-PLGA triblock copolymer was confirmed by NMR, GPC, DSC, and DLS. The copolymer was mixed with emulsomes to form thermoresponsive gels for the nasal delivery of OX. All of the prepared thermoresponsive gels exhibited a reversible thermogelling behavior with visible precipitation of the copolymer at elevated temperatures. Both copolymer and emulsome concentrations contributed, to the formation of thermogels with high viscosities. Sequestration of emulsomes in 30% thermogel resulted in retardation of OX release, increased gel matrix viscosity, but did not affect mucoadhesive properties as compared to thermogel alone. The OX-emulsome thermogel dramatically increased the systemic OX absorption but did not improve the OX brain concentration in terms of C_{max} and AUC as compared to the OX-emulsomes alone. However, the emulsomal thermogel, extended the presence of OX in the brain to up to 48 h, which could offer a better control of seizures for a longer time period. A fact that needs to be investigated further.

Supplementary Materials: The following are available online at http://www.mdpi.com/1999-4923/10/4/217/s1, Figure S1. Synthesis of PLGA-PEG-PLGA triblock copolymer by ring opening polymerization of glycolide, D,L-lactide and polyethylene glycol (PEG); Figure S2. ^{1}H-NMR spectrum of PLGA-PEG-PLGA tri-block copolymer with (a) and (d) pertaining to lactide methyl and methane protons, (b) pertaining to ethylene oxide methene protons and (c) pertaining to glycolide methene protons; Figure S3. GPC chromatograms of PEG and PLGA-PEG-PLGA copolymer; Figure S4. DSC thermograms of PEG polymer and the synthesized PLGA-PEG-PLGA tri-block copolymer; Figure S5. Size distribution of PLGA-PEG-PLGA micellar solution (20% *w/v* in deionized water) measured at temperatures in the range of 10 to 45 °C; Figure S6. (A)Temperature sweep data that shows variation in viscosity and phase angle with temperature for PLGA-PEG-PLGA copolymer samples prepared in concentrations of 15, 20, and 25% *w/v* in deionized water (B) Time sweep data that shows variation in elastic modulus, viscous modulus and viscosity of PLGA-PEG-PLGA copolymer sample with time (C) Frequency sweep data that shows variation in elastic and viscous modulus with frequency for PLGA-PEG-PLGA copolymer samples prepared in concentrations of 15, 20, and 25% *w/v* in deionized water.

Author Contributions: Conceptualization, L.C., M.E.S and G.A.S.A.; methodology, L.C., M.E.S., G.M.E.-Z. and M.C.; formal analysis and investigation L.C., G.M.E.-Z., S.M., M.C. and M.E.S.; resources, L.C., G.F.P. and G.A.S.A.; writing—original draft preparation, L.C., S.M., M.E.S. and M.C.; writing—review and editing, L.C., M.E.S., L.I. and G.A.S.A.; funding acquisition, L.C., G.F.P. and G.A.S.A.

Funding: This research received no external funding and the APC was funded by Luca Casettari.

Acknowledgments: The authors wish to thank Fabio De Belvis for the design and realization of the graphical abstract.

Conflicts of Interest: The authors declare no conflict of interest.

References

1. Yan, H.; Fujiwara, H.; Sasaki, K.; Tsujii, K. Rapid Swelling/Collapsing Behavior of Thermoresponsive Poly(*N*-isopropylacrylamide) Gel Containing Poly(2-(methacryloyloxy)decyl phosphate) Surfactant. *Angew. Chem.* **2005**, *44*, 1951–1954. [CrossRef] [PubMed]
2. Bae, S.J.; Suh, J.M.; Sohn, Y.S.; Bae, Y.H.; Kim, S.W.; Jeong, B. Thermogelling poly (caprolactone-b-ethylene glycol-b-caprolactone) aqueous solutions. *Macromolecules* **2005**, *38*, 5260–5265. [CrossRef]
3. Ji, S.; Ding, J. A Macroscopic Helix Formation Induced by the Shrinking of a Cylindrical Polymeric Hydrogel. *Polym. J.* **2001**, *33*, 701–703. [CrossRef]
4. Nayak, S.; Lyon, L.A. Photoinduced phase transitions in poly(*N*-isopropylacrylamide) microgels. *Chem. Mater.* **2004**, *16*, 2623–2627. [CrossRef]
5. Kim, H.-J.; Lee, J.-H.; Lee, M. Stimuli-Responsive Gels from Reversible Coordination Polymers. *Angew. Chem.* **2005**, *44*, 5810–5814. [CrossRef] [PubMed]
6. Suri, J.T.; Cordes, D.B.; Cappuccio, F.E.; Wessling, R.A.; Singaram, B. Continuous Glucose Sensing with a Fluorescent Thin-Film Hydrogel. *Angew. Chem.* **2003**, *42*, 5857–5859. [CrossRef] [PubMed]
7. Zentner, G.M.; Rathi, R.; Shih, C.; McRea, J.C.; Seo, M.-H.; Oh, H.; Rhee, B.; Mestecky, J.; Moldoveanu, Z.; Morgan, M. Biodegradable block copolymers for delivery of proteins and water-insoluble drugs. *J. Control. Release* **2001**, *72*, 203–215. [CrossRef]
8. Tiller, J.C. Increasing the Local Concentration of Drugs by Hydrogel Formation. *Angew. Chem.* **2003**, *42*, 3072–3075. [CrossRef] [PubMed]
9. Zhang, Y.; Zhu, W.; Wang, B.; Ding, J. A novel microgel and associated post-fabrication encapsulation technique of proteins. *J. Control. Release* **2005**, *105*, 260–268. [CrossRef] [PubMed]
10. Beebe, D.J.; Moore, J.S.; Bauer, J.M.; Yu, Q.; Liu, R.H.; Devadoss, C.; Jo, B.-H. Functional hydrogel structures for autonomous flow control inside microfluidic channels. *Nature* **2000**, *404*, 588–590. [CrossRef] [PubMed]

11. Eeckman, F.; Moës, A.J.; Amighi, K. Synthesis and characterization of thermosensitive copolymers for oral controlled drug delivery. *Eur. Polym. J.* **2004**, *40*, 873–881. [CrossRef]
12. Casey, D.J.; Jarrett, P.K.; Rosati, L. Diblock and Triblock Copolymers. Patents US4716203A, 29 December 1987.
13. Cerrai, P.; Tricoli, M.; Andruzzi, F.; Paci, M.; Paci, M. Polyether-polyester block copolymers by non-catalysed polymerization of ε-caprolactone with poly (ethylene glycol). *Polymer* **1989**, *30*, 338–343. [CrossRef]
14. Youxin, L.; Kissel, T. Synthesis and properties of biodegradable ABA triblock copolymers consisting of poly (L-lactic acid) or poly (L-lactic-*co*-glycolic acid) A-blocks attached to central poly (oxyethylene) B-blocks. *J. Control. Release* **1993**, *27*, 247–257. [CrossRef]
15. Jeong, B.; Bae, Y.H.; Kim, S.W. Drug release from biodegradable injectable thermosensitive hydrogel of PEG–PLGA–PEG triblock copolymers. *J. Control. Release* **2000**, *63*, 155–163. [CrossRef]
16. Jeong, B.; Lee, K.M.; Gutowska, A.; An, Y.H. % Thermogelling Biodegradable Copolymer Aqueous Solutions for Injectable Protein Delivery and Tissue Engineering. *Biomacromolecules* **2002**, *3*, 865–868. [CrossRef] [PubMed]
17. Kim, H.-J.; Lee, J.-H.; Lee, M. Stimuli-responsive gels from reversible coordination polymers. *Angew. Chem.* **2005**, *117*, 5960–5964. [CrossRef]
18. Ruel-Gariepy, E.; Leroux, J.-C. In situ-forming hydrogels—Review of temperature-sensitive systems. *Eur. J. Pharm. Biopharm.* **2004**, *58*, 409–426. [CrossRef] [PubMed]
19. Katakam, M.; Ravis, W.R.; Banga, A.K. Controlled release of human growth hormone in rats following parenteral administration of poloxamer gels. *J. Control. Release* **1997**, *49*, 21–26. [CrossRef]
20. Wenzel, J.G.; Balaji, K.S.; Koushik, K.; Navarre, C.; Duran, S.H.; Rahe, C.H.; Kompella, U.B. Pluronic® F127 gel formulations of Deslorelin and GnRH reduce drug degradation and sustain drug release and effect in cattle. *J. Control. Release* **2002**, *85*, 51–59. [CrossRef]
21. Huh, K.M.; Cho, Y.W.; Park, K. PLGA-PEG block copolymers for drug formulations. *Drug Dev. Deliv.* **2003**, *3*, 1–11.
22. Zhang, J. *Switchable and Responsive Surfaces and Materials for Biomedical Applications*; Elsevier: New York, NY, USA, 2014.
23. Nguyen, M.K.; Lee, D.S. Injectable biodegradable hydrogels. *Macromol. Biosci.* **2010**, *10*, 563–579. [CrossRef] [PubMed]
24. Shim, M.S.; Lee, H.T.; Shim, W.S.; Park, I.; Lee, H.; Chang, T.; Kim, S.W.; Lee, D.S. Poly (D,L-lactic acid-*co*-glycolic acid)-*b*-poly (ethylene glycol)-*b*-poly (D,L-lactic acid-*co*-glycolic acid) triblock copolymer and thermoreversible phase transition in water. *J. Biomed. Mater. Res. A* **2002**, *61*, 188–196. [CrossRef] [PubMed]
25. Lee, A.L.; Venkataraman, S.; Fox, C.H.; Coady, D.J.; Frank, C.W.; Hedrick, J.L.; Yang, Y.Y. Modular composite hydrogels from cholesterol-functionalized polycarbonates for antimicrobial applications. *J. Mater. Chem. B* **2015**, *3*, 6953–6963. [CrossRef]
26. Karavasili, C.; Fatouros, D.G. Smart materials: In situ gel-forming systems for nasal delivery. *Drug Discov. Today* **2016**, *21*, 157–166. [CrossRef] [PubMed]
27. Toledano, R.; Gil-Nagel, A. Adverse effects of antiepileptic drugs. *Semin. Neurol.* **2008**, *28*, 317–327. [CrossRef] [PubMed]
28. Minn, A.; Leclerc, S.; Heydel, J.-M.; Minn, A.-L.; Denizot, C.; Cattarelli, M.; Netter, P.; Gradinaru, D. Drug transport into the mammalian brain: The nasal pathway and its specific metabolic barrier. *J. Drug Target.* **2002**, *10*, 285–296. [CrossRef] [PubMed]
29. Chandrika, M.V.; Babu, M.K. Design and development of Candesartan cilexetil emulsomal drug delivery systems for the effective management of cardiovascular diseases. *Indian J. Res. Pharm. Biotechnol.* **2014**, *2*, 1283.
30. Ucisik, M.H.; Küpcü, S.; Schuster, B.; Sleytr, U.B. Characterization of CurcuEmulsomes: Nanoformulation for enhanced solubility and delivery of curcumin. *J. Nanobiotechnol.* **2013**, *11*, 37. [CrossRef] [PubMed]
31. Kumar, D.; Sharma, D.; Singh, G.; Singh, M.; Rathore, M.S. Lipoidal soft hybrid biocarriers of supramolecular construction for drug delivery. *ISRN Pharm.* **2012**, *2012*, 474830. [CrossRef] [PubMed]
32. Chen, Y.-C.; Hsieh, W.-Y.; Lee, W.-F.; Zeng, D.-T. Effects of surface modification of PLGA-PEG-PLGA nanoparticles on loperamide delivery efficiency across the blood–brain barrier. *J. Biomater. Appl.* **2013**, *27*, 909–922. [CrossRef] [PubMed]
33. Ding, M.; Li, J.; Tan, H.; Fu, Q. Self-assembly of biodegradable polyurethanes for controlled delivery applications. *Soft Matter* **2012**, *8*, 5414–5428. [CrossRef]

34. Duvvuri, S.; Janoria, K.G.; Mitra, A.K. Development of a novel formulation containing poly (D, L-lactide-*co*-glycolide) microspheres dispersed in PLGA–PEG–PLGA gel for sustained delivery of ganciclovir. *J. Control. Release* **2005**, *108*, 282–293. [CrossRef] [PubMed]

35. Senesi, A. *Analysis of Rheological Properties of Thermogel Copolymers Based PLGA-PEG1500-PLGA: Effect of the Molecular Weight of the Side Chains*; University of Camerino: Camerino, Italy, 2013.

36. Ghahremankhani, A.A.; Dorkoosh, F.; Dinarvand, R. PLGA-PEG-PLGA tri-block copolymers as an in-situ gel forming system for calcitonin delivery. *Polym. Bull.* **2007**, *59*, 637–646. [CrossRef]

37. Song, Z.; Feng, R.; Sun, M.; Guo, C.; Gao, Y.; Li, L.; Zhai, G. Curcumin-loaded PLGA-PEG-PLGA triblock copolymeric micelles: Preparation, pharmacokinetics and distribution in vivo. *J. Colloid Interface Sci.* **2011**, *354*, 116–123. [CrossRef] [PubMed]

38. Gao, Y.; Ren, F.; Ding, B.; Sun, N.; Liu, X.; Ding, X.; Gao, S. A thermo-sensitive PLGA-PEG-PLGA hydrogel for sustained release of docetaxel. *J. Drug Target.* **2011**, *19*, 516–527. [CrossRef] [PubMed]

39. Paliwal, R.; Paliwal, S.R.; Mishra, N.; Mehta, A.; Vyas, S.P. Engineered chylomicron mimicking carrier emulsome for lymph targeted oral delivery of methotrexate. *Int. J. Pharm.* **2009**, *380*, 181–188. [CrossRef] [PubMed]

40. El-Zaafarany, G.M.; Soliman, M.E.; Mansour, S.; Awad, G.A.S. Identifying lipidic emulsomes for improved oxcarbazepine brain targeting: In vitro and rat in vivo studies. *Int. J. Pharm.* **2016**, *503*, 127–140. [CrossRef] [PubMed]

41. Khodaverdi, E.; Hadizadeh, F.; Tekie, F.S.M.; Jalali, A.; Mohajeri, S.A.; Ganji, F. Preparation and analysis of a sustained drug delivery system by PLGA–PEG–PLGA triblock copolymers. *Polym. Bull.* **2012**, *69*, 429–438. [CrossRef]

42. Basu, S.; Bandyopadhyay, A.K. Development and characterization of mucoadhesive in situ nasal gel of midazolam prepared with Ficus carica mucilage. *AAPS PharmSciTech* **2010**, *11*, 1223–1231. [CrossRef] [PubMed]

43. Patel, V.M.; Prajapati, B.G.; Patel, M.M. Formulation, evaluation, and comparison of bilayered and multilayered mucoadhesive buccal devices of propranolol hydrochloride. *AAPS PharmSciTech* **2007**, *8*, E147–E154. [CrossRef] [PubMed]

44. Gabal, Y.M.; Kamel, A.O.; Sammour, O.A.; Elshafeey, A.H. Effect of surface charge on the brain delivery of nanostructured lipid carriers in situ gels via the nasal route. *Int. J. Pharm.* **2014**, *473*, 442–457. [CrossRef] [PubMed]

45. Qiao, M.; Chen, D.; Ma, X.; Liu, Y. Injectable biodegradable temperature-responsive PLGA–PEG–PLGA copolymers: Synthesis and effect of copolymer composition on the drug release from the copolymer-based hydrogels. *Int. J. Pharm.* **2005**, *294*, 103–112. [CrossRef] [PubMed]

46. Shit, S.C.; Maiti, S. Application of NMR spectroscopy in molecular weight determination of polymers. *Eur. Polym. J.* **1986**, *22*, 1001–1008. [CrossRef]

47. Perinelli, D.; Bonacucina, G.; Cespi, M.; Naylor, A.; Whitaker, M.; Palmieri, G.; Giorgioni, G.; Casettari, L. Evaluation of P (L) LA-PEG-P (L) LA as processing aid for biodegradable particles from gas saturated solutions (PGSS) process. *Int. J. Pharm.* **2014**, *468*, 250–257. [CrossRef] [PubMed]

48. Kwon, G.S.; Cho, H. Thermogel Formulation for Combination Drug Delivery. Patents US20150025106, 22 July 2014.

49. Chen, Y.; Li, Y.; Shen, W.; Li, K.; Yu, L.; Chen, Q.; Ding, J. Controlled release of liraglutide using thermogelling polymers in treatment of diabetes. *Sci. Rep.* **2016**, *6*, 31593. [CrossRef] [PubMed]

50. Yu, L.; Zhang, Z.; Ding, J. Influence of LA and GA sequence in the PLGA block on the properties of thermogelling PLGA-PEG-PLGA block copolymers. *Biomacromolecules* **2011**, *12*, 1290–1297. [CrossRef] [PubMed]

51. Chen, L.; Ci, T.; Yu, L.; Ding, J. Effects of molecular weight and its distribution of peg block on micellization and thermogellability of plga–peg–plga copolymer aqueous solutions. *Macromolecules* **2015**, *48*, 3662–3671. [CrossRef]

52. Jeong, B.; Kim, S.W.; Bae, Y.H. Thermosensitive sol–gel reversible hydrogels. *Adv. Drug Deliv. Rev.* **2012**, *64*, 154–162. [CrossRef]

53. Guo, X.; Cui, F.; Xing, Y.; Mei, Q.; Zhang, Z. Investigation of a new injectable thermosensitive hydrogel loading solid lipid nanoparticles. *Die Pharmazie* **2011**, *66*, 948–952. [PubMed]

54. Yang, Y.; Wang, J.; Zhang, X.; Lu, W.; Zhang, Q. A novel mixed micelle gel with thermo-sensitive property for the local delivery of docetaxel. *J. Control. Release* **2009**, *135*, 175–182. [CrossRef] [PubMed]

55. Gwaltney, J.J.M.; Hendley, J.O.; Phillips, C.D.; Bass, C.R.; Mygind, N.; Winther, B. Nose blowing propels nasal fluid into the paranasal sinuses. *Clin. Infect. Dis.* **2000**, *30*, 387–391. [CrossRef] [PubMed]

56. Clarot, T.; Hensley, C. System for Delivering a Composition to the Nasal Membrane and Method of Using Same. U.S. Patent US20060275343A1, 7 December 2006.

57. Hsu, Y.Y.; Gresser, J.D.; Stewart, R.R.; Trantolo, D.J.; Lyons, C.M.; Simons, G.A.; Gangadharam, P.R.; Wise, D.L. Mechanisms of isoniazid release from poly (*d*, *l*-lactide-*co*-glycolide) matrices prepared by dry-mixing and low density polymeric foam methods. *J. Pharm. Sci.* **1996**, *85*, 706–713. [CrossRef] [PubMed]

58. Athanasiou, K.A.; Niederauer, G.G.; Agrawal, C.M. Sterilization, toxicity, biocompatibility and clinical applications of polylactic acid/polyglycolic acid copolymers. *Biomaterials* **1996**, *17*, 93–102. [CrossRef]

59. Sawant, D.; Dandagi, P.M.; Gadad, A.P. Formulation and evaluation of sparfloxacin emulsomes-loaded thermosensitive in situ gel for ophthalmic delivery. *J. Sol-Gel Sci. Technol.* **2016**, *77*, 654–665. [CrossRef]

60. Khodaverdi, E.; Tekie, F.S.M.; Mohajeri, S.A.; Ganji, F.; Zohuri, G.; Hadizadeh, F. Preparation and investigation of sustained drug delivery systems using an injectable, thermosensitive, in situ forming hydrogel composed of PLGA–PEG–PLGA. *AAPS PharmSciTech* **2012**, *13*, 590–600. [CrossRef] [PubMed]

61. Jones, D.S.; Woolfson, A.D.; Djokic, J.; Coulter, W. Development and mechanical characterization of bioadhesive semi-solid, polymeric systems containing tetracycline for the treatment of periodontal diseases. *Pharm. Res.* **1996**, *13*, 1734–1738. [CrossRef] [PubMed]

62. Jones, D.S.; Woolfson, A.D.; Brown, A.F.; Coulter, W.A.; McClelland, C.; Irwin, C.R. Design, characterisation and preliminary clinical evaluation of a novel mucoadhesive topical formulation containing tetracycline for the treatment of periodontal disease. *J. Control. Release* **2000**, *67*, 357–368. [CrossRef]

63. Eouani, C.; Piccerelle, P.; Prinderre, P.; Bourret, E.; Joachim, J. In-vitro comparative study of buccal mucoadhesive performance of different polymeric films. *Eur. J. Pharm. Biopharm.* **2001**, *52*, 45–55. [CrossRef]

64. Yu, T.; Wang, Y.-Y.; Yang, M.; Schneider, C.; Zhong, W.; Pulicare, S.; Choi, W.-J.; Mert, O.; Fu, J.; Lai, S.K. Biodegradable mucus-penetrating nanoparticles composed of diblock copolymers of polyethylene glycol and poly (lactic-*co*-glycolic acid). *Drug Deliv. Transl. Res* **2012**, *2*, 124–128. [CrossRef] [PubMed]

65. Carvalho, F.C.; Bruschi, M.L.; Evangelista, R.C.; Gremião, M.P.D. Mucoadhesive drug delivery systems. *Braz. J. Pharm. Sci.* **2010**, *46*, 1–17. [CrossRef]

66. Soane, R.; Frier, M.; Perkins, A.; Jones, N.; Davis, S.; Illum, L. Evaluation of the clearance characteristics of bioadhesive systems in humans. *Int. J. Pharm.* **1999**, *178*, 55–65. [CrossRef]

67. Gao, K.; Jiang, X. Influence of particle size on transport of methotrexate across blood brain barrier by polysorbate 80-coated polybutylcyanoacrylate nanoparticles. *Int. J. Pharm.* **2006**, *310*, 213–219. [CrossRef] [PubMed]

68. Zhou, X.; Chen, Z. Preparation and performance evaluation of emulsomes as a drug delivery system for silybin. *Arch. Pharm. Res.* **2015**, *38*, 2193–2200. [CrossRef] [PubMed]

69. Shorvon, S. Oxcarbazepine: A review. *Seizure* **2000**, *9*, 75–79. [CrossRef] [PubMed]

70. Hellewell, J.S. Oxcarbazepine (Trileptal) in the treatment of bipolar disorders: A review of efficacy and tolerability. *J. Affect. Disord.* **2002**, *72*, S23–S34. [CrossRef]

71. Martinez, W.; Ingenito, A.; Blakeslee, M.; Barkley, G.L.; McCague, K.; D'Souza, J. Efficacy, safety, and tolerability of oxcarbazepine monotherapy. *Epilepsy Behav.* **2006**, *9*, 448–456. [CrossRef] [PubMed]

72. Kaur, I.P.; Bhandari, R.; Bhandari, S.; Kakkar, V. Potential of solid lipid nanoparticles in brain targeting. *J. Control. Release* **2008**, *127*, 97–109. [CrossRef] [PubMed]

73. Jin, K.; Xie, L.; Childs, J.; Sun, Y.; Mao, X.O.; Logvinova, A.; Greenberg, D.A. Cerebral neurogenesis is induced by intranasal administration of growth factors. *Ann. Neurol.* **2003**, *53*, 405–409. [CrossRef] [PubMed]

74. Kumar, M.; Misra, A.; Mishra, A.; Mishra, P.; Pathak, K. Mucoadhesive nanoemulsion-based intranasal drug delivery system of olanzapine for brain targeting. *J. Drug Target.* **2008**, *16*, 806–814. [CrossRef] [PubMed]

75. Jain, N.; Akhter, S.; Jain, G.K.; Khan, Z.I.; Khar, R.K.; Ahmad, F.J. Antiepileptic intranasal Amiloride loaded mucoadhesive nanoemulsion: Development and safety assessment. *J. Biomed. Nanotechnol.* **2011**, *7*, 142–143. [CrossRef] [PubMed]

76. Perucca, E. Extended-release formulations of antiepileptic drugs: Rationale and comparative value. *Epilepsy Curr.* **2009**, *9*, 153–157. [CrossRef] [PubMed]

77. Steinhoff, B.; Stefan, H.; Schulze-Bonhage, A.; Hueber, R.; Paulus, W.; Wangemann, M.; Elger, C. Retardiertes vs. schnell freisetzendes Oxcarbazepin bei therapierefraktärer fokaler Epilepsie. *Der Nervenarzt* **2012**, *83*, 1292–1299. [CrossRef] [PubMed]

78. Moffatt, S.; Cristiano, R.J. Uptake characteristics of NGR-coupled stealth PEI/pDNA nanoparticles loaded with PLGA-PEG-PLGA tri-block copolymer for targeted delivery to human monocyte-derived dendritic cells. *Int. J. Pharm.* **2006**, *321*, 143–154. [CrossRef] [PubMed]

79. Chang, C.-W.; Choi, D.; Kim, W.J.; Yockman, J.W.; Christensen, L.V.; Kim, Y.-H.; Kim, S.W. Non-ionic amphiphilic biodegradable PEG–PLGA–PEG copolymer enhances gene delivery efficiency in rat skeletal muscle. *J. Control. Release* **2007**, *118*, 245–253. [CrossRef] [PubMed]

80. Chang, G.; Li, C.; Lu, W.; Ding, J. N-Boc-Histidine-Capped PLGA-PEG-PLGA as a Smart Polymer for Drug Delivery Sensitive to Tumor Extracellular pH. *Macromol. Biosci.* **2010**, *10*, 1248–1256. [CrossRef] [PubMed]

81. Castrén, K.; Pienimäki, P.; Arvela, P.; Vähäkangas, K. Metabolites and DNA-binding of carbamazepine and oxcarbazepine in vitro by rat liver microsomes. *Hum. Exp. Toxicol.* **1996**, *15*, 577–582. [CrossRef] [PubMed]

82. Aktaş, Z.; Cansu, A.; Erdoğan, D.; Take, G.; Goktas, G.; Ozdek, S.; Serdaroglu, A. Retinal ganglion cell toxicity due to oxcarbazepine and valproic acid treatment in rat. *Seizure* **2009**, *18*, 396–399. [CrossRef] [PubMed]

pharmaceutics

Article

Enhanced Delivery of Imatinib into Vaginal Mucosa via a New Positively Charged Nanocrystal-Loaded in Situ Hydrogel Formulation for Treatment of Cervical Cancer

Li-qian Ci [1,2,†], Zhi-gang Huang [1,†], Feng-mei Lv [2], Jun Wang [2], Ling-lin Feng [3], Feng Sun [4], Shui-juan Cao [5], Zhe-peng Liu [2], Yu Liu [1,*], Gang Wei [1] and Wei-yue Lu [1]

[1]   Department of Pharmaceutics, School of Pharmacy, Fudan University & Key Laboratory of Smart Drug Delivery (Fudan University), Ministry of Education, Shanghai 201203, China; ciliqian@foxmail.com (L.-q.C.); 16211030018@fudan.edu.cn (Z.-g.H.); weigang@shmu.edu.cn (G.W.); wylu@shmu.edu.cn (W.-y.L.)
[2]   School of Medical Instrument and Food Engineering, University of Shanghai for Science and Technology, Shanghai 200093, China; 15216806348@163.com (F.-m.L.); doudou19940424@163.com (J.W.); zhepengliu@126.com (Z.-p.L.)
[3]   NHC Key Laboratory of Reproduction Regulation (Shanghai Institute of Planned Parenthood Research), Fudan University, Room 904, No 1 Research Building, 2140 Xietu Road, Shanghai 200032, China; fenglinglinxin@163.com
[4]   Chinese Academy of Sciences Shanghai Institute of Materia Medica, Shanghai 201203, China; sunfengbbb@simm.ac.cn
[5]   Experimental Teaching Center, School of Pharmacy, Fudan University, Shanghai 201203, China; chaoshui2011@126.com
*   Correspondence: liuyu@fudan.edu.cn; Tel.: +86-21-5198-0090
†   Equally contributing authors.

Received: 14 November 2018; Accepted: 9 December 2018; Published: 4 January 2019

Abstract: The present study was carried out to investigate the potential of cationic functionalization on imatinib nanocrystals to improve the mucoadhesiveness and, thus, delivery to the lesion of cervicovaginal tumors. Amino-group-functionalized imatinib nanocrystals (NC@PDA-NH$_2$) were prepared with near-spheroid shape, nanoscale size distribution, positive zeta potential, and relatively high drug content with the aid of the polydopamine-coating technique. Efficient interaction between NC@PDA-NH$_2$ and mucin was proven by mucin adsorption which was related to the positive zeta-potential value of NC@PDA-NH$_2$ and the change in the size distribution on mixing of NC@PDA-NH$_2$ and mucin. Cellular uptake, growth inhibition, and apoptosis induction in cervicovaginal cancer-related cells demonstrated the superiority of NC@PDA-NH$_2$ over unmodified nanocrystals. For practical intravaginal administration, NC@PDA-NH$_2$ was dispersed in Pluronic F127-based thermosensitive in situ hydrogel, which showed suitable gelation temperature and sustained-release profiles. In comparison with unmodified nanocrystals, NC@PDA-NH$_2$ exhibited extended residence on ex vivo murine vaginal mucosa, prolonged in vivo intravaginal residence, and enhanced inhibition on the growth of murine orthotopic cervicovaginal model tumors indicated by smaller tumor size, longer median survival time, and more intratumor apoptosis with negligible mucosal toxicity. In conclusion, cationic functionalization endowed NC@PDA-NH$_2$ significant mucoadhesiveness and, thus, good potential against cervicovaginal cancer via intravaginal administration.

Keywords: mucoadhesiveness; cervicovaginal tumors; cationic functionalization; imatinib; nanocrystals; in situ hydrogel

1. Introduction

Cervical cancer is the fourth most common cause of death from cancer in women [1]. With the development and popularization of regular Papanicolaou (Pap) tests, the majority of cervical cancer patients can be diagnosed in the early stages when the tumor is small in size and confined to the cervix. Nevertheless, the current treatment for early-stage cervical cancer usually involves significant adverse side effects. Surgery and radiation therapy are associated with increased risks of future negative gynecological and obstetric outcomes, including impaired sexual function, infertility, preterm delivery, and low birth weight. Systemic pharmacotherapy is generally the last option because only a negligible proportion of the drug reaches the vaginal mucosal epithelium. Now, clinicians are realizing that cervicovaginal tumors may represent the most important potential field needing good vaginal formulations [2]. Sustained and localized drug delivery in the female reproductive tract may avoid adverse effects associated with systemic administration, improve efficacy by assuring adequate local drug concentration, and allow convenient self-administration [3]. For example, the first tyrosine kinase inhibitor, imatinib, was reported to prevent the activation of platelet-derived growth factor receptor (PDGFR), which is often overexpressed in cervical cancer [4], thus inhibiting cervical cancer cell proliferation. In a study which screened carbo- and cisplatin, topotecan, paclitaxel, imatinib, gefitinib, cetuximab, and trastuzumab on freshly isolated tumor cells of 16 patients, 66% of tumor samples were sensitive to imatinib [5]. When administered orally, it worked effectively in the clinic, possibly due to its high plasma protein binding and insufficient drug delivery to the vaginal mucosal epithelium. It is reasonable to expect a positive outcome for imatinib if vaginal formulations with adequate vaginal mucosal delivery efficiency are available.

Recently, nanocrystals (NC) drew increasing interest in field of delivery of poorly soluble drugs [6–8] for their nanoscale and high drug content. These properties seem to be attractive for vaginal formulations. Only nanocrystals with suitable mucoadhesive modification can overcome the self-cleaning mechanism of the vagina, assure prolonged contact time with mucosa, and avoid multiple daily doses [9]. One of the most promising mucoadhesive strategies is cationic modification, which is based on the electrostatic interaction with negatively charged mucin in the mucus, as well as mucosal epithelial cells. The most exciting recent advance is positively charged 10-hydroxycamptothecin-loaded nanogels for intravesical instillation which successfully prolonged intravesical residence time, improved penetration into the vesical mucosa, and enhanced the anti-tumor efficacy in a murine orthotopic bladder cancer model [9]. Cationic functionalization was also applied in vaginal formulations. We previously synthesized a cationic derivative of Pluronic F127 to prepare a new type of thermosensitive/mucoadhesive in situ hydrogel, which significantly prolonged intravaginal drug residence and improved mucosal penetration [10]. Similar benefits were also reported for imiquimoid-loaded nanocapsules [11].

Being highly dispersed in nature, NCs are thermodynamically unstable, necessitating surface modification to prevent possible particle growth. In the meantime, surface modification can change the in vivo performance of nanocrystals. Polyethylene glycol (PEG)ylated paclitaxel nanocrystals showed good stability and in vivo tumor inhibition efficacy [12]. Albumin-stabilized paclitaxel nanocrystals showed enhanced uptake by SPARC$^+$ B16F10 melanoma cells and in vivo anti-tumor efficacy [13], and albumin-stabilized hydroxycamptothecin nanocrystals showed enhanced intratumor accumulation and prolonged survival time in MCF-7 model tumor-bearing mice [14]. Pluronic F68-stabilized paclitaxel nanocrystals exhibited elevated interaction with cancer cells and intratumor accumulation [15,16]. Pluronic F68 and soybean lecithin-stabilized 7-ethyl-10-hydroxycamptothecin nanocrystals inhibited the growth of MCF-7 model tumors more efficiently [17]. The abovementioned surface modification examples for nanocrystals are mainly based on either physical adsorption of stabilizers or chemical derivatization of the prototype drug.

Alternatively, polydopamine (PDA) coating may provide another choice. In a weak basic environment, dopamine can self-polymerize on the surface of solid materials to form a PDA layer which can subsequently react with thiol or amine groups at *o*-quinone moieties [18]. Since the pioneer work of Messersmith's group [19], this property of PDA attracted increasing interest for its good biocompatibility and capability of forming of nanostructures [20,21] or their surface functionalization [22,23]. Liang et al. recently reported the promising performance of tumor-targeting modified PDA-coated camptothecin nanocrystals [24].

Herein, positively charged polydopamine-coated imatinib nanocrystals (NC@PDA-NH$_2$) were prepared and characterized with respect to basic physicochemical properties, drug content and release, and in vitro interaction with mucin and cervical cancer-related cell lines. NC@PDA-NH$_2$ was further dispersed in a Pluronic F127-based in situ hydrogel vehicle to allow adequate interaction time between nanocrystals and mucosa. The NC@PDA-NH$_2$-loaded Pluronic F127-based in situ hydrogel (NC@PDA-NH$_2$/FG) was optimized based on rheological and release profiles and characterized with respect to ex vivo residence on mouse vaginal mucosa, in vivo intravaginal retention, and anti-tumor efficacy in a murine orthotopic cervicovaginal tumor model.

2. Methods

2.1. Materials and Animals

Imatinib (IMN), 1,1'-dioctadecyl-3,3,3',3'-tetramethylindotricarbocyanine iodide (DiR), 2-(4-amidinophenyl)-6-indolecarbamindine dihydrochloride (DAPI), and 6-coumarin (C6) were purchased from Meilun Biotechnology Ltd. Co. (Dalian, Liaoning, China). Pluronic F127 (F127) was purchased from BASF Ltd. Co. (Ludwigshaften, Germany). Optical coherence tomography (OCT) was purchased from Sakura Finetek Inc. (Torrrance, CA, USA). Porcine gastric mucin (PGM) was purchased from Sigma-Aldrich Ltd. Co. (St Louis, MO, USA) and purified as described in previous literature [23]. All other chemicals were of analytical grade, purchased from Sinopharm Reagent Ltd. Co. (Shanghai, China) and used as received. Two cervical cancer-related cell lines, TC-1 and SiHa, were purchased from Fu-Heng Cell Center (Shanghai, China).

Female C57BL/6 mice were provided by Shanghai Laboratory Animal Center (Shanghai, China). All animals were allowed free access to standard food and tap water and acclimated for at least one week before use. All animal experiments were carried out in accordance with the guidelines evaluated and approved by the Ethics Committee of the School of Pharmacy, Fudan University (2015-O3-YJ-LY-0D approved on 4 March 2015).

2.2. Preparation of NC, NC@PDA, and NC@PDA-NH$_2$

NC@PDA-NH$_2$ was prepared by three steps. Firstly, a mixture of imatinib (3.5 mg) and stabilizers (3.8 mg TPGS and 7.5 mg citrate acid) was fully dissolved in 3 mL of ethanol in a round-bottom flask. Ethanol was evaporated with a rotary evaporator at 40 °C to form a thin film on the wall of the flask. Then, 5 mL of 35 mM NaHCO$_3$ aqueous solution was added to the film at room temperature. After hydration by gentle mixing, NCs were formed. Secondly, 5 mg of dopamine was added to 5 mL of the abovementioned NC suspension and incubated at room temperature for 10 min on a rotating rocker. Then, the suspension was centrifuged at 4448× *g* for 15 min at room temperature to remove unreacted dopamine and obtain NC@PDA. Thirdly, the pellet was re-suspended in 5 mL of pure water containing appropriate amounts of Boc-NHCH$_2$CH$_2$-NH$_2$ to react for at least 3 h. Then, the suspension was centrifuged at 4448× *g* for 15 min at room temperature to remove unreacted Boc-NHCH$_2$CH$_2$-NH$_2$ and was deprotected in 3 M HCl for 3 h to obtain NC@PDA-NH$_2$. DiR- or C6-labeled nanocrystals were similarly prepared except that DiR or C5 (5 μg/mL) was included in the initial mixture in the first step.

2.3. Characterization of NC, NC@PDA, and NC@PDA-NH$_2$

For determination of drug loading (DL) and encapsulation efficiency (EE), lyophilized nanocrystals with a premeasured mass were dissolved in acetonitrile (ACN), filtered with a 0.45-μm syringe filter, diluted if necessary, and submitted to HPLC analysis on an Agilent 1100 HPLC system (Palo Alto, CA, USA) equipped with an Xtimate ® C18 column (25 cm × 4.6 mm, particle size: 5 μm;

Welch Technology, Shanghai, China) with a mobile phase 45:55 (v/v) mixture of ACN/ammonium acetate buffer solution (10 mM, pH 10) at a flow rate 0.7 mL/min and a detection wavelength of 272 nm.

EE and DL were respectively calculated according to the following equations:

$$EE(\%) = \frac{\text{Amount of drug in nanocrystals}}{\text{Total amount of feeding drug}} \times 100\%,$$

$$DL(\%) = \frac{\text{Amount of drug in nanocrystals}}{\text{Total mass of nanocrystals}} \times 100\%.$$

In vitro release of imatinib from nanocrystals was investigated using the dialysis bag method with vaginal fluid simulant (VFS) as the release medium, prepared as reported previously [25] The morphology of various nanocrystals was observed using a transmission electron microscope (TEM, JEM-2100F, JEOL Co., Tokyo, Japan). The size distribution and zeta potential of nanocrystals were measured at 37 °C using dynamic light scattering (DLS) with a Zetasizer (ZS-10-82, Malvern Instruments Ltd. Co., Malvern, UK).

X-ray powder diffraction (XRPD) of nanocrystals was analyzed with a D2 Phaser diffractometer (BrukerCorp., Billerica, MA, USA) with a Cu-Kα radiation source and a LYNXEYE™-compound silicon strip detector. The powder patterns were obtained from 1 to 40° 2θ at a scan speed of 5°/min and a step size of 0.02°. The voltage and current used were 40 kV and 44 mA, respectively.

Differential scanning calorimetry (DSC) was carried out using a Perkin-Elmer Pyris 1 DSC instrument (Waltham, MA, USA) equipped with an intra-cooler 2P cooling accessory. Accurately weighed samples were separately sealed in standard aluminum pans and scanned from 20 to 300 °C at a heating rate of 10 °C/min with a nitrogen purge of 10 mL/min.

2.4. Interaction between Mucin and Nanocrystals

To investigate the change in the size distribution after mixing mucin and nanocrystals, purified PGM was mixed with NC@PDA-NH$_2$ or NC at the weight ratio of 2:1 in citrate buffer (0.1 M, pH 5, the physiological vaginal pH) for DLS measurements.

For determination of the adsorption amount (AA) of mucin by nanocrystals, purified PGM was mixed with NC@PDA-NH$_2$ with different positive surface charges (see Supplementary Materials) or NC at the weight ratio of 2:1 in citrate buffer (0.1 M, pH 5), incubated at 37 °C for 1 h and then centrifuged at 6672× g for 10 min (H1650-W centrifuge, Xiang-yi Instrument Inc., Changsha, China). The concentration of PGM in the supernatant was measured using Pierce® BCA Protein Assay Kits (Thermo Scientific, Rockford, IL, USA) to calculate AA according to the following equation:

$$AA = \frac{\text{initial amount of PGM} \ - \text{amount of PGM after adsorption}}{\text{Amount of nanocrystals}}.$$

2.5. Interaction of Nanocrystals with Cervicovaginal-Related Cell Lines

TC-1 and SiHa cells were grown in RPMI-1640 medium and DMEM medium, respectively, both containing 10% fetal bovine serum (FBS) and penicillin (100 IU/mL) and streptomycin (100 μg/mL).

For intracellular localization of nanocrystals, TC-1 cells were seeded in a 35-mm dish with a glass window (MatTek, Ashland, MA, USA) at a density of 4 × 10^4 cells per dish. After 24 h, the medium was replaced with fresh medium. Cells were incubated with LysoTracker Red DND-99 (25 nM) for 30 min and then incubated with C6-labeled NC@PDA-NH$_2$, NC, or free probe C6 for 2 h. Following washing with PBS, the cells were fixed with 4% paraformaldehyde in PBS for 20 min. After nucleus staining with DAPI, fluorescent images were taken with a Zeiss AXIO Observer Z1 confocal microscope (ZEISS LSM710, Zeiss, Athens, German). The fluorescence intensity of the cells was quantitatively analyzed using FCM analysis (BD FACSCalibur, Sparks, MD, USA) at the excitation wavelength (Ex) of 466 nm and emission wavelength (Em) of 504 nm using a Flow Cytometry System (BD FACSCalibur, Sparks, MD, USA).

For quantitative comparison of intracellular drug content, TC-1 cells were seeded in a 12-well plate at a density of 1.2 × 10^5 cells per well. After overnight incubation, the cell culture medium was replaced with fresh medium containing NC@PDA-NH$_2$, NC, or free imatinib (firstly dissolved in DMSO and then diluted in PBS) with the final concentration equivalent of imatinib at 120 µg/mL. After 4 h, cells were washed with PBS and collected for determination of the intracellular imatinib amount by HPLC as described in Section 2.3.

The cytotoxicity of NC@PDA-NH$_2$, NC, or free IMN on TC-1 or SiHa cells over a range of imatinib concentrations for 72 h was measured using the standard MTT method. Half maximal inhibitory concentration (IC$_{50}$) was calculated using GraphPad Prism 6 (La Jolla, CA, USA).

Apoptosis of TC-1 or SiHa cells induced by NC@PDA-NH$_2$, NC, or free IMN after incubation for 48 h was compared using flow cytometry after standard Annexin V-FITC/propidium iodide (PI) staining.

2.6. Preparation and Characterization of NC@PDA-NH$_2$/FG

NC@PDA-NH$_2$/FG was prepared by dissolving an appropriate amount of Pluronic F127 in the corresponding nanocrystal suspension at 4 °C. NC-loaded F127 in situ hydrogel (NC/FG) was prepared similarly. Free imatinib/FG was prepared using the thin film-cold method as described in previous literature [10].

The rheology of NC@PDA-NH$_2$/FG with three different F127 concentration was investigated using a rotatory rheometer (Bohlin Gemini II, Malvern Instruments Ltd. Co., Malvern, UK) equipped with a parallel plate in the oscillation mode from 15–40 °C at a heating rate of 1 °C/min with a fixed frequency of 1 Hz and a fixed strain of 0.01. In vitro release of PC@PDA@NC/FG was evaluated using the membraneless method using vaginal fluid simulant (VFS) as the release medium. The concentration of imatinib in release samples was measured by HPLC as described in Section 2.3.

2.7. Ex Vivo and In Vivo Evaluation of the Mucoadhesiveness of NC@PDA-NH$_2$/FG

For suitable gelation temperature, a weight concentration of 17.5% of F127 was selected for further investigation. Ex vivo adhesion on murine vaginal mucosa, intramucosal penetration of fluorescent-labeled NC@PDA-NH$_2$/FG, NC/FG, and corresponding free probe/FG, and the intravaginal drug placement of NC@PDA-NH$_2$/FG, NC/FG, and free IMN/FG were compared with methods similar to our previous work [10] in healthy C57BL/6 female mice.

For ex vivo adhesion evaluation, C57BL/6 female mice were sacrificed with excess inhalation of ether to get the vagina mucosa. Onto the freshly prepared vagina mucosa which was smoothed out and fixed on a plastic card, 10 µL of corresponding tested formulation was dropped with a pipette. These tissues were kept at 37 °C under repeated flushing with 10 µL of VFS every 10 min with a pipette. Near-infrared fluorescent (NIR) images were obtained every hour for 8 h with a whole-mouse fluorescent imaging system (IVIS spectrum, PerkinElmer, Santa Clara, CA, USA) at Ex 748 nm and Em 780 nm.

For in vivo intramucosal penetration, 10 µL of tested formulation per mouse was intravaginally administered to female ICR mice by a microliter syringe with a blunt needle. Three mice were randomly selected from each group and sacrificed with excess inhalation of ether to get the vaginal tissue which was fixed in paraformaldehyde for 24 h, dehydrated in sucrose solution, embedded in OCT, sectioned on a freezing microtome, stained with DAPI, and observed under a fluorescence microscope (DMI 4000, Leica Camera Co., Wetzlar, Germany).

For quantitation of intravaginal drug placement, healthy mice (24 mice per group) were intravaginally administered with NC@PDA-NH2/FG, NC/FG, or free drug (suspended imatinib powder)/FG, as described in Section 2.5. At every pre-determined time point (immediately, 2 h, 4 h, 6 h, and 8 h after administration), six mice were randomly selected from each group to perform vaginal lavage in which the vagina was thoroughly lavaged by normal saline as previously reported. Imatinib concentration in the vaginal lavage and mucosa was determined as described in Section 2.3.

2.8. In Vivo Efficacy against the Orthotopic Cervicovaginal Tumor Model in Mice

An orthotopic cervicovaginal TC-1 tumor model was established in female C57BL/6 mice according to the method of Yang et al. [26]. Mice (6–8 weeks old) were subcutaneously treated with medroxyprogesterone acetate (2.5 mg per mouse per day) for a consecutive seven days prior to tumor inoculation. Then, mice were anesthetized to gently disrupt their cervicovaginal epithelia with a cytobrush. TC-1 cells were inoculated by vaginal instillation (1×10^5 cells per mouse) three days prior to day 0. Following day 0, intravaginal administration began. The formation and growth of tumor was preliminarily confirmed by palpation, as well as anatomical and histological examination, which found that TC-1 tumors grew along the length of the cervicovaginal tract and extended laterally toward surrounding tissues.

To compare the tumor growth inhibition effect of NC@PDA-NH$_2$/FG vs. NC/FG at three imatinib dosages (2, 4, and 8 mg/kg), 160 tumor-bearing mice were divided into eight groups (20 mice per group) including NC@PDA-NH$_2$/FG (8 mg/kg), NC@PDA-NH$_2$/FG (4 mg/kg), NC@PDA-NH$_2$/FG (2 mg/kg), NC/FG (8 mg/kg), NC/FG (4 mg/kg), NC/FG (2 mg/kg), free imatinib/FG (4 mg/kg), and normal saline intravaginally administered every other day. The animal number for each group was set at 20 to ensure that at least six animals survived by day 21 for all groups, especially for the normal saline control group. On day 21, mice were sacrificed for resection of uterus, cervix, and vagina to take photographs, weighing the tumors, and performing further microscopic examination for H&E staining or TUNEL assay (DeadEnd^{TM} Fluorometric TUNEL system, Promega, Madison, WI, USA). The change in the body weight was also monitored.

2.9. Statistical Analysis

All statistical analysis was performed with GraphPad Prism 6. Data were analyzed with one-way ANOVA test to determine the difference of means among groups. The logrank (Mantel-Cox) test was used to compare survival curves. A value of $p < 0.05$ was considered statistically significant.

3. Results and Discussion

3.1. Preparation and Characterization of NC@PDA-NH$_2$

As depicted by Scheme 1, the core NCs were prepared by film hydration. Subsequently, dopamine was added to self-polymerize on the surface of NCs to obtain PDA-coated NCs (NC@PDA). The PDA coating provided the reacting platform for Boc-NH-CH$_2$CH$_2$-NH$_2$. Finally, the Boc groups were removed by acidic treatment to provide positive charges on the surface of NC@PDA-NH$_2$. NC@PDA-NH$_2$ could be prepared with a relative high drug content of $76.84 \pm 1.78\%$ (Table 1).

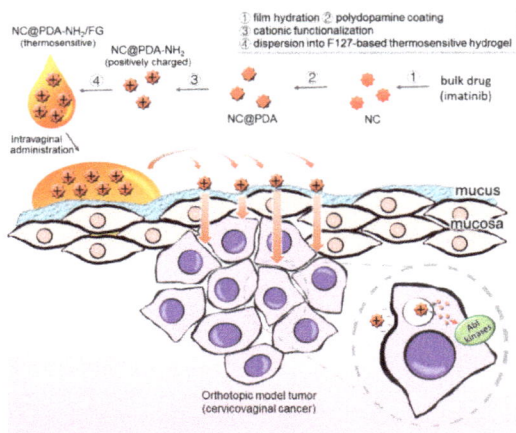

Scheme 1. Illustration of the preparation and in vivo fate of amino-group-functionalized polydopamine (PDA)-coated imatinib nanocrystals (NC) dispersed in F127 (FG) hydrogel (NC@PDA-NH$_2$/FG) in the orthotopic mouse cervicovaginal cancer model after intravaginal administration.

NC, NC@PDA, and NC@PDA-NH$_2$ all showed a near-spheroid shape (Figure 1A) with nanoscale size (Figure 1B). The zeta potentials of NC and NC@PDA were -14.9 ± 2.7 mV and -44.0 ± 3.4 mV, respectively, while that of NC@PDA-NH$_2$ was $+27.2 \pm 2.9$ mV (Figure 1C), indicating the success of cationic modification. The size distribution of NC@PDA-NH$_2$ remained basically unchanged after one month, while the size of unmodified NC increased after only several days, which may be attributed to the electrostatic expulsion among positively charged NC@PDA-NH$_2$.

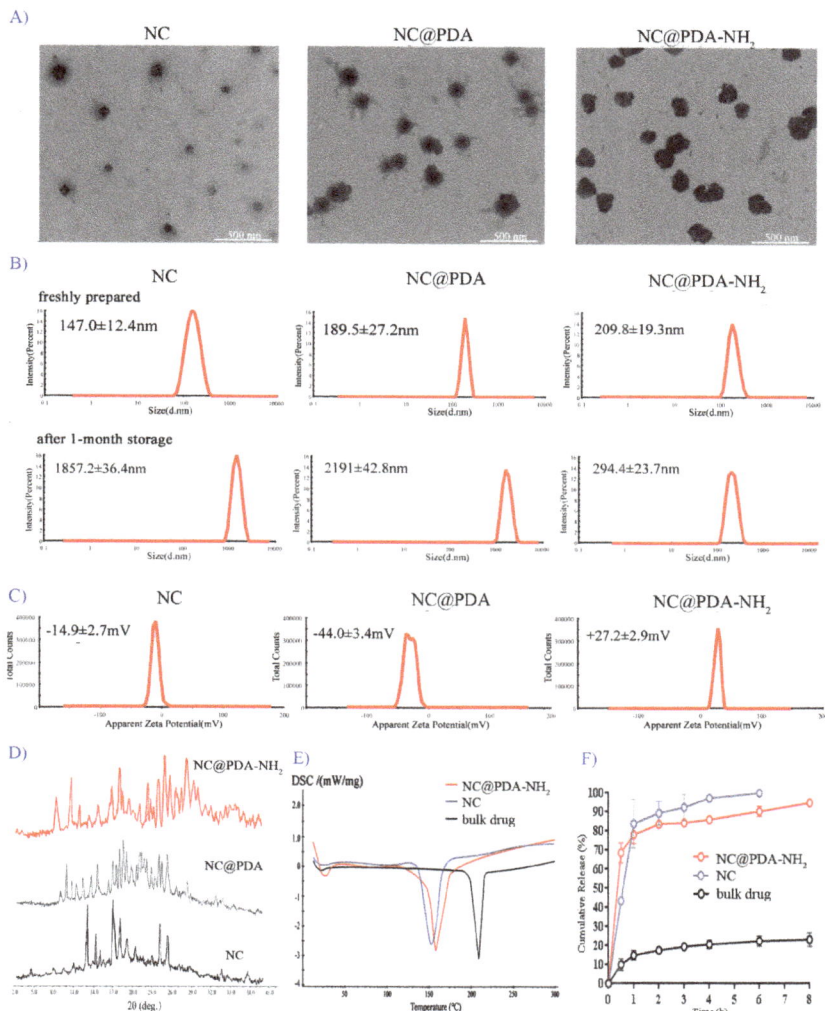

Figure 1. Characterization of NC, NC@PDA, and NC@PDA-NH$_2$. (**A**) TEM images. (**B**) size distribution measured by dynamic light scattering (DLS). Upper panels: freshly prepared; lower panels: after one month of storage. (**C**) Zeta-potential measured by DLS. (**D**) X-ray diffraction (XRD) patterns. (**E**) Differential scanning calorimetry (DSC) curves. (**F**) In vitro release profiles in vaginal fluid simulant (VFS) ($n = 3$, mean $\pm$ SD).

The XRPD patterns of bulk drug displayed peaks at 12.96°, 14.13°, 17.1°, 18.7°, 20.9°, 24.4°, and 25.2° (2θ), consistent with previous reports for I-type crystalline imatinib. By contrast, the patterns of NC and NC@PDA-NH$_2$ both showed distinct peaks at 15.0°, 17.2°, 18.1°, 18.7°, and 21.1°, characteristic of G-type crystalline [27] (Figure 1D). The DSC curves also indicated changes in the crystalline type from bulk drug to nanocrystals (Figure 1E).

In vitro release from NC and NC@PDA-NH$_2$ was much faster than that of bulk drug, perhaps related to their small size. This may be beneficial because most of the imatinib could remain in nanocrystals during the penetration across the mucus, as well as upon interaction with mucosa and entering tumor cells.

Table 1. Drug loading (DL) and entrapment efficiency (EE) for nanocrystal (NC), polydopamine (PDA)-coated NC (NC@PDA), and amino-group-functionalized NC@PDA (NC@PDA-NH$_2$) ($n = 3$, mean ± SD).

	Drug Loading (DL) (%)	Entrapment Efficiency (EE) (%)
NC	94.47 ± 2.85	94.45 ± 4.81
NC@PDA	82.72 ± 3.66	83.55 ± 12.01
NC@PDA-NH2	76.84 ± 1.78	87.11 ± 11.43

3.2. Cationic Functionalization Favored Interaction of Nanocrystals with Mucin

Adsorption of mucin is a widely used parameter in the evaluation of mucoadhesiveness [28]. NC@PDA-NH$_2$ with different positive surface charges was prepared (Figure S2, Supplementary Materials) and compared with respect to the capability of adsorbing mucin (Figure 2A). It is clear that the amount of mucin adsorption was directly correlated with the value of positive surface charge, indicating the important role of cationic functionalization in mucin adsorption by NC@PDA-NH$_2$. The interaction between NC@PDA-NH$_2$ and mucin was further proven by the increase in size after mixing NC@PDA-NH$_2$ and mucin (Figure 2B). A similar change in the particle size of mucin was also observed in the presence of positively charged polymers, including chitosan and amino-functionalized poloxamer 407, indicative of the interaction between positively charged polymers and mucin [29].

A)

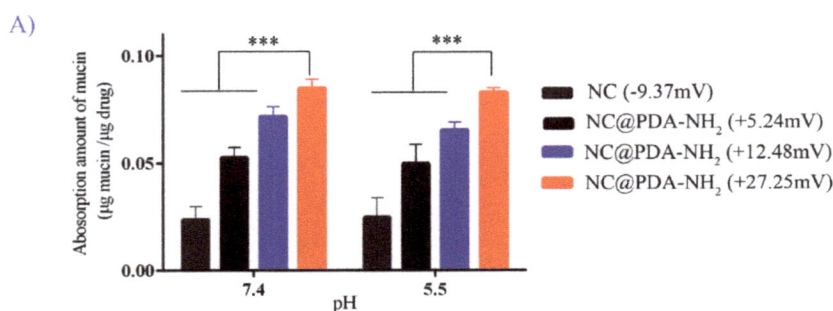

Figure 2. *Cont.*

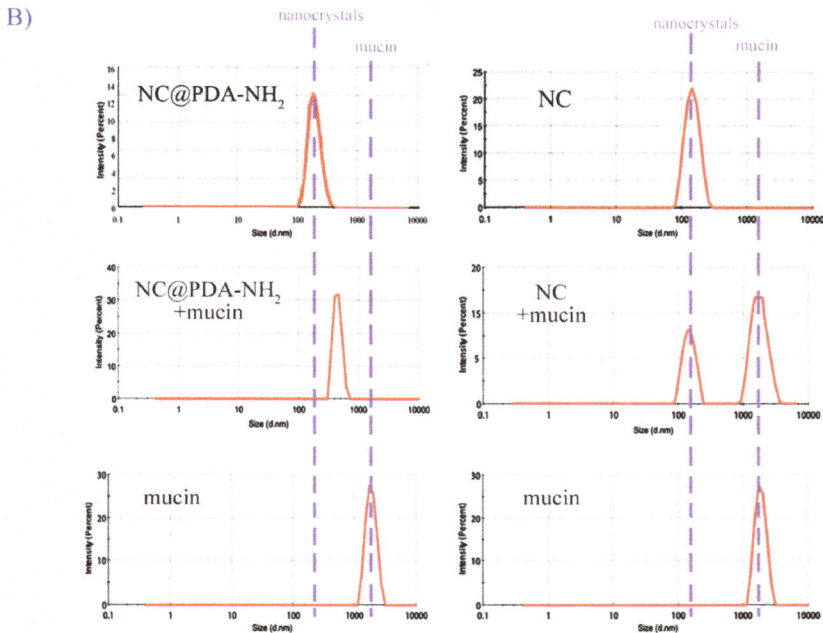

Figure 2. Interaction between NC@PDA-NH$_2$ and mucin. (**A**) Adsorption of mucin by NC@PDA-NH$_2$ with different surface charges or NC (n = 3, mean ± SD). (**B**) Change in size distribution of NC@PDA-NH$_2$ (or NC) after mixing with mucin. *** indicates $p < 0.001$.

3.3. Cationic Functionalization Favored Interaction of Nanocrystals with Cells

Investigation into the interaction between NC@PDA-NH$_2$ and cervical cancer-related cells was performed on TC-1 cells, which are immortalized murine epithelial cells transformed to express human papillomavirus (HPV)-16 E6/E7 and activated human c-Ha-ras oncogene, and exhibit similar genetic traits to human papillomavirus (HPV)-induced cervical tumors [26]. Both CLSM images (Figure 3A) and flow cytometry data (Figure 3B) demonstrated more cellular uptake of NC@PDA-NH$_2$ than NC, attributable to the electrostatic interaction between the positive charges on NC@PDA-NH$_2$ and the negative charges on the cell membrane. The intracellular fluorescent signal of NC@PDA-NH$_2$ overlapped with that of LysoTracker with a Pearson's correlation coefficient (R) of 0.80, suggesting possible involvement of the endocytosis pathway. Further investigation into the cellular uptake mechanism will be included in future work. Quantitative measurements of intracellular IMN concentration further confirmed that more imatinib entered cells after incubation with NC@PDA-NH$_2$ than NC or free imatinib (Figure 3C). The above enhanced cellular uptake was in accordance with the prolonged adhesion on the surface of cellular monolayers of positively charged liposomes than negatively charged or neutral liposomes [30].

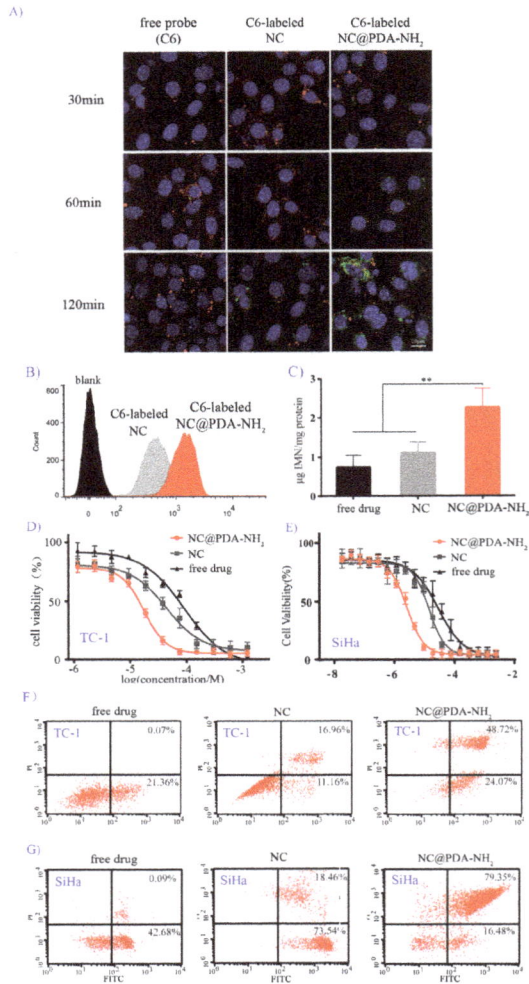

Figure 3. Cellular uptake and cytotoxicity in cervical cancer-related cell lines. (**A**) Representative CLSM images of TC-1 cells co-incubated with 6-coumarin (C6)-labeled NC@PDA-NH$_2$, NC, or free probe C6 (green signal). The nucleus was stained with 2-(4-amidinophenyl)-6-indolecarbamindine dihydrochloride (DAPI; blue) and the lysosomes were stained with LysoTracker Red. (**B**) Flow cytometry analysis on the fluorescent intensity of cells after co-incubation for 2 h with C6-labeled NC@PDA-NH$_2$, NC, or free probe in TC-1 cells. (**C**) Intracellular drug content after co-incubation for 72 h with NC@PDA-NH$_2$, NC, or free imatinib in TC-1 cells ($n = 5$, mean $\pm$ SD, ** represents $p <$ 0.01). (**D,E**) In vitro cytotoxicity of NC@PDA-NH$_2$, NC, or free imatinib after 48 h of co-incubation in TC-1 cells (**D**) or SiHa cells (**E**). (**F,G**) Apoptotic cell populations determined by flow cytometry with Annexin V-FITC and propidium iodide (PI) staining after co-incubation with NC@PDA-NH$_2$, NC, or free imatinib in TC-1 cells (**E**) or SiHa cells (**G**). The lower-left (Q3), lower-right (Q4), upper-right (Q2), and upper-left (Q1) quadrants in each panel indicate the populations of normal, early, and late apoptotic, and apoptotic necrotic cells, respectively.

As shown by the MTT results (Figure 3D), enhanced cellular growth inhibition was observed with NC@PDA-NH$_2$. The IC$_{50}$ values of NC@PDA-NH$_2$, NC, and free drug were 16.8 μM, 39.3 μM, and 84.9 μM, respectively. Such enhanced cellular growth inhibition of NC@PDA-NH2 compared to NC and free drug might be relevant with the different uptake and, thus, different intracellular drug accumulation.

More cellular apoptosis was also observed with NC@PDA-NH$_2$. NC@PDA-NH$_2$, NC, and free drug resulted in 24.07%, 11.16%, and 21.36% early apoptotic cells in the fourth quadrant (Q4) and 48.7%, 16.96%, and 0.07% late apoptotic cells in Q1, respectively. Similar trends were also observed in MTT and apoptosis results with another cervical cancer-related cell line (SiHa cells).

3.4. Cationic Functionalization Prolonged Intravaginal Retention and Enhanced Mucosal Penetration

Before ex vivo and in vivo application, NC@PDA-NH$_2$ was dispersed in Pluronic F127-based thermosensitive hydrogel (FG) to avoid leakage which might happen if administered as a simple aqueous dispersion, and enough time was allowed for nanocrystals to interact with the mucosa. Other vehicles for nanoparticles were also reported for vaginal use, such as hydroxypropyl methylcellulose/poly(vinyl alcohol) films [31] and poly(vinyl alcohol) nanofibers [32]. FG was also applied as a vaginal formulation vehicle with good safety for many therapeutic agents. Due to its lack of mucoadhesive properties, FG may serve as an ideal vehicle for the evaluation of NC@PDA-NH$_2$.

Consistent with previous reports on FG [33], the phase transition temperature and in vitro drug release rate of NC@PDA-NH$_2$-containing FG (NC@PDA-NH$_2$/FG) were both dependent on the concentration of Pluronic F127 (Figure 4). A concentration of 17.5% (*w*/*w*) was selected for Pluronic F127 to assure easy administration and moderate dispersion into vaginal fluid.

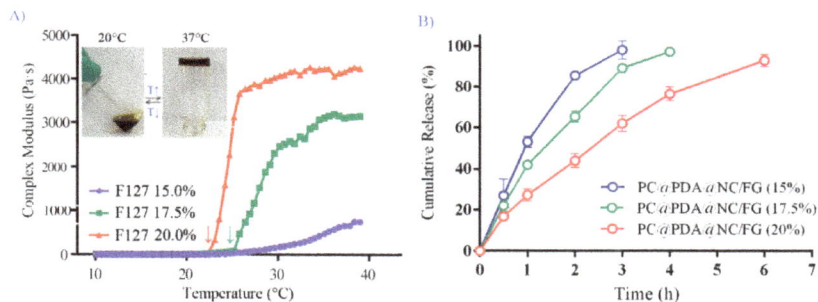

Figure 4. Rheological and in vitro release profiles of NC@PDA-NH$_2$/FG. (**A**) Temperature-dependent rheological profiles of NC@PDA-NH$_2$/FG with different F127 concentration (15.0%, 17.5%, and 20.0%, *w*/*w*). The red and green arrows denote the gelation temperature for 20.0% and 17.5%, respectively, while the thermal phase transition was not obvious for 15.0%. The insert is the typical photograph of NC@PDA-NH$_2$/FG (17.5%) at storage (20 °C) or body temperature (37 °C). (**B**) Release profiles from NC@PDA-NH$_2$/FG at different F127 concentration (15.0%, 17.5% and 20.0%, *w*/*w*) at 37 °C in VFS (*n* = 3, mean ± SD).

When dropped on ex vivo murine vagina mucosa and continuously flushed with VFS for 8 h, NC@PDA-NH$_2$/FG resulted in significantly longer residence of fluorescent signal than NC/FG or free probe/FG (Figure 5A,B). When observed microscopically, prolonged, more, and deeper fluorescence was found in the vaginal mucosa of mice administered with NC@PDA-NH$_2$/FG, suggesting improved accessibility and penetration into vaginal mucosa. Quantitative measurements of intravaginal imatinib amount further confirmed the superiority of NC@PDA-NH$_2$/FG with respect to intravaginal residence (Figure 5D).

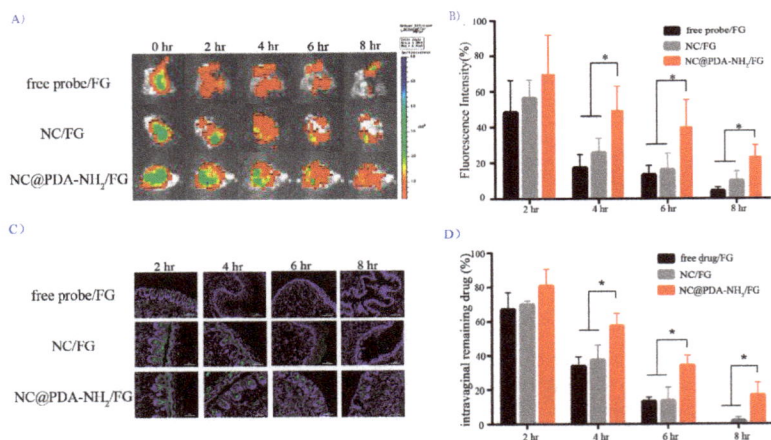

Figure 5. Ex vivo mucoadhesiveness and in vivo placement. (**A**) Typical fluorescent images, and (**B**) semi-quantitative fluorescent intensity (n = 6, mean ± SD) for the ex vivo residence of 1,1′-dioctadecyl-3,3,3′,3′-tetramethylindotricarbocyanine iodide (DiR)-labeled NC@PDA-NH$_2$/FG, NC/FG, or free probe DiR/FG on the surface of ex vivo vaginal mucosa of healthy mice during flushing by VFS at 37 °C. (**C**) Fluorescent microscopic images (green signal for C6, blue signal for DAPI; scale bar = 100 μm), and (**D**) intravaginal residence percentage of imatinib in healthy mice vaginally administered with NC@PDA-NH$_2$/FG, NC/FG, or free imatinib/FG (n = 6, mean ± SD); * indicates $p < 0.05$.

3.5. Cationic Functionalization Improved Tumor Inhibition in the Orthotopic TC-1 Cervical Cancer Model

The orthotopic TC-1 model was reported to represent a stringent model for cervicovaginal cancer within a short time frame and localized similarly to the anatomy of cervical tumors. In addition, this model is suitable for testing mucoadhesive formulations because it features the cervicovaginal mucus layer that acts as a barrier to particle penetration [26].

The tumor growth inhibition effect was firstly investigated after daily intravaginal administration treatment with NC@PDA-NH$_2$/FG or NC/FG for three weeks at three different doses (2, 4, and 8 mg/kg/2 d) by observing the tumor size by the end (Figure 6A). The inhibition effects of NC@PDA-NH$_2$/FG and NC/FG were both dose-dependent. More importantly, NC@PDA-NH$_2$/FG inhibited the growth of model tumors more effectively. This might be explained by more accessibility of NC@PDA-NH$_2$ to the vaginal mucosal as indicated by the semi-quantitative analysis of optical density of fluorescent microscopic images.

More and deeper fluorescence was found in the vaginal mucosa bearing model tumors for fluorescent-labeled NC@PDA-NH$_2$/FG (Figure 6B). Based on the Kaplan–Meier survival curves at the dosage of 4 mg/kg/2 d, NC@PDA-NH$_2$/FG prolonged the median survival time, 7.0-fold that of free drug/FG (35 d vs. 20 d) and 2.1-fold that of NC/FG group (35 d vs. 26 d). More apoptosis areas were also observed in the microscopic sections from the NC@PDA-NH$_2$/FG group than the NC/FG group (Figure 6E).

The safety of NC@PDA-NH$_2$/FG was evaluated by monitoring the change in the animal body weight during the abovementioned three-week treatment and histological examination of the vaginal mucosa by the end. As shown in Figure 6E, the body weight of mice in the NC@PDA-NH$_2$/FG group slowly increased, reflecting their relatively good health state. By contrast, the body weight continuously decreased in the free drug/FG or control groups (normal saline).

H&E staining sections (Figure 6F) also demonstrated the maximal anti-tumor efficiency and minimal mucosal toxicity for the NC@PDA-NH$_2$/FG group. The mucosal epithelium was destructed and compressed by the prosperous tumor tissues in the control group, while the mucosal epithelium partially recovered in the NC@PDA-NH$_2$/FG group.

As the TC-1 model tumor grew, elevated interstitial pressure within tumor tissue impaired intratumor penetration and made complete tumor eradication ultimately difficult for free drug [34]. It is encouraging that NC@PDA-NH$_2$/FG effectively suppressed the growth of TC-1 model tumors. Future studies using other murine cervical tumor models which are less aggressive and resemble the slow tumor progression in humans will further substantiate the effectiveness of NC@PDA-NH$_2$/FG.

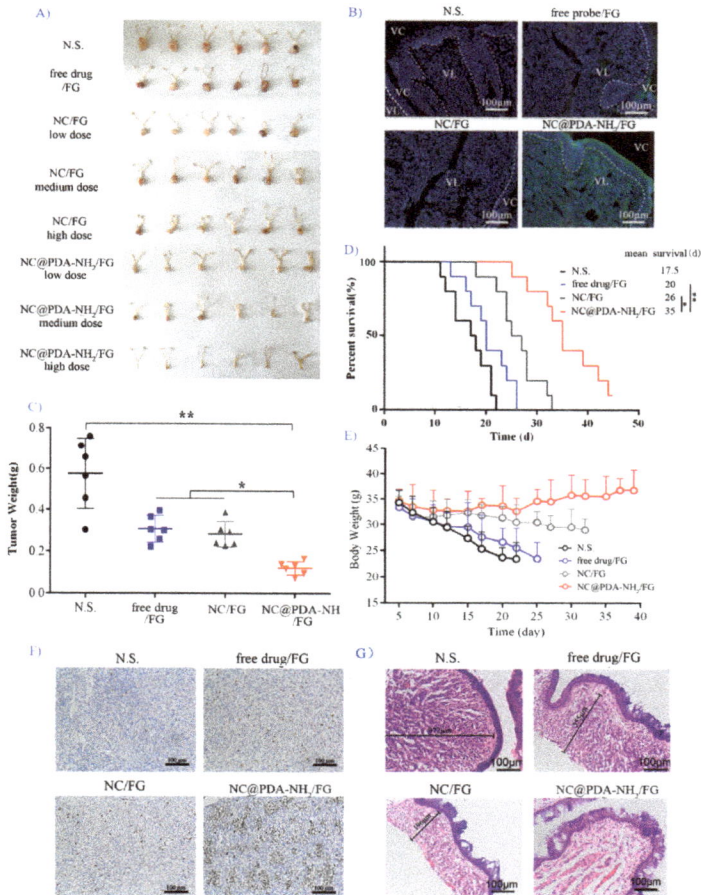

Figure 6. In vivo evaluation in orthotopic TC-1 cervicovaginal model tumor-bearing mice after intravaginal administration of different formulations every other day. (**A**) Dose-dependent inhibition on the tumor size after three-week treatment (dose: 2, 4, and 8 mg/kg/2 d). (**B**) Penetration of fluorescent signal into the vaginal mucosa (4 h after administration). (**C**) Tumor weights after treatment for three weeks (dose: 4 mg/kg/2 d; $n = 6$). (**D**) Survival time (dose: 4 mg/kg/2 d; $n = 10$). (**E**) Change in anima body weight (dose: 4 mg/kg/2 d; $n = 10$). (**F**) Representative immunohistochemical microphotographs of tumor sections stained for apoptosis after three-week treatment (dose: 4 mg/kg/2 d). (**G**) Representative H&E microphotographs of tumors and vagina after three-week treatment (dose: 4 mg/kg/2 d). * indicates $p < 0.05$, ** indicates $p < 0.01$.

4. Conclusions

In summary, positively charged NC@PDA-NH$_2$ significantly interacted with mucin in vitro and resulted in more cellular uptake, cellular growth inhibition efficacy, and induction of apoptosis. NC@PDA-NH$_2$/FG exhibited good ex vivo and in vivo mucoadhesiveness, as well as improved anti-tumor efficacy in the murine orthotopic cervicovaginal cancer tumor model. In conclusion, cationic functionalization endowed imatinib nanocrystals good potential as a novel mucoadhesive approach for intravaginal treatment of cervicovaginal cancer. Our work also reveals the good potential of surface functionalization based on polydopamine coating on nanocrystals, which appear to be a good nanoscale drug delivery system with high drug content for poorly soluble drugs.

Supplementary Materials: The following are available online at http://www.mdpi.com/1999-4923/11/1/15/s1, Figure S1: Influence of reaction time on the size distribution and zeta potential of resulted nanocrystals measured by dynamic light scattering. Left: reaction time of PDA@NC with Boc-NHCH$_2$CH$_2$NH$_2$; right: deprotection time in acidic environment, Figure S2: NC@PDA-NH2 with different zeta potentials for comparison of mucin adsorption, Figure S3: Size distribution and zeta potentials of C6-labeled NC, NC@PDA, and NC@PDA-NH2, Figure S4: Typical chromatograph for imatinib (1 ug/mL, LLOQ), Figure S5: Typical chromatograph of vaginal lavage samples after intravaginal administration of NC@PDA-NH2/FG.

Author Contributions: L.-q.C. and Z.-g.H. were responsible for the acquisition of data. F.-m.L. and J.W. substantially helped in the animal experiments. L.-l.F. and F.S. helped in the analysis of data. S.-j.C. established the tumor-bearing animal model. Z.-p.L. drafted the work. Y.L. designed the work. G.W. and W.-y.L. substantively revised it.

Funding: This research was funded by China Nature Science Foundation (81573361 and 81102385), Program of Shanghai Academic Research Leader (18XD1400500), the Open Project Program of Key Lab of Smart Drug Delivery (Fudan University), Ministry of Education, China and the Open Project Program of Key Laboratory of Contraceptives and Devices Research (NPFPC) (Shanghai Institute of Planned Parenthood Research, China).

Conflicts of Interest: The authors declare no conflict of interest.

Abbreviations

PDA	polydopamine
NC	nanocrystals
NC@PDA-NH2	cationic functionalized polydopamine-coated imatinib nanocrystals
NC@PDA	polydopamine-coated imatinib nanocrystals
F127	Pluronic F127
FG	Pluronic F127-based in situ hydrogel
TKI	tyrosine kinase inhibitors
IMN	imatinib
C6	6-coumarin
DiR	1,1'-dioctadecyl-3,3,3',3'-tetramethylindotricarbocyanine iodide
OCT	optical coherence tomography
DAPI	2-(4-amidinophenyl)-6-indolecarbamindine dihydrochloride
PGM	porcine gastric mucin
DL	drug loading
EE	encapsulation efficiency
TEM	transmission electron microscope
DLS	dynamic light scattering
XRPD	X-ray powder diffraction
DSC	differential scanning calorimetry
VFS	vaginal fluid stimulant

References

1. Bernard, W.S.; Christopher, P.W. *World Cancer Report 2014*; World Health Organization: Switzerland, Geneva, 2014.
2. Major, I.; McConville, C. Vaginal drug delivery for the localised treatment of cervical cancer. *Drug Deliv. Transl. Res.* **2017**, *7*, 817–828. [CrossRef] [PubMed]
3. Cook, M.T.; Brown, M.B. Polymeric gels for intravaginal drug delivery. *J. Control. Release* **2018**, *270*, 145–157. [CrossRef] [PubMed]
4. Taja-Chayeb, L.; Chavez-Blanco, A.; Martínez-Tlahuel, J.; González-Fierro, A.; Candelaria, M.; Chanona-Vilchis, J.; Robles, E.; Dueñas-Gonzalez, A. Expression of platelet derived growth factor family members and the potential role of imatinib mesylate for cervical cancer. *Cancer Cell Int.* **2006**, *6*, 22. [CrossRef]
5. Kummel, S.; Heidecke, H.; Brock, B.; Denkert, C.; Hecktor, J.; Koninger, A.; Becker, I.; Sehouli, J.; Thomas, A.; Blohmer, J.U.; et al. Imatinib—A possible therapeutic option for cervical carcinoma: Results of a preclinical phase I study. *Gynakol. Geburtshilfliche Rundsch.* **2008**, *48*, 94–100.
6. Gao, L.; Liu, G.; Ma, J.; Wang, X.; Zhou, L.; Li, X. Drug nanocrystals: In vivo performances. *J. Control. Release* **2012**, *160*, 418–430. [CrossRef] [PubMed]
7. Müller, R.H.; Gohla, S.; Keck, C.M. State of the art of nanocrystals: Special features, production, nanotoxicology aspects and intracellular delivery. *Eur. J. Pharm. Biopharm.* **2011**, *78*, 1–9. [CrossRef] [PubMed]
8. Lu, Y.; Li, Y.; Wu, W. Injected nanocrystals for targeted drug delivery. *Acta Pharm. Sin. B* **2016**, *6*, 106–113. [CrossRef]
9. Guo, H.; Xu, W.; Chen, J.; Yan, L.; Ding, J.; Hou, Y.; Chen, X. Positively charged polypeptide nanogel enhances mucoadhesion and penetrability of 10-hydroxycamptothecin in orthotopic bladder carcinoma. *J. Control. Release* **2017**, *259*, 136–148. [CrossRef]
10. Ci, L.Q.; Huang, Z.G.; Liu, Y.; Liu, Z.P.; Wei, G.; Lu, W.Y. Amino-functionalized poloxamer 407 with both mucoadhesive and thermosensitive properties: Preparation, characterization and application in vaginal drug delivery system. *Acta Pharm. Sin. B* **2017**, *7*, 593–602. [CrossRef]
11. Frank, L.A.; Chaves, P.S.; D'Amore, C.M.; Contri, R.V.; Frank, A.G.; Beck, R.C.; Pohlmann, A.R.; Buffon, A.; Guterres, S.S. The use of chitosan as cationic coating or gel vehicle for polymeric nanocapsules: Increasing penetration and adhesion of imiquimod in vaginal tissue. *Eur. J. Pharm. Biopharm.* **2017**, *114*, 202–212. [CrossRef]
12. Zhang, H.; Hu, H.; Zhang, H.; Dai, W.; Wang, X.; Wang, X.; Zhang, Q. Effects of PEGylated paclitaxel nanocrystals on breast cancer and its lung metastasis. *Nanoscale* **2015**, *7*, 10790–10800. [CrossRef] [PubMed]
13. Park, J.; Sun, B.; Yeo, Y. Albumin-coated nanocrystals for carrier-free delivery of paclitaxel. *J. Control. Release* **2017**, *263*, 90–101. [CrossRef] [PubMed]
14. Zhang, L.; Wei, W.; Ma, G. HSA induced HCPT nanocrystal for high-performance antitumor therapy. *J. Control. Release* **2017**, *259*, e82. [CrossRef]
15. Gao, W.; Chen, Y.; Thompson, D.H.; Park, K.; Li, T. Impact of surfactant treatment of paclitaxel nanocrystals on biodistribution and tumor accumulation in tumor-bearing mice. *J. Control. Release* **2016**, *237*, 168–176. [CrossRef] [PubMed]
16. Gao, W.; Lee, D.; Meng, Z.; Li, T. Exploring intracellular fate of drug nanocrystals with crystal-integrated and environment-sensitive fluorophores. *J. Control. Release* **2017**, *267*, 214–222. [CrossRef] [PubMed]
17. Chen, M.; Li, W.; Zhang, X.; Dong, Y.; Hua, Y.; Zhang, H.; Gao, J.; Zhao, L.; Li, Y.; Zheng, A. In vitro and in vivo evaluation of SN-38 nanocrystals with different particle sizes. *Int. J. Nanomed.* **2017**, *12*, 5487–5500. [CrossRef]
18. Zhang, C.; Gong, L.; Xiang, L.; Du, Y.; Hu, W.; Zeng, H.; Xu, Z. Deposition and Adhesion of Polydopamine on the Surfaces of Varying Wettability. *ACS Appl. Mater. Interfaces* **2017**, *9*, 30943–30950. [CrossRef]
19. Lee, H.; Dellatore, S.M.; Miller, W.M.; Messersmith, P.B. Mussel-Inspired Surface Chemistry for Multifunctional Coatings. *Science* **2007**, *318*, 426–430. [CrossRef]
20. Liu, Y.; Ai, K.; Liu, J.; Deng, M.; He, Y.; Lu, L. Dopamine-melanin colloidal nanospheres: An efficient near-infrared photothermal therapeutic agent for in vivo cancer therapy. *Adv. Mater.* **2013**, *5*, 1353–1359. [CrossRef]

21. Li, Y.; Jiang, C.; Zhang, D.; Wang, Y.; Ren, X.; Ai, K.; Chen, X.; Lu, L. Targeted polydopamine nanoparticles enable photoacoustic imaging guided chemo-photothermal synergistic therapy of tumor. *Acta Biomater.* **2017**, *47*, 124–134. [CrossRef]

22. Zeng, X.; Tao, W.; Liu, G.; Mei, L. Polydopamine-based surface modification of copolymeric nanoparticles as a targeted drug delivery system for cancer therapy. *J. Control. Release* **2017**, *259*, e150–e151. [CrossRef]

23. Xue, P.; Sun, L.; Li, Q.; Zhang, L.; Guo, J.; Xu, Z.; Kan, Y. PEGylated polydopamine-coated magnetic nanoparticles for combined targeted chemotherapy and photothermal ablation of tumour cells. *Colloids Surf. B Biointerfaces* **2017**, *160*, 11–21. [CrossRef] [PubMed]

24. Zhan, H.; Jagtiani, T.; Liang, J.F. A new targeted delivery approach by functionalizing drug nanocrystals through polydopamine coating. *Eur. J. Pharm. Biopharm.* **2017**, *114*, 221–229. [CrossRef] [PubMed]

25. Owen, D.H.; Katz, D.F. A vaginal fluid simulant. *Contraception* **1999**, *59*, 91–95. [CrossRef]

26. Yang, M.; Yu, T.; Wang, Y.Y.; Lai, S.K.; Zeng, Q.; Miao, B.; Tang, B.C.; Simons, B.W.; Ensign, L.M.; Liu, G.; et al. Vaginal delivery of paclitaxel via nanoparticles with nonmucoadhesive surfaces suppresses cervical tumor growth. *Adv. Healthc. Mater.* **2014**, *3*, 1044–1052. [CrossRef] [PubMed]

27. Novartis, A.G. Crystalline F, G, H, I and K type of Imatinib Mesylate. CN Patent 2006800440007.7, 26 November 2008.

28. Prosperi-Porta, G.; Kedzior, S.; Muirhead, B.; Sheardown, H. Phenylboronic-acid-based polymeric micelles for mucoadhesive anterior segment ocular drug delivery. *Biomacromolecules* **2016**, *17*, 1449–1457. [CrossRef]

29. Nikogeorgos, N.; Efler, P.; Kayitmazer, A.B.; Lee, S. "Bio-glues" to enhance slipperiness of mucins: Improved lubricity and wear resistance of porcine gastric mucin (PGM) layers assisted by mucoadhesion with chitosan. *Soft Matter* **2015**, *11*, 489–498. [CrossRef]

30. Adamczak, M.I.; Hagesaether, E.; Smistad, G.; Hiorth, M. An in vitro study of mucoadhesion and biocompatibility of polymer coated liposomes on HT29-MTX mucus-producing cells. *Int. J. Pharm.* **2016**, *498*, 225–233. [CrossRef]

31. Büyükköroğlu, G.; Şenel, B.; Başaran, E.; Yenilmez, E.; Yazan, Y. Preparation and in vitro evaluation of vaginal formulations including siRNA and paclitaxel-loaded SLNs for cervical cancer. *Eur. J. Pharm. Biopharm.* **2016**, *109*, 174–183. [CrossRef]

32. Ci, T.; Yuan, L.; Bao, X.; Hou, Y.; Wu, H.; Sun, H.; Cao, D.; Ke, X. Development and anti-*Candida* evaluation of the vaginal delivery system of amphotericin B nanosuspension-loaded thermogel. *J. Drug Target.* **2018**, *26*, 829–839. [CrossRef] [PubMed]

33. Liu, Y.; Yang, F.J.; Feng, L.L.; Yang, L.; Chen, L.Y.; Wei, G.; Lu, W.Y. In vivo retention of poloxamer-based in situ hydrogels for vaginal application in mouse and rat models. *Acta Pharm. Sin. B* **2017**, *7*, 502–509. [CrossRef] [PubMed]

34. Lin, K.Y.; Guarnieri, F.G.; Staveley-O'Carroll, K.F.; Levitsky, H.I.; August, J.T.; Pardoll, D.M.; Wu, T.C. Treatment of Established Tumors with a Novel Vaccine That Enhances Major Histocompatibility Class II Presentation of Tumor Antigen. *Cancer Res.* **1996**, *56*, 21–26. [PubMed]

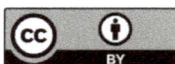

MDPI

St. Alban-Anlage 66

4052 Basel

Switzerland

Tel. +41 61 683 77 34

Fax +41 61 302 89 18

www.mdpi.com

Pharmaceutics Editorial Office

E-mail: pharmaceutics@mdpi.com

www.mdpi.com/journal/pharmaceutics